UNDERSTANDING TUBERCULOSIS – GLOBAL EXPERIENCES AND INNOVATIVE APPROACHES TO THE DIAGNOSIS

Edited by **Pere-Joan Cardona**

Understanding Tuberculosis – Global Experiences and Innovative Approaches to the Diagnosis
Edited by Pere-Joan Cardona

Published by InTech

Janeza Trdine 9, 51000 Rijeka, Croatia

Publishing Process Manager Marija Radja

Technical Editor Teodora Smiljanic

Cover Designer InTech Design Team

Additional hard copies can be obtained from orders@intechopen.com

Understanding Tuberculosis – Global Experiences and Innovative Approaches to the Diagnosis, Edited by Pere-Joan Cardona
p. cm.
ISBN 978-953-307-938-7

For EU product safety concerns:
IN TECH d.o.o., Prolaz Marije Krucifikse Kozulić 3, 51000 Rijeka, Croatia,
info@intechopen.com or visit our website at intechopen.com.

Meet the editor

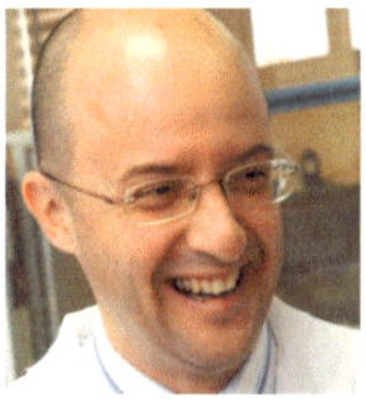

After obtaining his MD at the Universitat Autònoma de Barcelona, Pere-Joan Cardona started an internship in Clinical Microbiology in 1994, in the Hospital Germans Trias i Pujol, where he was familiarized with the problem of TB in its clinical and diagnostic challenges. Invited by Ian Orme at CSU, he was trained on the development of TB experimental models. PhD was obtained in 1999. He became Head of the Experimental Tuberculosis Unit at the Institut Germans Trias i Pujol of Badalona and Assistant Professor of Microbiology at UAB. He has been involved for the last 15 years in the study of the pathophysiology of TB infection. Additionally, he has authored 70 peer-reviewed publications in the field and is responsible for the development of different experimental models in mice, guinea pigs, goats and mini-pigs, and in the development of new drug regimens and vaccines against TB.

Contents

Preface

Mycobacterium tuberculosis is a disease that is transmitted through aerosol. This is the reason why it is estimated that a third of humankind is already infected by *Mycobacterium tuberculosis*. The vast majority of the infected do not know about their status. *Mycobacterium tuberculosis* is a silent pathogen, causing no symptomatology at all during the infection. In addition, infected people cannot cause further infections. Unfortunately, an estimated 10 percent of the infected population has the probability to develop the disease, making it very difficult to eradicate. Once in this stage, the bacilli can be transmitted to other persons and the development of clinical symptoms is very progressive. Therefore the diagnosis, especially the discrimination between infection and disease, is a real challenge. In this book, we present the experience of worldwide specialists on the diagnosis, along with its lights and shadows.

Dr. Pere-Joan Cardona
Institut Germans Trias i Pujol (IGTP)
Catalunya, Spain

Part 1

Experience on Laboratory Diagnosis Around the World

1

Clinical Laboratory Diagnostics for *Mycobacterium tuberculosis*

N. Esther Babady[1] and Nancy L. Wengenack[2]
[1]*Memorial Sloan-Kettering Cancer Center, New York, New York,*
[2]*Mayo Clinic, Rochester, Minnesota,*
USA

1. Introduction

This chapter highlights current state-of-the-art methods for the detection and identification of *Mycobacterium tuberculosis* (*Mtb*) complex in the clinical diagnostic laboratory. Methods discussed include stain and culture which traditionally would have been followed by phenotypic-based identification methods. At this point in time however, molecular methods are considered the gold standard for both the rapid detection of *Mtb* directly from patient specimens as well as for the identification of *Mtb* following growth in culture. There are also instances where speciation of *Mtb* in order to distinguish it from other members of the *Mtb* complex is clinically important and these will be discussed. In addition, this chapter provides an overview of methods used in the clinical laboratory for *Mtb* drug resistance testing and suggests what the future might hold for *Mtb* diagnostics.

2. *M. tuberculosis* and biosafety in the clinical laboratory

M. tuberculosis presents a risk of laboratory-acquired infection due to its transmission via aerosol routes, ability to withstand common laboratory processing techniques such as heat-fixation or frozen section preparation and a extremely low ID_{50} of <10 bacilli. The United States Centers for Disease Control and Prevention (CDC) estimates that laboratory workers are three times more likely than non-laboratory workers to become infected with *Mtb*. Therefore, biological safety organizations have defined a number of safety practices and procedures that must be strictly followed when working with *Mtb* which is classified as a risk group 3 organism. Specimens and cultures of unknown isolates shall be handled as if they contain *Mtb* until proven otherwise. Only non-aerosol generating processes such as accessioning of specimen or reading of acid-fast smears can be done under BSL-2 conditions outside of a BSC. All other specimen-handling including opening/closing of tubes, pipeting and transfer must be done in a BSC. Personnel must exercise caution to avoid aerosol generation. More specifically, smear preparation, culture decontamination and concentration, and culture plating must be done inside a BSC with the possible exception of the centrifugation step. However, centrifugation must be done using aerosol-proof containers which are opened, loaded and closed inside the BSC to reduce the risk of personnel exposure. All laboratory surfaces must be decontaminated with a tuberculocidal reagent before and after working with specimens and cultures. Propagation and manipulation of *Mtb* complex cultures (e.g., identification and susceptibility testing) requires BSL-3 practices, equipment and facilities. Clinical laboratories without BSL-3 facilities must refer all positive mycobacterial cultures to another laboratory with BSL-3 capabilities for identification and, if necessary, susceptibility testing. Acid-fast smears must not be prepared from positive mycobacterial cultures of unknown identity without BSL-3 facilities. Identification methods (e.g., biochemical analysis, nucleic acid hybridization probes, sequencing, PCR) required initial specimen processing under BSL-3 conditions until any viable mycobacteria have been rendered non-viable by heating and/or lysis via chemical or physical means. Laboratories must verify that their processing methods are effective in rendering *Mtb* nonviable prior to conducting any activities outside of a BSL-3 laboratory.

BSL-3 facilities have highly specialized requirements some of which include restricted laboratory access, self-closing double door entry, directional airflow with a specified number of air exchanges over time, BSCs exhausted to the outside, and posted signage regarding the hazard (in this case *Mtb*). Class II BSCs are one of the most important pieces of equipment in the mycobacteriology laboratory and they must be maintained in good working order at all times. Frequent (at least daily) checks of function by means such as magnehelic gauge monitoring is needed. Regular maintenance and certification programs must be undertaken and documentation of cabinet performance must be maintained by the laboratory. Specimens should be covered before transport and should be transported in well-sealed, leak-proof containers. All biohazard waste should be autoclaved prior to leaving the facility.

BSL-3 personnel safety practices include the use of fluid-resistant, cuffed, solid-front gowns, gloves, eye protection, respiratory protection (N-95 or better fitted respirator or powered air purifying respirator (PAPR)). Each laboratory must perform a risk assessment to define the personal protective equipment, facilities and engineering practices that are appropriate for their institution and that comply with applicable regulations. The risk assessment is the responsibility of the laboratory director but it should be done in collaboration with institutional biosafety officials as this is helpful in making certain that no safety practice has been overlooked. A sample risk assessment is provided in Table 1 but each laboratory must perform their own assessment as situations may differ between laboratories. The laboratory must have a written spill procedure and must review the procedure with lab staff regularly to assure competency. Spill "drills" in which staff physically respond to a simulated spill are highly recommended as they routinely point out any potential gaps in procedures or staff knowledge.

Strict regulations exist in many countries concerning the shipping and transportation of diagnostic specimens that are known to contain or that potentially contain *Mtb* complex and for shipment of known *Mtb* complex isolates. Personnel who package these specimens and isolates must have specialized training that is updated at prescribed intervals. Packaging materials must be leak-proof, able to withstand unpredictable handling throughout the transportation chain and must be properly labeled in order to alert transportation workers of hazards contained within the package. Individuals involved in the shipping of specimens and isolates should be knowledgeable about the regulations within their country and if, sending specimens or isolates internationally, within the destination country.

Procedure	Aerosol Potential	Biosafety Level Required	Personal Protective Equipment Required	Engineering Controls Required	Special Practices or Equipment Required
Reading of smears (AR, Kinyoun, Modified Acid Fast)	Slight	BSL 2	Gown, gloves	May be done on bench top	
Manipulation of mycobacterial cultures for identification (e.g. subculturing)	Significant	BSL 3	Gown, shoe covers, eye protection, gloves and respirator/head cover or PAPR	Work in biological safety cabinet	Use disposable loops; Use racks to prevent tipping/spilling; Work over disinfectant-soaked towel
Susceptibility testing of mycobacteria	Significant	BSL 3 for setup BSL 2 for incubation and reading of closed bottles/ plates/ tubes	Setup - Gown, shoe covers, eye protection, gloves and respirator/head cover or PAPR	Work in biological safety cabinet to inoculate bottles, tubes or plates with organism	Use extreme care to avoid aerosol generation when inoculating bottles/plates/tubes

Table 1. Sample partial risk assessment – this table is intended as an example of one style of risk assessment that can be developed. Each laboratory must develop a laboratory-specific risk assessment in conjunction with their institutional safety officer(s).

3. Stains for mycobacteria

Mycobacteria, including *Mtb* complex, can be rapidly and inexpensively detected directly from pretreated and concentrated respiratory specimens, body fluids, and tissue using acid-fast stains. A Gram stain is not able to reliably detect mycobacteria which can appear as non-stained "ghosts" or as beaded Gram-positive bacilli. Therefore, acid-fast stains, such as the Ziehl-Neelsen stain or the fluorescent auramine-rhodamine stain are recommended for mycobacteria. The acid-fast stain forms a complex between the unique mycolic acids of the mycobacterial cell wall and the dye (e.g., fuchsin). Complex formation makes the mycobacteria resistant to destaining by acid-alcohols providing the basis for the "acid-fast" terminology. Non-acid fast bacteria do not retain the acid-fast dye in the presence of the acid-alcohol decolorizer and are often stained in a subsequent step using a counterstain such as methylene blue. Commonly utilized acid-fast stains contain carbol-fuchsin dye and are the Ziehl-Neelsen stain which utilizes phenol plus heat to aid in dye penetration, and the Kinyoun stain which uses phenol in the absence of heat. The Ziehl-Neelsen stain is considered the more sensitive of the two (Somoskovi et al., 2001). Fluorescent stains such as auramine O are also used alone or in combination with rhodamine B. The fluorescent stains exhibit increased fluorescence upon binding DNA and RNA providing enhanced sensitivity for examining concentrated direct specimens by staining the bacilli while avoiding non-specific staining of artifacts and background more typical of the non-fluorescent stains.

Mycobacteria appear as long slender rods (1-10μm long x 0.2-0.6μm wide) and are often slightly curved or bent. At least 300 fields should be examined under high power (1000X) when using a carbol-fuchsin stain and light microcopy. The fluorochrome stain can be examined using a lower power (250X) and a minimum of 30 fields should be examined under the lower power (Pfyffer & Palicova, 2011). When positive, an indication of the quantity of acid-fast bacilli present should be provided. Factors which influence the sensitivity of acid-fast smears include the amount of acid-fast bacilli present in the specimen, the experience of the reader, the stain used, the number of fields examined, the type of specimen (e.g., generally respiratory specimens have higher yield than non-respiratory), the patient population being examined, volume of the specimen and smear pre-treatment (direct vs. pre-treated, concentrated). Rigid quality control processes must be followed to prevent cross-contamination and false results. Laboratories should use a positive and negative control slide for each batch of acid-fast smears prepared and should have a second reader confirm positive results and at least 10% of negative slides to reduce the potential for incorrect results. Staining jars or dishes should not be used to prevent potential cross-contamination and care should be taken to avoid the transfer of bacilli via the microscopy oil used for examining the slide. Laboratories must also participate in a proficiency testing programs (e.g., College of American Pathologists) to ensure continued competency.

Acid-fast stains lack sensitivity and a large number of bacilli (10^4-10^6/mL) are required for a positive stain. Therefore, a positive stain from a respiratory specimen is typically thought to correlate with a higher infectivity potential and patients are routinely placed in airborne isolation rooms until their acid-fast smears convert to negative. Immunocompromised individuals often present with lower bacterial loads making detection by smear difficult (Chegou et al., 2011). Up to 30% of persons (commonly children) are unable to produce sputum for a smear requiring the use of more invasive methods (gastric washing, bronchoalveolar lavage, etc). Smears can be used to follow the response to treatment in smear-positive individuals. A concentration step provides increase sensitivity over direct smear microscopy (Steingart et al., 2006).

Acid-fast stains are also non-specific and the reader cannot determine the species of mycobacteria present in a positive smear. Mycobacteria tend to clump and produce cord-like strands of bacilli and there may be some indication of which species is present based on characteristic cording but this is highly subjective and not recommended as a routine method of determining species (Attorri et al., 2000; Julian et al., 2010).

4. Culturing of *M. tuberculosis*

The growth of *Mtb* in culture is considered the gold standard for identification of a case of tuberculosis. The sensitivity of culture is much better than an acid-fast smear with only 10-100 viable organisms/mL of specimen required for a positive culture. Media for the growth of *Mtb* is the same as that used for other mycobacteria species and generally includes both a solid and a liquid-based medium. Solid media utilized is typically either egg-based such as the Lowenstein-Jensen (L-J) medium or agar-based such as Middlebrook 7H10 medium.

Antimicrobial agents can be added to help with elimination of contaminating organisms which may have a more rapid growth rate than *Mtb* and which may therefore obscure any *Mtb* present on the plate. In general, *Mtb* colonies are seen more rapidly on agar-based medium (10-12 days) as opposed to egg-based medium (18-24 days) (Liu et al., 1973). Care must be taken to protect Middlebrook medium from excessive light and heat which results in breakdown of the medium and release of a formaldehyde byproduct which is toxic to *Mtb* (Miliner et al., 1969). Use of Middlebrook 7H11 medium containing casein is reported to improve the recovery of isoniazid-resistant isolates of *Mtb* (Pfyffer & Palicova, 2011). Broth medium such as Middlebrook 7H9 medium is reported to provide a more rapid recovery of *Mtb* compared with solid medium. There are several commercially-available semi-automated broth culture systems for mycobacteria including *Mtb* complex. The BACTEC 460 radiometric and BACTEC 960 Mycobacterial Growth Indicator Tube (MGIT) fluorimetric systems (Becton, Dickinson, Sparks, MD) and the VersaTREK culture system (TREK Diagnostics Systems, Cleveland, OH) are FDA-cleared in the United States. The BACTEC 460 system is currently being phased out by the manufacturer in favor of the non-radiometric MGIT system. Other culture systems include Septi-Chek biphasic System (Becton, Dickinson,) and the MB/BacT Alert 3D system (bioMérieux, Marcy l'Etoile, France) which has a colorimetric CO_2-based sensor to detect mycobacterial growth. There are numerous publications in the literature which compare the performance of the commercially-available broth systems but in general, these systems have a sensitivity of 88-93% for the detection of *Mtb* complex (Cruciani et al., 2004).

Cultures for *Mtb* complex should be incubated at 35-37°C in an atmosphere of 5-10% CO_2 for primary cultures on solid medium. Since *Mtb* complex grows slowly in culture, many laboratories choose to examine culture plates for growth twice per week during early stages of growth and then weekly for older cultures. The advantage of semi-automated broth systems such as the MGIT and VersaTREK are that CO_2-supplementation is not generally required and the cultures are continuously monitored without the need for laboratory technologist intervention unless a culture is flagged by the instrument as positive. After either a solid or broth culture shows growth, the presence of acid-fast bacilli must be confirmed as described below in order to rule out non-mycobacterial contaminants.

5. Identification of *M. tuberculosis* from culture isolates

5.1 Microscopy

The first step in the examination of organisms growing on either solid media or liquid media is to confirm their identity using various staining methods as discussed in section 3. Depending on the stain used, the identification of *Mycobacterium* bacilli is done using either a light microscope under 100 x oil immersion objective or a fluorescent microscope under 25x or 40x objective. Microscopy however is not specific and cannot differentiate *Mtb* from other *Mycobacterium* and further analysis is required for final identification which can take up to 4-6 weeks.

Recently, the Microscopic Observation Drug Susceptibility (MODS) assay has been reported for the detection of *Mtb* complex in liquid culture through microscopic observation of characteristic cording and this method is characterized as in "late stage development/evaluation" for use in high TB burden settings by the World Health

Organization (WHO) (Caviedes & Moore, 2007; Moore, 2007; WHO, 2008; Ha et al., 2009; Limaye et al., 2010).

5.2 Biochemical analysis

Following microscopic and microscopic examination of culture isolates, final identification to the species level of *Mtb* complex is performed using a set of conventional biochemical reactions in combination with growth temperature. Although conventional biochemical assays are relatively inexpensive and simple to perform, they are time-consuming due to required incubation periods of up to 4 weeks, resulting in major delays in identification. Furthermore, with greater than 130 mycobacterial species identified to date, the use of phenotypic methods is limited and biased to identify only the most common species of mycobacteria, underestimating the complexity of the genus and resulting in misidentification of unfamiliar species (Kirschner et al., 1993; Springer et al., 1996). *M. tuberculosis*, as with other members of the *Mtb* complex, is a slow growing mycobacterium, requiring in general 15 days to 40 days to grow in culture. The optimal isolation temperature for the organism is 35-37°C and the organism does not produce pigmentation even following exposure to light (non-chromogen). The most useful biochemical tests used for identification of a nonchromogenic, slow-growing mycobacterium such as *Mtb* complex includes: niacin accumulation, nitrate reduction, pyrazinamidase activity, inhibition of thiophene-2-caroxylic acid hydrazide, urease activity and catalase activity. Other tests that can provide additional information include tellurite reduction, Tween 80 hydrolysis, the arylsulfatase test, iron uptake and NaCl tolerance. In general, a mature growth (2-3 weeks) is required for biochemical tests, they are often performed on a LJ slants and require up to 3 weeks for final read of results.

5.2.1 Niacin accumulation

Niacin (nicotinic acid) is produced by all species of mycobacteria and further metabolized to nicotinamide adenine dinucleotide (NAD). However, *Mtb* complex, *M. simiae* and some strains of *M. chelonae, M. bovis,* and *M. marinum* do not have the enzyme responsible for metabolizing niacin, resulting in its accumulation in the culture media. A water extract is prepared by adding 1 mL of sterile water to the surface of an LJ slant with a growth of mycobacteria species at least three weeks-old. An aliquot of this extract is then added to a tube containing a niacin strip, incubated for up to 30 minutes with gentle shaking. A positive reaction (presence of niacin) is read as the development of a yellow color. Since species other than *Mtb* complex can accumulate niacin, additional biochemical testing is required for the final identification of *Mtb* complex.

5.2.2 Nitrate reduction

M. tuberculosis complex contains the enzyme nitroreductase which is able to reduce nitrate (NO_3) into nitrite (NO_2). This reaction is detected in the laboratory by inoculating a nitrate broth with a loopful of a 3-4 weeks old mycobacterial culture and α-napthalamine, and sulfanilic acid that will react with the released NO_2 to produce a red or pink color. A negative result (lack of color) is further confirmed by the addition of zinc dust. If a red color (nitrate reduced) develops following addition of zinc dust, then the original result is confirmed as negative.

5.2.3 Pyrazinamidase

The deamination of pyrazinamide into pyrazinoic acid and ammonia by the enzyme pyrazinamidase (PZA) is an essential test to distinguish *Mtb* complex (PZA positive) from *M. bovis* (PZA negative). Other non-tuberculous mycobacteria species including *M. marinum* and *M. avium* complex can also be positive for PZA. The test is performed by inoculating two LJ slants with the mycobacterium species and incubating them for 4 days at 35-37°C in a non-CO_2 incubator. After 4 days, 1% ferric ammonium sulphate is added to one of the tube and incubated at room temperature for 30 minutes. The PZA reaction is positive if a pink band forms on the surface of the LJ slant. If the reaction is negative, the LJ slant is incubated for an additional 4 hours at 2-8 °C and observed for the appearance of the pink band. If the test is still negative after 4 hours, the second tube will be tested on day 7 to finalize the test.

5.2.4 Urease

The presence of urease, the enzyme that hydrolyzes urea into ammonia and carbon dioxide, can be detected in mycobacterial species by incubating an actively growing culture to a urea broth for up to 7 days at 35-37°C in a non-CO_2 incubator, with readings done at days 1, 3 and 7. *M. tuberculosis* complex is positive for urease and will produce a dark pink to red color following incubation in urea broth.

5.2.5 Inhibition of thiophene-2-caroxylic acid hydrazide (TCH)

M. tuberculosis complex can be differentiated from *M. bovis* by its ability to grow in the presence of TCH, a property shared by most mycobacteria species except for *M. bovis*. This test uses quadrant Petri dishes with one of the quadrant containing TCH. A dilute suspension of the mycobacterial growth (10^{-3} to 10^{-4} in sterile water) is added to each quadrant and the plate incubated for 3 weeks at 35-37°C in a 10 % CO_2 incubator. A resistant organism shows greater than 1% growth in the TCH quadrant when compared to growth in the control quadrant.

5.2.6 Arylsulfatase test

Arylsulfatase is an enzyme that hydrolyzes free phenolphthalein from the tri-potassium salt of phenolphthalein disulfite. A suspension of a pure mycobacterium culture in sterile water is incubated with phenolphthalein in oleic acid agar for either 3 days (rapid growers) or 14 days (slow growers) at 35-37°C in a non-CO_2 incubator. The appearance of a pink or red color after addition of sodium bicarbonate (Na_2CO_3) indicates a positive reaction. All members of the *Mtb* complex lack the arylsulfatase enzyme and are therefore negative for that reaction (Koneman, 2006; Lee, 2010).

5.2.7 Catalase test

Catalase is an enzyme that splits hydrogen peroxide (H_2O_2) into water (H_2O) and oxygen (O_2). Unlike the catalase assay used to identify for other types of bacteria (i.e. *Streptococcus* spp.), the catalase assay for mycobacteria is performed using 30% H_2O_2 (Superoxol) in 10% Tween-80 and the test performed both at 22-25°C and 68°C. *M. tuberculosis* complex has catalase activity at 22-25°C but not at 68°C (ie., heat-labile catalase). In addition to determining catalase activity at 68°C, the strength of the catalase reaction is also evaluated to differentiate *Mtb* complex from other mycobacteria. This semiquantitative test is performed by adding Superoxol to a 2-weeks-old culture of mycobacteria growing on a Lowenstein-Jensen slant at 37°C. Five minutes after addition of the Superoxol, the strength of the catalase reaction is determined by measuring the height of the bubbles, characteristic of the catalase reaction, in the tube. If the height of the bubbles is > 45 mm, the reaction is considered high and if the height of the bubbles is < 45 mm, the reaction is considered low. *M. tuberculosis* complex has low catalase activity.

5.2.8 Iron uptake

Only a few mycobacteria species are able to take up iron from ferric ammonium citrate and convert it to iron oxide (rust). This biochemical reaction is mainly used to identify *M. fortuitum* which when incubated with 20% ferric ammonium citrate for up to 3 weeks on a Lowenstein-Jensen slant at 28-30°C will turn a dark, rusty brown color. *M. tuberculosis* complex does not take up iron.

5.2.9 NaCl tolerance

The ability to grow on media containing 5% NaCl differentiates the slow growing mycobacteria from the rapid growers as only *M. triviale* (a slow grower) can grow on this media and only *M. chelonae* and *M. mucogenicum* (rapid growers) fails to grow in the presence of this salt concentration. The test is performed by inoculating an LJ slant containing 5% NaCl with a 1 MacFarland concentration of a mycobacterial culture and incubating it at 28°C in a 5-10% CO_2 incubator for up to 4 weeks (Witebsky & Kruczak-Filipov, 1996; Lee, 2010). *M. tuberculosis* complex does not grow on LJ slant containing 5% NaCl.

5.2.10 Tellurite reduction

Most mycobacterium can reduce potassium tellurite to metallic tellurium in liquid broth within 3 days. The test is performed by inoculating a Middlebrook 7H9 liquid medium containing Tween 80 with a heavy concentration of organisms and incubating at 37°C in a 5-10% CO_2 incubator for up to 7 days. After 7 days, a solution of potassium tellurite is added to the liquid culture and further incubated for 3 days. A positive reaction shows a black precipitate (metallic tellurium) at the bottom of the tube. This test is often used to identify MAC. *M. tuberculosis* complex is negative for tellurite reduction (Witebsky & Kruczak-Filipov, 1996; Lee, 2010).

5.2.11 Tween 80 hydrolysis

This assay tests for the presence of the enzyme lipase which can cleave the oleic acid from the detergent Tween 80 (polyoxyethylene sorbitan monooleate). The release of the oleic acid from Tween 80 results in a change of color of the neutral indicator from yellow to red within 5-10 days after incubation of Tween-80 with a mycobacterium at 37°C in a 5-10% CO_2 incubator. *M. tuberculosis* complex is negative for Tween 80 hydrolysis.

The use of conventional methods for the initial identification of *Mtb* complex is not ideal. This section provided a review of the most common tests used traditionally but the combined use of these various assays results in a significant delay in identification of up to one month after growth of the culture in the laboratory. The following sections will cover the more rapid methods currently in use in most mycobacteriology laboratory for identification of *Mtb* complex.

Biochemical Test	**Reaction**
niacin accumulation	Positive
nitrate reduction	Positive
pyrazinamidase activity	Positive
urease activity	Positive
inhibition of thiophene-2-caroxylic acid hydrazide (TCH)	Positive
arylsulfatase test	Negative
catalase test	Negative (heat-labile)
iron uptake	Negative
NaCl tolerance	Negative
tellurite reduction	Negative
Tween 80 hydrolysis	Negative

Table 2. Biochemical tests for identification of *Mycobacterium tuberculosis* complex from a culture isolate

5.3 High-Performance Liquid Chromatography

High-performance liquid chromatography (HPLC) of mycolic acids was first proposed for use as a standard test in mycobacteria species identification by the CDC in 1985. This technique had been widely used by clinical chemistry laboratories for the separation and identification of drug compounds (Butler & Guthertz, 2001). HPLC can be used to differentiate mycobacteria based on differences in their mycolic acid profiles. Mycolic acids are high-molecular weight fatty acids with long carbon side chains present in abundance in the cell wall of mycobacteria and other organisms including *Corynebacterium, Dietzia, Rhodococcus, Nocardia, Gordonia, Williamsia, Skermania,* and *Tsukamurella* species with *Mycobacterium* species containing the longest carbon chain (60-90) (Butler & Guthertz, 2001). Mycolic acids samples are prepared through a series of steps involving saponification of the mycobacteria, organic solvent extraction and derivatization of the mycolic acids to UV-adsorbing *p*-bromophenacyl (PBPA) esters (Durst et al., 1975; Butler et al., 1991). The derivatized mycolic acids solution is then separated on a HPLC instrument and the resulting chromatogram interpreted based on the peak pattern which is specific for each species of mycobacterium (Butler et al., 1991; Butler & Guthertz, 2001).

Although sensitive and specific when compared to biochemical tests and other molecular assays, with agreement ranging from 90-99% depending on the mycobacterial species (Guthertz et al., 1993; Thibert & Lapierre, 1993), HPLC is a technically demanding method which is not easily implemented in routine diagnostic laboratories. This method requires a high level of expertise for recognition of species based on the HPLC chromatogram and therefore only limited to a few reference laboratories including the CDC in Atlanta, GA. A commercial HPLC assay, the Sherlock Mycobacteria Identification HPLC system (SMIS; MIDI Inc., Newark, DE), was developed to simplify use of HPLC in the clinical laboratories through automated recognition of mycobacterial species based on software that analyzes HPLC peak patterns comparing them to a library containing several *Mycobacterium* species chromatograms (Kellogg et al., 2001; LaBombardi et al., 2006). Of the 370 isolates tested in a multicenter study by SMIS, 327 (88%) were identified to the species level by the SMIS software with 279 (75%) correctly identified (Kellogg et al., 2001). The sensitivity of the SMIS identification could be increased to 98.9% (366/370) by manual calculation of relative peak height ratios and relative retention times and additional biochemical properties. In another study by LaBombardi et al. (LaBombardi et al., 2006), the SIMS correctly identified 61/90 isolates (67.8%) growing on Middlebrook 7H11 plates (BBL, Sparks, MD) and 73/161 (45.3%) isolates growing in VersaTREK Myco bottles (TREK Diagnostic Systems, Cleveland, OH). This performance was increased by used of a modified library to 91% for isolates growing on solid media and 83.2% for isolates recovered from liquid culture. In both studies, no *Mtb* complex isolates were misidentified and the sensitivity ranged from 83-100% (Kellogg et al., 2001; LaBombardi et al., 2006). Of note, although HPLC is a faster and more sensitive technology than conventional biochemical testing, this method cannot be used directly on clinical specimen and is not able to differentiate between members of the *Mtb* complex, except for the *M. bovis* BCG strain (Butler et al., 1991; Floyd et al., 1992).

5.4 Nucleic acid hybridization probes

The introduction of nucleic acid hybridization probes in the clinical laboratory significantly impacted the turn-around time and workload for identification of mycobacteria species. Nucleic acid hybridization probes are single-stranded or double-stranded DNA/RNA fragments, labeled with a radioactive, chemiluminescent or a fluorescent marker, that are complementary to a target DNA or RNA sequence (Wetmur, 1991). In clinical microbiology, nucleic acid hybridization probes often target ribosomal RNA (rRNA) because of their high copy number present in organisms growing in culture. The first nucleic acid hybridization probes from Gen-Probe (San Diego, CA) for rapid identification of *M. avium* complex and *Mtb* complex were labeled with I^{125} radioactive isotope. Labeled DNA-RNA complexes were separated from non-hybridized DNA using an adsorption suspension containing hydroxyapatite and the I^{125} in the adsorbed labeled complex was counted using a gamma counter. Results were calculated as percentage of input probe hybridized (Drake et al., 1987; Kiehn & Edwards, 1987; Ellner et al., 1988; Musial et al., 1988; Peterson et al., 1989). The introduction of these radioactive probes resulted in a significant decrease in the turn-around time for identification of both *M. avium* complex and *Mtb* complex from weeks to approximately 2 hours with sensitivity and specificity ranging from 83-100% and 99.2-100% respectively (Drake et al., 1987; Kiehn & Edwards, 1987; Ellner et al., 1988; Musial et al., 1988; Peterson et al., 1989).

The I^{125} probes were eventually replaced with non-radioactive probes to reduce staff potential for exposure to radioactive materials. Two types of non-isotopic probes were introduced, the synthetic nucleic acid probes (SNAP) (Syngene, Inc., San Diego, CA) and the AccuProbes (Gen-Probe, San Diego, CA). The SNAP probes utilized DNA probes labeled with alkaline-phosphatase and was performed by spotting the isolate to be tested on a nylon membrane and incubating the membrane with the labeled probes, followed by incubation in a solution of nitroblue tetrazolium chloride, 5-brom-4-chloro-3- indolyphosphate substrates and alkaline phosphatase buffer. A positive reaction was read as the presence of a blue or purple color on the nylon membrane within a few hours (Lim et al., 1991; Woodley et al., 1992). Although 100% sensitive, cross-reactivity was detected with SNAP probes between *Mtb* complex and *M. terrae*, requiring the 68°C catalase test to be performed to differentiate between the two species (Lim et al., 1991; Ford et al., 1993).

AccuProbes are labeled with acridinium ester and hybridization is measured by chemiluminescence following hydrolysis of the label upon addition of H_2O_2 and NaOH. The chemiluminescence is measured using a luminometer and expressed as RLU (relative light units). Unlike the previous version with the I^{125} isotope, no wash steps are necessary as non-hybridized probes are chemically degraded and only acridinium ester-labeled, hybridized probes can produce measurable chemiluminescence (Goto et al., 1991). The AccuProbe for *Mtb* complex can be performed on culture growing from both liquid and solid media and will detect all members of the *Mtb* complex (Gen-Probe, 2011). The sensitivity and specificity of the acridinium ester labeled probes was comparable to that of the radioisotope labeled probes (Goto et al., 1991; Lebrun et al., 1992). Similar to the SNAP probes, detection of some strain of *M. terrae* by *Mtb* complex probes was also observed (Lim et al., 1991; Ford et al., 1993), although increased stringency in the detection method resolved the false-positive detection of *M. terrae* by AccuProbes *Mtb* complex probes.

Although the use of nucleic acid probes has allowed same day identification of *Mtb* complex from culture, the sensitivity of these probes is not high enough for detection of the organisms directly from clinical specimens, which still limits the rapid identification to the time it takes for the organisms to grow in either liquid or solid media. Furthermore, the *Mtb* complex AccuProbes do not distinguish amongst members of the *Mtb* complex.

5.5 Line Probe assays

Line Probe assays were developed to expand the range of mycobacterium species identified using nucleic acid probes since those were only available for *Mtb* complex, *M. avium*, *M. intracellulare*, *M. kansasii* and *M. gordonae* (Gen-Probe, San Diego, CA). The first commercially available LineProbe assay, the INNO LiPa Mycobacteria (Innogenetics, Ghent, Belgium), uses reverse hybridization technology in which probes are immobilized as parallel lines on a membrane strips as opposed to being in solution as is the case with AccuProbes. Amplified, biotinylated DNA fragments of the 16-23S rRNA spacer region of mycobacterial organisms are incubated with the labeled strips; addition of streptavidin-alkaline phosphatase and a chromogenic substrates results in the formation of a precipitate on the membrane where hybridization as occurred (Scarparo et al., 2001; Tortoli et al., 2001). The LiPa assay is able to detect up to 14 different species of mycobacteria (Table 3) and results are interpreted according to a flowchart decision scheme (Tortoli et al., 2001). A multicenter evaluation of LiPa assay conducted in Italy tested 238 mycobacterial organisms from both solid and liquid media as well as two Nocardia strains (Tortoli et al., 2001). All 238 mycobacterial strains reacted with the genus specific probes for a sensitivity of 100% and 61 of the 238 strains were identified to the species level. The other 177 strains were outside of the detection range of the LiPa assay. Additional studies using only liquid culture media, MB/BacT Alert 3D (Organon Teknika, Boxtel, The Netherlands), and BACTEC 12B Bottles (BACTEC; Becton Dickinson, Sparks, MD), showed similar sensitivity of 100% for detection of mycobacterial strains by the genus specific probes as well as correct identification at the species levels and specificity of 100% (Miller et al., 2000; Scarparo et al., 2001).

The LiPa test is a more complex assay than the AccuProbe, requiring highly skilled technologists and has a turn-around time of at least 6 hours, including a PCR amplification step. Furthermore, control of the hybridization temperature is key to preventing formation of non-specific bands. However, in addition to its ability to detect several mycobacterial species compared to AccuProbes, the Inno-LiPa assay has the advantage of being able to detect mixed mycobacterial infections which often results in decreased sensitivity of the AccuProbes (Scarparo et al., 2001). Both assays still have to be performed from organisms growing in culture and are not able to differentiate among the members of the *Mtb* complex.

Another line probe assay, the GenoType Mycobacterium (Hain, Nehren, Germany) was developed and made available in two different kit formats. One kit, the Genotype Mycobacterium CM (Common Mycobacteria) was designed to detect the most frequently isolated mycobacteria species in clinical laboratories while the other kit, the Genotype Mycobacterium AS (Additional Species), was designed for the detection of less frequently encountered mycobacteria species (Makinen et al., 2006; Richter et al., 2006; Russo et al., 2006). Russo and colleagues tested 197 isolates including genera other than mycobacteria previously identified by conventional biochemical tests, HPLC, Inno-Lipa and 16S rRNA sequencing (Russo et al., 2006). The sensitivity of the assay for the mycobacterium genus was 98.9 and 99.4% for the CM and AS kits respectively with a specificity of 100% for the AS kit and 88.9% for the CM kit due to weak cross-reaction of several strains of the genus *Tsukamurella*. The overall sensitivity and specificity for species identification was 97.9% and 92.4% for the CM kit and 99.3% and 99.4% for the AS kit with all members of the *Mtb* complex correctly identified as *Mtb* complex by the CM kit and *Mtb* species by the AS kit. Similar performance were established in other independent studies evaluating the GenoType CM and AS kits, with the sensitivity and specificity for *Mtb* complex members approaching 100% when compared to 16S rRNA sequencing and biochemical testing (Makinen et al., 2006; Richter et al., 2006).

A third kit from Hain LifeScience, the Genotype MTBC DNA strip assay was designed specifically for the differentiation of members of the *Mtb* complex and identification of *M. bovis* BCG. Similar to the LiPa assay, the MTBC DNA strip assay uses reverse hybridization technology on a solid membrane matrix. The DNA probes immobilized on the membranes target polymorphisms in the *gyrB* DNA sequence of the *Mtb* complex and the RD1 deletion of *M. bovis* BCG (Richter et al., 2003). Ritcher and colleagues (Richter et al., 2003) evaluated the performance of the MTBC assay using well-characterized strains of *Mtb* complex including *Mtb*, *M. bovis* subsp. *bovis*, *M. bovis* subsp. *caprae*, *M. bovis* BCG, *M. africanum* subtype I , *M. africanum* subtype II , *M. canetti*, and *M. microti* as well as clinical isolates of *Mtb* complex identified by conventional methods and other molecular tests (PCR-Restriction fragment length polymorphism). The MTBC assay was able to differentiate all species of the *Mtb* complex except for separating *Mtb* from some strains of *M. africanum* subtype II and *M. canetti* (sensitivity of 94%). A similar study conducted by Neonakis and colleagues showed 100% agreement between conventional methods/AccuProbes and MTBC assay for the identification and differentiation of 120 clinical isolates of the *Mtb* complex (Neonakis et al., 2007).

Species	**AccuProbes**	**Inno-LiPa**	**GenoType CM**	**GenoType AS**	**GenoType MTBC**
Mycobacterium spp.		X	X		
M. tuberculosis complex	X	X	X		
M. tuberculosis					X
M. bovis subsp. *bovis*					X
M. bovis BCG					X
M. bovis subsp. *caprae*					X
M. africanum					X
M. microti					X
M. kansasii	X	X	X	X	
M. avium	X	X	X		
M. intracellulare	X	X	X		
MAI-X		X			
M. malmonense		X	X		
M. haemophilum		X		X	
M. scrofulaceum		X	X		
M. paratuberculosis		X			
M. silvaticum		X			
M. chelonae		X	X		
M. gastri		X		X	
M. xenopi		X	X		
M. gordonae	X	X	X		
M. abscessus			X		
M. fortuitum			X		
M. marinum			X		
M. ulcerans			X	X	
M. peregrinum			X		
M. simiae				X	
M. mucogenicum				X	
M. goodii				X	
M. celatum				X	
M. smegmatis				X	
M. genavense				X	
M. lentiflavum				X	
M. heckeshornense				X	
M. szulgai				X	
M. phlei				X	
M. asiaticum				X	
M. shimoidei				X	

Table 3. Mycobacterium species detected by commercially available probe assays

5.6 DNA sequencing

The first report of nucleic acid sequencing for the identification of mycobacteria appeared in the literature in the early 1990s. Rogall et al. (Rogall et al., 1990) described the use of a 1 kb gene fragment targeting the 5′ region of the 16S rRNA to detect and differentiate among the various species of mycobacteria, including the *Mtb* complex. In this study, amplified sequences were electrophoresed on a 6% sequencing gel, dried and the gel was exposed to X-rays film for 12 hours. Sequences obtained were then analyzed using a multisequence alignment algorithm from SAGE program (Rogall et al., 1990). This entire process was completed in approximately 2 days. Other nucleic acid targets were analyzed including the *rpoB* gene, encoding the β-subunit of the RNA polymerase, which had the added advantage of detecting rifampin resistance (Kim et al., 1999; Kasai et al., 2000), the 16-23S rDNA internal transcribed spacer (ITS) (Roth et al., 1998), the 32-kDa protein (Soini et al., 1994) and the 65 kDa heat shock protein (Kapur et al., 1995). Each of these targets presented advantages and disadvantages, mainly related to their ability to differentiate closely-related organisms. Today, sequencing of the 16S rDNA has become the gold standard for mycobacteria species identification. The process was eventually automated and commercialized (MicroSeq 500bp and 1500bp 16S rDNA Bacterial Sequencing Kits, Applied Biosystems, Carlsbad, CA), which resulted in standardization of the assay across laboratories. The MicroSeq 16S rDNA bacterial identification assay analyzes a larger portion of the 16S rDNA than the one described earlier by Rogall et al. (Rogall et al., 1990), resulting in increased discriminating power. The introduction of capillary electrophoresis and fluorescent dyes to replace the cumbersome sequencing gels and radioactive labels, the development of genetic analyzer and the National Center for Biotechnology Information (NCBI) tool, BLAST (Basic Local Alignment Sequence Tool), further improved on the use of sequencing for mycobacterial species identification.

DNA sequencing using the MicroSeq system is based on sequencing by capillary electrophoresis and consists of 4 steps: DNA extraction, amplification, sequencing and data analysis. Total genomic DNA extraction is performed simply by lysis of organisms in a chaotropic solution (PrepMan Ultra, Applied Biosystems), followed by heating at 95°C for 10 minutes to kill the organisms. Extraction is followed by 16S rRNA amplification, PCR products clean-up and sequencing PCR and analysis on a genetic analyzer. The sequence obtained is then analyzed against the MicroSeq database library and/or the BLAST database on the NCBI website (http://blast.ncbi.nlm.nih.gov/Blast.cgi).

Studies evaluating the performance of the MicroSeq systems for identification of mycobacteria have repeatedly shown the advantages of using this technique over traditional biochemical tests and with the increase in available and correct sequences in various database, the sensitivity of the assay continues to increase (Patel et al., 2000; Cloud et al., 2002; Hall et al., 2003; Woo et al., 2011). The main limitation of sequencing for identification of mycobacteria as discussed above remains the inability to distinguish several species of mycobacteria based solely on the 16S rRNA including *M. chelonae*, *M. abscessus*, and *M. immunogenum* and the various members of the *Mtb* complex (Hall et al., 2003; Woo et al., 2011). Alternative sequencing targets (eg., *rpoB*) can often be used to distinguish mycobacterial species which cannot be resolved using the 16S target.

5.7 PCR methods (conventional and real-time)

The pattern of resistance of pyrazinamide (PZA) is often used to distinguish between *Mtb* and *M. bovis/M. bovis* BCG strains (section 5.2.3). Only a few laboratory-developed tests (LDTs) have been designed to differentiate among members of the *Mtb* complex (Parsons et al., 2002; Huard et al., 2003; Pinsky & Banaei, 2008). Pinsky and Banaei (Pinsky & Banaei, 2008) reported a real-time PCR assay, using a series of different primer pairs targeting the RD (region of difference) 9 (present in all *Mtb* complex members), the RD1 (absent in *M. bovis* BCG strains), the RD4 (absent in *M. bovis*). This multiplex real-time PCR uses melt curve analysis from two separate PCRs to identify and distinguish between *Mtb, M. bovis,* and *M. bovis* BCG directly from isolates growing in culture. Similarly, although on a conventional PCR format, the RD1 sequence was used as a target for the differentiation of *Mtb, M. bovis,* and *M. bovis* BCG from culture isolates (Lee et al., 2010).

5.8 Immunoassay methods

There are several commercially-available immunoassay methods which allow the identification of *Mtb* complex from culture by detection of *Mtb*-specific antigens. These tests are rapid requiring only minutes to perform after growth of the organism but literature reports indicate variable performance (Martin et al., 2011; Said et al., 2011; Steingart et al., 2011; Yu et al., 2011)

6. Direct identification of *M. tuberculosis* from clinical specimens

6.1 Line probe assays

The INNO LiPa Mycobacteria (Innogenetics), described previously in section 5.5, has been evaluated for use directly on clinical specimens without waiting for growth of *Mtb* complex in culture. In a study by Perandin et al. (Perandin et al., 2006), the INNO Lipa Mycobacteria assay was evaluated, with slight modifications, on both pulmonary specimens and extrapulmonary specimens (stools, urines, lymph nodes, gastric fluids and pus). The overall sensitivity and specificity of the test was 79.5% and 84.6% respectively for pulmonary specimens and 71.4% and 100 %, respectively for extrapulmonary specimens. As expected the sensitivity and specificity of the assay was much lower when tested on specimens than culture isolates and the authors suggested this was due to the lower numbers of organisms present in specimens.

The INNO-LiPA Rif TB (Innogenetics) test, designed to detect *Mtb* complex and rifampin susceptibility in culture isolates, has also been tested on clinical specimens in multiple studies (Gamboa et al., 1998; de Oliveira et al., 2003; Johansen et al., 2003; Traore et al., 2006). In one of the largest studies, Traore and colleagues (Traore et al., 2006) evaluated the performance of the INNO-LiPA assay by testing 420 sputum samples from both treated and untreated patients, with 311 smear positive and 109 smear negative specimens. The assay detected *Mtb* complex DNA in 92% of smear positive specimens and 94.5% of smear negative specimens, a higher detection rate than culture which detected *Mtb* complex in 74.3% of all specimens.

An alternative version to the line assay GenoType Mycobacterium (Hain LifeScience), the GenoType Mycobacterium Direct Assay (Hain Lifescience) was designed to detect *Mtb* complex and *M. avium, M. intracellulare, M. kansasii,* and *M. malmoense* directly from clinical specimens. This assay is performed in three parts consisting of an RNA isolation and capture step, followed by an isothermal amplification of the 23S rRNA, and finally a reverse-hybridization of the amplified products on the membrane strips. Evaluation of this assay showed sensitivity and specificity ranging from 80.5-97% to 75-100% respectively when compared to culture (Franco-Alvarez de Luna et al., 2006; Seagar et al., 2008; Neonakis et al., 2009; Kiraz et al., 2010).

In general, the sensitivity of these line assays is lower when tested directly on clinical specimens as compared to their sensitivity when used on culture isolates. However, with a turn-around time of about 2 days compared to at least 6 weeks to obtain growth in culture, these assays, with their high specificity, provide information that is directly useful for clinical management of patients.

6.2 FDA-approved PCR methods

The first FDA-approved amplification test for diagnosis of *Mtb* complex was the Amplified Mycobacterium Tuberculosis Direct (MTD) test (Gen-Probe Inc, San Diego, CA). This assay was based on the amplification of *Mtb* complex rRNA followed by detection of the amplified rRNA by hybridization of chemiluminescent acridinium ester-labeled DNA probes. The sensitivity and specificity of the assay in earlier studies testing against N-acetyl-L-cysteine treated respiratory samples (smear positive and smear negative), was 91.9-100% and 97.6-100%, respectively when compared to culture (Abe et al., 1993; Pfyffer et al., 1994; Welch et al., 1995). The MTD test presented several advantages over traditional methods including the use of rRNA, which is present in several copies in *Mtb* complex, rapid turn-around time (day vs. weeks), single tube amplification and detection, although culture is still required for susceptibility testing of the organisms (Abe et al., 1993; Pfyffer et al., 1994). The MTD test is only FDA-approved for respiratory specimens; however, the assay performance in extrapulmonary specimens has also been evaluated by several investigators. Vlaspodler et al. (Vlaspolder et al., 1995) showed variable sensitivity for different specimens with detection in pleural fluids being as low as 20% (with specificity of 96%) and sensitivity and specificity in other specimens, including urines, lymph nodes, CSF, gastric fluids and lung biopsies, of 100% and 95% respectively. Similar results were obtained in other studies that included a greater numbers of non-respiratory specimens, with sensitivities ranging from 93-100% and specificities of 100% for both smear-positive and smear negative specimens (Chedore & Jamieson, 1999; Woods et al., 2001).

A second PCR assay approved by the FDA was the AMPLICOR *Mycobacterium tuberculosis* test (AMPLICOR MTB; Roche Diagnostic Systems, Somerville, N.J.). This assay targeted the 16S rRNA gene with colorimetric detection using probe hybridization (Piersimoni & Scarparo, 2003). In a study by D'Amato and colleagues, the sensitivity and specificity of the Amplicor MTB when compared to culture as the gold standard was: 55.3% and 99.6% from smear negative and 94.1% and 100% from smear positive respiratory specimens (D'Amato et al., 1995). Other studies showed sensitivity and specificity for the assay ranging from 70.4% to 79.5% with specificity greater than 98% when compared to culture and conventional microscopy (Schirm et al., 1995; Bergmann & Woods, 1996; Devallois et al., 1996) and sensitivity generally increasing 75-98 % for AFB positive specimens (Schirm et al., 1995; Bergmann & Woods, 1996). Testing of non-respiratory samples by the Amplicor MTB assay supported its use in diagnosis of extrapulmonary tuberculosis as the sensitivity and specificity varied from 76%-100% and 99.9-100%, respectively when compared to clinical diagnosis (Shah et al., 1998). These non-respiratory specimens included various tissue biopsies (lung, lymph nodes, liver) and various body fluids (pleural, ascites, CSF, synovial, gastric, pericardial and peritoneal).

A second version of the Amplicor assay, the Cobas Amplicor MTB-PCR (Roche Diagnostics) was developed as a semi-automated assay that combined the amplification, detection and reporting of results (Bodmer et al., 1997; Levidiotou et al., 2003). Evaluation of the new assay showed increased sensitivity over the manual assay with one study testing >1,000 respiratory specimens reporting a sensitivity and specificity of 91.3% and 99.6% (Bodmer et al., 1997) and the other reporting an overall sensitivity and specificity of 82.5% and 99.8% after testing greater than 7,000 specimens (respiratory and non-respiratory)(Levidiotou et al., 2003).

Both the MTD and the Amplicor assays were evaluated on broth samples including BACTECT 12B bottles (Becton Dickinson, Sparks, MD) and the ESP II (Trek Diagnostics, Westlake, OH), with sensitivity of greater than 90% for both assays in both media and specificity of 100% (Hernandez et al., 1997; Smith et al., 1997; Bergmann & Woods, 1999; Desmond & Loretz, 2001).

6.3 Laboratory-developed PCR methods

Several targets, including the 65-kD antigen of *Mtb* complex (Pao et al., 1990; Brisson-Noel et al., 1991; Totsch et al., 1994), the protein antigen B (Sjobring et al., 1990), the repetitive sequences IS6110 (Brisson-Noel et al., 1991; Eisenach et al., 1991; Sankar et al., 2010) and IS986 (Abe et al., 1993), have been used over the years for the detection of *Mtb* complex by LDTs. Earlier tests were based on conventional PCR, with a multi-step manual extraction process followed by amplification and detection of the amplified target on polyacrylamide gel. Depending on the target used, the sensitivity and specificity of these conventional PCR assays directly from respiratory specimens ranged from 84.2-100% and 62.6-100% with culture and clinical diagnosis used as a gold standard. However, due to limitations inherent with conventional PCR including high potential for cross-contamination, real-time PCRs, combined with automated extraction, have largely replaced these methods in clinical laboratories.

Real-time PCR is faster than conventional PCR and does not require post-amplification manipulation of the amplified DNA, reducing the potential for cross-contamination. Several real-time PCR LDTs have been developed for diagnosis of pulmonary tuberculosis. In one of the earlier studies by Miller et al (Miller et al., 2002), a real-time PCR assay was developed on the LightCycler platform (Roche Diagnostics, Indianapolis, IN) with primers targeting the internal transcribed spacer region of the mycobacterium genome with specific hybridization probes designed for the detection of *Mtb* complex. The sensitivity and specificity of this assay for smear-positive respiratory specimens was 98.1% and 100% respectively with a turn-around time of less than 5 hours (Miller et al., 2002). Other studies, with different targets, have reported similar results (Shrestha et al., 2003) and many have been designed as multiplex assays to differentiate *Mtb* complex from other non-tuberculosis mycobacteria based on melting curve analysis (Shrestha et al., 2003). Furthermore, these assays were often shown to be as sensitive and specific as the available commercial assays such as the Cobas Amplicor (Miller et al., 2002; Shrestha et al., 2003).

Both conventional and real-time PCRs have also been developed for the diagnosis of extrapulmonary tuberculosis using both fresh specimens and paraffin-embedded tissues. Some of the fresh specimens that have been evaluated by various PCR include fine needle aspirates and tissue biopsies of lymph nodes, blood, urines, bone marrow aspirates and skin biopsies with variable sensitivities and specificities (Hsiao et al., 2003; Bruijnesteijn Van Coppenraet et al., 2004; Chakravorty & Tyagi, 2005; Ritis et al., 2005; Torrea et al., 2005; Rebollo et al., 2006). Although paraffin-embedded tissues are not optimal samples for PCR, often, they are the only specimens available to rule out tuberculosis. The sensitivity and specificity of PCR assays, conventional and real-time, on paraffin-embedded tissues varies from 64-100% and 73- 100%, respectively (Beqaj et al., 2007; Baba et al., 2008; Nopvichai et al., 2009; Luo et al., 2010).

Unlike PCR assays previously mentioned for differentiation of members of *Mtb* complex, a real-time PCR assay, developed by Halse and colleagues (Halse et al., 2011) at the New York State Public Health Laboratory, showed the ability to differentiate among members of the *Mtb* complex directly from clinical specimens based on the detection of five targets including RD1, RD4, RD9, RD12 and a region external to RD9. The assay was able to detect 155 of 165 clinical specimens (94%) and 708/727 (97%) of positive BACTEC MGIT-960 bottles. Furthermore, this assay was able to distinguish not only *Mtb*, *M. bovis* and *M. bovis* BCG but also *M. africanum*, *M. microti*, and *M. canettii*.

7. Drug resistance testing for *M. tuberculosis*

The CDC published recommendations that drug susceptibility testing be performed on the first *Mtb* complex isolate from a each patient and also if a patient is failing therapy (based on clinical evidence or positive culture after three months on therapy) (MMWR, 1993). This recommendation was formulated following a resurgence in cases of tuberculosis from the mid-1980s to the early 1990s of up to 18% with resistance strains present in as high as 33% of cases in New York city (MMWR, 1993). Susceptibility testing is currently performed most commonly by traditional methods either agar-based or broth based methods with resistance defined as growth of greater than 1% of organisms tested against a specific drug (Canetti et al., 1963).

7.1 Indirect proportion method

Although patient specimens can be tested directly for drug susceptibility with the advantage of decreased time to results, this method is limited to smear-positive specimens and results may be difficult to interpret if contamination occurs (Woods, 2011). The 1% indirect proportion method is performed on Middlebrook 7H10 agar medium poured in a four-quadrant Petri dish with one quadrant serving as the control quadrant and containing no drug and the other three quadrants containing increasing concentration of the drug being tested. The inoculum is prepared using organisms growing on solid or liquid media adjusted to a 1.0 McFarland and diluted to 10^{-2} and 10^{-4}; 0. 1 mL of each dilution is then added to each quadrant of separate plate and incubated for up to three weeks at 37 ± 1°C in an atmosphere of 5 to 10% CO_2 (CLSI, 2003). The percentage of drug resistance is calculated by dividing the total colony count in a quadrant containing drug by the total colony count in the control quadrant (at least 50 colonies) and multiplying by 100. If the percentage is greater than 1%, then the organism is resistant and therapy with the drug tested is likely to fail (CLSI, 2008; Woods, 2011). This method is used primarily for susceptibility testing of the first line drugs, isoniazid (INH), rifampin (RIF) and ethambutol (EMB), as well as second line drugs, when resistance to RIF or two of the first-line drug is detected (CLSI, 2008).

7.2 Rapid broth methods

In order to circumvent the long turn-around time of the agar proportion methods and provide clinicians with timely drug susceptibility results, rapid broth methods were developed for both growth and susceptibility testing of *Mtb* complex. The first system, the BACTEC 460, was a based on measurement of radioactive $^{14}CO_2$ produced by metabolic breakdown of ^{14}C-labelled palmitic acid contained in a 7H12 liquid medium in the presence or absence of specific drugs (Middlebrook et al., 1977; Siddiqi et al., 1981; Snider et al., 1981; Laszlo et al., 1983). The agreement between the conventional and the radiometric susceptibility testing assays varied from 96.4-98% with most results obtained within 7 days (Siddiqi et al., 1981; Laszlo et al., 1983). Additionally, unlike the 1% indirect agar method, the radiometric method was conducive to testing of *Mtb* complex susceptibility against pyrazinamide (PZA), which requires an acidic environment not easily achievable on solid media. Heifets and Isman modified the radiometric method by lowering the pH with addition of phosphoric acid at the same time as PZA but after the growing culture had reached exponential phase (Heifets & Iseman, 1985). This initial study, with limited number of isolates, showed good correlation between PZA susceptibility as measured by the radiometric method and detection of the pyrazinamidase enzyme as described under biochemical testing (Heifets & Iseman, 1985). The method described by Heifets and Isman was further modified and proved useful in facilitating the measurement of PZA susceptibility of *Mtb* complex by the radiometric method (Tarrand et al., 1986; Salfinger & Heifets, 1988).

The BACTEC 460 radiometric method for susceptibility testing was eventually replaced with the fully automated Mycobacteria Growth Indicator tube (MGIT 960, Becton Dickinson, Sparks, MD), which had been introduced for broth culture of mycobacteria species from clinical specimens without the use of radioactive materials (Chew et al., 1998; Heifets et al., 2000). Each drug-containing MGIT bottle is inoculated with either 0.5 mL of a 1:100 dilution of a MGIT tube positive for 1-2 days, a 1:5 dilution of a MGIT tube positive for 3-5 days or a 0.5 McFarland if the inoculum is prepared from an organism growing on solid media (Siddiqi, 2010). The control, drug-free MGIT bottle is inoculated with a 1:100 dilution of the inoculum used for the drug-containing MGIT bottle. The MGIT 960 system automatically interprets the results of the test based on the growth unit (GU). If the GU is greater than 100 for a drug-containing MGIT bottle, the isolate is resistant and if the GU is less than or equal to 100 then the isolate is susceptible. However, for the test to be valid, the GU of the control bottle cannot reach 400 before 4 days or after 13 days, which suggests that the growth was too heavy or too light respectively (Woods, 2011). The MGIT 960 system is FDA-approved for susceptibility testing of *Mtb* complex against the first-line drugs including RIF (2 μg/ml), INH (0.4 μg/ml and 0.1 μg/ml), and EMB (7.5 μg/ml and 2.5 μg/ml), PYZ (100 μg/ml) and streptomycin (STR, 6.0 μg/ml and 2.0 μg/ml) (CLSI, 2008). Evaluation of the MGIT performance for the primary tuberculosis drugs showed results that were comparable to the BACTEC 460 radiometric methods as well as the agar proportion methods (>90% agreement) (Ardito et al., 2001; Adjers-Koskela & Katila, 2003; Scarparo et al., 2004), except for EMB and STR which had agreement varying from less than 80% to 98% (Adjers-Koskela & Katila, 2003; Scarparo et al., 2004; Hall et al., 2006; Garrigo et al., 2007). More recently, the MGIT 960 was evaluated for susceptibility testing of second-line drugs including levofloxacin, amikacin, capreomycin and ethionamide with overall agreement of 96% at critical concentrations when compared to the agar proportion method (Lin et al., 2009). Similar results were obtained in a study comparing the manual version of the MGIT to the agar method using the second-line drugs ofloxacin, kanamycin, ethionamide, and capreomycin (Martin et al., 2008). In both studies, the agreement between the two methods for ethionamide was markedly lower (86-88%) than for the other drugs (Martin et al., 2008; Lin et al., 2009).

Another fully automated broth system that is FDA-approved for susceptibility testing of *Mtb* complex is the VersaTREK instrument (TREK Diagnostics, Cleveland, OH). The VersaTREK (formerly ESP culture system II) is FDA-approved for susceptibility testing of *Mtb* complex against the first-line drugs including RIF (1 µg/ml), INH (0.4 µg/ml and 0.1 µg/ml), ETH (8 µg/ml and 5 µg/ml), and PZA (100 µg/ml) (CLSI, 2008). Drug susceptibility for each isolate tested is manually determined by comparing the time to detection of growth between the control bottle and the bottle containing the drug. If the difference is greater than three days or if the bottle remains negative, the isolate is considered susceptible. If the difference is less than or equal to 3 days, then the isolate is considered resistant. However, for the test to be valid, the time to growth in the control bottle has to be between 3 and 10 days following inoculation with 0.5 mL of a 1:10 dilution of a 1.0 McFarland inoculum (Bergmann & Woods, 1998; Ruiz et al., 2000). Evaluation of the VersaTREK instrument against the agar proportion method or the BACTEC 460 for susceptibility testing of *Mtb* against INH, RIF, ETB, and STR showed results similar to the MGIT 960, with agreement > than 95% for all drugs except ETB and STR (agreement between 90-95%) for which the VersaTrek generally called susceptible organisms that were resistant (Bergmann & Woods, 1998), although only a few isolates were tested in the study. Similar results were obtained by other investigators, except for STR, which unlike the previous study, had an agreement of 99.7% with the BACTEC 460 method (Ruiz et al., 2000).

7.3 Molecular detection of resistance markers

Although conventional methods described above are still the main-stay in detection of drug resistance in most laboratories, several studies have been conducted to developed more rapid and specific methods of detection of multi-drug resistance markers in *Mtb* complex. These assays are based on the detection of specific mutations in a variety of genes reported to confer resistance to several of the anti-tuberculosis drugs.

The Genotype MTBDR*plus* (Hain Lifescience) is a commercial line probe assay developed for the detection of INH and RIF resistance in *Mtb* complex isolates and smear-positive specimens (Hillemann et al., 2007). Resistance to INH results from mutations in genes whose products are involved in the activation and binding of INH including the *katG*, the *inhA*, the *ahpC-oxyR*, *ahpC* and *ndh* genes, while resistance to RIF is due mainly to mutation in the *rpoB* gene, which encodes the β-subunit of the DNA-dependent RNA polymerase, RIF binding target (Zhang & Yew, 2009).

The Genotype MTBDR*plus* assay detects the most common mutations found in the *rpoB*, *katG* and *inhA* genes, an improvement from other line-probe assays such as the INNO-LiPA Rif (Innogenetics) and the GenoType MTBDR (Hain Lifescience), which only target the *rpoB* mutation (INNO-LiPA Rif) or *rpoB* and *katG* mutations (GenoType MTBDR). Evaluation of the Genotype MTBDR*plus* assay by Hillemann et al (Hillemann et al., 2007) on clinical strains and smear-positive sputa revealed a detection rate of 98.7% (74/75) and 96.8% (30/31) of RIF resistance in clinical isolates and sputa specimens respectively. INH resistance was detected in 92% (69/75) and 90% (36/41) of clinical isolates and sputa specimens respectively. Similar detection rate were obtained by Barnard et al (Barnard et al., 2008) who tested 536 consecutive smear-positive sputum specimens with a sensitivity of 98.9% for detection of RIF resistance and 94.2% for the detection of INH resistance when compared to results obtained with conventional methods. Although the assay is limited to the detection of known mutations of RIF and INH, the high concordance rate with conventional methods and the rapid time to results makes the MTBDR*plus* assay a useful test for the management of multi-drug resistance tuberculosis.

Another version of the line probe assay, the GenoType MTBDR*sl* (second-line) (Hain Lifescience), was recently introduced for the detection of mutations in the *gyrA* gene, the 16S rRNA gene and the *embB* gene which confer resistance to fluoroquinolones, aminoglycosides and capreomycin, and ethambutol respectively (Hillemann et al., 2009). This assay shows variable performance characteristics when compared to phenotypic methods or sequencing, ranging from 75.6-90% for fluoroquinolones, 43-100% for aminoglycosides, 71.4-87.5% for capreomycin and suboptimal rate in all studies for ethambutol (38.5-64.2%) (Hillemann et al., 2009; Kiet et al., 2010; Huang et al., 2011; Kontsevaya et al., 2011).

Multiple home-brew PCR assays have been developed for the detection of the most common gene mutations conferring resistance to *Mtb* complex strains. A recent study reports the development of a multiplex real-time PCR assay to detect all known mutations in the *gyrA* gene responsible for conferring resistance to fluoroquinolones (Chakravorty et al., 2011). This assay is based on an asymmetrical PCR using sloppy molecular beacon probes that extends the entire quinolone resistance determining region (QRDR), a region of the *gyrA* gene containing most of the known mutations responsible for fluoroquinolones resistance (Takiff et al., 1994). This assay was 100% sensitive and 100% specific in detecting fluoroquinolones resistance in 92 clinical isolates of *Mtb* complex, when compared to sequencing.

As many as 21 mutations in the *katG* gene can cause decreased activity of INH against *Mtb* complex (Ando et al., 2010). Although several assays have focused on the S315T mutation of *KatG* (Mokrousov et al., 2002; Zhang et al., 2007; Tho et al., 2011), which is known to confer high-level resistance to INH and be present in as many as 90% of resistant *Mtb* isolates in Russia (Marttila et al., 1998; Mokrousov et al., 2002), the study by Ando and colleagues showed that other mutations in the *KatG* gene can cause high-level resistance and those should be included in molecular assays targeting the *katG* gene (Ando et al., 2010).

The utility of the assays is limited since they often target detection of resistance to one class of antimicrobial, depends on the available knowledge of current mutations conferring resistance, and as such, can only be use in conjunction with other assays. Several investigators have focused their efforts in developing assays similar to the MTBDR*plus* assay to include resistant marker to more than one class of antituberculosis drugs and for more than one mutation per gene target (Sekiguchi et al., 2007; Zhang et al., 2007; Ong et al., 2010; Pholwat et al., 2011).

Other molecular assays that have been developed for the detection of resistance markers have included locked nucleic acid probes (van Doorn et al., 2008) and multiplex PCR amplimer conformation analysis (Cheng et al., 2004), pyrosequencing (Marttila et al., 2009; Garza-Gonzalez et al., 2010; Halse et al., 2010), oligonucleotide microarray (Caoili et al., 2006), and mass spectrometry (Wang et al., 2011).

8. Future directions

Clinical diagnostics for *Mtb* continue to evolve (Wilson, 2011) and in some cases, the future may be at our fingertips (Van Rie et al., 2010). For example, the GeneXpert MTB/RIF PCR assay (Cepheid, Sunnyvale, CA) allows for the automated, direct detection of *Mtb* complex in respiratory specimens and it has been endorsed by the WHO for use in low-income countries (WHO, 2008). The Xpert assay provides excellent sensitivity and specificity from direct specimens while providing a same day turn-around time for results (Helb et al., 2010; Boehme et al., 2011; Marlowe et al., 2011; Rachow et al., 2011; Scott et al., 2011). In addition, the assay provides immediate information on RIF resistance and has recently been successfully evaluated using non-respiratory specimens (Ioannidis et al., 2011; Miller et al., 2011).

Older technologies utilized in new ways are also making inroads in *Mtb* diagnostics. The use of mass spectrometry for the identification of *Mtb* complex from culture isolates may replace current standards such as biochemical analysis, nucleic acid hybridization probes, and DNA sequencing due to the ability of mass spectrometry to rapidly and accurately identify *Mtb* in a cost-effective manner while minimizing technologist hands-on time and effort (Saleeb et al., 2011). Although still in it's infancy in the diagnostic microbiology laboratory, this technology may also have utility in predicting drug resistance patterns and evaluating epidemiologic groups (Bouakaze et al., 2011; Massire et al., 2011; Schurch et al., 2011).

Finally, new technologies such as next generation sequencing are still largely utilized for research purposes in microbiology but some authors have suggested that there may come a time when application of this powerful technology will find a niche in the diagnostic microbiology laboratory (Ansorge, 2009; Rogers & Bruce, 2010; Engelthaler et al., 2011; Pallen & Loman, 2011).

9. References

Abe, C., K. Hirano, et al. (1993). "Detection of Mycobacterium tuberculosis in clinical specimens by polymerase chain reaction and Gen-Probe Amplified Mycobacterium Tuberculosis Direct Test." *J Clin Microbiol* 31(12): 3270-3274.

Adjers-Koskela, K. & M. L. Katila (2003). "Susceptibility testing with the manual mycobacteria growth indicator tube (MGIT) and the MGIT 960 system provides rapid and reliable verification of multidrug-resistant tuberculosis." *J Clin Microbiol* 41(3): 1235-1239.

Ando, H., Y. Kondo, et al. (2010). "Identification of katG mutations associated with high-level isoniazid resistance in Mycobacterium tuberculosis." *Antimicrob Agents Chemother* 54(5): 1793-1799.

Ansorge, W. J. (2009). "Next-generation DNA sequencing techniques." *New biotechnology* 25(4): 195-203.

Ardito, F., B. Posteraro, et al. (2001). "Evaluation of BACTEC Mycobacteria Growth Indicator Tube (MGIT 960) automated system for drug susceptibility testing of Mycobacterium tuberculosis." *J Clin Microbiol* 39(12): 4440-4444.

Attorri, S., S. Dunbar, et al. (2000). "Assessment of morphology for rapid presumptive identification of Mycobacterium tuberculosis and Mycobacterium kansasii." *Journal of clinical microbiology* 38(4): 1426-1429.

Baba, K., S. Pathak, et al. (2008). "Real-time quantitative PCR in the diagnosis of tuberculosis in formalin-fixed paraffin-embedded pleural tissue in patients from a high HIV endemic area." *Diagn Mol Pathol* 17(2): 112-117.

Barnard, M., H. Albert, et al. (2008). "Rapid molecular screening for multidrug-resistant tuberculosis in a high-volume public health laboratory in South Africa." *Am J Respir Crit Care Med* 177(7): 787-792.

Beqaj, S. H., R. Flesher, et al. (2007). "Use of the real-time PCR assay in conjunction with MagNA Pure for the detection of mycobacterial DNA from fixed specimens." *Diagn Mol Pathol* 16(3): 169-173.

Bergmann, J. S. & G. L. Woods (1996). "Clinical evaluation of the Roche AMPLICOR PCR Mycobacterium tuberculosis test for detection of M. tuberculosis in respiratory specimens." *J Clin Microbiol* 34(5): 1083-1085.

Bergmann, J. S. & G. L. Woods (1998). "Evaluation of the ESP culture system II for testing susceptibilities of Mycobacterium tuberculosis isolates to four primary antituberculous drugs." *J Clin Microbiol* 36(10): 2940-2943.

Bergmann, J. S. & G. L. Woods (1999). "Enhanced Amplified Mycobacterium Tuberculosis Direct Test for detection of Mycobacterium tuberculosis complex in positive BACTEC 12B broth cultures of respiratory specimens." *J Clin Microbiol* 37(6): 2099-2101.

Bodmer, T., A. Gurtner, et al. (1997). "Evaluation of the COBAS AMPLICOR MTB system." *J Clin Microbiol* 35(6): 1604-1605.

Boehme, C. C., M. P. Nicol, et al. (2011). "Feasibility, diagnostic accuracy, and effectiveness of decentralised use of the Xpert MTB/RIF test for diagnosis of tuberculosis and multidrug resistance: a multicentre implementation study." *Lancet* 377(9776): 1495-1505.

Bouakaze, C., C. Keyser, et al. (2011). "Matrix-Assisted Laser Desorption Ionization-Time of Flight Mass Spectrometry-Based Single Nucleotide Polymorphism Genotyping Assay Using iPLEX Gold Technology for Identification of Mycobacterium tuberculosis Complex Species and Lineages." *J Clin Microbiol* 49(9): 3292-3299.

Brisson-Noel, A., C. Aznar, et al. (1991). "Diagnosis of tuberculosis by DNA amplification in clinical practice evaluation." *Lancet* 338(8763): 364-366.

Bruijnesteijn Van Coppenraet, E. S., J. A. Lindeboom, et al. (2004). "Real-time PCR assay using fine-needle aspirates and tissue biopsy specimens for rapid diagnosis of mycobacterial lymphadenitis in children." *J Clin Microbiol* 42(6): 2644-2650.

Butler, W. R. & L. S. Guthertz (2001). "Mycolic acid analysis by high-performance liquid chromatography for identification of Mycobacterium species." *Clin Microbiol Rev* 14(4): 704-726.

Butler, W. R., K. C. Jost, Jr., et al. (1991). "Identification of mycobacteria by high-performance liquid chromatography." *J Clin Microbiol* 29(11): 2468-2472.

Canetti, G., S. Froman, et al. (1963). "Mycobacteria: Laboratory Methods for Testing Drug Sensitivity and Resistance." *Bull World Health Organ* 29: 565-578.

Caoili, J. C., A. Mayorova, et al. (2006). "Evaluation of the TB-Biochip oligonucleotide microarray system for rapid detection of rifampin resistance in Mycobacterium tuberculosis." *J Clin Microbiol* 44(7): 2378-2381.

Caviedes, L. & D. A. Moore (2007). "Introducing MODS: a low-cost, low-tech tool for high-performance detection of tuberculosis and multidrug resistant tuberculosis." *Indian J Med Microbiol* 25(2): 87-88.

Chakravorty, S., B. Aladegbami, et al. (2011). "Rapid detection of fluoroquinolone-resistant and heteroresistant Mycobacterium tuberculosis by use of sloppy molecular beacons and dual melting-temperature codes in a real-time PCR assay." *J Clin Microbiol* 49(3): 932-940.

Chakravorty, S. & J. S. Tyagi (2005). "Novel multipurpose methodology for detection of mycobacteria in pulmonary and extrapulmonary specimens by smear microscopy, culture, and PCR." *J Clin Microbiol* 43(6): 2697-2702.

Chedore, P. & F. B. Jamieson (1999). "Routine use of the Gen-Probe MTD2 amplification test for detection of Mycobacterium tuberculosis in clinical specimens in a large public health mycobacteriology laboratory." *Diagn Microbiol Infect Dis* 35(3): 185-191.

Chegou, N. N., K. G. Hoek, et al. (2011). "Tuberculosis assays: past, present and future." *Expert review of anti-infective therapy* 9(4): 457-469.

Cheng, A. F., W. W. Yew, et al. (2004). "Multiplex PCR amplimer conformation analysis for rapid detection of gyrA mutations in fluoroquinolone-resistant Mycobacterium tuberculosis clinical isolates." *Antimicrob Agents Chemother* 48(2): 596-601.

Chew, W. K., R. M. Lasaitis, et al. (1998). "Clinical evaluation of the Mycobacteria Growth Indicator Tube (MGIT) compared with radiometric (Bactec) and solid media for isolation of Mycobacterium species." *J Med Microbiol* 47(9): 821-827.

CLSI (2008). Susceptibility Testing of Mycobacteria, Nocardiae, and Other Aerobic Actinomycetes; M24-A2, Approved Standard. Wayne, PA, Clinical and Laboratory Standards Institute.

Cloud, J. L., H. Neal, et al. (2002). "Identification of Mycobacterium spp. by using a commercial 16S ribosomal DNA sequencing kit and additional sequencing libraries." *J Clin Microbiol* 40(2): 400-406.

Cruciani, M., C. Scarparo, et al. (2004). "Meta-analysis of BACTEC MGIT 960 and BACTEC 460 TB, with or without solid media, for detection of mycobacteria." *J Clin Microbiol* 42(5): 2321-2325.

D'Amato, R. F., A. A. Wallman, et al. (1995). "Rapid diagnosis of pulmonary tuberculosis by using Roche AMPLICOR Mycobacterium tuberculosis PCR test." *J Clin Microbiol* 33(7): 1832-1834.

de Oliveira, M. M., A. da Silva Rocha, et al. (2003). "Rapid detection of resistance against rifampicin in isolates of Mycobacterium tuberculosis from Brazilian patients using a reverse-phase hybridization assay." *J Microbiol Methods* 53(3): 335-342.

Desmond, E. P. & K. Loretz (2001). "Use of the Gen-Probe amplified mycobacterium tuberculosis direct test for early detection of Mycobacterium tuberculosis in BACTEC 12B medium." *J Clin Microbiol* 39(5): 1993-1995.

Devallois, A., E. Legrand, et al. (1996). "Evaluation of Amplicor MTB test as adjunct to smears and culture for direct detection of Mycobacterium tuberculosis in the French Caribbean." *J Clin Microbiol* 34(5): 1065-1068.

Drake, T. A., J. A. Hindler, et al. (1987). "Rapid identification of Mycobacterium avium complex in culture using DNA probes." *J Clin Microbiol* 25(8): 1442-1445.

Durst, H. D., M. Milano, et al. (1975). "Phenacyl esters of fatty acids via crown ether catalysts for enhanced ultraviolet detection in liquid chromatography." *Anal Chem* 47(11): 1797-1801.

Eisenach, K. D., M. D. Sifford, et al. (1991). "Detection of Mycobacterium tuberculosis in sputum samples using a polymerase chain reaction." *Am Rev Respir Dis* 144(5): 1160-1163.

Ellner, P. D., T. E. Kiehn, et al. (1988). "Rapid detection and identification of pathogenic mycobacteria by combining radiometric and nucleic acid probe methods." *J Clin Microbiol* 26(7): 1349-1352.

Engelthaler, D. M., T. Chiller, et al. (2011). "Next-generation sequencing of Coccidioides immitis isolated during cluster investigation." *Emerg Infect Dis* 17(2): 227-232.

Floyd, M. M., V. A. Silcox, et al. (1992). "Separation of Mycobacterium bovis BCG from Mycobacterium tuberculosis and Mycobacterium bovis by using high-performance liquid chromatography of mycolic acids." *J Clin Microbiol* 30(5): 1327-1330.

Ford, E. G., S. J. Snead, et al. (1993). "Strains of Mycobacterium terrae complex which react with DNA probes for M. tuberculosis complex." *J Clin Microbiol* 31(10): 2805-2806.

Franco-Alvarez de Luna, F., P. Ruiz, et al. (2006). "Evaluation of the GenoType Mycobacteria Direct assay for detection of Mycobacterium tuberculosis complex and four atypical mycobacterial species in clinical samples." *J Clin Microbiol* 44(8): 3025-3027.

Gamboa, F., P. J. Cardona, et al. (1998). "Evaluation of a commercial probe assay for detection of rifampin resistance in Mycobacterium tuberculosis directly from respiratory and nonrespiratory clinical samples." *Eur J Clin Microbiol Infect Dis* 17(3): 189-192.

Garrigo, M., L. M. Aragon, et al. (2007). "Multicenter laboratory evaluation of the MB/BacT Mycobacterium detection system and the BACTEC MGIT 960 system in comparison with the BACTEC 460TB system for susceptibility testing of Mycobacterium tuberculosis." *J Clin Microbiol* 45(6): 1766-1770.

Garza-Gonzalez, E., G. M. Gonzalez, et al. (2010). "A pyrosequencing method for molecular monitoring of regions in the inhA, ahpC and rpoB genes of Mycobacterium tuberculosis." *Clin Microbiol Infect* 16(6): 607-612.

Gen-Probe (2011). AccuProbe: Mycobacterium Tuberculosis Complex Culture Identification Test.

Goto, M., S. Oka, et al. (1991). "Evaluation of acridinium-ester-labeled DNA probes for identification of Mycobacterium tuberculosis and Mycobacterium avium-

Mycobacterium intracellulare complex in culture." *J Clin Microbiol* 29(11): 2473-2476.

Guthertz, L. S., S. D. Lim, et al. (1993). "Curvilinear-gradient high-performance liquid chromatography for identification of mycobacteria." *J Clin Microbiol* 31(7): 1876-1881.

Ha, D. T., N. T. Lan, et al. (2009). "Microscopic observation drug susceptibility assay (MODS) for early diagnosis of tuberculosis in children." *PloS one* 4(12): e8341.

Hall, L., K. A. Doerr, et al. (2006). "Verification of antimicrobial susceptibility testing of Mycobacterium tuberculosis." *J Clin Microbiol* 44(5): 1921.

Hall, L., K. A. Doerr, et al. (2003). "Evaluation of the MicroSeq system for identification of mycobacteria by 16S ribosomal DNA sequencing and its integration into a routine clinical mycobacteriology laboratory." *J Clin Microbiol* 41(4): 1447-1453.

Halse, T. A., J. Edwards, et al. (2010). "Combined real-time PCR and rpoB gene pyrosequencing for rapid identification of Mycobacterium tuberculosis and determination of rifampin resistance directly in clinical specimens." *J Clin Microbiol* 48(4): 1182-1188.

Halse, T. A., V. E. Escuyer, et al. (2011). "Evaluation of a single-tube multiplex real-time PCR for differentiation of members of the Mycobacterium tuberculosis complex in clinical specimens." *J Clin Microbiol* 49(7): 2562-2567.

Heifets, L., T. Linder, et al. (2000). "Two liquid medium systems, mycobacteria growth indicator tube and MB redox tube, for Mycobacterium tuberculosis isolation from sputum specimens." *J Clin Microbiol* 38(3): 1227-1230.

Heifets, L. B. & M. D. Iseman (1985). "Radiometric method for testing susceptibility of mycobacteria to pyrazinamide in 7H12 broth." *J Clin Microbiol* 21(2): 200-204.

Helb, D., M. Jones, et al. (2010). "Rapid detection of Mycobacterium tuberculosis and rifampin resistance by use of on-demand, near-patient technology." *J Clin Microbiol* 48(1): 229-237.

Hernandez, A., J. S. Bergmann, et al. (1997). "AMPLICOR MTB polymerase chain reaction test for identification of Mycobacterium tuberculosis in positive Difco ESP II broth cultures." *Diagn Microbiol Infect Dis* 27(1-2): 17-20.

Hillemann, D., S. Rusch-Gerdes, et al. (2007). "Evaluation of the GenoType MTBDRplus assay for rifampin and isoniazid susceptibility testing of Mycobacterium tuberculosis strains and clinical specimens." *J Clin Microbiol* 45(8): 2635-2640.

Hillemann, D., S. Rusch-Gerdes, et al. (2009). "Feasibility of the GenoType MTBDRsl assay for fluoroquinolone, amikacin-capreomycin, and ethambutol resistance testing of Mycobacterium tuberculosis strains and clinical specimens." *J Clin Microbiol* 47(6): 1767-1772.

Hsiao, P. F., C. Y. Tzen, et al. (2003). "Polymerase chain reaction based detection of Mycobacterium tuberculosis in tissues showing granulomatous inflammation without demonstrable acid-fast bacilli." *Int J Dermatol* 42(4): 281-286.

Huang, W. L., T. L. Chi, et al. (2011). "Performance assessment of the GenoType MTBDRsl test and DNA sequencing for detection of second-line and ethambutol drug resistance among patients infected with multidrug-resistant Mycobacterium tuberculosis." *J Clin Microbiol* 49(7): 2502-2508.

Huard, R. C., L. C. Lazzarini, et al. (2003). "PCR-based method to differentiate the subspecies of the Mycobacterium tuberculosis complex on the basis of genomic deletions." *J Clin Microbiol* 41(4): 1637-1650.

Ioannidis, P., D. Papaventsis, et al. (2011). "Cepheid GeneXpert MTB/RIF assay for Mycobacterium tuberculosis detection and rifampin resistance identification in patients with substantial clinical indications of tuberculosis and smear-negative microscopy results." *J Clin Microbiol* 49(8): 3068-3070.

Johansen, I. S., B. Lundgren, et al. (2003). "Direct detection of multidrug-resistant Mycobacterium tuberculosis in clinical specimens in low- and high-incidence countries by line probe assay." *J Clin Microbiol* 41(9): 4454-4456.

Julian, E., M. Roldan, et al. (2010). "Microscopic cords, a virulence-related characteristic of Mycobacterium tuberculosis, are also present in nonpathogenic mycobacteria." *J Bacteriol* 192(7): 1751-1760.

Kapur, V., L. L. Li, et al. (1995). "Rapid Mycobacterium species assignment and unambiguous identification of mutations associated with antimicrobial resistance in Mycobacterium tuberculosis by automated DNA sequencing." *Arch Pathol Lab Med* 119(2): 131-138.

Kasai, H., T. Ezaki, et al. (2000). "Differentiation of phylogenetically related slowly growing mycobacteria by their gyrB sequences." *J Clin Microbiol* 38(1): 301-308.

Kellogg, J. A., D. A. Bankert, et al. (2001). "Application of the Sherlock Mycobacteria Identification System using high-performance liquid chromatography in a clinical laboratory." *J Clin Microbiol* 39(3): 964-970.

Kiehn, T. E. & F. F. Edwards (1987). "Rapid identification using a specific DNA probe of Mycobacterium avium complex from patients with acquired immunodeficiency syndrome." *J Clin Microbiol* 25(8): 1551-1552.

Kiet, V. S., N. T. Lan, et al. (2010). "Evaluation of the MTBDRsl test for detection of second-line-drug resistance in Mycobacterium tuberculosis." *J Clin Microbiol* 48(8): 2934-2939.

Kim, B. J., S. H. Lee, et al. (1999). "Identification of mycobacterial species by comparative sequence analysis of the RNA polymerase gene (rpoB)." *J Clin Microbiol* 37(6): 1714-1720.

Kiraz, N., I. Saglik, et al. (2010). "Evaluation of the GenoType Mycobacteria Direct assay for direct detection of the Mycobacterium tuberculosis complex obtained from sputum samples." *J Med Microbiol* 59(Pt 8): 930-934.

Kirschner, P., B. Springer, et al. (1993). "Genotypic identification of mycobacteria by nucleic acid sequence determination: report of a 2-year experience in a clinical laboratory." *J Clin Microbiol* 31(11): 2882-2889.

Koneman, E. W. (2006). Identification of Mycobacteria using Conventional Methods. *In Color Atlas and Textbook of Diagnostic Microbiology*. E. W. Koneman. Philadelphia, Lippincott: 1085-1090.

Kontsevaya, I., S. Mironova, et al. (2011). "Evaluation of Two Molecular Assays for Rapid Detection of Mycobacterium tuberculosis Resistance to Fluoroquinolones in High-Tuberculosis and -Multidrug-Resistance Settings." *J Clin Microbiol* 49(8): 2832-2837.

LaBombardi, V. J., R. Katariwala, et al. (2006). "The identification of mycobacteria from solid media and directly from VersaTREK Myco bottles using the Sherlock Mycobacteria Identification HPLC system." *Clin Microbiol Infect* 12(5): 478-481.

Laszlo, A., P. Gill, et al. (1983). "Conventional and radiometric drug susceptibility testing of Mycobacterium tuberculosis complex." *J Clin Microbiol* 18(6): 1335-1339.

Lebrun, L., F. Espinasse, et al. (1992). "Evaluation of nonradioactive DNA probes for identification of mycobacteria." *J Clin Microbiol* 30(9): 2476-2478.

Lee, H. R., S. Y. Kim, et al. (2010). "Novel multiplex PCR using dual-priming oligonucleotides for detection and discrimination of the Mycobacterium tuberculosis complex and M. bovis BCG." *J Clin Microbiol* 48(12): 4612-4614.

Lee, L. V. (2010). Convential Biochemicals. *Clinical Microbiology Procedures Handbook*. L. S. Garcia. Washington, D.C, American Society for Microbiology. 2: 7.6.1.1.-7.6.3.3.

Levidiotou, S., G. Vrioni, et al. (2003). "Four-year experience of use of the Cobas Amplicor system for rapid detection of Mycobacterium tuberculosis complex in respiratory and nonrespiratory specimens in Greece." *Eur J Clin Microbiol Infect Dis* 22(6): 349-356.

Lim, S. D., J. Todd, et al. (1991). "Genotypic identification of pathogenic Mycobacterium species by using a nonradioactive oligonucleotide probe." *J Clin Microbiol* 29(6): 1276-1278.

Limaye, K., S. Kanade, et al. (2010). "Utility of Microscopic Observation of Drug Susceptibility (MODS) assay for Mycobacterium tuberculosis in resource constrained settings." *The Indian journal of tuberculosis* 57(4): 207-212.

Lin, S. Y., E. Desmond, et al. (2009). "Multicenter evaluation of Bactec MGIT 960 system for second-line drug susceptibility testing of Mycobacterium tuberculosis complex." *J Clin Microbiol* 47(11): 3630-3634.

Liu, P. I., D. H. McGregor, et al. (1973). "Comparison of three culture media for isolation of Mycobacterium tuberculosis: a 6-year study." *Appl Microbiol* 26(6): 880-883.

Luo, R. F., M. D. Scahill, et al. (2010). "Comparison of single-copy and multicopy real-time PCR targets for detection of Mycobacterium tuberculosis in paraffin-embedded tissue." *J Clin Microbiol* 48(7): 2569-2570.

Makinen, J., M. Marjamaki, et al. (2006). "Evaluation of a novel strip test, GenoType Mycobacterium CM/AS, for species identification of mycobacterial cultures." *Clin Microbiol Infect* 12(5): 481-483.

Marlowe, E. M., S. M. Novak-Weekley, et al. (2011). "Evaluation of the Cepheid Xpert MTB/RIF assay for direct detection of Mycobacterium tuberculosis complex in respiratory specimens." *J Clin Microbiol* 49(4): 1621-1623.

Martin, A., D. Bombeeck, et al. (2011). "Evaluation of the BD MGIT TBc Identification Test (TBc ID), a rapid chromatographic immunoassay for the detection of Mycobacterium tuberculosis complex from liquid culture." *J Microbiol Meth* 84(2): 255-257.

Martin, A., A. von Groll, et al. (2008). "Rapid detection of Mycobacterium tuberculosis resistance to second-line drugs by use of the manual mycobacterium growth indicator tube system." *J Clin Microbiol* 46(12): 3952-3956.

Marttila, H. J., J. Makinen, et al. (2009). "Prospective evaluation of pyrosequencing for the rapid detection of isoniazid and rifampin resistance in clinical Mycobacterium tuberculosis isolates." *Eur J Clin Microbiol Infect Dis* 28(1): 33-38.

Marttila, H. J., H. Soini, et al. (1998). "A Ser315Thr substitution in KatG is predominant in genetically heterogeneous multidrug-resistant Mycobacterium tuberculosis isolates originating from the St. Petersburg area in Russia." *Antimicrob Agents Chemother* 42(9): 2443-2445.

Massire, C., C. A. Ivy, et al. (2011). "Simultaneous identification of mycobacterial isolates to the species level and determination of tuberculosis drug resistance by PCR followed by electrospray ionization mass spectrometry." *J Clin Microbiol* 49(3): 908-917.

Middlebrook, G., Z. Reggiardo, et al. (1977). "Automatable radiometric detection of growth of Mycobacterium tuberculosis in selective media." *Am Rev Respir Dis* 115(6): 1066-1069.

Miliner, R. A., K. D. Stottmeier, et al. (1969). "Formaldehyde: a photothermal activated toxic substance produced in Middlebrook 7H10 medium." *Am Rev Respir Dis* 99(4): 603-607.

Miller, M. B., E. B. Popowitch, et al. (2011). "Performance of Xpert MTB/RIF RUO Assay and IS6110 Real-Time PCR for Mycobacterium tuberculosis Detection in Clinical Samples." *J Clin Microbiol.*

Miller, N., T. Cleary, et al. (2002). "Rapid and specific detection of Mycobacterium tuberculosis from acid-fast bacillus smear-positive respiratory specimens and BacT/ALERT MP culture bottles by using fluorogenic probes and real-time PCR." *J Clin Microbiol* 40(11): 4143-4147.

Miller, N., S. Infante, et al. (2000). "Evaluation of the LiPA MYCOBACTERIA assay for identification of mycobacterial species from BACTEC 12B bottles." *J Clin Microbiol* 38(5): 1915-1919.

MMWR (1993). "Initial therapy for tuberculosis in the era of multidrug resistance. Recommendations of the Advisory Council for the Elimination of Tuberculosis." *MMWR Recomm Rep* 42(RR-7): 1-8.

Mokrousov, I., O. Narvskaya, et al. (2002). "High prevalence of KatG Ser315Thr substitution among isoniazid-resistant Mycobacterium tuberculosis clinical isolates from northwestern Russia, 1996 to 2001." *Antimicrob Agents Chemother* 46(5): 1417-1424.

Mokrousov, I., T. Otten, et al. (2002). "Detection of isoniazid-resistant Mycobacterium tuberculosis strains by a multiplex allele-specific PCR assay targeting katG codon 315 variation." *J Clin Microbiol* 40(7): 2509-2512.

Moore, D. A. (2007). "Future prospects for the MODS assay in multidrug-resistant tuberculosis diagnosis." *Future Microbiol* 2(2): 97-101.

Musial, C. E., L. S. Tice, et al. (1988). "Identification of mycobacteria from culture by using the Gen-Probe Rapid Diagnostic System for Mycobacterium avium complex and Mycobacterium tuberculosis complex." *J Clin Microbiol* 26(10): 2120-2123.

Neonakis, I. K., Z. Gitti, et al. (2009). "Evaluation of GenoType mycobacteria direct assay in comparison with Gen-Probe Mycobacterium tuberculosis amplified direct test and GenoType MTBDRplus for direct detection of Mycobacterium tuberculosis complex in clinical samples." *J Clin Microbiol* 47(8): 2601-2603.

Neonakis, I. K., Z. Gitti, et al. (2007). "Evaluation of the GenoType MTBC assay for differentiating 120 clinical Mycobacterium tuberculosis complex isolates." *Eur J Clin Microbiol Infect Dis* 26(2): 151-152.

Nopvichai, C., A. Sanpavat, et al. (2009). "PCR detection of Mycobacterium tuberculosis in necrotising non-granulomatous lymphadenitis using formalin-fixed paraffin-embedded tissue: a study in Thai patients." *J Clin Pathol* 62(9): 812-815.

Ong, D. C., W. C. Yam, et al. (2010). "Rapid detection of rifampicin- and isoniazid-resistant Mycobacterium tuberculosis by high-resolution melting analysis." *J Clin Microbiol* 48(4): 1047-1054.

Pallen, M. J. & N. J. Loman (2011). "Are diagnostic and public health bacteriology ready to become branches of genomic medicine?" *Genome Med* 3(8): 53.

Pao, C. C., T. S. Yen, et al. (1990). "Detection and identification of Mycobacterium tuberculosis by DNA amplification." *J Clin Microbiol* 28(9): 1877-1880.

Parsons, L. M., R. Brosch, et al. (2002). "Rapid and simple approach for identification of Mycobacterium tuberculosis complex isolates by PCR-based genomic deletion analysis." *J Clin Microbiol* 40(7): 2339-2345.

Patel, J. B., D. G. Leonard, et al. (2000). "Sequence-based identification of Mycobacterium species using the MicroSeq 500 16S rDNA bacterial identification system." *J Clin Microbiol* 38(1): 246-251.

Perandin, F., G. Pinsi, et al. (2006). "Evaluation of INNO-LiPA assay for direct detection of mycobacteria in pulmonary and extrapulmonary specimens." *New Microbiol* 29(2): 133-138.

Peterson, E. M., R. Lu, et al. (1989). "Direct identification of Mycobacterium tuberculosis, Mycobacterium avium, and Mycobacterium intracellulare from amplified primary cultures in BACTEC media using DNA probes." *J Clin Microbiol* 27(7): 1543-1547.

Pfyffer, G. E., P. Kissling, et al. (1994). "Direct detection of Mycobacterium tuberculosis complex in respiratory specimens by a target-amplified test system." *J Clin Microbiol* 32(4): 918-923.

Pfyffer, G. E. & F. Palicova (2011). Mycobacterium: General Characteristics, Laboratory Detection, and Staining Procedures. *Manual of Clinical Microbiology, 10th edition*. J. C. Versalovic, K.C.; Funke, G.; Jorgensen, J.H.; Landry, M.L.; and Warnock, D.W. Washington, DC, ASM Press: 472-502.

Pholwat, S., S. Heysell, et al. (2011). "Rapid first- and second-line drug susceptibility assay for Mycobacterium tuberculosis isolates by use of quantitative PCR." *J Clin Microbiol* 49(1): 69-75.

Piersimoni, C. & C. Scarparo (2003). "Relevance of commercial amplification methods for direct detection of Mycobacterium tuberculosis complex in clinical samples." *J Clin Microbiol* 41(12): 5355-5365.

Pinsky, B. A. & N. Banaei (2008). "Multiplex real-time PCR assay for rapid identification of Mycobacterium tuberculosis complex members to the species level." *J Clin Microbiol* 46(7): 2241-2246.

Rachow, A., A. Zumla, et al. (2011). "Rapid and accurate detection of Mycobacterium tuberculosis in sputum samples by Cepheid Xpert MTB/RIF assay--a clinical validation study." *PloS one* 6(6): e20458.

Rebollo, M. J., R. San Juan Garrido, et al. (2006). "Blood and urine samples as useful sources for the direct detection of tuberculosis by polymerase chain reaction." *Diagn Microbiol Infect Dis* 56(2): 141-146.

Richter, E., S. Rusch-Gerdes, et al. (2006). "Evaluation of the GenoType Mycobacterium Assay for identification of mycobacterial species from cultures." *J Clin Microbiol* 44(5): 1769-1775.

Richter, E., M. Weizenegger, et al. (2003). "Evaluation of genotype MTBC assay for differentiation of clinical Mycobacterium tuberculosis complex isolates." *J Clin Microbiol* 41(6): 2672-2675.

Ritis, K., S. Giaglis, et al. (2005). "Diagnostic usefulness of bone marrow aspiration material for the amplification of IS6110 insertion element in extrapulmonary tuberculosis: comparison of two PCR techniques." *Int J Tuberc Lung Dis* 9(4): 455-460.

Rogall, T., T. Flohr, et al. (1990). "Differentiation of Mycobacterium species by direct sequencing of amplified DNA." *J Gen Microbiol* 136(9): 1915-1920.

Rogers, G. B. & K. D. Bruce (2010). "Next-generation sequencing in the analysis of human microbiota: essential considerations for clinical application."*Mol Diagn Ther* 14(6): 343-350.

Roth, A., M. Fischer, et al. (1998). "Differentiation of phylogenetically related slowly growing mycobacteria based on 16S-23S rRNA gene internal transcribed spacer sequences." *J Clin Microbiol* 36(1): 139-147.

Ruiz, P., F. J. Zerolo, et al. (2000). "Comparison of susceptibility testing of Mycobacterium tuberculosis using the ESP culture system II with that using the BACTEC method." *J Clin Microbiol* 38(12): 4663-4664.

Russo, C., E. Tortoli, et al. (2006). "Evaluation of the new GenoType Mycobacterium assay for identification of mycobacterial species." *J Clin Microbiol* 44(2): 334-339.

Said, H. M., N. Ismail, et al. (2011). "Evaluation of TBc identification immunochromatographic assay for rapid identification of Mycobacterium tuberculosis complex in samples from broth cultures." *J Clin Microbiol* 49(5): 1939-1942.

Saleeb, P. G., S. K. Drake, et al. (2011). "Identification of mycobacteria in solid-culture media by matrix-assisted laser desorption ionization-time of flight mass spectrometry." *J Clin Micobiol* 49(5): 1790-1794.

Salfinger, M. & L. B. Heifets (1988). "Determination of pyrazinamide MICs for Mycobacterium tuberculosis at different pHs by the radiometric method." *Antimicrob Agents Chemother* 32(7): 1002-1004.

Sankar, S., B. Balakrishnan, et al. (2010). "Comparative evaluation of nested PCR and conventional smear methods for the detection of Mycobacterium tuberculosis in sputum samples." *Mol Diagn Ther* 14(4): 223-227.

Scarparo, C., P. Piccoli, et al. (2001). "Direct identification of mycobacteria from MB/BacT alert 3D bottles: comparative evaluation of two commercial probe assays." *J Clin Microbiol* 39(9): 3222-3227.

Scarparo, C., P. Ricordi, et al. (2004). "Evaluation of the fully automated BACTEC MGIT 960 system for testing susceptibility of Mycobacterium tuberculosis to pyrazinamide, streptomycin, isoniazid, rifampin, and ethambutol and comparison with the radiometric BACTEC 460TB method." *J Clin Microbiol* 42(3): 1109-1114.

Schirm, J., L. A. Oostendorp, et al. (1995). "Comparison of Amplicor, in-house PCR, and conventional culture for detection of Mycobacterium tuberculosis in clinical samples." *J Clin Microbiol* 33(12): 3221-3224.

Schurch, A. C., K. Kremer, et al. (2011). "Mutations in the regulatory network underlie the recent clonal expansion of a dominant subclone of the Mycobacterium tuberculosis Beijing genotype." *Infect Genet Evol: journal of molecular epidemiology and evolutionary genetics in infectious diseases* 11(3): 587-597.

Scott, L. E., K. McCarthy, et al. (2011). "Comparison of Xpert MTB/RIF with other nucleic acid technologies for diagnosing pulmonary tuberculosis in a high HIV prevalence setting: a prospective study." *PLoS medicine* 8(7): e1001061.

Seagar, A. L., C. Prendergast, et al. (2008). "Evaluation of the GenoType Mycobacteria Direct assay for the simultaneous detection of the Mycobacterium tuberculosis complex and four atypical mycobacterial species in smear-positive respiratory specimens." *J Med Microbiol* 57(Pt 5): 605-611.

Sekiguchi, J., T. Miyoshi-Akiyama, et al. (2007). "Detection of multidrug resistance in Mycobacterium tuberculosis." *J Clin Microbiol* 45(1): 179-192.

Shah, S., A. Miller, et al. (1998). "Rapid diagnosis of tuberculosis in various biopsy and body fluid specimens by the AMPLICOR Mycobacterium tuberculosis polymerase chain reaction test." *Chest* 113(5): 1190-1194.

Shrestha, N. K., M. J. Tuohy, et al. (2003). "Detection and differentiation of Mycobacterium tuberculosis and nontuberculous mycobacterial isolates by real-time PCR." *J Clin Microbiol* 41(11): 5121-5126.

Siddiqi, S. (2010). BACTEC MGIT 960 SIRE-Nonradiometric Susceptibility Testing for Mycobacterium tuberculosis. *Clinical Microbiology Procedures Handbook*. L. S. Garcia. Washington, D.C, American Society for Microbiology. 2: 7.8.5.1-7.8.5.5.

Siddiqi, S. H., J. P. Libonati, et al. (1981). "Evaluation of rapid radiometric method for drug susceptibility testing of Mycobacterium tuberculosis." *J Clin Microbiol* 13(5): 908-912.

Sjobring, U., M. Mecklenburg, et al. (1990). "Polymerase chain reaction for detection of Mycobacterium tuberculosis." *J Clin Microbiol* 28(10): 2200-2204.

Smith, M. B., J. S. Bergmann, et al. (1997). "Detection of Mycobacterium tuberculosis in BACTEC 12B broth cultures by the Roche Amplicor PCR assay." *J Clin Microbiol* 35(4): 900-902.

Snider, D. E., Jr., R. C. Good, et al. (1981). "Rapid drug-susceptibility testing of Mycobacterium tuberculosis." *Am Rev Respir Dis* 123(4 Pt 1): 402-406.

Soini, H., E. C. Bottger, et al. (1994). "Identification of mycobacteria by PCR-based sequence determination of the 32-kilodalton protein gene." *J Clin Microbiol* 32(12): 2944-2947.

Somoskovi, A., J. E. Hotaling, et al. (2001). "Lessons from a proficiency testing event for acid-fast microscopy." *Chest* 120(1): 250-257.

Springer, B., L. Stockman, et al. (1996). "Two-laboratory collaborative study on identification of mycobacteria: molecular versus phenotypic methods." *J Clin Microbiol* 34(2): 296-303.

Steingart, K. R., L. L. Flores, et al. (2011). "Commercial serological tests for the diagnosis of active pulmonary and extrapulmonary tuberculosis: an updated systematic review and meta-analysis." *PLoS medicine* 8(8): e1001062.

Steingart, K. R., M. Henry, et al. (2006). "Fluorescence versus conventional sputum smear microscopy for tuberculosis: a systematic review." *The Lancet Infect Dis* 6(9): 570-581.

Takiff, H. E., L. Salazar, et al. (1994). "Cloning and nucleotide sequence of Mycobacterium tuberculosis gyrA and gyrB genes and detection of quinolone resistance mutations." *Antimicrob Agents Chemother* 38(4): 773-780.

Tarrand, J. J., A. D. Spicer, et al. (1986). "Evaluation of a radiometric method for pyrazinamide susceptibility testing of Mycobacterium tuberculosis." *Antimicrob Agents Chemother* 30(6): 852-855.

Thibert, L. & S. Lapierre (1993). "Routine application of high-performance liquid chromatography for identification of mycobacteria." *J Clin Microbiol* 31(7): 1759-1763.

Tho, D. Q., N. T. Lan, et al. (2011). "Multiplex allele-specific polymerase chain reaction for detection of isoniazid resistance in Mycobacterium tuberculosis." *Int J Tuberc Lung Dis* 15(6): 799-803.

Torrea, G., P. Van de Perre, et al. (2005). "PCR-based detection of the Mycobacterium tuberculosis complex in urine of HIV-infected and uninfected pulmonary and extrapulmonary tuberculosis patients in Burkina Faso." *J Med Microbiol* 54(Pt 1): 39-44.

Tortoli, E., A. Nanetti, et al. (2001). "Performance assessment of new multiplex probe assay for identification of mycobacteria." *J Clin Microbiol* 39(3): 1079-1084.

Totsch, M., K. W. Schmid, et al. (1994). "Rapid detection of mycobacterial DNA in clinical samples by multiplex PCR." *Diagn Mol Pathol* 3(4): 260-264.

Traore, H., A. van Deun, et al. (2006). "Direct detection of Mycobacterium tuberculosis complex DNA and rifampin resistance in clinical specimens from tuberculosis patients by line probe assay." *J Clin Microbiol* 44(12): 4384-4388.

van Doorn, H. R., D. D. An, et al. (2008). "Fluoroquinolone resistance detection in Mycobacterium tuberculosis with locked nucleic acid probe real-time PCR." *Int J Tuberc Lung Dis* 12(7): 736-742.

Van Rie, A., L. Page-Shipp, et al. (2010). "Xpert((R)) MTB/RIF for point-of-care diagnosis of TB in high-HIV burden, resource-limited countries: hype or hope?" *Expert review of molecular diagnostics* 10(7): 937-946.

Vlaspolder, F., P. Singer, et al. (1995). "Diagnostic value of an amplification method (Gen-Probe) compared with that of culture for diagnosis of tuberculosis." *J Clin Microbiol* 33(10): 2699-2703.

Wang, F., C. Massire, et al. (2011). "Molecular characterization of drug-resistant Mycobacterium tuberculosis isolates circulating in China by multilocus PCR and electrospray ionization mass spectrometry." *J Clin Microbiol* 49(7): 2719-2721.

Welch, K., G. Brown, et al. (1995). "Performance of the Gen Probe amplified Mycobacterium tuberculosis direct test in a laboratory that infrequently isolates Mycobacterium tuberculosis." *Diagn Microbiol Infect Dis* 22(3): 297-299.

Wetmur, J. G. (1991). "DNA probes: applications of the principles of nucleic acid hybridization." *Crit Rev Biochem Mol Biol* 26(3-4): 227-259.

WHO (2008). New Laboratory Diagnostic Tools for Tuberculosis Control. Geneva, Stop TB Partnership and World Health Organization.

Wilson, M. L. (2011). "Recent advances in the laboratory detection of Mycobacterium tuberculosis complex and drug resistance." *Clin Infect Dis: an official publication of the Infectious Diseases Society of America* 52(11): 1350-1355.

Witebsky, F. G. & P. Kruczak-Filipov (1996). "Identification of mycobacteria by conventional methods." *Clin Lab Med* 16(3): 569-601.

Woo, P. C., J. L. Teng, et al. (2011). "Automated identification of medically important bacteria by 16S rRNA gene sequencing using a novel comprehensive database, 16SpathDB." *J Clin Microbiol* 49(5): 1799-1809.

Woodley, C. L., M. M. Floyd, et al. (1992). "Evaluation of Syngene DNA-DNA probe assays for the identification of the Mycobacterium tuberculosis complex and the Mycobacterium avium complex." *Diagn Microbiol Infect Dis* 15(8): 657-662.

Woods, G. L., J. S. Bergmann, et al. (2001). "Clinical Evaluation of the Gen-Probe amplified mycobacterium tuberculosis direct test for rapid detection of Mycobacterium tuberculosis in select nonrespiratory specimens." *J Clin Microbiol* 39(2): 747-749.

Woods, G. L. L., S-Y. G., Desmond, E.P. (2011). Susceptibility Test Methods: Mycobacteria, Nocardia, and Other Actinomycetes. *Manual of Clinical Microbiology*. J. C. Versalovic, K.C.; Funke, G.; Jorgensen, J.H.; Landry, M.L.; and Warnock, D.W. Washington, D.C., ASM Press. 1: 1215-1238.

Yu, M. C., H. Y. Chen, et al. (2011). "Evaluation of the rapid MGIT TBc identification test for culture confirmation of Mycobacterium tuberculosis complex strain detection." *J Clin Microbiol* 49(3): 802-807.

Zhang, S. L., J. G. Shen, et al. (2007). "A novel genotypic test for rapid detection of multidrug-resistant Mycobacterium tuberculosis isolates by a multiplex probe array." *J Appl Microbiol* 103(4): 1262-1271.

Zhang, Y. & W. W. Yew (2009). "Mechanisms of drug resistance in Mycobacterium tuberculosis." *Int J Tuberc Lung Dis* 13(11): 1320-1330.

2

Laboratory Diagnosis of Latent and Active Tuberculosis Infections in Trinidad & Tobago and Determination of Drug Susceptibility Profile of Tuberculosis Isolates in the Caribbean

Patrick Eberechi Akpaka and Shirematee Baboolal
Unit of Microbiology & Pathology, Department of Para Clinical Sciences, Faculty of Medical Sciences, The University of the West Indies, St. Augustine Trinidad & Tobago

1. Introduction

Tuberculosis (TB) is a life-threatening, infectious disease caused by the bacteria *Mycobacterium tuberculosis*. The disease has plagued human beings for many centuries as signs of tubercular damage have been found in Egyptian mummies and bones dating back at least 5,000 years ago **[1]**. Today, despite advances in diagnosis and treatment, TB is still a global pandemic, fueled by the spread of the Human Immunodeficiency Virus (HIV), the Acquired Immunodeficiency Syndrome (AIDS), poverty and a lack of proper health services in many developing countries **[2]**. As a developing nation, many of the Caribbean countries face serious challenges in the diagnosis, treatment, care and management of patients with TB. Some of these challenges include TB/HIV co-infection, drug resistance, inadequate laboratory services, growth of inequity stemming from rising poverty and the presence of weak health systems in many countries **[3]**. A major challenge that affects the Caribbean is the lack of proper facilities for laboratory diagnosis of TB; and there is a dire shortage of laboratory facilities and capability for culture and drug susceptibility testing. Because of this, many cases of TB with low bacillary load may be missed by smear microscopy if culture is not routinely performed. This is even more so in HIV/AIDS patients where smear microscopy may be negative due to the small numbers of bacilli being produced as a result of reduced pulmonary cavity formation **[4]**.

Weak laboratory service is one of the major obstacles to reducing the global burden of TB. The clinical mycobacteriology laboratory plays a major role in the prevention strategies and control measures of TB **[5]**. A wide spectrum of laboratory techniques has been developed to confirm the diagnosis of active and latent TB infection. No single laboratory test method is perfect, and unfortunately, some of the methods of diagnosis on which clinicians still rely on were developed more than a century ago.

It was based on these challenges that the aims of this study were conceived - to compare the available screening and investigative methods for detection of latent TB in Trinidad and Tobago; and also to evaluate methods for detection of drug resistance to *Mycobacterium tuberculosis* isolates recovered from clinical and cultured specimens from several Caribbean countries.

2. Materials and methods

Study setting and Site: The overall study design and methods have been described previously [6, 7]. Briefly, this prospective observational cross sectional population and laboratory based study was carried out at the Mycobacteriology laboratory at the Caribbean Epidemiology Centre (CAREC) in Trinidad and Tobago. The materials used for the study included individuals and clinical specimens from patients managed for TB infection in Trinidad and Tobago collected over a twelve month period as well as convenient clinical specimens and *M. tuberculosis* isolates from several countries in the Caribbean that were referred to CAREC for culture, identification and drug susceptibility testing over a twenty four month period.

Specimen collection: The specimens used included sputum and other clinical specimens from several Caribbean countries including Antigua, Belize, Dominica, Jamaica, Montserrat, St. Kitts, Nevis, St. Lucia, St. Vincent and the Grenadines, Trinidad and Tobago and Turks and Caicos Islands. While sputum and clinical specimens were referred from countries that did not perform culture or was not performing culture for TB during the study, cultures on Lowestein Jensen (LJ) slants were referred from countries that had the capability to perform culture for mycobacteria but were unable to perform identification and drug susceptibility testing. These countries included The Bahamas, Barbados, Trinidad and Tobago, Suriname and Guyana. For specimens coming from Trinidad and Tobago, both clinical specimens and cultures on LJ were included in the study. Diagnosis of latent TB infection was performed using the Quantiferon Gold Assay. For this test blood samples were collected in heparinized tubes. Individuals for this assay included contacts of confirmed tuberculosis patients, health care workers from the Caura Chest Hospital and the Chest Clinic at the Eric Williams Medical Sciences Complex, inmates of the maximum security prison (where a case of TB was identified) and HIV positive patients attending routine care and treatment clinic.

All specimens referred to CAREC over a two year period (September 2006 - August 2008) from the CAREC Member Countries except Trinidad and Tobago were included in the study. Only specimens from Trinidad and Tobago referred to CAREC over a one year period (September 2006 to October 2007) were included in the study. Clinical specimens were collected from hospitalized patients, chest clinics and sometimes from patients attending the offices of their private physicians and sent to the hospital laboratory or public health laboratory in each country for acid fast bacilli. For culture and drug susceptibility testing (DST), a portion of the specimen was referred, while for laboratories that are able to culture for mycobacteria, clinical specimens were processed using the N-acetyl-L-cysteine-sodium hydroxide (NALC-NaOH) method, inoculated and incubated until visible growth was seen on the LJ slants. Slants showing positive growth were then referred for identification and DST. Patients from Trinidad and Tobago in addition to giving blood specimens placed in heparin and transported at room temperature to the laboratory for detection of latent TB also had tuberculin skin tests (Mantoux test) administered on their forearm. Results of the reaction were was read after 72 hours.

Inclusion and exclusion criteria: (a) Only specimens showing positive growth on LJ or BACTEC 460 TB system were further analysed. (b) Repeat specimens or culture were not included. (c) Specimens without basic demographic data were excluded. (d) Cultures that showed growth of contaminating organisms were also not included in the study.

Data collection: For specimens originating from Trinidad & Tobago, a standardized questionnaire was used to obtain additional information of the test subjects. The questionnaire was divided into several sections including demographics, clinical information, medical history, laboratory investigation, radiographic findings, risk factors and treatment. Several methods were used to collate data, including going through the patient's file at the hospital and speaking to the County and the Public Health Nurses. Information (usually age, gender, type of specimen, HIV status and nationality) of specimens from other countries was taken from the patient's form that accompanied the specimens when they were received at the laboratory for culture, identification and DST. Information obtained was then entered into Excel spreadsheet for analysis.

Digestion and Decontamination of the specimens: All clinical specimens were processed in a Biological Safety Cabinet (BSC) using the NALC-NaOH method as previously described in literature **[8]**. Specimens on LJ slants were also processed in a BSC observing all safety precautions that are applicable when working with live tuberculosis cultures as has been described **[9]**. From the LJ slants colonies of growth were removed with a sterile disposable loop and placed in tubes containing glass beads and 0.5ml sterile distilled water. The tubes were vortexed for approximately 10 seconds to break up the large clumps of mycobacteria and then left undisturbed for 5-10 minutes. Following this, 0.1 ml portions of the supernatant were used to inoculate into BACTEC 12B vials only.

Processing of blood sample for latent TB detection: Blood specimens in heparin tubes were incubated overnight with antigens according to the manufacturer's (Cellestis Inc., USA) instructions. To do this the blood was mixed at least 20 times by gently inverting the tube, then in a 24 well culture plate 1.0ml of blood was placed in each of 4 wells. To each well 3 drops of the respective reagent was added; saline (NIL), early secretory antigen target-6 (ESAT-6), culture filtrate protein-10 (CFP-10) and phytohemaglutinin (Mitogen control), mixed thoroughly into the blood using a plate shaker for 1-2 minutes and then incubated overnight at 37°C. After overnight incubation, the plasma was removed from each well, placed in labeled tubes and stored at 4°C after which the enzyme linked immunosorbent assay (ELISA) test for the detection of IFN-γ was performed.

Culture of clinical specimens: Clinical specimens were cultured using two types of media, the LJ media and 12B media using the BACTEC 460 TB system (Becton Dickenson). For this 0.1 ml of sediments were added aseptically into each of these two media using a tuberculin syringe and needle. Supernatant from LJ cultures were only inoculated on 12B media as above. Both LJ slants and 12B vials were incubated at 37°C. 12B vials were read twice weekly for the first 2 weeks and then once a week for the next 6 weeks for the presence of growth while LJ slants were read weekly for up to 8 weeks. 12B cultures showing positive growth (between 50 to 100 growth units) or LJ slants showing colonies of mycobacteria were removed and identified using the NAP (p-nitro-α-acetylamino-β-hydroxyl-propiophenone) test. Cultures that showed growth of contaminating organisms were discarded. The supernatant was reprocessed and reinoculated. If the cultures were still contaminated, they were discarded.

Identification of mycobacteria using the NAP test: When mycobacterial growth was detected from either the 12B growth media or the LJ slants, each isolate was further identified using the NAP test. This test was performed by adding 1.0 ml of positive culture media to a vial containing p-nitro-α-acetylamino β-hydroxyl-propiophenone. This vial together with the original culture vial was incubated at 37^{0}C and read daily for 4 consecutive days. The culture was identified as *M. tuberculosis* Complex (MTBC) if the tube containing NAP did not allow growth of the mycobacteria while the original tube continued to grow. If growth was detected in both tubes, then the culture was identified as non-tuberculous mycobacteria (NTM); and these were further identified to species level using the Common Mycobacteria (CM) genotyping line probe assay from Hain Lifesciences (Germany). For quality control, a Clinical and Laboratory Standards Institute (CLSI) strain of *M. tuberculosis,* H37Rv was tested along with test specimens each week and for each new lot number of reagents that was used.

Drug Susceptibility Testing using BACTEC 460 TB System: Drug susceptibility tests (DSTs) using the BACTEC 460 TB system was performed on all isolates that belonged to the MTBC group. Only DST to 4 first line drugs and their concentrations - Streptomycin (2.0mg/L), Isoniazid (0.1mg/L), Rifampicin (2.0mg/L) and Ethambutol (2.5mg/L) were used for the study. For DSTs, 0.1 ml of broth from each positive specimen was inoculated to 12B vials containing fixed concentrations of the antibiotics listed above. A control vial without antibiotics was also inoculated with a 1:100 dilution of the respective growth media. All vials were incubated at 37°C and read daily in the BACTEC 460 machine until the control tube read 30 growth units.

The result of each test was determined as resistant if they were above or susceptible if below of the control GI reading. For quality control, once a month and when new antibiotics were prepared, cultures with known resistance patterns were tested along with the test specimens.

Identification of Mycobacteria using Hain Genotyping Assay: This procedure consisted of the following summarized steps: (a) DNA extraction from mycobacterial culture; (b) Preparation of Master Mix for PCR procedure; (c) Amplification Procedure; (d) Hybridization and Detection and; (e) Interpretation of results

DNA extraction: DNA extraction was performed using mycobacteria from liquid cultures (i.e. from positive 12B BACTEC culture vials). DNA extraction was performed when there was heavy growth of mycobacteria (when the liquid culture read at least 900 growth units). In a BSC 1.0ml of the culture was removed from the vial with a tuberculin needle and syringe and placed in a 2.5ml micro-centrifuge tube. The tube was then closed and centrifuged in a micro-centrifuge for 15 minutes at 13,000 r.p.ms. After centrifugation the supernatant was removed and the sediment re-suspended in 300μl molecular grade water. This suspension was then boiled at 96°C in a water bath for 15 minutes to lyse and inactivate the bacilli. After boiling the suspension was then placed in a sonicating water bath for a further 15 minutes. 5μl of this supernatant was used for the amplification reaction.

Preparation of Master Mix: In a sterile room specifically used for preparing master mixes, the master mix was prepared by combining the following reagents in a micro tube: 35μl of PNM (containing a mixture of triphosphate deoxynucleoside and primers marked with biotin). PNM is included in kit; 5µl of 10X buffer for polymerase incubation; 2.0µl of 2.5mM $MgCl_2$; 0.2µl of HotStart Taq polymerase (Qiagen, Germany); 2.0µl of distilled water. The final volume was 45µl and this is the amount used for 1 sample. This amount was multiplied by the number of samples and controls. After preparation, 45µl amounts of the master mix were aliquoted in 0.5ml centrifuge tubes and labeled with the specimen number before the addition of DNA.

Amplification Procedure: In another room and under a BSC, 5µl of each DNA solution was added to the respective labeled tube containing the master mix prepared above to reach a final volume of 50µl. After addition of the DNA, the tubes were mixed properly by vortexing for 10 seconds. Amplification was performed in a thermal cycler (Perkin Elmer 9600 thermal cycler; Applied Biosystem, CA, USA) using the following amplification protocol: one denaturation cycle of 15 min at 95°C, followed by 10 denaturation cycles of 30s at 95°C and ten elongation cycles of 2 min at 58°C, followed by 20 additional denaturations of 25s at 95°C and annealing of 40s at 53°C, continuing with an elongation step of 40s at 70°C and finishing with an extension cycle of 8 minutes at 70°C. After amplification the amplified DNA was kept at 4°C until hybridization was done.

Hybridization and Detection: Hybridization and detection were performed as described by the manufacturers using a semi-automated method in a TwinCubator (Hain Lifesciences, Nehren, Germany).

Reverse Hybridization Process: In the Reverse Hybridization process, each strip has a total of 17 reaction zones. The first band contains the conjugate control designed to indicate that the conjugate has been effectively united with the substrate, thereby facilitating correct visualization. The second band includes a universal control designed to detect all known mycobacteria and members of the group of gram-positive bacteria with a high G+C content. This band is used for checking the presence of the amplified product after hybridization. The third band contains a sequence that amplifies a fragment of the 23S rRNA region, which is common to all known members of the tuberculosis complex. Amplification bands 4-17 include probes specific for each of the mycobacteria species. A combination of these bands enables identification of the different species of mycobacteria, including *M. tuberculosis* complex.

Drug susceptibility using MTBDRplus (Line probe assay): This procedure was performed exactly as that for identification of mycobacteria except for the difference in the primers used and the type of specimen. While cultured material was used for the Common Mycobacterium CM assay, clinical specimens were used for the MTBDR*plus* assay. The primers used were specific to detect presence of wild types and mutations. Each strip contained bands that detected *M. tuberculosis* Complex, locus controls (*rpo*B, *kat*G and *inh*A) as well as Wild Types (WT) and mutations for *rpo*B, *kat*G and *inh*A. There were eight WT for *rpo*B gene (WT 1-8) and four mutations (MUT 1, 2A, 2B and 3). For *kat*G gene there was one WT and 2 mutations (MUT 1and 2) and for *inh*A gene 2 WT (1 and 2) and 4 mutations (MUT 1, 2, 3A and 3B). The isolate was identified as *M. tuberculosis* complex when the TUB band was present. Resistance was determined when a wild type was missing and or a mutation present for each of the gene on the strip.

ELISA test for detection of gamma interferon (IFN-γ): For each ELISA test run, two strips or 16 wells were required for standards and 4 wells were required for each patient sample.

All reagents except the conjugate were brought to room temperature before the test. For each run the required number of strips were removed from the kit and placed on a strip holder. The standard dilutions were prepared (8.0IU/ml - 0.125IU/ml) as well as the conjugate dilution (5µl conjugate concentrate to 1.0ml of diluent). To each well 50µl conjugate dilution was added followed by 50µl standard dilution and 50µl respective patient samples. The contents of the wells were mixed for 1-2 minutes using a plate shaker and then incubated for 2 hours at room temperature to enable the antigen-conjugate complex to adhere to the surface of the microwells. After incubation, the wells were washed with wash buffer 5 times using an automated plate washer to remove excess conjugate complex. This was followed by the addition of 100µl enzyme substrate (kit component). The wells were mixed as before and incubated for a further 30 minutes at room temperature. The reaction was stopped after this time with 50µl enzyme stop solution and the optical densities of each well measured using wavelengths of 450 and 620. Results were calculated by plotting the results on a graph using Microsoft Office Excel. Results greater than 0.35 in the ESAT-6 and CFP-10 wells were recorded as positive while results less than 0.35 were recorded as negative.

Data Analysis: Statistical analysis of results of culture, identification, DST as well as questionnaire information were performed using Epi Info 3.5.1 version, Centers for Disease Control & Prevention software **[10]** and Open Epi version 2.3 **[11]**. Associations between variables were assessed using Chi-square analysis and Fisher's exact test. *P*-values of ≤ 0.05 were considered statistically significant.

Ethical approval: The Ethics committee of the Faculty of Medical Sciences, The University of the West Indies, St. Augustine, Trinidad and Tobago, approved the study while written permission for use of the specimens was received from the Chief Medical Officers in the Ministry of Health from each of the countries represented in the study.

3. Results

Specimens and patients: A total of 1,262 specimens comprising 43% culture materials and 57% clinical samples obtained from 15 Caribbean countries were used for this study. The highest number of specimens 28% were obtained from Trinidad & Tobago and the least 0.2% was from Dominica as depicted on Table 1. For latent TB detection, 560 subjects were recruited from Trinidad and Tobago.

Culture and Identification: The BACTEC 460-TB culture method used for culturing the specimens yielded 773 positive cultures and from this, 79.04% (611/773) were identified to belong to the *Mycobacterium tuberculosis* complex group, while 20.96% (162/773) were NTMs using NAP test. The Hain Common Mycobacteria (CM) genotyping assay was used to further identify the NTMs isolates that consisted of *Mycobacterium fortuitium* (34.6%), followed by *Mycobacterium intracellulare* (12.3%), *Mycobacterium gordonae* (6.8%), and *Mycobacterium kansassi* (6.2%). The genotyping assay was unable to identify 16.7% of the NTMs, while 7.4% showed characteristics of mixed infection with *M. tuberculosis* and *M. fortuitium* (referred to Hain Lifesciences for confirmation). The distribution of the NTMs isolates from the various Caribbean countries is highlighted in Table 2.

Country	Specimens Clinical samples	 Culture materials	Total (%)
Antigua	3	-	3 (0.24)
Bahamas	-	28	28 (2.22)
Barbados	-	26	26 (2.06)
Belize	54	-	54 (4.28)
Dominica	2	-	2 (0.16)
Guyana	-	214	214 (16.96)
Jamaica	208	-	208 (16.48)
Montserrat	25	-	25 (1.98)
St. Kitts	3	-	3 (0.24)
Nevis	5	-	5 (0.40)
St. Lucia	77	-	77 (6.10)
St. V & G	7	-	7 (0.55)
Suriname	-	240	240 (19.02)
T&T	328	34	362 (28.68)
TCI	8	-	8 (0.63)
TOTAL	720 (57.05)	542 (42.95)	1,262 (100)

St. V&G = St. Vincent and the Grenadines, T&T = Trinidad & Tobago, TCI = Turks & Caicos Islands

Table 1. Distribution of specimens (clinical samples and cultures) received from fifteen (15) Caribbean countries used for this study (%).

Species	**N (%)**	**Countries**
M. fortuitium	56 (34.6)	BDS, BLZ, GUY, SUR, T&T
M. intracellulare	20 (12.3)	ANT, GUY, JAM, STL, SUR, T&T
M. gordonae	11 (6.8)	BRB, GUY, SUR
M. kansassi	10 (6.2)	BRB, JAM, T&T
M. abscessus	8 (4.9)	BRB, JAM, SUR
M. avium	6 (3.7)	JAM, SUR, TCI, NVS
M. intermedium	4 (2.5)	SUR
M. scrofoleceum	3 (1.9)	BLZ, SUR, T&T
M. interjectum	3 (1.9)	SUR, TCI
M. simiae	1 (0.6)	JAM
M. chelonae	1 (0.6)	SUR
Mycobacterium species	27 (16.7)	GUY, JAM, SUR, MNT
Mixed infection (MTB and *M. fortuitium*)	12 (7.4)	JAM, SUR
TOTAL	162(100)	

N = total number, MTB = Mycobacterium tuberculosis, T&T = Trinidad & Tobago, TCI = Turks and Caicos Islands, JAM = Jamaica, SUR = Suriname, GUY = Guyana, MNT = Montserrat, BLZ = Belize, NVS = Nevis, BRB = Barbados, ANT = Antigua

Table 2. Distribution of non tuberculosis mycobacteria (NTM) species identified in specimens from Caribbean countries using the Common Mycobacteria (CM) genotyping assay

3.1 Tuberculin Skin Test and QuantiFERON-TB Gold for the detection of Latent TB infection

A total of 560 subjects were recruited from Trinidad & Tobago for this component of the study. They all had blood samples drawn from them and equally had TST administered on their forearm. Of these 560, only 530 of the subjects met the study criteria and were therefore included in the final analysis of the results. Summary of the result of the detection of latent TB infection using the tuberculin skin test (TST) and the QuantiFERON-TB Gold assay is given on Table 3.

The majority of the subjects were males (73.5%) and between the ages of 40 and 49 years (32.8%), The TST results surprisingly revealed that only 1.8% (3/165) of the TB patient (control group) readings were <5 mm and only 3% (5/165) were 5-9 mm. As expected, 95.2% of the TB patients had a wheal reaction ≥10 mm. None of the HIV subjects had a reaction of ≥ 10 mm but most of them (90.6%) had a reaction < 5 mm; the rest (9.4%) had a reaction measuring 5-9 mm. Among the health care workers, there were no TST readings ≥ 15mm, but most (73.2%) were <5 mm. In Trinidad and Tobago, a TST reading ≥ 10 mm among uncompromised individuals is considered a positive result. For individuals with HIV or any other underlying condition, such as malignancy, the positive cutoff threshold drops to 5-9 mm. Therefore, the 9.4% of HIV-positive subjects in the current study with readings at that level were considered to have positive TST results. Cutoff thresholds for interpretation of actual TST results (which are not considered biologically meaningful) range from 5 mm to 15 mm, depending on the type of high-risk group being surveyed and the level of TB prevalence in the study setting. The positive cutoff values used in the current study are relatively high but did not affect the final study results due to the clustered distribution of the induration values described above.

The comparative results of the two test methods used for the diagnosis or screening for latent TB infection among high risk groups in Trinidad & Tobago (Table 3) revealed that the QFT-G assay detected a significantly higher proportion of latent TB infected individuals than the TST in all high-risk groups except TB patients (the study controls), among whom the TST appeared to be more effective. The differences were statistically significant among all target groups studied for each testing method.

There was no significant age difference between the TST positive subjects and those with positive results for the QFT-G assay, who ranged from 20 to 60 years and 21 to 59 years respectively (with a mean age of 33.1 versus 34.5 years; $p > 0.05$). Most of the HIV and TB positive subjects (68.8% and 69.7% respectively) were in the 30-59 year age group.

The average number of hours required to complete the TST was 70.1 hours versus 23.4 hours for the QFT-G assay ($p < 0.0001$). The average cost to perform each TST was US $3.70 (for a total cost of US $2,065.00), whereas US $18.60 was required to carry out the QFT-G assay (total cost of US $10,440.00). These differences were significant (US$3.70 versus US$18.60; $p = 0.0008$) and favored use of the TST method for latent TB infection (LTBI) detection.

When the results of both tests were combined, the rate of LTBI detection increased to 88.7%. In the prison inmate group, concomitant results for both tests were available for 62 subjects. Of these, 24.2% (15/62) tested positive based on the TST and 56.5% (35/62) tested positive based on the QFT-G assay. The rate of concordance between the two tests for this target group was 49.7% (32/62) for negative results, and 15.6% (10/62) for positive results, and overall agreement of 76%. For all discordant results, subjects were more likely to be TST-positive and QFT-G - negative (92.1%) versus TST-negative and QFT-G - positive (7.0%). Overall, 39.6% of all subjects had a positive TST result and 51.3% had a positive QFT-G assay result. The significant differences obtained for TAT favored the QFT-G assay, whereas the cost of material required to perform the tests favored the TST.

High risk group	N	No. cases detected (%)		P-value
		TST	QFT-G	
TB patients' contacts[a]	200	35 (17.5)	78 (39.0)	<0.001
Health Care Workers	40	3 (7.5)	15 (37.5)	<0.003
Prison inmates	62	15 (24.2)	35 (56.5)	<0.006
HIV+ patients	60	12 (20.0)	26 (43.3)	<0.0006
TB Patients (controls)	168	157 (93.5)	118 (70.2)	<0.008
Total	530	210 (39.6)	272 (51.3)	0.08
Cost per test[b]		$3.70	$18.60	<0.0008
Turnaround time[c]		70.0	23.0	<0.0001

N = total number of subjects tested. [a] Individuals who came into contact with active TB patients - friends and family members. [b] In 2010 US dollars ($1 = 6.35 TTD). [c] Average number of hours from time of intradermal injection of tuberculin on subjects' forearms to the time wheal reaction at puncture was read within 72 hours.

Table 3. Comparison of QuantiFERON® TB-Gold (QFT-G) assay and tuberculin skin test (TST) in diagnosis/screening for latent tuberculosis (TB) infection among high-risk groups from Trinidad & Tobago

The average number of hours required to complete the TST was 70.0 hours versus 23.0 hours for the QFT-G assay (p <0.0001). The average cost to perform each TST was US $3.70 (for a total cost of US $2,065.00), whereas US $18.60 was required to carry out the QFT-G assay (total cost of US $10,440.00). These differences were significant (US$3.70 versus US$18.60; p =0.0008) and favored use of the TST method for LTBI detection.

Drug Susceptibility Testing (DST): The BACTEC 460 TB System was used to successfully determine the drug susceptibility tests (DST) of 91.3% (558/611) cultures identified as *M. tuberculosis* Complex from 12 of the Caribbean countries as revealed on Table 4. Overall, a total of 42 (7.5%) isolates from 8 countries showed resistance to at least one or more anti-TB drugs.

Analysis of the susceptibility pattern to the anti TB agents revealed that 73.8% (31/42) of the isolates were resistant to isoniazid (INH), 66.7% (28/42) were resistant to rifampicin (RIF), 38.9 (16/42) were resistant to both RIF and INH while 28.6% (12/42) were either resistant to streptomycin or ethambutol. The highest number of isolates subjected to DST analysis were obtained from Trinidad & Tobago and then followed by Guyana. Although no multidrug resistance was seen in isolates from several of the Caribbean countries, the highest frequency of resistance and multidrug resistance were noted among isolates from Guyana.

The Hain Genotyping line probe assay (MTBDR*plus*) was further used to genotypically analyze a total of 33 isolates that had initially been identified to be resistant to INH (26 isolates) and/or RIF (24 isolates) by the phenotypic method. This result is shown on Table 5. Overall, of the 24 isolates showing resistance to RIF using the phenotypic method, 23 (95.8%) showed resistance with the genotypic method. Of the 26 isolates showing resistance to INH with the phenotypic method, 9 (34.6%) showed resistance with the genotypic method. Additionally, 2 isolates sensitive to INH with the phenotypic method showed resistance with the genotypic method and 1 isolate resistant to RIF with the phenotypic method was sensitive with the genotypic method.

Resistance to RIF was identified genotypically by the presence or absence of mutations in the *rpo*B gene, while resistance to INH was identified by the presence or absence of mutations in the *kat*G and *inh*A genes. The codons most frequently involved in RIF mutations were S-531L (57.1%) and codon S-516L (20%). Twenty (20) isolates carried the most common mutation, Ser531 → Leu. As for INH resistance, of the 9 isolates that the Genotype MTBDR*plus* detected, 78% of them carried mutation at S315T1 codon of the *kat*G gene, showing AGC → ACC mutation, and 22% showed AGC → ACA mutation. Equally, 64.7% of these mutation occurred at these bands at the *inh*A gene in the MDR isolates from the region.

Country	N	S	R	MDR
Bahamas	21	15	6 (14.3)	0
Barbados	14	12	2 (4.8)	1 (6.25)
Belize	5	3	2 (4.8)	1 (6.25)
Dominica	1	1	0	0
Guyana	141	117	24 (57.1)	13 (81.25)
Jamaica	95	92	3 (7.14)	0
St. Lucia	10	10	0	0
St. Kitts	2	2	0	0
St. V&G	6	6	0	0
Suriname	115	112	3 (7.1)	1 (6.25)
T&T	145	144	1 (2.4)	0
TCI	3	2	1 (2.4)	0
Total	558	516	42 (100)	16 (100)

N = number of isolates tested, S = isolates fully susceptibile to all first line drugs, R = isolates resistant to any of the first line drugs, MDR = isolates resistant to both isoniazid and rifampcin, T&T - Trinidad and Tobago, TCI - Turks and Caicos Islands, St. V&G - St. Vincent and the Grenadines.

Table 4. BACTEC 460 TB System susceptibility results of 558 TB isolates (patients) from the Caribbean (%)

BACTEC 460 MTBDRplus	rpoB		katG		InhA			
	MWT	Mut	MWT	Mut	MWT	Mut	RIF	INH
RIF	WT7	2A	-	-	-	-	R	-
R	WT8	3	-	-	-	-	R	-
R	N	2A, 3	-	-	-	-	R	-
R	WT8	3	-	-	-	-	R	-
R	WT8	3	-	-	-	-	R	-
RE	WT8	3	-	-	-	-	R	-
I	WT8	3	N	N	N	N	R	S
I	-	-	N	N	N	N	-	S
I	-	-	N	N	N	N	-	S
I	-	-	WT1	1	N	N	-	R
I	-	-	N	N	N	N	-	S
I	W3,4	-	N	N	N	N	R	S
I	-	-	N	N	WT1	1	-	R
IE	_	-	N	N	N	N	-	S
IR	WT8	3	N	N	N	N	R	S
IR	WT8	3	N	N	W	1	R	R
IR	WT4,5,7,8	N	N	N	N	N	R	S
IR	WT7	2B	N	N	N	N	R	S
IR	N	N	N	N	WT1	1	S	R
IR	WT8	3	N	N	N	N	R	S
IR	WT2.3	N	WT1	N	N	N	R	R
IRE	WT8	3	N	N	N	N	R	S
IRE	WT3.4	1	N	N	WT1	1	R	R
IRE	WT8	3	N	N	N	N	R	S
IRE	WT8	N	WT1	1	N	N	R	R
SIR	WT3, 4		N	N	N	N	R	S
SIRE	WT3, 4		1	N	N	N	R	S
SIRE	WT8	3	N	N	N	N	R	S
SIRE	WT8	N	WT1	1	N	N	R	R
IRE	WT8	N	WT1	1	N	N	R	S
SIR	WT3, 4		N	N	N	N	R	S
SIRE	WT3, 4		1	N	N	N	R	S
SIRE	WT8	3	N	N	N	N	R	S
SIRE	WT8	N	WT1	1	N	N	R	R

MWT = Missing wild type, MUT = mutation, N = none, R = resistant, S = susceptible, R-IRE = resistant to isoniazid, rifampicin and Ethambutol, R-SIRE = resistant to Streptomycin, isoniazid, rifampicin and ethambutol

Table 5. Results of MTBDR*plus* for isolates that showed resistance to INH and RIF using BACTEC 460 assay

4. Discussions

One of the major objectives of this study was to evaluate the tuberculin skin test (TST), the method currently being used in Trinidad & Tobago, with that of the Quantiferon TB-Gold Test (a new IFN-γ based test that has now been introduced in the market for LTBI detection) to determine the cost and efficiency of these methods in detecting latent TB infection (LTBI). Unlike the TST and IFN-γ analysis, most diagnostic assays for detecting *M. tuberculosis* infection are based on either isolation or identification of the bacteria, which makes them inapplicable for diagnosis of latent infection. The development of IFN-γ tests to detect T-cells specific for *M. tuberculosis* antigens addressed this important issue. The current study was carried out among individuals from various groups with a high risk of developing TB due to either exposure to or contact with TB patients, lack of isolation facilities, or weak infection control. In the current study, the two selected testing methods (QFT-G and TST) detected LTBI among the various target groups at different rates.

Among the TB patient [control] group, the rate of TB detection by the QFT-G assay (70.2%) was significantly different from that of the TST. This rate of detection was similar to that observed by Lee *et al.*, who reported a sensitivity of 70% among 87 patients diagnosed with TB **[12],** and higher than both the 64.4% rate of detection observed by Kobashi *et al.* in Japan **[13]** and the rate observed by Dewan *et al.*, who reported a sensitivity of 60% in culture-confirmed cases **[14].** However, the 70.2% rate was lower than that reported by both Kang *et al.* (81% sensitivity in 54 patients) and Mori *et al.* (89% sensitivity among 118 patients) **[15, 16].** More recently, Kobashi *et al.* demonstrated significant differences in the quantitative responses of IFN-γ to *M. tuberculosis* between patients with active TB disease and those with LTBI **[13].**

Combining the results for the QFT-G assay and the TST in the current study increased the overall sensitivity for detection of LBTI among the culture-confirmed TB-infected control group. This confirms and reinforces recommendations that negative results should not be used alone to exclude active TB but should be interpreted in conjunction with other clinical and diagnostic findings **[17].** It also underscores the fact that the QFT-G assay has a limited role in the evaluation of patients with culture-confirmed TB. The authors of the current study agree with Kobashi *et al.*'s conclusion that it would be difficult to use the QFT-G assay to completely discriminate active TB disease from LTBI **[13].**

In the current study, 43.3% of all HIV patients included in the analysis had a positive result for the QFT-G assay. This was in huge contrast to the earlier study by Kobashi *et al.* **[13],** in which all HIV patients produced QFT-G–positive results. The indeterminate or nonreactive results observed in some of the HIV-positive subjects in the current study also contrast with those found by Ferrara *et al.* **[17].** In the current study, the QFT-G assays were run several times to minimize the effect of laboratory and procedural errors. However, the indeterminate and nonreactive results persisted, with test results continuing to produce low mitogen levels. Although all indeterminate or nonreactive results were excluded from the final analysis, the QFT-G assay results should be interpreted with caution, bearing in mind the high prevalence of HIV in Trinidad & Tobago and the Caribbean region. Several possible explanations for a high rate of indeterminate and nonreactive results have been adduced and these include the presence of lymphocytopenia and/or inflammatory and immunosuppressive conditions, as well as hypoalbuminemia, which suggests poor nutritional status **[13]**, and there is a high probability that some of these conditions could have existed among the subjects of the current study. Lymphocytopenia (especially the CD4 strain) has been shown to depend on the elaboration of inflammatory cytokines by T-cells previously sensitized to *M. tuberculosis*–specific antigens in QFT-G assays. In the blood, mononuclear cells from peripheral blood are stimulated in vitro, and the production of IFN-γ from sensitized T-lymphocytes by *M. tuberculosis*–specific antigen is measured by ELISA in the QFT-G **[18,19]**.

In the current study, however, only 58% of TST-positive subjects had a positive QFT-G result. More than half of this group consisted of prison inmates with a documented TST > 10 mm. In Trinidad & Tobago, TST is likely to be a very good indicator of latent infection in recently exposed individuals because of the following reasons (a) most individuals under the age of 20 years did not receive the BCG vaccination, which was discontinued during the early 1990s, and (b) BCG vaccination has been observed to significantly increase the likelihood of a positive TST in subjects without LTBI.

Multiple outbreaks of TB, including those involving the multi-drug-resistant strain (MDR-TB), have been reported in prisons and jails, especially among HIV-infected inmates, a population regarded as having moderate risk of acquiring TB **[20]**. The results of the current study from this moderate-risk population show that prevalence of LTBI was 24.2% and 56.5% based on the TST and the QFT-G assay respectively. These values were quite high compared to those observed in correctional facilities in the United States, where prevalence was less than 10%. However, the QFT-G values obtained in the current study were in line with the current rate of TB in Trinidad & Tobago, which is estimated to be about 17 per 100 000 population **[21]**. It has been suggested that annual TB screening of prison inmates using the TST may account for the increase in the number of TST-positive results, due to the "boosting" effect caused by repeat use of the test. However, this type of screening is not carried out among prison inmates in Trinidad & Tobago. Therefore, the high rate of TST-positive results in the current study could be attributed mainly to exposure to the disease.

The prevalence of LTBI among health care workers using the TST in the current study was a mere 7.5%. This value was very low compared to those reported by studies in Portugal (33%) and Germany (10%)**[22, 23]**. The low value found in the current study may have been due to a smaller sample size and the use of a higher positive cutoff. Like the studies in Portugal and Germany, the current study showed that the QFT-G assay was more useful than the TST in identifying LTBI among health care workers. As this target group may be exposed to TB more frequently than the local population, screening of staff exposed to the disease is frequently recommended to identify infected individuals and treat them adequately and promptly. Because the QFT-G assay was more sensitive than the TST in detecting LTBI, the authors of the current study strongly support its use in screening health care workers in Trinidad & Tobago.

The TST may also be less desirable due to complications in interpreting its results caused by the above-mentioned boosting effect (from repeat testing) as well as conversions and reversions (changes in results from negative at baseline to positive and vice versa, respectively). In a study on health care workers in India, Pai *et al.* suggested that individuals with recent exposure to TB usually presented with large increases ($\geq$ 10 mm) in TST indurations that were always accompanied by substantial increases in IFN-γ **[24]**. This finding was in line with the results of the current study.

The QFT-G assay also fared better than the TST in terms of TAT. In terms of cost, however, the TST appears best suited for the resource-strapped environment of Trinidad & Tobago (if the calculation of this variable is based mainly on the cost of the materials required to perform the test versus the cost of labor and other inputs). This argument is partly supported by Pooran *et al.*, who concluded in a recent report that screening for LTBI using TST alone was the most cost-effective testing strategy but ultimately incurred the highest cost due to test inaccuracies **[25]**. Another factor that may make the TST less cost-effective over time is high replacement costs, since the Mantoux test solution is often not accessible in developing countries and would have to be replaced with the relatively labor-intensive IFN-γ release assay. Minimizing cost for TB testing has become increasingly important because prevalence of the disease has fallen dramatically in developed countries and more than 90% of all cases worldwide occur in resource-strapped developing countries **[26]**. However, as pointed out by both Diel *et al.* and Marra *et al.*, use of the IFN-γ release assay alone or in combination with the TST for screening close TB contacts prior to LTBI treatment is highly cost-effective in reducing the TB disease burden **[27, 28, 29]**.

4.1 Profiles of drug susceptibility patterns of *Mycobacterium tuberculosis* isolates encountered in the Caribbean

Drug resistance using the Hain Lifescience MTBDR*plus* line probe assay revealed that this method performed very well for the detection of RIF resistance isolates in the region. This is in agreement with the high sensitivity reported elsewhere [**30, 31, 32**]. However, the results for detection of resistance to INH were much lower using this assay. This observation is not unique since the molecular mechanisms for INH resistance are not fully understood and about 25-30% of phenotypic INH-resistance associated mutations are still unaccounted for [**32**].

This study revealed that the codon most frequently involved in the mutation was the S-531L of the *rpo*B gene among the RIF resistant isolates. Similar result has been reported by Cavusoglu *et al.*, 2007 [**34**], but Barnard *et al.*, 2008 [**35**], reported that most mutations in the isolates tested in their study occurred at several other codons. Also, a high proportion of the mutational changes were detected in the S-315T1 codon of the *kat*G gene for the INH and RIF monoresistant isolates in this study in contrast to regions reported elsewhere [**35**]. This was a trend reported in a high burden setting that seem to be a different trend among the *M. tuberculosis* isolates seen here in the Caribbean region.

The MTBDR*plus* genotype assay allowed for the rapid and specific detection of most mutations conferring resistance to RIF and to a lesser extent INH. Collective observations have indicated that mutations to the *rpo*B gene may account for the greater than 96% of the resistance to RIF [**30,35**]. This present study indicated that this is also true for Caribbean TB isolates that showed an overall resistance detection of 95.8% with the MTBDR*plus* assay.

Detection of INH resistance using the MTBDR*plus* assay for the *kat*G and *inh*A gene was disappointing. In this study, only 34.6% resistance to INH was detected using the MTBDR*plus* assay which is less than that reported by Johnson *et al.*, 2008 **[36]**. Other studies showed detection of 60-90% within the *kat*G gene and 15-43% within the *inh*A gene **[32, 31]**. Nonetheless, it must be kept in mind that the isolates used in this study were screened using the single drug concentration of 0.1µg/ml of INH in the BACTEC 460 TB system (which detects low levels of resistance to INH at this concentration, mainly useful for therapeutic purposes). The study did not discriminate between strains with low levels of INH resistance with those harboring a high level of resistance, a fact that may indirectly explain the poor agreement between the number of INH-resistant isolates detected using the gold-standard BACTEC 460 TB as compared to the MTBDR*plus* (26 instead of 9). In fact, it has been shown that the MTBDR*plus* assay was unable to detect low levels of INH resistance that was commonly detected using the BACTEC 460 TB system **[32]**.

Previous reports have confirmed that high INH concentration levels of more than 0.4µg/ml can be detected in the *kat*G genes among *M. tuberculosis* isolates that are resistant to the drug **[32]**. This detection of low INH resistance among the *M. tuberculosis* isolates seen in this study could perhaps be because of the low concentration of the INH drug used. In addition, the MTBDR*plus* assay only detects those resistances of *M. tuberculosis* that have their origins in the *rpo*B, *kat*G and *inh*A regions (MTBDR*plus* kit insert). Since resistance originating from mutations of other genes or gene regions as well as other RIF and INH mechanisms are not detected by the MTBDR*plus,* it could be that other mechanisms of resistance possessed by the isolates from the Caribbean were not detected. This will definitely require further studies since such was outside the scope of this study.

With the MTBDR*plus* assay, clinical specimens that are AFB positive with moderate to many AFBs, can be reliably tested for drug resistance. Furthermore, the genotypic DST method was able to detect drug resistance in samples that were contaminated as well as in those that had lost viability, circumventing the need to request follow-up sputum thus decreasing the time between specimen collection, results and treatment of the patient. This study also showed that less time was spent using the MTBDR*plus* in detecting INH and RIF resistance in TB isolates in the Caribbean. Using the BACTEC 460 TB system, the mean time for reporting results showing any drug-resistance was 32 days for cultures and 40 days for clinical specimens. This time represented repeating all drug-sensitivities for specimens showing any resistance. For specimens that were sensitive to anti-TB drugs, the mean time was 21 days for clinical specimens and 14 days for isolates.

Determination of drug resistance is difficult due to technical reasons and in several cases; these results are not always accurate **[37]**. In addition, it can take up to 6 weeks to get a phenotypic DST result and during this time many transmission events may take place. Therefore, alternative methods need to be evaluated to improve the speed of diagnosis especially drug resistant TB and this is what was achieved using the MTBDR*plus* assay in this study. With the BACTEC 460 system, culture material was not able to give results for non viable or contaminated materials; however in this study the MTBDR*plus* system gave identifiable results. This is in agreement with what has been reported as these tests are able to perform on specimens that contain non viable bacilli or from specimen that were contaminated by other bacteria and fungi **[32, 35, 36]**.

Although MTBDR*plus* assay has limitations as with any DNA-based screening nucleic acid sequence, it is possible that mutations that do not cause an amino acid exchange (silent mutations) will still produce the absence of one of the wild type probes. In addition, this assay only detects those resistance of the *M. tuberculosis* that have origins in the *rpo*B, *kat*G and *inh*A regions, yet the high sensitivity of RIF resistance detection is a plus point since this test can be used for detecting RIF resistance, a surrogate marker for multiple drug resistance in *M. tuberculosis* isolates. This assay is an excellent test to use on selected clinical samples because the amount of time required in generating a result was within 24 hours after receipt of specimen, culturing of the specimen is not required and contaminated as well as non-viable cultures can be used. Finally, the test method was also cheaper to use in resource-poor countries like in the Caribbean region.

Despite the global expansion in coverage of drug-resistance surveillance, data on drug resistance are still unavailable for more than 100 countries throughout the world **[38]**. Even in the Caribbean there is a paucity of information or data on the anti TB susceptibility pattern. This study was very important as it provided data on drug resistance that was lacking for most of the countries in the Caribbean. The level of drug resistance observed in most of the countries in this study was quite low with the exception of Guyana. Although drug resistance has been reported from several countries in the Caribbean, data reported to WHO on drug resistance is lacking as only Trinidad and Tobago reported 1 case of MDR-TB to the WHO in 2006 **[39]**.

In this study, resistance to anti-TB medications was seen in seven countries, five of which had >5 cases of TB/100,000 population and with one country (Guyana) accounting for 85% of the MDR-TB strains seen. This data confirms the continued existence of drug resistance in Guyana, as an earlier report by Menner *et al.*, 2005 **[40]** also reported a high frequency of drug resistance in this country with 22.2% of the isolates tested showing resistance to at least one anti-tuberculosis drug and 11.1% showing resistance to INH and RIF **[40]**. The reason for the continued persistence of MDR-TB in Guyana according to Menner *et al* is the lack of human resources to adequately follow up and monitor patient treatment as well as poor management of the tuberculosis control programme **[40]**. In this present study similar results were seen as 20.5% of isolates tested showed resistance to at least one anti-TB drug and 14.5% showed resistance to INH and RIF (MDR-TB).

Unlike previous studies from Africa, Haiti and Guyana that showed high levels of drug-resistance with high TB/HIV co-infection rates **[40, 41, 42, 43, 44]**, the moderate TB incidence seen in the rest of the Caribbean was not accompanied by any substantial level of drug-resistance. For example, there was no case of drug resistance among TB isolates from Trinidad and Tobago. This was very surprising especially with the high levels of TB/HIV co-infection (30.6% of the TB positive cases) and the high defaulter rate (22.7% of the TB positive cases). As reported in the literature, drug resistance was commonly seen in other countries where there was inadequate chemotherapy and also where HIV co-infections was present **[45, 46]**; but this is in contrast to Trinidad & Tobago where despite the high prevalence of HIV co-infection with TB, drug resistant cases were almost non- existent.

The absence of drug resistance in Trinidad and Tobago may be attributed to the excellent care and treatment TB programme such as direct observed treatment (DOT), adequate provision and supply of TB drugs that exists in the country. Additionally, all patients with tuberculosis are admitted and managed at the Caura Chest hospital until they become non-infectious, after which they are monitored on a regular basis by public health officials from the TB programme.

In Suriname drug resistance was rarely seen and when it occurred, only mono-resistance was seen. Mono-resistance was also recorded for isolates from Jamaica and The Bahamas, two countries where HIV infection is also relatively high and where low levels of resistance are seen. As in Trinidad and Tobago, the TB programmes in these countries are well managed and there is a very good collaboration between the TB and the HIV programmes.

A review of the literature for drug resistance in other parts of the Caribbean showed that similar low levels of drug resistance have been seen in the French Caribbean Islands of Guadeloupe and Martinique where there is significant migrant population from Haiti, an area of high drug resistance. The incidence of monoresistance in the French Caribbean Islands was 12.9%, however the incidence of MDR-TB was much lower with a rate of 0.9% **[47]**.

Limitations of the study: An inherent limitation designed to compare cost and turnround time against an imperfect conventional test such as TST is that no gold standard has been established for resolution of discordant results. The MTBDR*plus* assay has the limitation that as a DNA assay based procedure that screens for nucleic acid sequence and not amino acid sequence, it is possible that mutations that do not cause amino acid exchange (silent mutations) will result in the absence of one of the wild types probes. Besides the assay detects only resistance that originate in the *rpo*B, *kat*G and *inh*A regions of the *Mycobacterium tuberculosis*. Hence other regions where resistance occurs will completely be missed.

The lack of adequate facilities for manipulation of solid and liquid cultures of *M. tuberculosis* is a major challenge in the Caribbean. Because of this drug susceptibility testing information for proper management of patients infected with TB as well as identification of species is limited.

5. Conclusions

Despite the several constraints and limitations, this study demonstrated that the QFT-G test was more effective and a quicker turnaround time was achieved over the TST in detecting LTBI among several target groups in the population studied. However, because the QFT-G appears more costly as well as showing indeterminate and non reactive response for immuno-compromised subjects such as HIV positive patients, care must be taken when screening or making a diagnosis of LTBI based on QFT-G results in a poor resource and high HIV prevalence setting like Trinidad & Tobago or any other Caribbean country.

The turnaround time for results for line probe assays is also a major asset. Additionally, the identification of organisms and DST can be performed on contaminated as well as non-viable specimens. Finally, the cost of this assay makes it ideal for use as it is less than 2 times that of traditional culture methods.

Although the Quantiferon Gold TB test results were comparable in many aspects with other published international studies the use of this test for the Caribbean may still be limited due to the cost involved when compared to the Tuberculin Skin Test. This is so because of the cost of the kit, transportation issues and the laboratory component of the test.

6. Recommendations

The authors therefore support the recommendation that Quantiferon Gold TB test be used in conjunction with the well established TST for the screening of patients suspected of infection. Confirmation of positive TST can then be performed using the QFT-G test if warranted. In cases where the patient is co-infected with HIV, the interpretation of the test should be made in collaboration with the CD4+ count of the patient as this test is dependent on the reaction of T-cells and if the CD4 count is low then the result can be falsely negative.

7. Acknowledgement

The authors would like to express their gratitude to all the subjects who volunteered for this study, the staff at Caura Chest hospital, Eric Williams Medical Sciences, Complex, CAREC, Trinidad & Tobago Public health laboratory for all their technical assistance and support in several ways. Fund for the study was partly provided by the University of the West Indies, St. Augustine.

8. References

[1] New Jersey Medical School (NJMS), National Tuberculosis Centre [Online]. Brief History of Tuberculosis, July 23, 1996 [*Assessed online March 27, 2009* from: http://www.umdnj.edu-ntbcweb/history.html].

[2] World Health Organization. TB/HIV Research priorities in resource-limited setting: Report of an expert consultation, 2005. WHO/HTM/TB/2005.355.

[3] Health Agenda for the Americas 2008-2017. Text document distributed at the launching ceremony in Panama City, 3 June, 2007.

[4] Getahun, H., Harrington, M., O'Brien, R., Nunn, P. (2007). Diagnosis of smear-negative pulmonary tuberculosis in people with HIV infection or AIDS in resource-constrained settings: informing urgent policy changes. Available at www.thelancet.com. Published online on February 28, 2007. DOI:10.1016/S0140-6736(07)60284-0.

[5] Hale YM, Pfyffer GE and Salfinger M, 2001. Laboratory diagnosis of mycobacterial infections: new tools and lessons learned. Clin. Infect. Dis. 33:834-846.

[6] Akpaka PE; Baboolal S, Clarke D, Francis L, Rastogi N. (2008) Evaluation of methods for rapid detection of resistance to isoniazid and rifampicin in Mycobacterium tuberculosis isolates collected in the Caribbean. *Journal of Clinical Microbiology; 46 (10):3426-3428*

[7] Baboolal S, Ramoutar D, Akpaka PE. (2010). Comparison of QuantiFERON®-TB Gold assay and Tuberculin skin test to detect latent tuberculosis infection among among target groups in Trinidad & Tobago. *Pan American Journal of Public Health/ Rev Panam Salud Publica; 28(1):36-42*

[8] Mathew, P., Kuo, Y.H., Vazirani, B., Eng, R.H.K and Weinstein, M.P. (2000). Are Three Sputum Acid Fast Bacillus Smears Necessary for Discontinuing Tuberculosis Isolation? J Clin Microbiol 40(9) 3482-3484.

[9] Herman, P., Fauville-Dufaux, M., Breyer, D., van Vaerebergh, B., Pauwels, K., Dai Do Thi, Chuong., Sneyers, M., Wanlin, M., Snacken, R and Moens, W. (2006). Biosafety recommendations for the contained use of *Mycobacterium tuberculosis* complex isolates in industrialized countries. Royal Library of Belgium Deposit Number: D/2006/2505/22.175. Supply, P., Lesjean, S., Savine, E., Kremer, K., van Soolingen, D., Locht, C. (2001). Automated high-throughput genotyping genotyping for study of global epidemiology of *Mycobacterium tuberculosis* based on mycobacterial interspersed repetitive units. J. Clin. Microbiol. 39. 3563-3571.

[10] Centers for Diseases Control and Prevention. Epi Info 3.5.1 version software. Atlanta Georgia, USA

[11] Dean, A.G., Sullivan, K.M., Soe, M.M. OpenEpi. Open Source Epidemiologic Statistics for Public Health version 2.3. www.OpenEpi.com. Updated 2009/20/05

[12] Lee, J. Y., Choi, H. J., Park, I-N., Hong, S-B., Oh, Y-M., Lim, C-M., Lee, S. D., Koh, Y., Kim, W. S., Kim, D. S., Kim, W. D., Shim, T. S. (2006). Comparison of two commercial interferon-γ assays for diagnosing *Mycobacterium tuberculosis* infection. Eur Respir J; 28:24-30.

[13] Kobashi, Y., Mouri, K., Obase, Y., Fukuda, M., Miyashita, N., Oka, M. (2007). Clinical evaluation of QuantiFERON TB-2G test for immunocompromised patients. Eur Respir J; 30:945-950.

[14] Dewan, P. K., Grinsdale, J., Kawamura, L. M. (2007). Low Sensitivity of a Whole-Blood Interferon-γ Release Assay for Detection of Active Tuberculosis. Clin Infect Dis; 44:69-73.

[15] Kang, Y. A., Lee., H. W., Yoon, H. I., Cho, B. L., Han, S. K., Shim, Y-S., Yim, J-J. (2005). Discrepancy Between the Tuberculin Skin Test and the Whole Blood Interferon γ Assay for the Diagnosis of Latent Tuberculosis Infection in an Intermediate Tuberculosis-Burden Country. JAMA; 293:2756-2760.

[16] Mori, T., Sakatani, M., Yamagishi, F. et al. (2004). Specific detection of tuberculosis infection: an interferon-gamma-based assay using new antigens. Am J Resp Crit Care Med; 170:59-64.

[17] Ferrara, G., Losi, M., Meacci, M., Meccugni, B., Piro, R., Roversi, P., Bergamini, B. M., D'Amico, R., Marchegiano, P., Rumpianesi, F., Fabbri, L. M., Richeldi, L. (2005). Routine Hospital Use of a New Commercial Whole Blood Interferon-γ Assay for the Diagnosis of Tuberculosis Infection. Am J Respir Crit Care Med. 172:631-635.

[18] Stuck, A. E., Minder, C. E., Frey, F. J. (1989). Risk of infection complication in patients taking glucocorticosteroids. Rev Infect Dis; 11: 954–963.

[19] Andersen, P., Munk, M. E., Pollock, J. M., Doherty, T. M. (2000). Specific immune based diagnosis of tuberculosis. Lancet; 256:1099–1104.

[20] Porsa, E., Cheng, L., Seale, M. M., Delclos, G. L,. Ma, X., Reich, R., Musser, J. M., Graviss, E. A. (2006). Comparison of a New ESAT-6/CFP-10 Peptide-Based Gamma Interferon Assay and a Tuberculin Skin Test for Tuberculosis Screening in a Moderate-Risk Population. Clin Vaccine Immunol; 13:53-58.

[21] Francis, M. and Rattan, A. (2006). Tuberculosis in CAREC Member Countries. CAREC Surveillance Report, Vol 26; No. 3

[22] Torres Costa J, Sá R, Cardoso MJ, Silva R, Ferreira J, Ribeiro C, et al. Tuberculosis screening in Portuguese healthcare workers using the tuberculin skin test and the interferon-gamma release assay. Eur Respir J. 2009;34(6):1423–8.

[23] Schablon A, Harling M, Diel R, Nienhaus A. Risk of latent TB infection in individuals employed in the healthcare sector in Germany: a multicentre prevalence study. BMC Infect Dis. 2010;10(1):107.

[24] Pai, M., Kaustubh, G., Joshi, R., Dogra, S., Kalantri, S., Mendiratta, D.K., Narang, P., Daley, C.L., Granich, R.M., Mazurek, G.H., Reingold, A.L., Colford, J.M. (2005). *Mycobacterium tuberculosis* Infection in Health Care Workers in Rural India. Comparison of a Whole-Blood Interferon γ Assay with Tuberculin Skin Testing. JAMA; 293 (22):2746-2754.

[25] Pooran A, Booth H, Miller RF, Scott G, Badri M, Huggett JF, et al. Different screening strategies (single or dual) for the diagnosis of suspected latent tuberculosis: a cost effectiveness analysis. BMC Pulmo Med. 2010;10(1):7.

[26] Mathema, B., Kurepina, N.E., Bifani, J. and Kreiswirth, B.N. (2006). Molecular Epidemiology of Tuberculosis: Current Insights. Clin Microbiol Rev; 19(4):658-685.

[27] Diel, R., Wrighton-Smith, P. and Zellweger, J-P. (2007). Cost-effectiveness of interferon-c release assay testing for the treatment of latent tuberculosis. Eur Respir J; 30: 321-332.

[28] Marra F, Marra CA, Sadatsafavi M, Morán-Mendoza O, Cook V, Elwood RK, et al. Cost-effectiveness of a new interferon-based blood assay, QuantiFERON-TB Gold, in screening tuberculosis contacts. Int J Tuberc Lung Dis. 2008;12(12):1414–24.

[29] Pai, M., Riley, L.W., Colford, J.M. Jr. (2004). Interferon-gamma assays in the immune diagnosis of tuberculosis: a systematic review. Lancet Infect Dis; 4: 761–776.

[30] Hilleman, D., Rush-Gerdes, S., Richter, E. (2007). Evaluation of the GenoType MTBDRplus Assay for Rifampin and Isoniazid Susceptibility Testing for *Mycobacterium tuberculosis* strains and Clinical Specimens. J Clin Microbiol 45(8): 2635-2640.

[31] Somoskovi, A., Dormandy, J., Mitsani, D., Rivenburg, J., Salfinger, M. (2006). Use of smear-positive samples to assess the PCR-based Genotype MTBDR assay for rapid, direct detection of the *Mycobacterium tuberculosis* Complex as well as its resistance to Isoniazid and Rifampicin. J Clin Microbiol 44(12):4459-4463.

[32] Bang, D., Anderson, A.B., Thomsen, V.Q. (2006). Rapid Genotypic detection of Rifampin- and Isoniazid- resistant Mycobacterium tuberculosis directly in clinical specimens. J Clin Microbiol 44(7):2605-2608.

[33] Wade., M.M., Zhang, Y., (2004). Mechanisms of drug resistance in Mycobacterium tuberculosis. Front Biosci 9975-994.

[34] Cavusoglu, C., Turhan, K., Akinci, P., Soyler, I. (2007). Evaluation of the Genotype MTBDR assay for rapid detection of rifampin and isoniazid resistance in Mycobacterium tuberculosis isolates. J Clin Microbiol 44; 2338-2342.

[35] Barnard, M., Albert, H., Coetzee, G., O Brien, R., Bosman, M.E. (2008). Rapid Molecular screening for multidrug-resistant tuberculosis in a high-volume health laboratory in South Africa. Am J Respir Crit Care Med 177:787-792.

[36] Johnson, R., Jordaan, A.M., Warren, R., Bosman, M., Young, D., Nagy, J.N., Wain, J.R., van Helden, P.D., Victor, T.C. (2008). Drug susceptibility testing using molecular techniques can enhance tuberculosis diagnosis. J Inf dev Countries 240-45.

[37] Parsons, L.M., Salfinger, M., Clobridge, A., Dormandy, J., Mirabello, L., Polletta, V.L., Sanic, A., Sinyavskiy, O., Larsen, S.C., Driscole, J., Zickas, G., Taber, H.W. (2005). Phenotypic and molecular characterization of Mycobacterium tuberculosis isolates resistant to both Isoniazid and Ethambutol. JCM 49(6) 2218-2225.

[38] Zignol, M., Hosseini, M.S., Wright, A., Weezenbeek, C.L., Nunn, P., Watt, C.J., Williams, B.G. and Dye, C. (2006). Global Incidence of Multidrug-resistant tuberculosis. J. Infect Dis. 194:479-85.

[39] World Health Organization. Global Tuberculosis Control, Surveillance, Planning and Financing. WHO Report, 2008. WHO/HTM/TB/2008.393

[40] Menner, N., Gunther, I., Orawa, H., Roth, A., Rambajan, I., Wagner, J., Hahn, H., Persaud, S., Ignatius, R. (2005). High frequency of multidrug-resistance Mycobactium tuberculosis isolates in Georgetown, Guyana. Tropical Medicine and International Health 10 (12) 1215-1218.

[41] Diguimbaye, C., Hilty, M., Ngandolo, R., Mahamat, H.H., Pfyffer, G.E., Baggi, F., Tanner, m., Schelling, E, Zinsstag. J. (2006). Molecular characterization and drug resistance testing of *Mycobacterium tuberculosis* isolates from Chad. J Clin Microbiol 44:1575-1577.186. Ferdinand, S., Sola, C., Verdol, B., Legrand, E.Goh, K.S., Berchel, M., Aubery, A., Timothee, M., Joseph, P., Pape, J.W., Rastogi, N. (2003). Molecular characterization and drug resistance patterns of strains of *Mycobacterium tuberculosis* isolated from patients in an AIDS counselling center in Port-au-Prince, Haiti: a 1-year study. J Clin Microbiol 41(2):694-702.

[42] UNAIDS/WHO/ AIDS Epidemic Update (2009). www.unaids.org/en/knowledgeCentre/HIVData/EpiUpdate/EpiUpdArchive/2009. [downloaded 18/02/11]

[43] Pratt, R., Robinson, V., Navin, T. (2009). Trends in Tuberculosis - United States, 2008. JAMA 301 (18): 1869-1871.

[44] Streicher, E.M., Warren, R.M., Kewlwy, C., Simpson, J., Rastogi, N., Sola, C., van der Spuy, G.D., van Helden, P.D., Victor, T.C., 2004. Genotypic and phenotypic characterization of drug resistant *Mycobacterium tuberculosis* isolates from rural districts of Western Cape Province of South Africa. J Clin Microbiol. 42, 891-894.

[45] Zagar, E. M., Mc Nerney, R., 2008. Multidrug-resistant tuberculosis. BMC Infectious Diseases 8:10 doi:10.1186/47 1-2334-8-10.

[46] Khue, P.M., Phue, T.Q., Hung, N.V., Jarlier, V., Robert, J. (2008). Drug resistance and HIV co-infection among pulmonary tuberculosis patients in Haiphong City, Vietnam. Int J Tuberc Lung Dis 12(7): 763-768.

[47] Brudey, K., Driscoll, J.R., Rigouts, L., Prodinger, W.M., Gori, A., Al-Hajoj, S.A., Allix, C., Aristimuno, L., Arora, J., Baumanis, V.,et al (2006). *Mycobacterium tuberculosis* complex genetic diversity: mining the fourth international spoligotyping database (SpolDB4) for classification, population genetics and epidemiology. BMC Microbiol. 6:6-23.

3

Tuberculosis is Still a Major Challenge in Africa

Simeon I.B. Cadmus[1], Osman El Tayeb[2] and Dick van Soolingen[3,4]
[1]*Department of Veterinary Public Health and Preventive Medicine, University of Ibadan, Ibadan,*
[2]*Damien Foundation,*
[3]*Departments of Pulmonary Diseases and Medical Microbiology, Radboud University of Nijmegen Medical Centre, Nijmegen*
[4]*National Tuberculosis Reference Laboratory, National Institute for Public Health and the Environment (RIVM), Bilthoven,*
[1]*Nigeria*
[2]*Belgium*
[3,4]*Netherlands*

1. Introduction

Africa is constituted of 53 independent countries (taking both South and North Sudan as one), has a one billion population and provides home to about 11% of the world's population. The human population in Africa was projected to grow at the rate of 2.6% from the 770 million people in 2005 to 2 billion in 2050 (Shapley, 2008). It currently carries a huge burden of tuberculosis (TB), estimated at 30% of the total global number of cases in 2009, coming second only after Asia (50%). In the same vein, in 2009, approximately 41% (9/22) of the highest burdened countries (HBCs) with TB worldwide were found in Africa (WHO, 2010a). Similarly, the World Health Organization (WHO) in 2007 estimated that the average incidence of TB in African countries more than doubled between 1995 and 2005 (WHO, 2007).

Generally, the burden of TB in Africa is driven by a generalized HIV epidemic; and the African region accounted for approximately 80% of the estimated 11–13% of the TB deaths which were HIV-positive in 2009 (WHO, 2010a). This problem is compounded by the general weak health care systems, inadequate laboratories, and conditions that promote transmission of infection, resulting in the emergence of drug-resistant *Mycobacterium tuberculosis* strains (Chaisson and Martinson, 2008). Other compounding factors, apart from HIV, that have resulted in the increasing trend of TB in Africa are poverty, which is closely related to malnutrition, crowded living conditions, lack of access to free or affordable health care services, and dependence on traditional healers that can facilitate the transmission of tuberculosis (Parson *et al.*, 2011). Occasional wars and civil disturbances worsen this situation and this is even complicated by droughts and regular natural disasters. Other self inflicted problems are poor government funding of health care services, occasioned by massive corruption and leading to diversion of meager local and foreign resources.

Despite these gloomy outlooks, some African countries have achieved commendable landmarks in reversing the frightening global trend of TB. For example, Kenya and the

United Republic of Tanzania were among the 13 countries listed from the HBCs that achieved treatment success rate target of 85% set by WHO for new sputum smear-positive cases of pulmonary TB (WHO, 2010a). Therefore, with concerted efforts and co-ordination within the African continent, greater achievements can be recorded to curtail the scourge of TB which has inflicted so much pain in Africans. Finally, intensified efforts to reduce deaths among HIV/+ TB co-infected cases are needed, especially in sub-Saharan Africa.

2. Surveillance system

The bane of TB diagnosis in Africa has been attributed to poorly coordinated national tuberculosis programs (NTPs), culminating in weak health systems. As a result of this, individuals co-infected with TB/HIV are made to steer through the complicated, harrowing and weak local health systems in order to get medical care. Many shuffle between health clinics for TB medications and district hospitals for antiretroviral drugs in a system where TB and HIV treatment and care are disjointed and therefore disintegrated. While services and drugs are generally free or highly subsidized, patients still complain about the cost of laboratory examinations, hospitalization, and transportation. This arises because patients still have to pay for several other services like X-ray and hospitalization which are really exorbitantly expensive and out of reach for some of the patients. Since most patients have to visit clinics far from their homes, the cost of transportation is often unbearable and the distress of travel further discourages them. Furthermore, TB control relies on passive case finding among individuals self-presenting to health care facilities, followed by either diagnosis based on clinical symptoms or laboratory diagnosis using insensitive sputum smear microscopy. Since repeated visits have to be made because presentations of serial sputum specimens are required (one taken on the spot and the second brought in the following morning), there are generally high default rates due to cost of visits and logistics. As a result of the bottlenecks encountered, patients are reluctant to visit these health facilities, therefore resulting in poor case finding and ability to achieve effective diagnosis and accurate treatment.

Health seeking behavior and non-adherence to therapy has been cited as a major barrier to the control of TB control globally (Gopi *et al.*, 2007). There are reports from Nigeria and other developing countries that delay in TB diagnosis and treatment initiation is common (Salami and Oluboyo, 2002; Gopi *et al.*, 2007; Odusanya and Babafemi, 2004), and this has been ascribed to negligence's from both the patients and doctors. Delay in diagnosis may aggravate the disease, augment the risk of death and enhance person to person transmission in the community (Odusanya and Babafemi, 2004). In Tanzania, 15% of patients were found to report to a health facility within 30 days of the onset of symptoms (Wandwalo and Morkve, 2000) while studies from Nigeria reported 81% (Enwuru et al., 2002) and 83% (Odusanya and Babafemi, 2004) patients delay for more than one month. Reasons for this are patients visiting local and poorly equipped private medical facilities, chemists, prayer houses and traditional healers; coupled with these, are poor knowledge and awareness about the disease among Africans in general (Odusanya and Babafemi, 2004; Enwuru *et al.*, 2007; Okeibunor *et al.*, 2007).

3. Infrastructural facilities and laboratory services

"Lack of new diagnostic tools and inadequate laboratory capacity hinders timely detection and management of drug resistance, with catastrophic consequences when dealing with lethal forms of TB", says Bert Voetberg, a lead health specialist in the World Bank's Africa region. In most African countries, smear microscopy laboratories consist of single rooms and are understaffed. In addition, they generally possess poorly maintained microscopes, and some of these laboratories lack consistent sources of electricity and clean water (Parsons *et al.*, 2011). Thus, the critical factor in TB control regarding early diagnosis and treatment that should limit the spread of the disease and reduce mortality is still an enormous problem in Africa. According to Chaisson and Martinson (2008), throughout Africa, the vast majority of the diagnosis of TB rests on the microscopic detection of acid-fast bacilli in sputum; an insensitive technique that is particularly ill suited for the detection of TB in HIV-infected patients, who have fewer bacilli in their sputum and more frequently suffer from extra-pulmonary TB than HIV negative patients. In patients with active pulmonary TB, only an estimated 45% of infections are detected by sputum microscopy when compared to culture (Dye *et al.*, 2005). This test, first developed in the 1880s and basically unchanged today, has the advantage of being simple, but has very low sensitivity (especially among HIV-coinfected patients). It is also very dependent on the skills of the technician, and a single technician can only process a relatively small number of slides per day (Perkins *et al.*, 2006). In addition, this method cannot differentiate between drug-sensitive and drug resistant TB, nontuberculous mycobacteria, and other Ziehl-Neelsen positive micro-organisms like Nocardia and Rhodocossus species. Due to these limitations, a staggering three million people who present annually with suspected TB may not be properly and timely diagnosed, because their infection (so-called smear-negative disease) cannot be detected by sputum microscopy (Onyebujoh *et al.*, 2006). Moreover, a significant over and misdiagnosis is expected because a part of the ZN positives do not represent tuberculosis. Therefore, the timely introduction of the use of light-emitting diode (LED) fluorescence microscopes (FM) will go a long way in improving the shortcomings of the conventional smear diagnosis of TB (Cuevas *et al.*, 2011; Hung *et al.*, 2007). "The fact that LED microscopes are more affordable than conventional fluorescent microscopes, and can be powered by battery in some cases, makes fluorescent microscopy potentially more widely available, and this should result in a better diagnostic for TB," said lead author Dr. Andrew Whitelaw from the University of Cape Town based on a study carried out in South Africa. It is also believed that other high HIV and TB burden countries in Africa would benefit a lot from the LED microscopy.

Again, laboratories with the capacity to provide culture and (molecular) drug sensitivity test (DST) services are essential for the diagnosis of drug-resistant TB; culture services are also important for diagnosis of smear negative TB, especially in African countries where the prevalence of HIV is high. However, capacity to perform culture and DST is seriously limited in African countries (WHO, 2009). Since the standard of care for TB diagnosis recommended by WHO (2010a) is (i) sputum smear microscopy for all cases and (ii) expansion of the use of culture to diagnose all bacteriologically-positive (not just smear-positive) cases towards the ultimate goal of using culture (or equivalents such as molecular tests) in the diagnosis of all cases, it becomes obvious that most countries in Africa will never achieve this goal because of the serious deficits in both human and infrastructural capacities. This is apparent especially when the demands for a biosafety level 3 facility for culture of *M. tuberculosis* (MTB) is introduced which is out of reach in almost all settings. Currently, very few countries in Africa can effectively carry out culture to confirm cases of TB. As a result of limitation in *Mycobacterium* culture capability, barely 5% countries in Africa can independently carry out drug susceptibility testing for infected TB patients (Table 1). Consequently, accurate diagnosis for effective treatment of TB patients is heavily compromised.

Countries	Population (Million)	Burden of TB incidence (no. of cases /100,000 individuals/ yr)	% of TB patients that are HIV positive (%)	Mortality due to TB/100,000 population	Smear microscopy laboratories per 100,000 population	Culture labs per 5 million population	Drug susceptibility test (DST) labs/ 10 million population	Second line DST Available	Local TB Funding	National Reference TB Laboratory
Algeria	35	59	NA	2.4	0.7	3.7	0.9	In country	Poor	Yes
Angola	18	298	15	30	0.8	0.3	0.5	No	Fair	Yes
Benin	9	93	16	17	0.6	0.6	0.6	In country	Poor	Yes
Botswana	2	694	66	57	2.3	2.6	5.1	Outside	Poor	Yes
Burkina Faso	16	215	20	55	0.7	0	0	Outside	Poor	Yes
Burundi	8	348	46	77	2.0	0.6	0	No	Poor	Yes
Cameroon	20	182	40	17	NA	NA	NA	In and outside	Poor	Yes
Cape Verde	<1	148	20	27	3.2	0	0	Outside	Poor	Yes
Central African Republic	4	327	33	44	1.6	1.1	2.3	No	Very poor	Yes
Chad	11	283	-	63	0.5	0	0	No	Very poor	Yes
Comoros	<1	39	-	7.8	NA	NA	NA	No	Very poor	Yes
Congo,* Democratic Republic (DRC)	66	372	20	76	2.2	<0.1	0.2	No	Poor	Yes
Congo, Republic	4	382	48	43	0.7	0	0	Outside	Very poor	Yes
Cote d'Ivoire	21	399	30	85	0.5	0.2	0.5	No	Poor	Yes
Djiboutu	<1	620	10	77	1.9	5.8	0	Outside	Very poor	Yes
Egypt	83	19	0	1.1	0.3	1.1	0.1	In country	Fair/ Good	Yes
Equitorial Guinea	<1	117	17	5	4.3	0	0	No	Very Good	No
Eritrea	5	99	-	14	1.5	1.0	2.0	Outside	Poor	Yes
Ethiopia*	83	359	20	64	1.4	0.1	0.2	Outside	Good	Yes
Gabon	1	501	59	62	0.9	3.4	6.8	Outside	Poor	No
Gambia, The	2	269	16	48	1.9	2.9	5.9	No	Poor	Yes
Ghana	24	201	22	46	1.0	0.6	0.8	No	Fair	Yes
Guinea	10	3	24	72	0.5	0.5	1.0	In country	Poor	Yes
Guinea-Bissau	2	229	-	30	3.3	NA	NA	No	Poor	Yes
Kenya*	40	305	44	15	3.0	0.8	1.0	Outside	Poor	Yes
Lesotho	2	634	77	14 (9.5)	0.9	2.4	4.8	Outside	NA	No
Liberia	4	28	1	59	3.7	0	0	In country	Poor	No
Libya	6	40	15	4.1	0.4	2.3	3.1	No	Poor	Yes
Madagascar	20	261	-	57	1.3	0.3	0.5	In country	Poor	Yes
Malawi	15	304	64	25	1.3	0.7	0.7	Outside	Poor	Yes
Mali	13	324	16	88	0.6	0.8	1.5	Outside	Poor	Yes
Mauritania	3	330	12	90	2.2	1.5	3.0	No	Poor	Yes
Mauritius	1	22	6	<1	NA	NA	NA	Outside	NA	Yes
Morocco	32	92	NA	5.8	0.5	2.2	0.6	Outside	Poor	Yes
Mozambique*	23	409	66	38	1.9	0.2	0.4	Outside	Poor	Yes
Namibia	2	727	58	31	1.4	2.3	4.6	Outside country	Good	Yes

Countries	Population (Million)	Burden of TB incidence (no. of cases /100,000 individuals/ yr)	% of TB patients that are HIV positive (%)	Mortality due to TB/100,000 population	Smear microscopy laboratories per 100,000 population	Culture labs per 5 million population	Drug susceptibility test (DST) labs/ 10 million population	Second line DST Available	Local TB Funding	National Reference TB Laboratory
Niger	15	181	12	41	0.3	0	0	Outside country	Very poor	No
Nigeria*	155	295	26	73	0.7	0.1	0.2	Outside country	Fair	Yes
Rwanda	10	376	34	76	1.9	0.5	1.0	No	Poor	Yes
Sao Tome & Principe	<1	98	13	19	1.2	0	0	No	Poor	Yes
Senegal	13	282	7	72	0.7	1.2	2.4	In country	Poor	Yes
Seychelles	<1	31	-	2.6	NA	NA	NA	In and outside	Poor	No
Sierra Leone	6	644	11	158	2.0	NA	NA	No	Very poor	Yes
Somalia	9	285	NA	58	0.6	0	0	Non	Very poor	No
South Africa*	50	971	58	45	0.5	1.6	3.2	In and outside country	Excellent	Yes
Sudan	42	119	4	24	0.9	0.1	0.2	Non	Poor	Yes
Swaziland	1	1257	13	64	NA	NA	NA	Outside country	Good	Yes
Tanzania*	44	183	37	9	1.6	0.1	0.2	Outside country	Poor	Yes
Togo	7	446	25	113	1.7	0.8	1.5	Non	Very poor	Yes
Tunisia	10	24	2	1.8	0.6	3.4	4.9	In country	Excellent	Yes
Uganda*	33	293	54	29	2.5	0.9	1.2	In country	Poor	Yes
Zambia	13	433	67	27	1.7	NA	2.3	Non	Poor	Yes
Zimbabwe*	13	742	78	82	1.0	0.4	0.8	Non	Poor	Yes

*African countries listed among the 22 high TB burdened nations in the world

Table 1. Showing the burden and challenges of TB in African countries

To respond to the urgent need for simple and rapid diagnostic tools at the point of treatment in HBCs, the Xpert MTB/RIF assay (GeneXpert, Cephied), a rapid molecular test for TB and rifampicin (RIF) resistance was recently developed. Though relatively new, this molecular assay has been described as one of the most promising in routine diagnosis in developing countries owing to its high sensitivity (98.2%), specificity (99.2%) and short turn-around time (2 hours) (Van Rie *et al.*, 2010). With regards to the detection of RIF resistance, the assay was reported to be highly sensitive (≥97.6%) and specific (≥98.1%), with performance characteristics which are superior to drug susceptibility testing by conventional culture-based assays and line probe assays (Boehme *et al.*, 2010). The rapid detection of MTB in sputum and RIF- resistance allows the physician to make critical patient management decisions regarding therapy during the same medical encounter. As conventional sputum smear microscopy has limited sensitivity and culture takes at least 4–6 weeks to produce result, the Xpert MTB/RIF assay seems a major improvement in African countries where proper facilities are scarce and rates of loss to follow-up are high. The additional advantage of the Xpert MTB/RIF assay is that when performed correctly, it is not associated with a measurable infection risk and results in a lower biohazard compared with conventional smear microscopy, making the assay suitable for point-of-care (POC) use in the typical African setting where bio-containment facilities are not readily available (Banada *et al.*, 2010).

4. Co-morbidities of TB and HIV/AIDS

Globally, an estimated 11-13% of the newly diagnosed TB patients are HIV positive and approximately 80% of these cases are in Africa (WHO, 2010a). The HIV infection is an established epidemiological factor causing additional challenges to the diagnosis of TB; hence, a major contributor to the increased incidence of TB across the world. Infection with HIV-1 increases the risk of reactivating latent TB infection by 80- to 100-fold, and HIV patients who acquire new TB infections also have higher rates of disease progression (Parson *et al.*, 2011). Tuberculosis can occur at all points in the immunosuppressive spectrum of HIV disease, with variable presentations, and, particularly in African countries, where TB is always a major indicator of HIV. Multiple studies have shown that fatality rates are higher for HIV-TB-co-infected patients who are on anti-TB treatment but not antiretroviral therapy (16 to 35%) than for treated TB patients who are HIV negative (4 to 9%) (Mukardi *et al.*, 2001). The study carried out by Ackah *et al*, (1995), in Abidjan, Co^te d'Ivoire, indicated that the highest death rates occurred in co-infected patients with the lowest CD4 cell counts. This is the same picture in most areas in Africa where HIV is prevalent. Unfortunately, despite the scale up of TB treatment in South Africa, the epidemic of HIV in that country has grievously compromised TB care and control. This scenario has manifested in increased incidence of multidrug resistance TB (MDR-TB) and extensively drug-resistant TB (XDR-TB). The sequel of all these compounding scenarios is a situation in which TB and HIV synergistically potentiates each other in the affected patients leading to difficulties in the accurate diagnosis of TB and eventually in increased rate of mortalities in the region.

Notwithstanding the huge funds expended to fight AIDS, TB and Malaria by the Global Fund and PEPFAR in Africa, the bulk of these funds have been spent on AIDS, therefore leaving a huge deficit in the area of TB. Consequently, most attention in the past was diverted at building both human and infrastructural capacities for AIDS prevention; while that for TB was scarcely given the needed support. This has led to limited diagnostic capacity for TB despite the prompt diagnosis of HIV in some cases; hence, leading to most patients dying of TB. Therefore, the parlance "living with HIV, dying of TB" has become a recurrent decimal in most African countries where TB and HIV are endemic (Parson *et al.*, 2011; Dorman and Chaisson, 2007; Gandhi *et al.*, 2006).

5. Newer diagnostics

In the face of various diagnostic challenges of TB due to compounding factors like poverty, HIV/AIDS and lately, the MDR-TB and XDR-TB infections in some African countries like South Africa, an urgent need has arisen for newer technologies to facilitate prompt diagnosis of TB. Clinical management of TB in African countries is hampered by the lack of rapid, simple and effective diagnostic tests. Correct diagnosis of TB is needed to improve treatment, reduce transmission, and control development of drug resistance.

6. Public-private collaborations

The internationally recommended DOTS strategy has been successfully implemented in the public sector by many National Tuberculosis Programs (NTPs), but in the private sector the quality of care is generally very poor (Uplekar and Rangan, 1993; Uplekar *et al.*, 1998). Since the situation of the NTPs in Africa is far from perfect, the problem has been further complicated by the poor operation of the DOTS program in the expanding private sector that is supposed to be a major TB care provider. Resulting from the weak link between the public and private practitioners in terms of complementary activities, funding and operational researches, several TB programs that are of immense benefits to the patients are denied. This is particularly worrisome in the area of TB diagnosis were limited facilities are available for patient care. Because of the very weak interactions, only few private practitioners in the urban settings provide quality diagnostic services that can support patient care. Moreover, only few of these private care givers are accessible to foreign agencies that can support in the scale up TB diagnosis. The resultant effect of this is a huge gap in TB diagnosis and therefore increased burden of the disease especially among rural dwellers that rely mostly on traditional healers who are not normally integrated into healthcare systems by government establishments. Obviously, these practitioners usually do not work according to the national guidelines for the treatment of TB.

Since traditional practices are common place in Africa and majority of Africans still live in rural settings with low literacy rate, many patients patronize local herbalists and quacks who pretend to be physicians and health givers. Traditionally, since herbal centers are not as expensive as most government health clinics, they are the first point of call for patients. Here, local herbs and other ritual concoctions are given, which in some cases worsen the patients health and this could be on for several weeks to years. Sadly, some of these patients die and some infect their relatives before recourse to government clinics/hospitals when complications would have set in. However, recent findings in the area of ethno-medicine have shown that some of the herbal medications have promising anti-tuberculosis activities. A lot therefore needs to be done by government and private research agencies to look into these assertions and see how traditional health care providers can be integrated into supporting TB care in rural settings in Africa.

Both formal and informal private practitioners comprise the health sector, working on voluntary basis or for profit. The number of professional societies, private hospitals, corporate health providers as well as community and traditional healing homes is fast growing. Therefore, mechanisms for collaboration between the public and private health sectors should be established. In order to promote compliance with treatment guidelines, private care providers should be involved in their development, or checks on the adherence to treatment and cure should be organized by the public sector. They should also be empowered to facilitate training within the sector. Improved program coverage, patient access to diagnostic and treatment services, increased case detection and treatment outcomes, and improved overall quality of care are some of the potential benefits of involving private health providers in delivery of services (Uplekar and Shepards, 1991; Pathania *et al.*, 1997). A model of successful public-private sector collaboration in TB control that is commendable in Africa is exemplified by the activities of the Damien Foundation, Belgium, a voluntary non-profit private TB support agency in Nigeria. This collaboration has over the years led to the achievement of about 85% TB active case finding and establishment of the first MDR-TB treatment Center in Nigeria. Though such other agencies abound in other African countries, however, more demonstrable milestones in terms of TB control coverage has to be set and seen to be achieved to justify the huge money said to be expended by these agencies in Africa.

7. Funding of TB control programs

With the gross domestic product (GDP) of the entire African continent valued at $2.2 million (World Bank, 2011) as against that of the US which is estimated at between $14.6-14.7 trillion (World Bank 2011; BEA, 2011), it is obvious that the continent will be unable to effectively finance and take care of its huge health burden. This is more obvious since the highest placed economy in Africa, Egypt is rated 25 globally with GDP of $467, 000 and the lowest country, Sao Tome and Principe rated 177 globally with GDP of $300. With the myriad of diseases, wars natural disasters and massive corruption in the continent, it will be difficult to fund TB care and especially the diagnostic component given the huge resources required both in human and infrastructural capacities. From the recently released WHO 2010 TB report, nearly all countries in the region relied on external funding and support for its DOTS program (WHO, 2010a). Consequently, TB program across the continent is poorly funded; with only about 5-15% barely in a situation to fund their program domestically (Table 1). Unfortunately, due to the recent global recession seriously having its unprecedented effects on the economy of western nations, the budgets of most donor agencies are grossly reduced, leaving great deficits and reduction in TB control support in Africa.

8. Political commitment

Most African countries are politically unstable and bereft of governments that can provide long term policies to sustain the health system. Given these political challenges, and problems of incessant wars, it is difficult to implement and sustain successful DOTS programs. Of particular reference is Somalia that has been deprived of stable government for almost two decades; therefore, it has no political commitment that will help facilitate any national TB control program. This is evident from the absence of a national TB reference laboratory and a non-existent platform (either local or foreign) to screen for drug resistant TB (WHO, 2010a). Unfortunately however, due to ignorance and lack of political will, some African countries fail to acknowledge the burden of MDR-TB despite the overwhelming evidence that points at this. Fortunately though, after so much foot dragging, some countries in Africa have finally set up mechanisms to carry out national MDR-TB surveys in collaboration with Global fund, Center for Disease Control (CDC) and WHO. One of such countries is Nigeria, and preliminary findings from the survey conducted indicate a high rate of MDR-TB (unpublished personal communication).

In other African countries with apparently stable governments, they are faced with self made problems like corruption, civil unrest that discourage full implementation of the TB control programs. Of particular importance again is the epidemic of HIV/AIDS which has incapacitated Africa, and leaving most governments with no option than to tackle the greater evil and leaving others like TB and Malaria for later days.

Despite the challenges African governments are responsible for; it is most unfortunate that most have only paid lips service to tackling the problem of TB. Sadly enough, they are only gored on by the carrot and stick approaches of the western nations and agencies before they made the little commitment seen so far. It is obvious that a larger role of the African Union (AU) is needed to tackle the challenges of TB. In this direction, there is a need for an AU Blue Print on the policy, mechanism, funding and achievable milestones within a practicable timeframe to reduce the burden of TB comparable to rates seen in Europe and other areas of the world with low burden of the disease.

9. Operational research

The fact that new technologies regarding TB diagnosis and control have been successful in western nations and regions of the world, does not necessarily translate to its success in Africa. In theory, biosafety level 3 laboratories are needed to conduct culture of MTB, however, so far such highly expensive and technically demanding facilities are very scarce in Africa. But also the recently developed molecular techniques that in principle do not need such expensive facilities are not as simple to implement in Africa as some assume. For example, despite the promise of the Xpert MTB/RIF assay in clinical trials, evidence has shown that knowledge to support the broader dissemination and implementation of those interventions (e.g., cost and financing of the intervention, provider training, availability of resources, monitoring the quality of intervention delivery) has limited the successful implementation of such innovations. Our previous experience has shown that substantial barriers have existed to limit prior attempts at implementing new technologies, such as the microscopic observation drug susceptibility assay (MODS) and the nitrate reductase assay (NRA). Accordingly, none of these techniques have been successfully integrated into the diagnostic algorithm for TB in Africa. Since no empirically-supported models exist to guide the dissemination and implementation of some of these technologies, sound operational feasibility projects are required before they are integrated into TB programs in Africa. Failure to carry out these assessments in the past, have lead to serious dire consequences in TB diagnosis despite huge resources that has been expended.

In order to make adequate use of promising pilot research findings, especially translational researches are required in African countries before new techniques are rolled out on a large scale. Of great importance here are translational researches bothering on the use of stool for prompt diagnosis of pediatric TB (Cadmus *et al.*, 2009), adaptation of the front loading smear microscopy (Ramsay et al., 2009), and the use of light emitting diode (LED) microscopes (Cuevas *et al.*, 2011) to mention a few. These translational researches are urgently needed giving the advantages they may offer in combating TB in the continent.

10. Role of international agencies

International agencies have played leading roles in the prevention and control of TB in most African countries in the past 50 years. Therefore, most diagnostic improvements experienced in Africa are driven by foreign donors and expertise. For example, the United States Government through its President's Emergency Plan for AIDS Relief (PEPFAR) spent about $307 million in 15 African countries between 2005 and 2008 for TB/HIV co-infected persons covering 367,000 patients (TTGHC, USA, 2009). Principally, the cost covered among other things routine TB screening in HIV infected people and improving laboratory surveillance systems in order to detect outbreaks of MDR- and XDR-TB. However, judging from the enormity of the burden of TB in the continent, it is obvious that the funds from the US and agencies from other western nations are not sufficient; hence, more needs to be done. This is particularly important in the areas of massive laboratory scale up and quality personnel that will operate the various laboratories since all these are grossly inadequate.

Currently, in Nigeria with the support of the PEPFAR program sponsored by the US government, the University of Maryland, through its Institute of Human Virology (IHV), center in Nigeria is supporting the Nigerian TB program in setting up a TB training school with a biosafety level 3 facility in northern Nigeria. The center has the capacity to carry out

LED fluorescence microscopy, culture and molecular techniques like the Hain assays as well as ancillary HIV diagnostic tests. Though similar sophisticated facilities abound in other African countries like Gambia, Mali, South Africa and Tanzania, they remain highly inadequate. Unfortunately, some of these facilities are merely for research and information gathering, rather than large scale use for TB control in such countries. However, since each program is handled by specific interest, there is limited coverage and sometimes no coordination even at the national level.

In other to facilitate effective TB care in African countries, there is a need for coalition of foreign donors to achieve optimal TB control platform for diagnosis and treatment. A step towards this direction is the formation of "The Tuberculosis Coalition for Technical Assistance (TBCTA). The coalition is guiding TB CARE I which is a USAID five year cooperative agreement (2010-2015) that has been awarded to TBCTA with KNCV Tuberculosis Foundation of the Netherlands as the lead partner. TBCTA is a unique coalition of the major international organizations in TB control. The coalition includes American Thoracic Society (ATS), FHI 360, International Union Against Tuberculosis and Lung Disease (The Union), Japan Anti-Tuberculosis Association (JATA), KNCV Tuberculosis Foundation, Management Sciences for Health (MSH), World Health Organization (WHO). The aim of TB CARE is to contribute to reaching the following specific USAID goals in the TB CARE countries (some African countries inclusive) with significant investment. It aims at (1) Sustaining or exceeding 84% case detection rate and 87% treatment success rate; (2). Treat successfully 2. 55 million new sputum-positive TB cases; (3). Diagnose and treat 57,200 new cases of multi-drug resistant (MDR) TB. Finally, TB CARE focuses on five priority areas that are needed for TB control in Africa namely: increasing political commitment for DOTS; strengthening and expanding DOTS Programs; increasing public and private sector partnerships; strengthening TB and HIV/AIDS collaboration; improving human and institutional capacity. With this anticipated initiative getting fully implemented in Africa, it is envisaged, that there will be a major turn-around in TB care through accurate diagnosis and treatment of patients.

11. Recommendations

To optimize TB control in the African continent, major changes are needed. The local political engagement needs to be enforced, not only to regulate the delicate relationship between the weak public Health care system and the expanding private sector, but also to stimulate international involvement in addressing the challenges faced. If more funding would be available, the implementation of new approaches in the diagnosis and treatment of TB should be considered a scientific discipline in itself; with serious considerations given to the integration of new methods and technologies before they are rolled out in Africa.

12. References

Ackah AN, Digbeu H, Daillo K, Greenberg AE, Coulibaly D, Coulibaly IM, Vetter KM, de Cock KM (1995). Response to treatment, mortality, and CD4 lymphocyte counts in HIV-infected persons with tuberculosis in Abidjan, Coˆte d'Ivoire. Lancet 345:607–610.

Banada PP, Sivasubramani SK, Blakemore R, Boehme C, Perkins MD, Fennelly K, Alland D. (2010). Containment of bioaerosol infection risk by the Xpert MTB/RIF assay and its applicability to point-of-care settings. Journal of Clinical Microbiology, 48: 3551-3557.

Boehme CC, Nabeta P, Hillermen D, Nicol MP, Shenai S, Krapp F, Allen J, Tahirli R, Blakemore R, Rustomjee R, Milovic A, Jones M, O'Brien SM, Persing DH, Ruesch-Gerdes S, Gotuzzo E, Rodrigues C, Alland D, Perkins MD (2010). Rapid Molecular Detection of Tuberculosis and Rifampin Resistance. New England Journal of Medicine 363;11: 1005-1015.

Bureau of Economic Analysis, US. Department of Commerce (2010). Gross Domestic Product Fourth Quarter and Annual 2010 (Advance Estimate) (Accessed August, 6 2011 http://www.bea.gov/newsreleases/national/gdp/2011/pdf/gdp4q10_adv.pdf

Cadmus SIB, Jenkins AO, Godfroid J, Osinusi K, Adewole IF, Murphy RL, Taiwo BO (2009). *Mycobacterium tuberculosis* and *Mycobacterium africanum* in Stools from Children in an Immunization Clinic in Ibadan, Nigeria. International Journal of Infectious Disease 13: 740-744.

Chaisson RE, Martinson NA (2008). Tuberculosis in Africa – Combating an HIV-Driven Crisis: New England Journal of Medicine 358;11: 1089-1092.

Cuevas LE, Al-Sonboli N, Lawson L, Yassin MA, Arbide I, Al-Aghbarim N, Sherchand JB, Al-Absi A, Emenyonu EN, Merid Y, Okobi MI, Onuoha JO, Aschalew M, Aseffa A, Harper G, Cuevas RMA, Theobald SJ, Nathanson C-M, Joly J, Faragher B, Squire SB, Ramsay A (2011). LED Fluorescence Microscopy for the Diagnosis of Pulmonary Tuberculosis: A Multi-Country Cross-Sectional Evaluation. PLoS Med 8(7): e1001057. doi:10.1371/journal.pmed.1001057

Dye C, Watt CJ, Bleed DM, Hosseini SM, Raviglione MC (2005). Evolution of tuberculosis control and prospects for reducing tuberculosis incidence, prevalence, and deaths globally. JAMA 2005; 293: 2767-2775.

Enwuru, CA., Idigbe, EO., Ezeobi, NV, Otegbeye, AF (2002). Care seeking behavioural patterns, awarness and diagnostic process in patients with smear- and culture-positive pulmonary tuberculosis in Lagos, Nigeria. Transactions of the Royal Society of Tropical Medicine and Hygiene 96, 614-616.

Gandhi NR, Moll A, Sturm AW, Pawinski R, Gavender T, Lalloo U, Zeller K, Andrews J, Friedland G (2006). Extensively drug-resistant tuberculosis as a cause of death in patients co-infected with tuberculosis and HIV in a rural area of South Africa. Lancet 368:1575–1580.

Gopi PG, Vasantha M, Muniyandi M, Chandrasekaran V, Balasubramanian R, Narayanan PR (2007). Risk factors for non-adherence to directly observed treatment (DOT) in a rural tuberculosis unti, Sounth India. Indian Journal of Tuberculosis 54:66-70.

Hung NV, Sy DN, Anthony RM, Cobelens FG, van Soolingen D (2007). Flourescence microscopy for tuberculosis diagnosis. Lancet Infectious Disease 7; 4: 238-239.

Mukadi YD, Maher D, Harries A (2001). Tuberculosis case fatality rates in high HIV prevalence populations in sub-Saharan Africa. AIDS 15:143–152.

Odusanya OO, Babafemi JO (2004). Patterns of delays amongst pulmonary tuberculosis patients in Lagos Nigeria. BMC Public Health 2(18): http://www.biomedcentral.com/1471-2458/4/18.

Okeibunor JC, Onyneho NG, Chukwu JN, Post E (2007). Where do tuberculosis patients go for treatment before reporting to DOTS clinics in southern Nigeria? Tanzania Health Research Bulletin 9;2: 94-101.

Onyebujoh P, Rodriguez W, Mwaba P (2006). Priorities in tuberculosis research. Lancet 367: 940-942.

Parsons LM, A´kos SA, Gutierrez C, Lee E, Paramasivan CN, Abimiku A, Spector S, Roscigno, G, Nkengasong, J (2011). Laboratory Diagnosis of Tuberculosis in Resource-Poor Countries: Challenges and Opportunities. Clinical Microbiology Reviews, 24: 314–350.

Pathania V, Almeida J, Kochi A (1997). TB patients and for profit health care providers in India.WHO/TB/97.223. 1997. Geneva.

Perkins MD, Roscigno G, Zumla A (2006). Progress towards improved tuberculosis diagnostics for developing countries. Lancet 367: 942-943.

Ramsay A, Yassin MA, Cambanis A, Hirao S, Almotawa A, Gammo M, Lovett Lawson L, Arbide I, Al-Aghbari N, Al-Sonboli N, Sherchand JB, Gauchan P, Cuevas LE (2009) Front-Loading SputumMicroscopy Services: An Opportunity to Optimise Smear-Based Case Detection of Tuberculosis in High Prevalence Countries. Tropical Medicine 2009. doi:10.1155/2009/398767.

Salami AK, Oluboyo PO (2002). Hospital prevalence of pulmonary tuberculosis and co-infection with human immunodeficiency virus in Ilorin; a review of nine years (1991-1999). West Afr J Med 21:24-7.

Shapley D (2008). Africa's population "emergency" Study: continent continuing population boom ((Accessed August 14, 2011 http://thedailygreen.com/environmental-news/latest/a).

Testimony on Tuberculosis before the Subcommittee on Africa and Global Health, Committee on Foreign Affairs, House of Representatives (2009) (Accessed August 1, 2011 http://2006-2009. pepfar.gov/press/101387.htm).

Uplekar M, Juvekar S, Morankar S, Rangan S, Nunn P (1998). Tuberculosis patients and practitioners in private clinics in India. International Journal of Tuberculosis and Lung Disease 2:324–9.

Uplekar MW, Rangan S (1993). Private doctors and tuberculosis control in India. Tuberculosis Lung and Disease. 1993; 74:332–7. doi: 10.1016/0962-8479(93)90108-A.

Uplekar MW, Shepard DS (1991). Treatment of tuberculosis by private general practitioners in India. Tubercle 1991; 72: 695-702.

Van Rie, A., Page-Shipp, L., Scott, L., Sanne, I. and Stevens, W (2010) Xpert® MTB/RIF for point-of care diagnosis of TB in high-HIV burden, resource-limited countries: hype or hope? Expert Review of Molecular Diagnostics 10, 937–946.

Wandwalo ER, Morkve O: Delay in tuberculosis case finding and treatment in Mwanza, Tanzania. International Journal of Tuberculosis and Lung Disease 2000, 4:133-8.

WHO, 2010a. Global tuberculosis control: WHO report 2010.

WHO 2010b. Stop TB Partnership and World Health Organization. Global Plan to Stop TB 2011-2015. WHO, Geneva: 2010

WHO report 2007: global tuberculosis control: surveillance, planning, finances Geneva: World Health Organization, 2007. (WHO/HTM/TB/2007.376.).

WHO. Global tuberculosis control: epidemiology, strategy, financing: WHO report 2009. (Accessed May, 13 2010, at http://www.who.int/tb/publications/global_report/2009/en/index.html

World Bank 2010. World Bank PPP GDP 2009 (Accessed August, 6 2011, at http://siteresources.worldbank.org/DATASTATISTICS/Resources/GDP_PPP.pdf).

4

Tuberculosis in Saudi Arabia

Sahal Al-Hajoj
Biological and Medical Research Department
King Faisal Specialist Hospital and Research Centre
Kingdom of Saudi Arabia

1. Introduction

1.1 Demography of Saudi Arabia

Saudi Arabia is the third-largest country in the Middle East by land area, constituting the bulk of the Arabian Peninsula, and the third-largest Arab country. It is bordered by Jordan and Iraq to the north and northeast, Kuwait, Qatar and the United Arab Emirates to the east, Oman in the southeast, and Yemen in the south. It is also connected to Bahrain by the King Fahad Causeway. The Persian Gulf lies to the northeast and the Red Sea to its west. The size of Saudi Arabia is approximately 2,149,690 square kilometers (830,000 sq mi). The total population is 27,136,977 as of the April 2010 census (18,707,576 Saudi nationals and 8,429,401 non-nationals). Until the 1960s, most of the population was nomadic or semi nomadic; due to rapid economic and urban growth, more than 95% of the population is now settled. Some cities and oases have densities of more than 1,000 people per square kilometer (2,600/mile^2). Saudi Arabia's population is characterized by rapid growth and a large cohort of youth.

2. National Tuberculosis Program (NTP) and Directly Observed Therapy (D.O.T.S)

In 1992, the Ministry of Health established a National Tuberculosis Control Committee to implement a control program throughout Saudi Arabia, and in 1999 the committee decided to implement D.O.T.S. The NTP in Saudi Arabia constitutes a manual, recording and reporting system, training, laboratory and X-ray services. Treatment services, drug and equipment supply is funded by the Ministry of Health. In Saudi Arabia there are several institutions providing healthcare for patients with tuberculosis; National Guard hospitals, Military hospitals, Security Forces hospitals and Ministry of Health hospitals. Patients attending private hospitals suspected of having TB are referred to government hospitals. There is no central system of record keeping, such that a patient currently receiving treatment at one institution may present to another with tuberculosis and be recorded as a new case (Al-Hajoj and Alrabiah). All institutions should report to the Ministry of Health, the body responsible for collecting data on Tuberculosis, but we believe that this is not being adhered to (Al-Hajoj and Alrabiah). Saudi Arabia's D.O.T.S success rate is comparatively well below international levels (Al-Hajoj and Alrabiah).

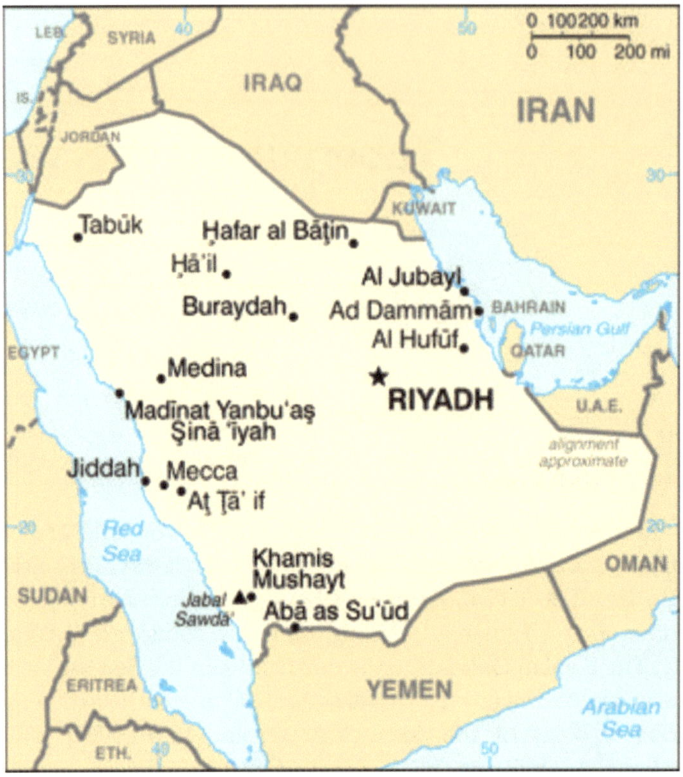

Fig. 1. Map of Saudi Arabia showing the total area, major cities and the borders with other countries.

3. Epidemiology of Tuberculosis world wide

According to a recent report by the World Health Organization (W.H.O); the estimated figure for the global burden of TB in 2009 reached 9.4 million cases and the total deaths hit 1.3 million among HIV-negative people and 0.38 million deaths among HIV-positive people. The report shows that most of the cases were in the South-East Asia, African and Western Pacific regions (35%, 30% and 20%, respectively).

4. Epidemiology of TB in Saudi Arabia

Tuberculosis in Saudi Arabia is still not fully controlled despite the huge efforts exerted by the government, represented by the Ministry of Health. According to the National TB Programs to eradicate the disease, TB continues to cause problems even with the implementation of D.O.T.S. It was anticipated that this program would bring the disease under control, but unfortunately the success has been limited (Al-Hajjaj 2000).

The first nationwide community-based survey of the epidemiology of tuberculosis was conducted by Al-Kassimi et al in 1990. In this study 7,721 subjects were screened in the 5 provinces. Prevalence of positive Mantoux test in non BCG vaccinated subjects and prevalence of bacillary cases on sputum culture were investigated. The authors found that the prevalence of positive Mantoux reaction in children aged 5-14 years was 6% +/- 1.8; higher in urban areas (10%), and lower in rural areas (2%). Yet there were higher prevalence of Mantoux reaction in the urban communities in the Western province (20% +/- 8.7 urban; 1% +/- 1.9 rural). Therefore the authors concluded that Saudi Arabia is among the middle prevalence countries (al-Kassimi, Abdullah et al.). The skin test conversion rate in unvaccinated Saudi Arabian children is about 0.5% per year, lower than in sub-Saharan countries (2%) but higher than in Europe (estimated at 0.1%) (el-Kassimi, Abdullah et al.). Another epidemiological study of tuberculosis infection was carried out between January 1987 and February 1990. In this study a proportional to population size sampling method was used for the whole country. A total of 1,933 subjects were screened and a pre-designed questionnaire was used to collect details of BCG scar, age, sex, residence area, nationality, education, occupation, and a tuberculosis test was done. A number of statistically significant association was found between positive tuberculin test (> 10mm) and age ($p < 0.0001$), sex ($p = 0.018$), nationality ($p = 0.009$), residence area ($p = 0.05$) and occupation ($p = 0.0003$) (Bener and Abdullah). In addition. The W.H.O 2007 estimation of the incidence of TB new cases was 46/100 000 population/year, the incidence of new smear positive cases was 21/100 000 population/year and the estimated prevalence of all forms of TB cases was 65/100 000 population/year. (WHO) report http://www.who.int/tb/country/data/download/en/index1.html. Contrary to W. H. O. report recent data showed that the total cases for the year 2008 was 3,918 in a population of approximately 27,136,977. Therefore according to this report, the incidence of all cases was estimated at 15.8/100 000 and the incidence of smear-positive tuberculosis was 8.2/100 000. However it is believed that the incident rate of TB varies from one region to another and between citizens and expatriates. For instance in Jeddah province (Western Province) Zaman et al studied epidemiology and incidence of Mycobacterium tuberculosis and other mycobacterial species infections in a wide cross-section of population over two (2) years (1987–1989). The study showed that incidence was highest among young adults and varied between Saudi and non-Saudi patients (Zaman). Anther study showed that in Jeddah (Western Province) the rate reached 64 cases per 100,000 compared with 32 per 100,000 in Riyadh (Central Province) (Al-Kassimi 1993; Qari 2002). The childhood and adolescents tuberculosis along with adult tuberculosis are on a rapid increasing phase in the country as per the available published data from the MOH statistics during the last few years (http://www.moh.gov.sa/statistics/index.html) with alarming rate (20%) of high prevalence of MDRTB was reported from Western region of KSA during 2001(M Y Khan 2001).

5. Drug resistance TB in Saudi Arabia

Empirical anti-tuberculosis therapy used in Saudi Arabia usually includes three to four first line drugs including isoniazid, rifampicin, ethambutol, pyrazinamide and streptomycin. Despite the implementation of the D.O.T.S, the number of patients effectively treated in Saudi Arabia has fallen below the WHO target of 85%, (Al-Hajjaj; Alrajhi, Abdulwahab et al.; Samman, Krayem et al.). A retrospective study was conducted which included 147 patients with culture proven diagnosis of tuberculosis seen at the King Khalid National Guard Hospital, Jeddah, between June 1993 and June 1999. One hundred and twenty six patients completed treatment and treatment success was 102/147 (69.4%) and failure 45/147 (30.6%). Noncompliance and drug resistance were considered the main two factors which are significantly associated with treatment failures (Samman, Krayem et al.). Abu-Amero KK reviewed data available for the last 10 years and he showed that the prevalence of single-drug-resistant tuberculosis ranged from 3.4% to 41% for isoniazid, 0% to 23.4% for rifampicin, 0.7% to 22.7% for streptomycin and 0% to 6.9% for ethambutol. However, the prevalence of multi drug-resistant tuberculosis (defined by WHO as resistance to two or more first-line anti tuberculosis drugs) ranged from 1.5% to 44% in different regions (Abu-Amero). Another study on 764 *M. tuberculosis* isolates obtained from 764 patients; resistance was noted in 65 (8.5%). Resistance to isoniazid was the highest, noted in 54 (7.1%); resistance to rifampicin, streptomycin and ethambutol was found to be 21 (2.7%), 29 (3.8%) and 12 (1.6%) isolates respectively. Poly resistance was noted in eight (1%) isolates and mono resistance in 38 (5%) isolates. Multi-drug-resistant *M. tuberculosis* was found in 19 (2.5%) isolates. There were 54 primary resistant isolates (7.6%), and 11 (22%) with acquired resistance. Resistance to at least one agent of the first-line anti-tuberculosis agents was 18.4%. Mono resistance to a single first-line agent was found in 10.9%, while poly resistance was noted in 7.6%. Multi-drug-resistant *tuberculosis* was noted in 5.7% of all isolates. Resistance to isoniazid was most commonly noted in 11% of isolates. Resistance rates to other agents were: rifampin 9.7%, streptomycin 9.1%, pyrazinamide 3.1%, and ethambutol 2.5%. Al-Hajoj et al summarized all available studies as it shown in table-1. However, the author insisted that these studies should be treated with extreme caution as many of them are old, no standardized technique, small and fragmented studies as they were carried out in a single hospital.

	Drug resistance					MDR-TB	Reference
City	**RIF**	**INH**	**PZA**	**ETB**	**STR**	%	
Jeddah	20.8	28.7	7.9	6.9	22.8	25	(al-Mazrou, Khoja et al.)
Riyadh	2.8	9.1	5	2.8	1.6	11.8	(Arya)
Jizan (South)	43	80	S	NA	53	44	(Ellis, al-Hajjar et al.)
Dammam	0.2	6	S	S	0.7	7	(Al-Rubaish, Madania et al.)

The above table is a summary of studies from different regions showing the percentage of drug resistance TB for single and multi anti-TB agents. It is not clear which method/s was used in each study. RIF-rifampicin, INH-isoniazid, PZA-pyrazinamide, ETB-ethambutol, STR-streptomycin, MDR-TB multi drug resistant tuberculosis.

Table 1. MDR-TB. Profile cities within the kingdom of Saudi Arabia

Recently, the King Faisal Specialist Hospital and Research Centre (KFSH&RC) TB-research unit undertook the responsibility to study drug resistance rate in the country. This study was planned with the help of W.H.O experts and in collaboration with the Ministry of Health. This study was funded by King Abdulaziz City for Science and Technology (KACST) under project # AT26-110. This study was the first of its type as it covered the whole country and in prospective mannar. The design of the study was to collect all isolates from all regional laboratories for one year. This was in concordance with W.H.O recommendation as there were no data to do cluster collection. All isolates with their epidemiological and clinical data were collected for one year starting from 01 June 2009 until

31 May 2010. A total of 2,842 were collected from 9 regions. 248 and 192 were removed from the total number as we found them to be NTM and repeated cultures respectively. Therefore the DST was carried out for 1904 isolates representing the whole country. A summary of the main findings are in table-2.

Drug	No. of resistant isolates	Rate of resistance
Any drug resistance	537	28.3%
Streptomycin	228	12%
Isoniazid	160	8.42%
Rifampicin	15	0.78%
Ethambutol	58	3.05%
Multi drug resistance	76	4%

Table 2. Summary of finding of an ongoing drug resistance surveillances.

6. Pulmonary and Extra-pulmonary Tuberculosis (EPTB)

11.7%. EPTB was reported in 1991. EPTB rates believed to be varies from one hospital to another and from one region to another (Bukhary and Alrajhi). Between 1979 and 1981 Froude and Kingston reviewed 162 cases diagnosed with EPTB from KFSH&RC. The ratio of pulmonary and extra-pulmonary TB was 1:1 during the 27-month period of the study (Froude and Kingston 1982). In 2001, extra-pulmonary TB was culture-confirmed in 2 out of every 3 cases of TB at KFSH&RC (Alrajhi, Abdulwahab et al. 2002). However, KFSH&RC is known to be a tertiary hospital and may be very selective and as a result this percentage has to be treated with extreme caution. In another hospital in Riyadh TB cases for 9 months between 1981 and 1982 was reviewed by Shanks et al. Out of 47 cases, pulmonary TB was documented in 57% of cases, and 43% were EPTB (Shanks, Khalifa et al. 1983). Mokhtar and Salman studied the details of 125 TB patients. EPTB was found in 15% of all cases identified (Mokhtar and Salman 1983). Onther study showed that EPTB accounted for 59% of all cases between 1987-1989, (Zaman 1991). However, it is worth mentioning that all the above studies may do not reflect the real picture of the incidences of EPTB. All these studies were carried out either at a tertiary hospital or in regional hospital, therefore, we recommend treating these data with extreme caution. For this reason we conducted a nation wide surveillance project to determine the rate of drug resistance in the country. In this project the whole country in a prospective manner was covered. All isolates with their epidemiological and clinical data were collected from all 9 centers where TB specimens are cultured. The total number of isolates collected was 2842. Upon classification of the type of the disease, we found that pulmonary cases form 82.4% while extra-pulmonary cases are at 17.6% (manuscript under preparation).

7. Mycobacteria other than TB

Non-tuberculous mycobacteria (NTM), also known as environmental mycobacteria or atypical mycobacteria or mycobacteria other than tuberculosis (MOTT), are mycobacteria which do not cause tuberculosis or Leprosy. As the incidence of tuberculosis fell slightly, infection by those mycobacteria became more readily recognized around the world. There is a worldwide increase in infections with non-tuberculous mycobacteria due to the emergence of the human immunodeficiency virus (HIV)-epidemic and other factors such as immunosuppressive therapy, malnutrition, and protracted treatment with broad-spectrum antibiotics. Non-tuberculous mycobacteria (NTM) are increasingly recognized as pathogens capable of causing extra-pulmonary disease, especially in immunocompromised individuals. The pathogenecity and clinical relevance of many NTM remain poorly understood. In addition, the optimal treatment of infections caused by many NTM is undefined due to interspecies and intraspecies variabilities, drug resistance, and limited literature describing disease caused by less common organisms.

Nontuberculous mycobacteria (NTM) are common inhabitants of the environment and have been cultured from water, soil, and animal sources worldwide. Human disease is believed to be acquired from environmental exposures, and unlike tuberculosis and leprosy, there has been no evidence of animal-to-human or human-to-human transmission of NTM.

NTM mainly involves the species *M.avium complex [MAC], M. abscessus, M.Chelonae M. fortuitum, M. scrofulaceum, M. marinum and M. kansasii* and there are many other species which is clinically relevant as a pathogen.

However, as tuberculosis declined and modern microbiological methods were developed, the importance of NTM in human disease became increasingly evident. NTM cause four distinct clinical syndromes.

1. Progressive pulmonary disease, especially in older persons caused primarily by *M. avium complex* (MAC) and *M. kansasii.*
2. Superficial lymphadenitis, especially cervical lymphadenitis, in children caused mostly by *MAC, M. scrofulaceum, M. malmoense* and *M. haemophilum.*
3. Disseminated disease in severely immunocompromised patients.
4. Skin and soft tissue infection usually as a consequence of direct inoculation.

NTM are opportunistic pathogens, mostly affecting patients with preexisting pulmonary disease such as chronic obstructive pulmonary disease [COPD] or tuberculosis (TB), or those with systemic impairment of immunity. The latter group includes those with HIV infection, immunosuppressive drugs users, and leukemia patients. NTM are very common in the environment and resistant to commonly used disinfectants, so they can be present in non-sterile patient material such as sputum and contaminated medical equipment (bronchoscope washers or samples in the laboratory) and consequently cause pseudo infection (Griffith DE 2007). Without evidence of person-to-person transmission of NTM, it is proposed that humans are infected from environmental sources that may include aerosols, soil, food, water and equipment. When NTM are isolated from a usually sterile site (e.g., blood, bone marrow, lymph nodes, synovial fluid), diagnosis of true disease is generally straightforward. However, when NTM are isolated from non-sterile sources, such as sputum or bronchoalveolar lavage samples, the diagnosis is less definitive, especially when the colony numbers are low or NTM are isolated from only one cultured specimen. Therefore, it is a challenge to differentiate true NTM lung disease from contamination and colonization. Thus, finding AFB by microscopy of respiratory specimens or by culture may pose a diagnostic problem for the clinician (Society. 1997).

In recent years, non-tuberculous mycobacteria (NTM) have emerged as an important cause of opportunistic nosocomial infections, but there is little known about the isolation and identification of NTM in Saudi Arabia. Larger, multicenter regional studies or mandatory reporting will be required to better understand the changing epidemiology of NTM in patients with or without HIV infection. There are many cases of NTM infections reported from different regions of Saudi Arabia but the actual numbers of cases are still unknown. However, there are scattered studies about the prevalence of NTM in Saudi Arabia. BaHammam et al showed that NTM is about 9% (BaHammam, Kambal et al.). A nation wide population-based survey however, revealed a much lower figure of 0.004% (Alrajhi and Al-Barrak; Baharoon; Bukhary and Alrajhi; Bukhary and Alrajhi; Sanai and Bzeizi). Recent collection of more than 3000 isolates from all regions in the country revealed that NTM cases are at 10% of total cases. Further study is needed to gain insight into the nature of NTM cases. In year 2010, a new species of NTM which resembled TB in terms of clinical features and response to the treatment was identified in collaboration work between the TB research unit at king Faisal Specialist Hospital and Research Centre and international collaborators. This species was called Riyadhense.

Mycobacterium abscess also was found to cause infection in an immune competent patients (Al-Hajoj et al 2012).

8. Childhood TB

Childhood TB (CHTB) is a neglected aspect of the TB epidemic, despite constituting 20% or more of the TB case-load in many countries with high TB incidence. CHTB is a significant child health problem, but is neglected because it is usually smear-negative and thus it's considered to make a relatively minor contribution to the spread of TB. Perhaps most importantly, there is a real need for prospective epidemiological studies to determine the true burden of TB among children in a wide spectrum of settings worldwide. Recent guidance has already taken a significant step in this direction by recommending NTPs record childhood TB cases by age category and clinical syndrome (WHO 2007).

As children acquire infection with *Mycobacterium tuberculosis* from adults in their environment, the epidemiology of childhood tuberculosis follows TB in adults. While global burden of childhood tuberculosis is unclear, in developing countries the annual risk of tuberculosis infection in children is 2-5 per cent. Nearly 8-20 per cent of the deaths caused by tuberculosis occur in children. It has been suggested that BCG vaccination is responsible for decrease in the occurrence of disseminated and severe disease (S.K. Kabra 2004). Crucially, a definitive microbiological diagnosis of CHTB is achieved in only a minority of cases, as young children rarely develop cavitatory lung disease or expectorate sputum, and a greater proportion of cases are extra-pulmonary. Diagnosis therefore usually relies on poorly validated clinical case definitions, and both under and over-diagnosis of pediatric TB are common, with potentially tragic consequences for children who are not diagnosed (Brent, Anderson et al. 2008). Neonates have the highest risk of progression to disease, and in infancy miliary and meningeal involvement is common. Children from 5 to 10 years of age are less likely to develop disease than other age groups, and adolescent patients can present with progressive primary tuberculosis or cavitary disease (Engelbrecht, Marais et al. 2006). Most children who develop disease do so within 2–12 months of initial infection, with pulmonary TB accounting for 60–80% of all cases. The two most common forms EPTB found in children are Lympho-hematogenous disease with multiple organ involvement and Tuberculous Meningitis [TBM]. The TBM is the most serious complication with involvement of the central nerves system and with a high mortality rate. The TBM is common in children compared to adults and its diagnosis is difficult because signs and symptoms are vague (Anna M M 2005) (Starke JR 2002). The prevalence of MDRTB in children probably reflects the level of primary drug resistance among organisms currently circulating in the community. Comprehensive studies on resistance to anti TB drugs in children are limited. It has been demonstrated that patient with MDRTB cause similar rates of infection and disease among household contacts as do the patients with drug susceptible tuberculosis.(H.Simon Schaaf 2001).

The diagnostic difficulties make to give only a little attention to children with MDRTB or children in contact with it. In controlled studies it has been shown that the rate of infection is even higher in childhood contact as compared to drug sensitive cases. The transmission of MDRTB is higher than that of sensitive TB. Treatment of MDRTB is expensive and associated with lower treatment completion and cure rates. Isoniazid is the effective drug for prophylactic therapy in children with an index case, but Rifampicin is an alternative in cases of Isoniazid resistance. In cases of MDRTB there is no proved regimen of treatment for children. The drug toxicity is much higher with second line and third line drugs regimen when treating MDRTB, multi drug regimen usually necessitating hospitalization and gradual build up of drug dosages and schedules. The treatment for MDRTB is challenging in a child and unfortunately most of the second line drugs do not have pediatric formulations (Ejaz A Khan 2002). Interruption in the transmission of *Mycobacterium tuberculosis* is one of the primary goals of TB control programs. The ability to track specific strains of *M. tuberculosis* improves the understanding of transmission and pathogenesis in a community and helps to control transmission with properly designed strategies (Kathryn DeRiemer 2004). The most common extrathoracic manifestation of TB in children is cervical lymphadenitis. A simple clinical algorithm that identified children with a persistent (longer than 4 weeks) cervical mass of 2×2cm or more, without a visible local cause or response to first-line antibiotics, showed excellent diagnostic accuracy in an area with endemic TB (Marais, Wright et al. 2006). At a global level, the WHO currently reports only smear-positive cases by age. The International Union Against TB and Lung Disease (IUATLD) currently recommends stratifying the reporting of smear-positive cases into two age categories: younger than 15 years of age and 15 years of age and older (D A Enarson 2000).

Reporting of smear-positive cases is considered a practical strategy that complements the Directly Observed Therapy (D.O.T.S) strategy. Nonetheless, an estimated 1.2 cases of smear-negative TB occur for every smear-positive case of TB. Furthermore, approximately 95 percent of cases in children younger than 12 years of age are smear-negative. Thus, the W.H.O policy of reporting only smear-positive cases by age causes a gross underestimation of the burden of TB in children (J.A. Jereb 1993). Childhood TB is a direct reflection of the incidence of adult disease within a community. A case of TB in a child usually represents primary disease transmitted from an infectious adult or adolescent and is considered a sentinel event in public health. In response to a case of childhood TB, local TB control programs ideally will conduct an investigation to identify the potential source of infection and additional cases. Due to limited resources, these investigations are not implemented in many parts of the world (Anna M M 2005). A positive culture is regarded as the 'gold standard test' to establish a definitive diagnosis of TB in a symptomatic child. It is, however, limited by the fact that organisms may be isolated from non-diseased (asymptomatic) children shortly after primary infection, during the initial period of organism multiplication and/or occult dissemination. In addition, traditional culture methods are limited by suboptimal sensitivity, slow turnaround times, excessive cost (automated liquid broth systems) and the low bacteriological yields achieved in children with active TB. It is important to point out that adolescent children (over 10 years of age) frequently develop sputum smear-positive disease that may be diagnosed using traditional methods (B.J. Marais 2005).

As childhood tuberculosis is a sensitive marker for ongoing transmission within a community, control programs should focus on children because they are the reservoirs of future disease (Lalitkanth 2001). Most children with TB in the world are not recorded in the national surveillance systems, even though they are the ones most likely to suffer severe complications of the disease. While there are many challenges in the diagnosis and treatment of TB in children, perhaps the greatest challenge globally is to begin to identify the extent of disease in this forgotten group (Shingadia. 2004). In Saudi Arabia childhood TB is also receiving little attention. However, despite this some cases are getting reported. For instance Peritoneal tuberculosis is relatively rare compared to adults but cases are reported from two regions of Saudi Arabia in children below 12 years (Saleh 1997). Primary tuberculosis of the penis with associated bilateral inguinal lymph node enlargement and a discharging sinus is described in an infant from the Abha Region (Annobil S H 1990). Banjar et al in a controlled study of 151 cases of non cystic fibrosis bronchiectasis conducted in a tertiary care centre in Riyadh among Saudi children, showed TB form 2% of the total cases (Banjar 2007). A case of congenital transmission of tuberculosis is reported from Riyadh region as a cutaneous disease with multiple abscess and resistance to primary antibiotics (Yousef A. Al-Katawee 2007). The central nervous system tuberculosis among children is reported from different regions of the country with considerable mortality rate and diagnostic and treatment problems (Bahemuka M 1989; Al-Deeb SM 1992). In a study of causes of uveitis conducted in an ophthalmology referral centre in Riyadh, it highlighted tubercular uveitis among children during 2002 (Islam and Tabbara).

9.Factors influencing the molecular epidemiology of tuberculosis in Saudi Arabia

9.1 Hajj

Saudi Arabia is a unique place as it is the place for the two holy mosques located in Mecca and Al-Madinah. The two holy mosques are the target for the one billion Muslims from all over the world. Thus every year the two cities Mecca and Al-Madinah receive more than three million for Hajj and visits to the holy mosque in Al-Madinah. The intense congestion of Hajjies, the majority of whom are coming from high endemic places, overcrowds and the close proximity furnish the grounds for infectious diseases transmission including TB. Other factors may influence the transmission including aging pilgrims whom may suffer from underlining disease such as immunological disorders, less hygiene among some of the pilgrims and the physical efforts exerted by pilgrims. As a matter of fact several studies showed that Hajj is an opportunity for TB transmission. Wilder-Smith et al conducted a prospective study to assess the risk of *M. tuberculosis* infection among Hajj pilgrims. He found high risk of *Mycobacterium tuberculosis* infection during the Hajj pilgrimage. In his study he showed that among 357 Singaporean pilgrims; 10% showed a substantial rise in immune response to the QuantiFERON TB assay antigens post-Hajj when compared to a pre-Hajj test (Wilder-Smith, Foo et al. 2005). Alzeer et al studied cases of pneumonia admitted to two hospitals during the 1994 pilgrimage (Hajj) season to Mecca. Sixty-four patients were enrolled in the study, of which 47 (75%) were men with a mean age of 63 years (range 21-91). Nearly all were from developing countries. Diagnosis was established in 46 patients (72%) with *Mycobacterium tuberculosis* being the commonest causative organism (20%) (Alzeer, Mashlah et al. 1998). The main finding of this study is that *Mycobacterium tuberculosis* is a common cause of pneumonia during Hajj season. As a matter of fact the variation of TB incidence among Saudi cities and in favor of Western province was attributed to Pilgrims influx.

9.2 Omra

Omra is another Islamic ritual through which individuals from all over the world target once again Mecca and Al-Madinah. The two holy mosques receive all year long hundreds of thousands whom again do come from endemic places. During the holy month of Ramadan the number of visitors to the two mosques peak again as it reaches up to three million in Mecca and may be another one million at Al-Madinah mosque. During the last 10 days of the holy month of Ramadan the majority of visitors do what is called Etekaf, during which people do not leave the grand mosques. The scene is overwhelming as a person can see individuals are sleeping and sitting next to each others. We believe such circumstances make these places fertile land for transmission of TB.

9.3 Expatriates

Saudi Arabia accommodates 8,429,401 expatriates scattered all over the country. They are in the country for work purposes. In addition considerable unknown numbers are moving around illegally and hide in farms and in houses. Unfortunately the majority of those expatriates are from endemic places; therefore they are forming a source of infection as they do not visit hospitals when they become diseased, fearing deportation after treatment.

9.4 Travelling

The Saudi national nowadays travels around the globe. Also we have a considerable number of students (more than 250 thousand including families members) studying abroad and scattered all over the world including countries where TB is high like India, Philippines and East Europe. We believe that the above mentioned factors are playing a major role in making TB spread and transmitted to the country and to outside of the country. This is supported by our recent finding of molecular epidemiology.

10. Molecular epidemiology of TB in Saudi Arabia

In 2007 we published some data on the molecular epidemiology in Saudi Arabia. A total of 1,505 clinical isolates of *M. tuberculosis*, the isolates were collected over a three year period from seven regions of Saudi Arabia and were genotyped using spoligo and MIRU -VNNTR techniques. A total of 387 individual patterns were obtained (clustering rate of 86.4%, 182 clusters containing between 2 to 130 isolates per cluster). A total of 94% of the strains matched to the spoligotype patterns in an international database. Majority of the isolates (81%) were imported strains including Central Asian-CAS 22.5%, ill-defined T clade 19.5%, East African Indian-EAI 13.5%, Haarlem 7.5%, Latin American Mediterranean-LAM 7.2%, Beijing 4.4%, Manu 2.7%, X 0.9%, and Bovis 0.9%. In addition two clonal complexes with unique spoligotyping signatures (octal codes 703777707770371, and 467777377413771) were specific to Saudi Arabia. Another on going study is taking place in Eastern province, which is a major industrial zone of the country and thus the immigrant population is high (Al-Hajoj et al.). According to the latest census reports, 2.7 million of citizens and 0.8 million of immigrants are living in the Eastern province (Statistics Department 2010). In this study a total of 533 TB isolates were collected with their epidemiological data. All the isolates were genotyped and lineages were assigned by using the online databasewww.miruvntrplus.org. There were 14 lineages identified among the study groups and 24 (4.5%) cases belonged either to undefined lineage or *M. bovis*. Among the total cases, Delhi/CAS (32%) and EAI (21.3%) are dominating, followed by Ghana (9.9%) and Haarlem (9.3%). TB population of the Saudi patients showed a higher predominance of Delhi/CAS (71/33.3%), followed by EAI (32/15%) and Ghana (24/11.3%). On the other hand, the non-Saudi isolates showed the domination of Delhi/CAS (100/31%) and EAI (82/25.5%), followed by Ghana (29/9%). The total numbers of undefined lineages were 17, and *M. bovis* (7 cases) was circulating only among Saudis. Cluster analysis showed 28 clusters of 148 isolates with a size of 2-18. Major clustering was found among the lineages Delhi/CAS (7 clusters) and EAI (6 clusters).

The study showed that some clades are circulating among Saudi only, others circulating among non-Saudi, and the rest circulating among both Saudi and non-Saudi (manuscript under preparation).

11. BCG vaccination

In Saudi Arabia BCG vaccine is given to every born baby as mandatory policy trying to protect the population against TB infection. It is believed that BCG is protecting against TB infection and may protect against Miliary Tuberculosis. BCG vaccination is being debated nowadays in Saudi Arabia as whether to continue to give the vaccine, delay it or stop it all together. Three years ago King Faisal Specialist Hospital and Research Centre held a conference on "Infections in Immunocompromised host" (18-19 November 2008). In this symposium, many specialists expressed their reservations about administering tuberculosis vaccine (BCG vaccine) to newborn children. They pointed out that in some cases of pediatrics with immune deficiencies, it is very important to delay the vaccination plan until the possibility of genetic immune deficiency has been ruled out. This is due to the complication of the vaccine and the dissemination of the disease. In addition, the country lacks data regarding the efficiency of BCG vaccination. In other words, we do not know whether BCG vaccine is protecting or not. Therefore the question is can we stop giving BCG vaccine to our babies? The philosophy behind this question is that BCG vaccine may not protect against TB; otherwise, why do we have up to 4000 cases yearly (according to a recent report by the Ministry of Health) despite the fact that all our babies are vaccinated at birth? BCG vaccination may cause confusion when skin test is carried out. Interpretation of skin test is extremely difficult in light of the fact that the protein used in skin test is shared by many species of mycobacteria. Shared protein is the main cause of the confusion (Mittrucker, Steinhoff et al.). Therefore positive skin test means i) exposure to real infection, ii) exposure to environmental mycobacterium or iii) reaction due to BCG vaccine itself. BCG vaccination causes a particular problem when it comes to diagnosing dormant TB using TST. It is for this reason that the BCG vaccine is not given in many countries such as The Netherlands, UK, and recently France; yet these countries have better control over tuberculosis when compared to many countries, including Saudi Arabia, where BCG vaccine is mandatory.

To role out the confusion caused by BCG vaccination we either have to stop BCG vaccination all together or introduce Interferon-γ tests (interferon gamma release assays, IGRAs) as additional diagnostic tools. IGRAs are based on the ability of the *Mycobacterium tuberculosis* antigens for early secretory antigen target 6 (ESAT-6) and culture filtrate protein 10 (CFP-10) to stimulate host production of interferon-gamma. Because these antigens are not present in nontuberculous mycobacteria or in BCG vaccine, these tests can distinguish between latent tuberculosis infection in asymptomatic patients and exposure to BCG or nontuberculous mycobacteria. The test is approved for diagnosis of latent tuberculosis and has also been used in patients with pulmonary tuberculosis (Al-Orainey; Stephan, Wolf et al.). We fully approve of the establishment of such diagnostic tools everywhere in the country. It is an expensive test at this particular stage but it is worth using, as delay in diagnosing difficult cases such as extra-pulmonary is more costly to the patients (as it might cost them their lives). In addition treating dormant tuberculosis, particularly when it comes to close contact individuals, is far cheaper than treating patients after they show full symptoms of the disease. On the other hand, it is a very bad practice to give prophylaxis to treat dormant tuberculosis based on skin test results as the test has proved its inability to distinguish real infection from exposure to environment tuberculosis or BCG vaccine. Also, giving a prophylaxis indiscriminately based on skin test gives a chance for drug resistance to develop. We believe it is the right time now to review our policy of giving BCG vaccine to our newly born babies as it is creating more confusion rather than providing protection: It causes diseases in immunocompromised patients. BCG vaccine causes confusion when it comes to interpretation of skin test results. Also, it gives false-positive and false-negative results.

12. HIV and TB in Saudi Arabia

Saudi Arabia started surveillance for HIV in 1984. Clinical suspicion, screening of contacts of HIV infected patients, routine screening of blood and organ donors, prisoners ,intravenous drug users, patients with other sexually transmitted infections, expatriates pre-employment testing are among reasons for HIV testing. All cases from 1984 through 2001 were reviewed. A total of 6,046 HIV infections were diagnosed, of which 1,285 (21.3%) of cases were Saudi citizens. HIV infections among Saudi citizens gradually increased over 18 year period, and jumped from 84 to 142 cases per year. The number of cases per 100,000 populations varied widely between regions. The infection was most common in the age group 20-40 years. The modes of transmission among Saudi citizens and expatriates were heterosexual contact, blood transfusion, perinatal transmission, homosexual contact, intravenous drugs, and bisexual contact. A total of 514/1285 (40%) Saudi patients died by year 2001.

TB infection is found to be associating with HIV infection like anywhere in the world. Alrajhi et al reviewed retrospectively medical charts of 437 patients diagnosed with tuberculosis from 1995-2000 in Riyadh. He found that screening was done for 178 (41%) patients: 2 (1.1%) of these were found to be HIV positive.In Saudi Arabia, screening for HIV in tuberculosis patients remains underutilized (Omair, Al-Ghamdi et al.).

217 new adult patients joined the HIV program between 1997 and 2007. TB was diagnosed in 16 patients (7.4%), all of whom had acquired immune-deficiency syndrome at the time of TB diagnosis. Seven developed extra-pulmonary disease (44%), six had pulmonary TB (37%), while three had both (19%). The TB incidence rate was 1,354 per 100,000 among the HIV-infected cohort. The incidence rate of pulmonary TB was 762/100,000 and for extra-pulmonary TB it was 592/100,000. Among pulmonary TB with HIV infection in Saudi Arabia, TB incidence is 30 times higher than in the general population, with significant mortality despite early diagnosis, treatment and tertiary care support (Al-Mazrou, Al-Jeffri et al.; Alrajhi; Alrajhi, Halim et al.; Alrajhi, Halim et al.; Alrajhi, Nematallah et al.; Edathodu, Halim et al.; Kordy, Al-Hajjar et al.; Madani; Madani, Al-Mazrou et al.; Memish and Osoba).

13. References

"Saudi Gazette: Nov. 24, 2010 - Census shows Kingdom's population at more than 27 million" [1]

Siraj Wahab (30 July 2009). "It's another kind of Saudization". Arab News. http://archive.arabnews.com/?page=1&section=0&article=124999&d=30&m=7&y=2009. Retrieved 13 January 2011.

Seok, Hyunho (1991). "Korean migrant workers to the Middle East". In Gunatilleke, Godfrey (ed.). Migration to the Arab World:

Abu-Amero, K. K. "Status of antituberculosis drug resistance in Saudi Arabia 1979-98." East Mediterr Health J 2002 Jul-Sep;8(4-5):664-70.

Al-Deeb SM, Y. B., Sharif HS, Motaery KR. (1992). "Neurotuberculosis: a review." Clin Neurol Neurosurg. 94: S30-3.

Al-Hajjaj, M. S. "The outcome of tuberculosis treatment after implementation of the national tuberculosis control program in Saudi Arabia." Ann Saudi Med. 2000 Mar;20(2):125-8.

Al-Hajjaj, M. S., and I.M Al-Khatim (2000). "High rate of non-compliance with anti-tuberculosis treatment despite a retrieval system:a call for implementation of directly observed therapy in Saudi Arabia." Int J Tuberc Lung Dis 4(4): 345-349.

Al-Hajoj, S. A. "Can we change the way we look at BCG vaccine?" Ann Thorac Med. 2009 Apr;4(2):92-3; author reply 93-4.

Al-Hajoj, S. A. and F. A. Alrabiah "Role of tuberculosis laboratories in Saudi Arabia. A call to implement standardized procedures." Saudi Med J. 2004 Nov;25(11):1545-8.

Al-Hajoj, S. A. and F. A. Alrabiah "Role of tuberculosis laboratories in Saudi Arabia. A call to implement standardized procedures." Saudi Med J 2004 Nov;25(11):1545-8.

Al-Hajoj Sa Fau - Zozio, T., F. Zozio T Fau - Al-Rabiah, et al. "First insight into the population structure of Mycobacterium tuberculosis in Saudi Arabia

Mycobacterium tuberculosis complex genetic diversity: mining the fourth international spoligotyping database (SpolDB4) for classification, population genetics and epidemiology." (0095-1137 (Print)).

Al-Kassimi, A. K. A., MS Al-Hajjaj, IO Al-Orainey, EA Bamgboye and MN Chowdhury (1993). "Nationwide community survey of tuberculosis epidemiology in Saudi Arabia." Tuber.Lung.Dis 74: 254-260.
al-Kassimi, F. A., A. K. Abdullah, et al. "Nationwide community survey of tuberculosis epidemiology in Saudi Arabia." Tuber Lung Dis 1993 Aug;74(4):254-60.
Al-Mazrou, Y. Y., M. H. Al-Jeffri, et al. "HIV/AIDS epidemic features and trends in Saudi Arabia." Ann Saudi Med. 2005 Mar-Apr;25(2):100-4.
al-Mazrou, Y. Y., T. A. Khoja, et al. "High proportion of multi-drug resistant Mycobacterium tuberculosis in Saudi Arabia." Scand J Infect Dis 1997;29(3):323.
Al-Orainey, I. O. "Diagnosis of latent tuberculosis: Can we do better?" Ann Thorac Med. 2009 Jan;4(1):5-9.
Al-Rubaish, A. M., A. A. Madania, et al. "Drug resistance pulmonary tuberculosis in the Eastern Province of Saudi Arabia." Saudi Med J 2001 Sep;22(9):776-9.
Alrajhi, A. A. "Human immunodeficiency virus in Saudi Arabia." Saudi Med J. 2004 Nov;25(11):1559-63.
Alrajhi, A. A., S. Abdulwahab, et al. "Risk factors for drug-resistant Mycobacterium tuberculosis in Saudi Arabia." Saudi Med J. 2002 Mar;23(3):305-10.
Alrajhi, A. A., S. Abdulwahab, et al. (2002). "Risk factors for drug-resistant *Mycobacterium tuberculosis* in Saudi Arabia." Saudi Med J 23(3): 305-10.
Alrajhi, A. A., M. A. Halim, et al. "Mode of transmission of HIV-1 in Saudi Arabia." AIDS. 2004 Jul 2;18(10):1478-80.
Alrajhi, A. A., M. A. Halim, et al. "Presentation and reasons for HIV-1 testing in Saudi Arabia." Int J STD AIDS. 2006 Dec;17(12):806-9.
Alrajhi, A. A., A. Nematallah, et al. "Human immunodeficiency virus and tuberculosis co-infection in Saudi Arabia." East Mediterr Health J. 2002 Nov;8(6):749-53.
Alzeer, A., A. Mashlah, et al. (1998). "Tuberculosis is the commonest cause of pneumonia requiring hospitalization during Hajj (pilgrimage to Makkah)." J Infect 36(3): 303-6.
Anna M M, J. R. S. (2005). "Current concepts of childhood tuberculosis." Seminars in pediatric infectious diseases. 16: 93-104.
Annobil S H , A.-H., Kazi T (1990). "Primary tuberculosis of the penis in an infant." Tubercle 71(3): 229-230.
Arya, S. C. "Drug resistant Mycobacterium tuberculosis in Saudi Arabia." Saudi Med J 2002 Apr;23(4):475.
B.J. Marais, R. P. G., A.C. Hesseling and N. Beyers, (2005). "Adult-type pulmonary tuberculosis in children 10–14 years of age." Pediatr Infect Dis 24: 733-744.
BaHammam, A., A. Kambal, et al. "Comparison of clinico-radiological features of patients with positive cultures of nontuberculous mycobacteria and patients with tuberculosis." Saudi Med J. 2005 May;26(5):754-8.
Bahemuka M, M. J. (1989). "Tuberculosis of the nervous system. A clinical, radiological and pathological study of 39 consecutive cases in Riyadh, Saudi Arabia." J Neurol Sci 90(1): 67-76.
Banjar, H. H. (2007). "Clinical profile of Saudi children with Bronchiectasis." inddian J of Pediatrics. 74(2): 149-152.
Bener, A. and A. K. Abdullah "Reaction to tuberculin testing in Saudi Arabia." Indian J Public Health. 1993 Oct-Dec;37(4):105-10.
Brent, A. J., S. T. Anderson, et al. (2008). "Childhood tuberculosis: out of sight, out of mind?" Transactions of the Royal Society of Tropical Medicine and Hygiene 102(3): 217-218.

Bukhary, Z. A. and A. A. Alrajhi "Extrapulmonary tuberculosis, clinical presentation and outcome." Saudi Med J. 2004 Jul;25(7):881-5.

D A Enarson, H. L. R., T Amadotir (2000). "Management of tuberculosis: a guide for low-income countries." International Union Against Tuberculosis and Lung Disease, Paris, France

Edathodu, J., M. M. Halim, et al. "Mother-to-child transmission of HIV: experience at a referral hospital in Saudi Arabia." Ann Saudi Med. 2010 Jan-Feb;30(1):15-7.

Ejaz A Khan, M. H. (2002). "Recognition and management of tuberculosis in children." Current Pediatrics(12): 545-550.

el-Kassimi, F. A., A. K. Abdullah, et al. "Tuberculin survey in the Eastern Province of Saudi Arabia." Respir Med. 1991 Mar;85(2):111-6.

Ellis, M. E., S. al-Hajjar, et al. "High proportion of multi-drug resistant Mycobacterium tuberculosis in Saudi Arabia." Scand J Infect Dis 1996;28(6):591-5.

Engelbrecht, A. L., B. J. Marais, et al. (2006). "A critical look at the diagnostic value of culture-confirmation in childhood tuberculosis." Journal of Infection 53(6): 364-369.

Froude, J. R. and M. Kingston (1982). "Extrapulmonary tuberculosis in Saudi Arabia, a review of 162 cases." King Faisal Specialist Hospital Medical Journal 2: 85-95.

Griffith DE, A. T., Brown-Elliot BA, Catanzaro A, Daley C, Gordin F, et al. (2007). "An official ATS/IDSA statement: diagnosis, treatment, and prevention of nontuberculous mycobacterial diseases." Am J Respir Crit Care Med. 175: 367-416.

H.Simon Schaaf, R. P. G., Magdalene Kennedy, Nulda Beyers, Peter B Hesseling and Peter R Donald (2001). "Evaluation of young children in contact with adult multi-drug resistant pulmonary tuberculosis: A 30-month follow-up. ." Pediatrics 109(5): 765-771. http://www.moh.gov.sa/statistics/index.html.

Islam, S. M. and K. F. Tabbara "Causes of uveitis at The Eye Center in Saudi Arabia: a retrospective review." Ophthalmic Epidemiol. 2002 Oct;9(4):239-49.

J.A. Jereb, G. D. K. a. D. S. P. (1993). "The epidemiology of tuberculosis in Children." Pediatr Infect Dis 1993(4): 220-231.

Kathryn DeRiemer, C. L. D. (2004). "Tuberculosis transmission based on molecular epidemiologic research. ." Seminars in respiratory and critical care medicine 25(3): 297-306.

Kordy, F., S. Al-Hajjar, et al. "Human immunodeficiency virus infection in Saudi Arabian children: transmission, clinical manifestations and outcome." Ann Saudi Med. 2006 Mar-Apr;26(2):92-9.

Lalitkanth (2001). "Childhood Tuberculosis increasing: But neglected. ." Indian Journal of Tuberculosis. 48(1): 1-2.

M Y Khan, A. J. K., A O Osoba, S WAli, Y Samman, Z Memish (2001). "Increasing resistance of M.tuberculosis to anti-TB drugs in Saudi Arabia. ." Int.journal of Antimicrobial Agents(17): 415-418.

Madani, T. A. "Sexually transmitted infections in Saudi Arabia." BMC Infect Dis. 2006 Jan 10;6:3.

Madani, T. A., Y. Y. Al-Mazrou, et al. "Epidemiology of the human immunodeficiency virus in Saudi Arabia; 18-year surveillance results and prevention from an Islamic perspective." BMC Infect Dis. 2004 Aug 6;4:25.

Marais, B. J. M. F. C. P. M., C. A. M. F. F. F. Wright, et al. (2006). "Tuberculous Lymphadenitis as a Cause of Persistent Cervical Lymphadenopathy in Children From a Tuberculosis-Endemic Area." Pediatric Infectious Disease Journal 25(2): 142-146.

Memish, Z. A. and A. O. Osoba "International travel and sexually transmitted diseases." Travel Med Infect Dis(2005 Aug 18): 2006 Mar;4(2):86-93.

Mittrucker, H. W., U. Steinhoff, et al. "Poor correlation between BCG vaccination-induced T cell responses and protection against tuberculosis." Proc Natl Acad Sci U S A(2007 Jul 18): 2007 Jul 24;104(30):12434-9.

Mokhtar, A. and K. Salman (1983). "Extrapulmonary tuberculosis." Saudi Med J 4: 317-322.

Omair, M. A., A. A. Al-Ghamdi, et al. "Incidence of tuberculosis in people living with the human immunodeficiency virus in Saudi Arabia." Int J Tuberc Lung Dis. 2010 May;14(5):600-3.

Qari, F. A. (2002). "The spectrum of tuberculosis among patients of the King Abdul Aziz University Hospital, Jeddah, Saudi Arabia." Southeast Asian J Trop Med Public Health 33(2): 331-337.

S.K. Kabra, R. L. V. S. (2004). "Some current concepts on childhood tuberculosis." Indian J Med Res 120(October 2004): pp 387-397.

Saleh, M. A.-F. A.-Q., Abdulaziz; Larbi, Emmanuel; Al-Fawaz, Ibrahim; Taha, Omar; Satti, Mohammed B. (1997). "Tuberculous Peritonitis in Children: Report of Two Cases and Literature Review." Journal of Pediatric Gastroenterology & Nutrition 24(2): 222-225.

Samman, Y., A. Krayem, et al. "Treatment outcome of tuberculosis among Saudi nationals: role of drug resistance and compliance." Clin Microbiol Infect. 2003 Apr;9(4):289-94.

Shanks, N. J., I. Khalifa, et al. (1983). "Tuberculosis in Saudi Arabia." Saudi Med J 4: 151-156.

Shingadia., T. W. a. D. (2004). "Global epidemiology of Paediatric tuberculosis." Journal of Infection. 48: 13-22.

Society., A. T. (1997). "Diagnosis and treatment of disease caused by nontuberculous mycobacteria." Am J Respir Crit Care Med. 156: s21-25.

Starke JR, J. H., Baltimore RS, Ed. (2002). Tuberculosis Infection. Pediatric diseases: Principles and practice. . Philadelphia, WB Saunders.

Statistics Department, M. (2010). Health Statistical Year book., Ministry of Health, Saudi Arabia.: 52-53.

Stephan, C., T. Wolf, et al. "Comparing QuantiFERON-tuberculosis gold, T-SPOT tuberculosis and tuberculin skin test in HIV-infected individuals from a low prevalence tuberculosis country." AIDS. 2008 Nov 30;22(18):2471-9.

WHO (2007). "A research agenda for childhood tuberculosis." World Health Organization WHO/HTM/TB/2007.381.

Wilder-Smith, A., W. Foo, et al. (2005). "High risk of Mycobacterium tuberculosis infection during the Hajj pilgrimage." Trop Med Int Health 10(4): 336-9.

Yousef A. Al-Katawee, L. A. A.-M., Abdulrahman S. Al-Showaier (2007). "Congenital tuberculosis presenting as cutaneous disease in a premature infant." Saudi Med. J 28(11): 1739-1740.

Zaman, R. "Tuberculosis in Saudi Arabia: epidemiology and incidence of Mycobacterium tuberculosis and other mycobacterial species." Tubercle 1991 Mar;72(1):43-9.

Zaman, R. (1991). "Tuberculosis in Saudi Arabia: epidemiology and incidence of Mycobacterium tuberculosis and other mycobacterial species." Tubercle 72(1): 43-9.

5

Diagnosis of *Mycobacterium tuberculosis*

Faten Al-Zamel
King Saud University
Saudi Arabia

1. Introduction

Tuberculosis (TB), caused by the intracellular bacterium, *Mycobacterium tuberculosis* (Mtb), has been a major health concern since it plagued ancient Egypt 5 thousand years ago. TB infects 9 million people every year, most of them children (especially in endemic areas), and it leads to approximately 2 million deaths annually (World Health Organization [WHO], 2008; Kabra & Lodha, 2004; Marais & Pai, 2007). These numbers are expected to increase in the coming years because of (1) the AIDS pandemic—a high percentage of the patients with human immunodeficiency virus (HIV) are co-infected with Mtb, and (2) the emergence of drug-resistant strains of the TB organisms (Corbett et al., 2003; Raviglione, 2003; WHO, 1994). This alarming increase in morbidity and mortality highlights the need to strengthen control measures. Accurate and rapid diagnosis is essential for controlling the disease, yet the traditional tests for TB produce results that are either inaccurate or take too long to be definitive. A fast and reliable diagnostic method that could differentiate between active and latent TB infection is lacking as well.

The current routine diagnostic tests for TB: sputum smear microscopy, chest X-ray, Mtb culture, tuberculin skin test, acid-fast staining, and serological tests—all have their limitations. Sputum smear microscopy can produce false negative results, whereas the acid-fast staining requires a large number of bacteria in the sputum to give an accurate reading; a chest X-ray alone is inconclusive; Mtb culture takes too long to produce a result; the tuberculin skin test lacks specificity and reliability; and serological tests, which use different TB antigens to detect Mtb infection, are fast but they lack the necessary sensitivity.

The only available TB vaccine is the bacille Calmette Géurin (BCG) vaccine, which is uneven in its efficacy. Various reports have indicated variable levels of protection ranging from 0 percent to 80 percent in different populations (Fine, 1995; Tuberculosis Research Centre [ICMR], 1999). Therefore, despite the fact that most people in developing countries are vaccinated with BCG at birth, TB is still a major public health problem. The prevalence of TB infection is reported as being as high as 40 percent worldwide, and the annual risk of infection is 2–4 percent worldwide (Anil, 1995).

Clinically, TB has two forms: An active form and a latent form (which is asymptomatic and non-contagious). If undiagnosed and untreated, a patient with active pulmonary TB will transmit the infection to 10–15 people each year (WHO, 2006). However, active TB is also fueled by the vast reservoir of latent TB infections that become reactivated. Immunocompetent individuals latently infected with Mtb have a 10 percent lifetime risk of developing active TB (Syblo, 1980; Harada, 2006). Data show that 5 percent of latently infected individuals will progress to active TB in the first 2 years after acquiring the infection, and an additional 5-10 percent of infected people will develop the active disease later in their lives (Comstock et al., 1974). This risk increases for people co-infected with HIV—especially children, for whom diagnosis of TB is even more challenging (Corbett et al., 2004).

If diagnosed, latent TB infected individuals can be cured with anti-tuberculosis treatment, which prevents progression to the active form of the disease. Because effective TB control can only be achieved with the accurate diagnosis and treatment of both active and latent infections, modern TB control programs require the identification of latent TB infection to the highest clinical standards. Accurate diagnosis and preventive treatment of latently infected individuals can substantially decrease the chance of development into active TB (Cohn, 2000). Delayed diagnosis, because of inaccuracy or the unavailability of diagnostic requirements—including the availability of rapid and accurate diagnostic methods—can preclude timely therapy, which may result in increasing morbidity and mortality, greater lung damage resulting in chronic disability, and higher health care costs (Kehinde et al., 2005; WHO, 2009).

The diagnosis dilemma for clinical TB continues to be a global issue. For pulmonary TB, it can be difficult to obtain robust respiratory specimens from the elderly, the young, and immuno-compromised patients. For those with extra-pulmonary TB, tissue biopsy is essential for histopathological and microbiological diagnosis (Bukhary & Alrajhi, 2004), yet techniques to obtain and examine biopsies are not available in all hospitals and may be associated with complications. A simple, noninvasive, rapid, and accurate method of diagnosis needs to be developed for successful treatment of both active and latent TB; with such a method, person-to person transmission of the disease would be greatly reduced, which would have a major impact on TB morbidity and mortality worldwide (Cambanis et al., 2007).

1.1 Specimen collection

For the detection of pulmonary and/or extrapulmonary TB, tests usually require sputum, gastric lavage, blood, urine, or other bodily fluids (such as cerebrospinal fluid, pleural, or ascetic fluid); in addition, tissue biopsy specimens are collected for the diagnosis of extrapulmonary TB. One of the objectives of developing TB biochemical markers and immunological assays is to replace the need for collecting tissue biopsy specimens from TB patients for diagnosis of the disease. Likewise, the development of immunochromatography tests (ICT), for which urine is used as a specimen, is an attempt to make diagnostic tests less invasive and costly, more rapid, and patient friendly. Up until now, regardless of which test is used, that test is usually accompanied by microbiological tests (smear microscopy and mycobacterial culture of sputum) to diagnose pulmonary TB and to determine the treatment be used. Sputum samples, after being collected, are decontaminated by using normal sodium hydroxide-N-acetyl-L-cystein (NaOH-NALC) and then sometimes centrifuged to get a better yield of the organisms (Kent & Kubica, 1985). Often three sputum samples are collected, including a "spot" specimen collected on the first day (first sputum); a morning (second sputum); and "spot" specimen (third sputum) collected on the second day. However, collecting adequate amount of sputum from patients is not always possible, especially in children younger than 10 years old or in adults who cannot produce enough sputum. In situations like these, procedures to stimulate cough with an aerosol solution and/or bronchoalveolar or gastric lavage can be used (Capelozzi et al., 2011; Mohan et al., 1995; Somu et al.,1995).

2. Traditional TB diagnostic tests and their associated problems

Traditional TB diagnosis usually requires high clinical presentation, laboratory materials, and methods for sputum smear microscopy (acid-fast bacilli), culture on solid and/or liquid media, chest radiography, and the tuberculin skin test. Tissue sampling is usually needed to confirm preliminary results in cases of extra-pulmonary TB. All of these tests have their respective shortcomings.

2.1 Sputum smear microscopy

Sputum-smear microscopy is 100 years old, but it is still the primary, easy to use, and affordable test for the confirmation of pulmonary TB at the lower level of health services. Acid-fast bacilli smear Ziehl-Neelsen (ZN) microscopy, which is prepared from unconcentrated sputum (direct smear), is the main laboratory tool supporting case detection. It is inexpensive and is relatively specific in settings where tuberculosis is endemic. However, direct smear microscopy can produce false-negative results, which have been observed in more than 30–50 percent of adult patients (Miorner et al., 1994; Daniel 1990), particularly in high HIV-prevalent settings (Elliot et al., 1993; Frieden et al., 2003; American Thoracic Society Workshop, 1997), and 85–90 percent of infected children (Newton et al., 2008). The acid-fast bacilli false-negative result rate is attributable, in part, to the low sensitivity of the test, which requires more than 10,000 bacilli per milliliter of sputum for reliable detection (Perkins, 2000). Obtaining good sputum samples can be difficult, and the studious attention of trained and motivated technicians (who are not always available) is necessary.

Many attempts have been made to improve and optimize the performance of smear microscopy, including with new technologies (Mase et al., 2007; Bonnet et al., 2007; Ramsay et al., 2009; Mabaera et al., 2007; Van Deun et al., 2004), such as fluorescence microscopy, which uses inexpensive light-emitting diodes (LED) as an alternative for conventional ZN microscopy. This substitution increases the sensitivity of the test and is easy to use, even in peripheral laboratories where culture facilities are not available (Hooja et al., 2011; Steingart et al., 2006a; Steingart et al., 2006b; Steingart et al., 2007; Van Deun et al., 2008; Trusov et al., 2009; Minion et al., 2009; Bonnet et al., 2011). In fact, the World Health Organization (WHO) Strategic and Technical Advisory Group (STAG) for TB recommended that fluorescence microscopy be phased in as an alternative for ZN (WHO, 2009), because it can be used even in low-income, high TB burden settings. It has been reported that LED fluorescence microscopy, either alone or in combination with single-specimen tests, could increase considerably the identification of smear-positive cases (Cattamanchi et al., 2010).

A wide variety of stains or fluorescence quenchers have been used with the LED fluorescence microscopy; however potassium permanganate at 0.5 percent in water is the stain most frequently used. Although potassium permanganate can produce very good results with the classical fluorescence microscopy systems (using mercury vapor lamps and epifluorecence), the very dark background sometimes makes it difficult to focus. Methylene blue (Mblue) is an alternative to potassium permanganate, which yields comparable results (Van Deun et al., 2010).

In an attempt to improve the performance of smear microscopy, sputum processing methods using household bleach (NaOCl), followed by a specimen concentration step (such as centrifuge or sedimentation, mentioned above), can be done in any laboratory setting before smear microscopy is used (Steingart et al., 2006; Angeby et al., 2004; Annam et al., 2009). However, some reports indicate that NaOCl sedimentation did not improve the performance of LED fluorescence microscopy in the diagnosis of pulmonary TB at low levels of health service in resource-poor countries (Bonnet et al., 2011).

Because the acid-fast bacilli smear is based on sputum, extra-pulmonary TB detection varies with the cytomorphology of inflammation at the site of infection, which is limited and may not exceed 40 percent (Nigussie et al., 2010; Gangane et al., 2008). The sputum smear microscopy test may also identify certain types of bacteria that are not Mtb, thus yielding a false-positive result for TB. The WHO estimates sputum smear microscopy only identifies 35 percent of patients with TB (Harris, 2004; Thornton et al., 1998). Furthermore, the 2010 WHO report indicated that in 2009, 43 percent of the 4.6 million reported new cases of pulmonary TB were diagnosed without microbiological confirmation (WHO, 2010). The failure to confirm TB infection can delay initiation of the appropriate therapy to adequately treat cases, which could prevent the further spreading of the disease (Cambanis et al., 2007).

2.2 Solid or liquid cultures

Solid or liquid cultures are still seen as the gold standard for TB detection because they are sensitive to live Mtb in the sputum sample; they can also provide data on the likely effectiveness of certain chemotherapeutic agents against TB. However, there are serious drawbacks to this test, such as the time needed to obtain the result (3–8 weeks). Clinical and therapeutic decisions are often made before the culture results are available. However, few facilities in low-income settings use culture for the diagnosis of TB; for those facilities the main method of diagnosis is sputum microscopy with acid. When culture *is* used in these settings, the Löwenstein-Jensen solid, egg-based, and agar-based Middlebrook 7H10 media are the ones used to recover mycobacteria from clinical materials (Metchock et al., 1999; Murray et al., 1998); these can take weeks to show results.

2.2.1 Advantages and disadvantages of cultures

A number of manual and automated systems have been developed to reduce the detection time of mycobacteria in clinical specimens. Both the biphasic Septi-chek acid-fast bacilli (Becton Dickinson, Sparks, MD) and the MB-Redox (BiotestAG, Dreieich, Germany) are examples of the manual systems. Advances in technology have led to the development of the automated systems such as radiometric BACTEC 460TB (Becton Dickinson), the fluorometric BACTEC MB9000 and BACTECMGIT (Mycobacteria Growth Indicator Tube), 960 systems (Becton Dickinson), the carbon dioxide–sensing MB/BacT ALERT 3D System (Organon Teknika, Durham, NC), and the pressure-sensing ESP Culture System II (Trek Diagnostic Systems, Westlake, OH). Detection time and isolation of Mtb were considerably improved (7–21 days) with the use of liquid media, such as the radiometric BACTEC 460 TB broth-based system. However, this procedure still requires trained technicians and special attention to safety issues regarding radioisotopes (Salfinger & Pfyffer, 1994; Laszlo et al., 1983). Another disadvantage of the BACTEC 460 TB system is the increased cost of radioactive waste disposal, an issue that encouraged manufacturers to develop a better alternative. The fully automated BACTEC Mycobacteril Growth Indicator Tube (MGIT) liquid medium system with early growth indicators (the BACTEC MGIT 960 system), is faster and more sensitive than both LJ and BACTEC 460 TB for testing the susceptibility of antituberculosis agents, and it is more effective in diagnosing the disease in smear-negative samples; this feature shows great potential to reduce the mortality rate from TB (Lu et al., 2002; Gérôme et al., 2009; Sinirtas et al., 2009; Morcillo et al., 2010).

The BACTEC MGIT 960 system is a high-capacity, fully automated continuous-monitoring system, which can test up to 960 samples for the rapid detection of mycobacteria, making it suitable for those laboratories dealing with a large number of specimens (Somoskovi et al., 2000; Hanna et al., 1999; Tortoli et al., 1999; Lee et al., 2003). In the determination of the early bactericidal activity in the clinical studies of new anti-tuberculosis agents, it has been found that the time of detection of MGIT 960 is better than colony-forming units of Mtb on solid media (Diacon et al., 2010).

Although the WHO recently recommended the expanded use of liquid culture systems, such as MGIT, in resource-constrained settings (WHO, 2007), historically these systems have not been used because of the high cost of the tests and the culture contamination rates (Chihota et al., 2010). The relatively high contamination rates of the MGIT culture has been reported to range from 5.5 to 15 percent in high-income settings, and as high as 29.3 to 33 percent in resource-constrained settings (Chien et al., 2000; Lee et al., 2003; Hanna et al., 1999; Somoskvi et al., 2000; Chihota et al., 2010).

2.2.2 New approaches to cultures

Using simple and inexpensive monoclonal assays, such as the Capilia TB assay (a rapid and low-technology method), which uses monoclonal antibodies to detect a secreted mycobacterial protein (MPB64) during culturing (solid or liquid culture) allows it to differentiate Mtb from non-TB mycobacteria (Muyoyeta et al., 2010; Ngamlert et al., 2009). To shorten the time required for bacterial growth detection, Mtb can be isolated in both liquid- and solid-media cultures (Lu et al., 2002).

Although automated systems such as BACTEC 460 TB, BACTEC 9000, and MGIT can be used to accelerate the growth of the bacteria, they can also produce inaccurate results (Daniel, 1987). Plus, it is not always possible to obtain bacteria in the sputum sample. False-positives, which range from 0.1 percent to 65 percent because of laboratory contamination is another concern with the culture technique (Ruddy et al., 2002). Viable organisms can present additional problems, especially in patients who have started treatment. Therefore, even though culture has thus far been considered the gold standard for TB diagnosis, it still lacks the desired accuracy; it has been estimated that no more than 81 percent of the confirmed TB cases can be detected by culture (API, 2006).

2.3 Tuberculin Skin Test (TST)

Tuberculin skin testing (TST), also known as the Mantoux test or Heaf test, remains in widespread use for both the diagnosis of active TB and the detection of latent TB, and for the identification of TB in health care workers, for whom the incidence of TB is higher than in the general population (Harries et al., 1997; Barrett et al., 1979) and who require routine checkups for accidental acquisition of TB infection and chemoprophylaxis. The TST is a delayed type hypersensitivity skin test: an induration develops and is measured 48 to 72 hours after the intradermal inoculation of purified protein derivatives. It is generally accepted that in adults a TST response greater than or equal to a 10-millimeter induration is indicative of TB infection; however in children, the gauge differs in different settings. Importantly, the TST is still used as an epidemiological tool to screen for TB and to calculate the annual risk of TB through data generated by TST surveys. TST surveys are useful for detection of TB in communities with low case-detection rates, to assess the effect of HIV infection on a TB epidemic, and to better understand the effect of both diseases on children (Farhat et al., 2006).

2.3.1 Limitations of the tuberculin skin test

Although the TST is inexpensive, easily available, and is the preferred test in most TB-prevalent settings, it has a number of limitations. The TST is not patient friendly, in that it requires two visits to the health facility: the first visit is when the test is administered; and the second visit, 2 - 3 days later, is to assess the skin's reaction. It is estimated that one third of the people tested never return after the 48- to 72-hour waiting period to have their tests read (ATS, 2000; Lee & Holzman, 2002).

2.3.2 False positives

Purified protein derivatives contain more than 200 antigens shared with the BCG vaccine and many of the non-TB environmental mycobacteria, which can result in low specificity of the TST (Huebner et al., 1993; Dacso 1990; Diel et al., 2009; Pai et al., 2008). This cross-reactivity results in false-positive reporting for a large percentage of the world's population. Some reports indicate that BCG vaccination can present TST false-positive results for up to 15 years after vaccination (Wang et al., 2002). These variables contribute to the false positive results: (1) the strain and dose of BCG inoculated (Wang et al., 2002; Davids et al., 2006); (2) the method of vaccine administration (Davids et al., 2006); (3) the time since vaccination (Menzies, 2000); (4) the number of BCG scars (Babayigit et al., 2011); and (5) the weight and age at the time of vaccination (Newort et al., 2004). If the BCG vaccine was received in infancy, the impact on TST results is minimal, especially 10 or more years after vaccination. A person's nutrition at the time of vaccination as well as genetic factors can also have an impact on the outcome of the TST results later on (Newport et al., 2004). More frequent, more persistent, and larger TST reactions were observed in individuals who had received the BCG vaccine later in life, ie, after infancy (Pérez-Then et al., 2007; Farhat et al., 2006). Sometimes TST indurations between 5–10 millimeters can still develop for up to 25 years after vaccination (Miret-Cuadras et al., 1996). The TST false positive reaction was not associated with a family history of tuberculosis, with exposure to cigarette smoke, number of household family members, and the presence of respiratory allergic diseases (Babayigit et al., 2011). A number of additional factors can contribute to false-positive results including inaccuracy of reading and documenting the results (Mancuso et al., 2008).

Furthermore, the TST does not distinguish between individuals infected with Mtb, vaccinated with BCG, or infected with environmental non-TB mycobacteria— almost one third of the people who test positive on the TST do not have a TB infection (American Thoracic Society [ATS], 2000; Huebner et al.,1993; von Reyn et al., 2001). Clinically non-TB mycobacteria rarely causes TST false-positives in low-prevalence settings of TB infection, however it does have an effect on the false-positive results of populations with a high prevalence of non-TB mycobacteria (Farhat et al., 2006). This lack of specificity (high rate of false-positive) in diagnosing both active and latent TB (WHO, 1995) is considered the TST's major drawback.

2.3.3 False negatives

The TST can also produce false-negative readings, and these can be product-related (associated with improper storage or handling). The number of tuberculin units inoculated and the type of tuberculin can have an effect on TST reactivity (Farhat et al., 2006). The sensitivity of the test is affected by the immunomodulation of the skin; the DTH response is influenced by illness or immunosuppression, and factors such as HIV infection or a young child's age can result in even lower sensitivity of the test for both latent and active TB (Swaminathan et al., 2008; Selwyn et al., 1992; Pesanti, 1994; Madariaga et al., 2007; Moreno et al., 2001).

2.3.4 The boosting effect

Other disadvantages associated with the TST include the "boosting effect," a phenomenon in which multiple TST administrations over time yield a false positive. The increased tuberculin reaction is seen in some individuals when a second skin test is administered 1 week to 1 year after administration of a first skin test that is nonreactive. This could be explained as an anamnestic recall of immune response that occurs in individuals with remote exposure to mycobacterial antigens. This phenomenon is a problem for people who are regularly screened for TB infection using the TST (for example, health care workers, hemodialysis patients, etc.) and become immunized to purified protein derivatives by the repeated administrations of the test (Dogan et al., 2005; Cengiz & Seker, 2006). Persistent negative TST in latent TB-infected individuals, despite the continued exposure, has been reported. It has been shown that this reaction can be attributed to genetic factors. These genetic factors not only influence the interaction between humans and Mtb but they can affect the outcome of the exposure: exposure but no infection, infection without progression, or progression to disease (Stein et al., 2008). Subjectivity and inter-individual variability, in the administration and reading of the TST can be added to the disadvantages and resultant errors, because it is difficult to administer small amounts of the protein uniformly; that is, the amount of purified protein derivatives delivered in the TST may vary, and this affects the size of the reaction (Chaparas et al., 1985).

Further research is needed to determine the best cut-offs for TST sensitivity, the optimal time for testing candidates, especially for people that need to be tested periodically (such as health care workers), and the cost-effectiveness of the test, given its limitations (Khawcharoenporn et al., 2011).

2.4 Chest X-ray

Chest radiography can be a useful tool to confirm TB when combined with a patient's history, physical exam, and laboratory tests in symptomatic and even smear-negative patients. Pulmonary TB almost always shows abnormalities on the chest radiograph; the pulmonary cavities and lesions are smaller when infected with TB than those caused by other chest health problems.

2.4.1 Disadvantages of chest X-ray

A chest X-ray cannot alone confirm a TB diagnosis. In many cases (40 percent), the infection is not in the lungs; radiography may not detect the early stages of TB disease, because the damage to the lungs may not yet be sufficiently marked to be detectable by a chest X-ray. Also, scarring in the lungs may be detected if previous TB disease has occurred (even if the patient is completely cured), and thus it is difficult to distinguish past cured TB from current TB disease.

2.4.2 Computerized Tomography (CT)

When both chest X-ray and computerized tomography were used to screen for latent TB in pre-transplant patients, abnormal findings were only detected on the chest CT (the chest X-ray results were normal), which indicates that chest CTs can detect latent TB better than chest X-rays (Lyu et al., 2011). Many studies have confirmed that CT has detected pulmonary TB cases that were missed by chest radiographs. Furthermore, high resolution CT alone, or CT together with the TST and INF-γ release assays, were effective in the differentiation between active TB and latent TB (Lee et al., 2010; Boloursaz, 2010). Even in sputum smear-negative sittings, high-resolution CT findings, such as tree-in bud appearance, lobular consolidation, and large nodules, accurately predicted the risk for pulmonary TB with reproducible results (Nakanishi et al., 2009).

2.5 Nucleic acid amplification test

The nucleic acid amplification test detects the nucleic acid specific to Mtb using an amplification technique (Noordhoek et al., 1995; Kadival et al., 1995; Nagi et al., 2007). Nucleic acid amplification is a relatively new assay for TB diagnosis that is available only in specialized, advanced laboratories (ATS, 2000). DNA amplification offers a fairly specific and sensitive diagnostic method in both pulmonary and extra-pulmonary TB, and most studies have shown it to be more sensitive than sputum smear microscopy, but less sensitive than microbial culture (Pfyffer, 1999; Magana-Arachchi et al., 2008). The specificity (ruling in disease) of the nucleic acid amplification test is high when applied to body fluids (extra-pulmonary), such as meningitis and pleural TB).

2.5.1 Limitations of the nucleic acid amplification test

The sensitivity (ruling out disease) can be compromised especially in respiratory specimens, where it can be highly variable and more inconsistent than specific (it is only about 60 percent effective under optimal conditions). This variability can be explained by the use of different cut-off values used in the different studies (Dinnes et al., 2007; Daley & Pai, 2007), in addition to the sequence variation in both commercial and in-house assays (Whilley et al., 2008).

Evaluation of commercial nucleic acid amplification tests in both pulmonary TB and extra-pulmonary TB indicated that nucleic acid amplification tests have high, consistent specificity and positive predictive values in smear-positive patients (Ling et al., 2008; Piersimoni et al., 2002; Reischl et al., 1998; Caruyvels et al., 1996; Coll et al., 2003; Goessens et al., 2005; Miragliotta et al., 2005; Ozkutuk et al., 2006; Guerra et al., 2007; Franco-Alvarez et al., 2006); however, in smear-negative cases, when a rapid diagnostic test is needed, the accuracy of the test is more modest and variable, and the results may be influenced by patient selection and the clinical setting in which the tests are carried out (Brown et al., 1999; Barnes, 1997).

Similar results were obtained when the clinical impact of the nucleic acid amplification test systems were evaluated in low-income countries that have a high burden of TB and HIV. The nucleic acid amplification test assays used in these studies had moderate sensitivity and high specificity for TB in a predominantly HIV-seropositive population with negative sputum-smear (Davis et al., 2011; WHO, 2010).

Different laboratories report significant variability in the reproduction of this test, which can lead to false-positive results (Chedore et al., 2006); this is a major concern because of the DNA contamination of assay reagents. Even though nucleic acid amplification test techniques can amplify a small amount of genetic material, the sample must still contain a certain number of TB bacteria to be effective, and this collection is not always possible, particularly with nonpulmonary TB (Haldar et al., 2007). Therefore, it has been suggested that nucleic acid amplification tests should be combined with other diagnostic tests (for example, tests detecting INF-γ) in order to increase the sensitivity of the test (Dinnes et al., 2007). Another disadvantage of the nucleic acid amplification test is that the assay cannot distinguish dead from viable organisms, so a positive result may indicate active disease even though the TB has been cured (Manjunath et al., 1991).

Although the test itself takes little time to administer, the time required to obtain the results is considerable. Laboratories often culture the sample first, to allow the bacteria to multiply (which takes a few weeks), before carrying out the nucleic acid amplification test. The nucleic acid amplification test method requires some level of technical skill (invasive procedures are sometimes necessary to obtain samples), and is prone to cross contamination. In order to provide valid results, the nucleic acid amplification test must be run in an environment that minimizes and detects cross-contamination and test-appropriate controls. Nucleic acid amplification tests can be expensive, and in underdeveloped countries where the high-burden TB exists, commercial nucleic acid amplification tests are rarely used because of cost and complexity. Although some studies suggest that nucleic acid amplification tests are cost-effective in diagnosing TB even in low-income countries (van Cleeff et al., 2005; Dowdy et al., 2008), their use has been limited. In-house techniques that might be substituted for commercial assays often produce results that can't be validated (Daley et al., 2007). When molecular methods were compared with conventional diagnostic procedures, mostly microscopic detection, it was found that the microscopic method on its own is better than the molecular method, because of the extra care needed to interpret the results (Runa et al., 2011).

2.5.2 New approach to the nucleic acid amplification test

A more recent commercial nucleic acid amplification test (the hyplex TBC test), which meets the demand for a low-cost system, has been introduced. The hyplex test is a qualitative system for the detection of members of the Mtb complex, and it is based on a multiplex polymerase chain reaction followed by reverse hybridization to specific oligonucleotide probes and enzyme-linked immunosorbent assay (ELISA) detection. In comparison to other commercial nucleic acid amplification test systems, the hyplex TBC shows good specificity but lower sensitivity, especially with smear-negative TB specimens; it also gives false-negative results, which puts it in the same class as the other nucleic acid amplification test assays (Hofmann-Thiel et al., 2010).

These observations indicate that commercial nucleic acid amplification tests cannot replace conventional tests and cannot be used alone to confirm TB. Improvement of this technique, especially its sensitivity, is required in order for it to be beneficial for the diagnosis of TB in low-resource countries where the prevalence of disease is higher than in other parts of the world.

3. New, more specific tests

3.1 Antibody-based diagnosis assay (TB ELISA)

Recently, many new serological procedures have been evaluated for diagnosing TB. Enzyme-linked immunosorbent assays (ELISA) theoretically represent attractive serodiagnostic methods, because they are simple, rapid, inexpensive, and do not require much training or sophisticated equipment. Several researchers have tried to develop ELISA tests utilizing different antigens, such as culture filtrate, purified extracts of glycolipid, and mycobacterial sonication antigens, as well as more specific mycobacterial non-recombinant and recombinant antigens of Mtb (Daniel et al., 1986; Escamilla et al., 1996; Laal et al., 1997). Tests using such antigens were designed to detect immunoglobulins IgG, IgM, or IgA against these TB-specific antigens in whole blood, plasma, or serum of both pulmonary and extra-pulmonary TB patients (Imaz et al., 2001; Raja et al., 2002, 2004; Ramalingam et al., 2002; Zheng et al., 1994; Patil et al., 1996). Antigens from mycobacteria other than Mtb (*M. habana*) were also evaluated for their ability to diagnose extra-pulmonary TB using ELISA, and these antigens were found to be effective (Chaturvedi & Gupta 2001). To date, the 38-kDa antigen is the best candidate for the ELISA technique for diagnosing TB in actively infected individuals—but it is not reliable in extra-pulmonary or TB-HIV co-infected patients (Abebe et al., 2007). Because the available ELISA tests cannot achieve a high sensitivity, these tests are unacceptable as single diagnostic tools for TB detection (Chiang et al., 1997; Ravn et al., 2005; Weldingh et al., 2005; Araujo et al., 2004; Raja et al., 2002). The use of relatively low pure Mtb antigens has contributed to the low sensitivity of the test.

Different studies have suggested that a combination of several key antigens (antigen cocktail) may result in better sensitivity. These antigens are presumably the specific, antigens to detect the latent and early stages of the active infection in both pulmonary TB as well as extra-pulmonary TB (Houghton et al., 2002). In order to develop a successful serodiagnostic method for TB, several factors must be considered: antigen recognition by infected individuals varies depending on the stage of the disease; the heterogeneity of human leukocyte antigen in different populations; bacterial load; and the immunological status of the patient (Abebe et al., 2007).

3.1.1 New approaches to ELISA

Recently, an ELISA test (lipoarabinomannan [LAM] antigen-detection assay) that uses urine as a sample has been developed, standardized, and is commercially available (Clearview® TB ELISA) (Boehme et al., 2005; Hamasur et al., 2001; Tessema et al., 2001). This test has many advantages: it is non-invasive, patient friendly, simple (dipstick prototype form of the test is available), rapid (requires 15 minutes to perform), easy to use, and it uses urine, which is a sterile biological fluid that is easier to obtain than sputum, which some patients have difficulties producing. Moreover, the test can be used with other body fluids, including sputum (Dheda, et al., 2010) cerebral-spinal fluid (Patel et al., 2009), and pleural fluid (Dheda K et al., 2009). However, the preliminary data indicate that the sensitivity of the urine LAM, although better than sputum microscopy in HIV-infected patients (Lawn et al., 2009), is still not adequate to replace mycobacterial culture in TB-infected patients, and the diagnostic efficacy is limited and requires further study (Gounder et al., 2011).

A promising, more rapid, and cost-effective form of ELISA has been developed: the Immunochromatographic (ICT) Test Kits; these kits detect serum antibodies against Mtb-specific antigens that are secreted by Mtb during active infection. The high sensitivity, specificity, and positive predictive values suggest that these kits are useful and simple diagnostic tools, especially for resource-poor diagnostic centers (Kumar et al., 2011).

3.2 Interferon-Gamma Release Assays (IGRAs)

Effector T cells of the cell-mediated immune response are normally present as a result of recent host encounters with antigen. T effector cells are short-lived and die off when the antigen is cleared from the host. Due to the short life of the effector T cells, their continued presence indicates that the cellular immune response is fighting a pathogen somewhere in the body. Therefore, diagnosis of an acute infection can be made by noting the presence of the antigen-specific effector T cells in a patient's blood or serum sample and by measuring the release of cytokines by the T effector cells when re-exposed to antigen in vitro. It has been shown recently that TB-specific Th1, Th22, and Th17 cells have an essential role in the immunity against TB infection; this provides a potential target for diagnosis and therapeutic intervention in TB disease (Qiao et al., 2011; Wozniak et al., 2010).

Th1 cells, which secrete INF-γ, are known to protect the body against the Mtb infection. This fact provides a unique way to examine the TB disease for diagnosis, prognosis, and treatment monitoring (Flynn et al., 1993; Boom, 1996; Gallegos et al., 2008). The production of INF-γ is influenced by many external factors, such as TB infection, and internal factors, such as interleukin (IL)-10, IL-12, IL-18, and IL-23 (Yu et al., 2011; Zhang J, et al., 2011; Han et al., 2011; Sahiratmadja et al., 2006). In fact some studies have suggested that some cytokines such as TNF-alpha, IL-2, IL-12, and IL-17 can be used to discriminate between active and latent TB disease (Sutherland et al., 2010; Schauf et al., 1993); however the exact role of each of these cytokines is not fully understood and needs to be investigated further.

Different reports have shown that the peripheral-blood mononuclear cells from patients infected with TB release INF-γ when exposed to Mtb-specific antigens *in vitro* (Ravn et al., 1999; Ulrichs et al., 1998; Lalvani et al., 2001 Mori et al., 2004). Based on these findings, different diagnostic assays have been developed to measure INF-γ released by peripheral-blood mononuclear cells cells in response to Mtb-specific antigens. Two such antigens are the early secreted antigenic target 6-kDa (ESAT-6) protein and culture filtrate protein 10-kDa (CFP-10) (Andersen et al., 2000; Tully et al., 2005). Both antigens have been shown to be important for the growth, survival, and pathogenesis of Mtb (Brodin et al., 2005; Munk et al., 2001). These proteins are secreted by Mtb in great quantities during the infection or when the bacteria are cultured *in vitro* (Andersen et al., 2000; Behr et al., 1999; Pai et al., 2004). Both ESAT-6 and CFP-10 are encoded within the region of deletion 1 (RD1) and are more specific to the organism because they are present in Mtb but are not shared with the BCG vaccine or with most of the environmental mycobacteria (Goletti et al., 2006; Sorensen et al., 1995; Harboe et al., 1996).

3.2.1 The interferon-gamma release assay tests

These discoveries have resulted in the development of two promising, blood-based, commercially available INF-γ release assay tests that have been approved for clinical use for the diagnosis of TB infection, and that use ESAT-6 and CFP-10 antigens: (1) QuantiFERON-TB Gold (QFT-G), which has been replaced in many parts of the world by a safer and simpler test method, QFT-G in-tube assay (QFT-IT) (Cellestis Limited Carnegie, Victoria, Australia) in which an additional Mtb-specific antigen TB7.7 is incorporated into the test (Syed et al., 2009; Stavri et al., 2009); and (2) T-SPOT.TB assay (Oxford Immunotech, Oxford, United Kingdom). Although the two tests share common features, they also have some technical distinctions (Richeldi, 2006). The two INF-γ release assays are designed to measure INF-γ production (INF-γ release assays) in two different ways, from peripheral-blood mononuclear cells of TB patients when exposed *in vitro* to ESAT-6 and CFP-10 proteins. QFT-G measures the quantity of INF-γ secreted by T cells, and T-SPOT.TB assay enumerates the number of TB-specific T cells secreting INF-γ after exposure to TB-specific antigens. Both of the INF-γ release assays require only a single patient visit, and the test results are available within 24 hours (Hill et al., 2004; Richeldi et al., 2004).

Many studies have shown that the QFT-G test is fairly accurate and has modest sensitivity to detect active TB (Kobashi et al., 2006; Kang et al., 2007; Pai et al., 2007). The QFT-G offers specificity of up to 97 percent in clinical trials, sensitivity of up to 89 percent, and provides clinicians with an accurate, reliable, and convenient TB diagnostic tool (Mori et al., 2004; Kobashi et al., 2006).

QFT-G has been useful for the diagnosis and differentiation between pulmonary TB and other pulmonary diseases; however it too has its limitations. Because the results depend on the clinical condition of the patients and the presence of immunosuppressive diseases, patients with localized lesions of TB infection and the elderly can sometimes get false-negative results (Kobashi et al., 2008; Kawabe, 2007).

The T-SPOT.TB test, on the other hand, quantifies the number of the INF-γ-producing TB-specific cells using a technology known as the Enzyme Linked Immunosorbent Spot (ELISPOT) assay, which is widely recognized as the most sensitive technique to measure antigen-specific T cell function. In the T-SPOT.TB assay, recently developed by Lalvani and coworkers, individual T cells specific for the two antigens (ESAT-6 and CFP-10) are enumerated (Lalvani, Pathan et al., 2001; Lalvani, Nagvenkar et al., 2001). With this technique, peripheral-blood mononuclear cells from infected individuals are cultured overnight (16-20 hours) with ESAT-6 and CFP-10 antigens to allow the release of INF-γ by the sensitized T cells (Lalvani & Hill, 1998; Lalvani et al., 1998). A single T cell produces a dark spot, which is the footprint of an individual Mtb-specific T cell, and the number of spots is quantified.

The T-SPOT.TB technique has an estimated pooled specificity of 93 percent and up to 90 percent sensitivity for patients with culture-confirmed TB from low-incidence countries; its sensitivity, therefore, is higher than the TST (Lalvani, Pathan et al., 2001; Lalvani, Nagvenkar et al., 2001), and it has a better performance than the TST in detecting active TB (Ozekinci et al., 2007).

In addition, T-SPOT.TB detects specific T cells at frequencies as low as 1 cell per 300,000 bystander cells (Heeger et al., 2001), making the assay very sensitive for detecting immune responses even in immunosuppressed individuals actively or latently infected, in very young children, in those on anti-TNF-α treatment, in transplant and renal dialysis patients, and in pregnant women (Gebauer et al., 2002; Piana et al., 2007).

Therefore, although QFT-G has some advantages over T-SPOT.TB; for instance, it is relatively easy to perform, requires fewer steps and less-expensive equipment—which makes it more suitable for "on-filed" usage in settings with limited resources—it has been shown in different reports to be less sensitive than the T-SPOT.TB assay (Adetifa et al., 2007). It is notable that the INF-γ release assays may vary in different populations depending on various factors, including genetic background, disease epidemiology, prevalence of HIV infection, exposure to environmental mycobacteria that have similar antigens, malnutrition, and other factors (Pai et al., 2004; Dinnes et al., 2007).

3.2.2 Interferon-gamma release assays: A tool to monitor TB chemotherapy

The response of INF-γ-producing T-cells in INF-γ release assays might be related to bacterial load (Hill et al., 2005); therefore, it could be used as a quantitative surrogate marker to monitor TB chemotherapy and drug efficacy during treatment, progression, or relapses (Komiya et al., 2011; Takayanagi et al., 2011; Ribeiro et al., 2009). In addition, a strong association between the T-SPOT.TB score and the degree of sputum positivity in patients has been reported (Oni et al., 2010).

It has been suggested that INF-γ release assays can provide useful, accurate, and rapid support in the diagnosis of extra-pulmonary TB (Lai et al., 2011; Patel et al., 2010; Lai et al., 2010). Although INF-γ release assays have higher sensitivity and specificity than conventional methods, further studies are needed to evaluate their role in diagnosing children and extra-pulmonary TB infections, especially in high TB-endemic settings (Amdekar et al., 2010).

3.2.3 A comparison of the interferon-gamma release assays with the tuberculin skin test

Both INF-γ release assays (QuantiFERON and T-SPOT.TB)are beginning to replace the TST, and both assays have been approved recently for clinical use in the United States, Europe, and Japan (FDA, 2005; Lalvani, Pathan, 2001). It has been shown that the INF-γ release assays have many advantages over the TSTs in the diagnosis of active as well as latent TB, especially in low-TB-endemic countries (Pai et al., 2004; Dinnes et al., 2007; Fukazawa, 2007; Kang et al., 2007; Ozekinic et al., 2007; Bartu et al., 2008; (Harada et al., 2008; Kabeer et al., 2010; Pia et al., 2008; Diel et al., 2009; Park et al., 2009; Toshiyama et al., 2010; Latorre et al., 2009). Since both assays are specific to Mtb and are not affected by previous exposure to environmental mycobacteria or vaccination with BCG, they have greater specificity and sensitivity than the TST in the diagnosis of latent TB in adults (Ewer et al., 2003; Shams et al., 2005; Kang et al., 2005).

In the majority of studies that compare the performance of INF-γ release assays with TSTs, INF-γ release assays seem to be significantly more accurate than TSTs and have poor agreement with it (I mean the TST), for the diagnosis of active or latent TB, in both immunocompetent or HIV-infected individuals (Rangaka et al., 2007; Mandalakas et al., 2008; Stephan et al., 2008; Jiang et al., 2009; Cağlayan et al., 2011; Cesur et al., 2010). In fact, moderate to poor diagnostic agreement between the different INF-γ release assays tests themselves has been observed (Richeldi et al., 2009; Talati et al., 2009; Latorre et al., 2010).

Nevertheless, determining the accuracy of either one of the INF-γ release assay tests to detect latent infections presents a challenge, because there is no gold standard available (Newton et al., 2008), and the only criteria that can be used is the patient's history of exposure to the disease (if known). Therefore, the accuracy and reliability of the estimated number of the global latent TB cases remains uncertain (Wiker et al., 2010). When INF-γ release assays were compared with TSTs in different longitudinal studies, INF-γ release assays may have a higher predictive value regarding the development of future TB, and unlike the TST, the INF-γ release assays (QFTGIT) results are not affected by gender or age of participants (Bakir et al., 2008; Legesse et al., 2011). Nevertheless, the decision to use INF-γ release assays instead of TSTs is often based on country guidelines and resource and logistics considerations (Cattamanchi et al., 2011).

3.2.4 The indeterminate response of interferon-gamma release assays

All INF-γ release assays are designed to include mitogen stimulation of tested cells as a positive control, along with the different TB-specific antigens used in the tests, to measure the ability of the harvested cells to produce INF-γ; when cells from tested individuals fail to respond sufficiently to either TB-specific antigens or, more specifically to the used mitogen control, the results are considered indeterminate. The indeterminate response can be explained by an error in specimen collection and handling or by the performance of the assay or T-cell anergy, which result in an inadequate response (Papay et al., 2011; Kobashi et al., 2009).

Among the different forms of the INF-γ release assays, QFT-IT has a lower rate of indeterminate results compared with T-Spot.TB, because of the simplicity of the in-tube form, which does not require as many steps as T-Spot.TB, and the fact that there is no storage of blood. T cells interact with antigens as soon as blood is collected into the QFT tubes, minimizing the potential loss of activity during storage of blood specimen.

Differences in indeterminate results have been observed among the different INF-γ release assay tests given to children; with children, both QFT-G and QFT-IT (ELISA-based assays) are significantly more affected by indeterminate results than T-SPOT.TB (ELISPOT-based assay) (Bergamini et al., 2009). These indeterminate results can be minimized by applying the assays after acute inflammation is resolved; this later application also reduces the cost of retesting (Zrinski et al., 2011).

3.2.5 Interferon-gamma release assays and detection of TB in children

Uncertainty about the sensitivity of INF-γ release assays to detect TB in children remains an issue; the use of INF-γ release assays to detect active and latent TB infection in children, seem to perform differently. Some studies have shown that the QFT-IT has a high sensitivity and less indeterminate rates in nonimmunosuppressed children of all age groups (from 1 month to 18 years old) (Zrinski et al., 2011). However, others have shown that both forms of QuantiFERON-TB tests (QFT-G and QFT-IT) were less sensitive and can give more indeterminate results than T-SPOT.TB in children younger than 4 years old (Bergamini et al., 2009; Nicol et al., 2009; Takamatsu, 2008).

It is a priority to detect and contain the disease in this age group. Because young children have a higher chance of developing active TB than older children, as a consequence of an impaired T-cell response (Lewinsohn et al., 2004), the American Academy of Pediatrics has recently recommended that the TST continue to be used to diagnose TB in children younger than 5 years old, and that INF-γ release assays be used for children older than 5 years old (Starke, 2009; Mazurek et al., 2010). However, because of the high risk in the 5-and-under age group, it has been suggested that both tests (QFT and the TST) be used in combination, whenever it is possible. This combination of tests would improve the diagnosis of TB, and the child would be considered infected if either or both are positive (Debord et al., 2011; Pavic et al., 2011). Other studies with children older than five, HIV-infected children, or nonimmunosuppressed children, indicated that indeterminate results with QFT-G, QFT-IT, or T-SPOT.TB—were undetected or uncommon (Bergamini et al., 2009; Mandalakas et al., 2008; Tsiouris et al., 2006).

The variation in the level of cytokines (INF- γ and IL-2) released by cells after stimulation with QFT antigens in children, is age dependent; it can identify those children with latent TB who are younger than 5 years old from those older than 5 years old (Lighter-Fisher et al., 2010).

3.2.6 Interferon-gamma release assays for testing TB in children with cancer

Both the TST and the INF-γ release assays were used to detect TB in children with cancer before their initial chemotherapy. All tests performed suboptimally, and therefore none of them can be used individually to confirm or disprove TB infection (Stefan et al., 2010).

3.2.7 Interferon-gamma release assays and screening for latent TB

In adult patients, latent TB can be detected more effectively with INF-γ release assays than with the TST; QFT-G and QFT-IT can be used for diagnosis and T-SPOT.TB for exclusion (Chang & Leung 2010). However, in some settings, both tests are used to screen for TB (Torres Costa et al., 2011; Katsenos et al., 2011).

Although INF-γ release assays are affected by cellular immune statutes and age, they demonstrate low agreement with the TST and perform better in detecting latent TB in adult patients (Santín Cerezales 2011; Zhao et al., 2011). Both of the INF-γ release assays (T-SPOT.TB and QFT) require only a single patient visit, and the test results are available within 24 hours (Hill et al., 2004; Richeldi et al., 2004).

The Centers for Disease Control and Prevention, USA, recommend that INF-γ release assays can replace the TST (single screening strategy) in all settings (Mazurek et al., 2005). However, recent UK TB guidelines advise screening for latent TB using the TST, followed by INF-γ release assays if the TST is positive (dual screening) (Leyten et al., 2007; Sauzullo et al., 2011; Dosanjh et al., 2008;148: Ritz et al., 2011). The dual screening strategy has been reported to be more cost-effective than the single screening strategy (INF-γ release assay or TST alone) for screening latent TB; however this conclusion and the interpretation of results is relative to the prevalence of TB in the setting as well as the length of contact with the infection (Pooran et al., 2010).

3.2.8 Drawbacks of interferon-gamma release assays

One limitation of the INF-γ release assays is that they are inconsistent in detecting TB in HIV patients. Some reports indicate that they are not the best tools for diagnosing TB among HIV-infected individuals with advanced immunodeficiency diseases, because of low sensitivity resulting from the low T-cell count (Chen et al., 2011). However, other studies reported that the sensitivity of the T-SPOT.TB assay in detecting TB in active HIV disease may be not highly impaired by advanced immunosuppression (Oni et al., 2010).

Another limitation of INF-γ release assays is their inability to distinguish active from past-treated TB infections (Kim et al., 2011; (Kim et al., 2010). The role of INF-γ release assays to distinguish between latent TB and active TB and their predictive ability of the progression of latent TB to active TB infection needs to be studied further, especially in high-burden settings (Dheda et al., 2009). Therefore, although INF-γ release assays have been approved in many countries to diagnose latent TB, especially in adults, this test still has little clinical value in the diagnosis of active TB (Dominguez et al., 2009). Nevertheless, growing evidence supports the idea that recruiting Mtb-specific T cells in active TB from fluids at the "local" sites of infection, such as pleural effusion (Wilkinson et al., 2005; Barnes et al., 1993; Barnes et al., 1989), cerebrospinal fluid (Thomas et al., 2008), ascites (Wilkinson et al., 2005), pericardial fluid (Biglino et al., 2008), and bronchoalveolar lavage (BAL) (Jafari et al., 2006; Jafari et al., 2009) is more effective than blood, in the diagnosis of extra-pulmonary TB. In this way the INF-γ release assays are looking at the "local " site of infection rather than "systemic" Mtb-specific immune response in blood, which may only provide background information about effector memory T-cells in active TB. This provides a promising approach to distinguish active TB from latent TB in routine clinical practice (Jafari et al., 2009).

The cut-off values currently recommended by the manufacturers are being disputed in some studies (Soysal et al., 2008). Consideration of new (low) cut-off values for both T-SPOT.TB and QFT, which may improve the assays' sensitivity, are now recommended, especially in intermediate- and high-endemic areas of TB and HIV (Soysal et al., 2008; Kanunfre et al., 2008; Legesse et al., 2010). The relative complexity of the INF-γ release assays can result in technical errors at many levels, resulting from insufficient cells, reduced cells activated due to prolonged transport or storage of blood, improper handling of specimens, the presence of INF-γ antibodies, and the incorrect addition of mutagen. Any of these technical problems can contribute to the invalidity and inaccuracy (unusual INF-γ measurements) of the test results, adding to its potential disadvantages (Kampmann et al., 2005; Powell et al., 2011).

The level of complexity mentioned above in addition to the requirement for special equipment, skilled laboratory personnel, and the high cost of the INF-γ release assays are among the limitations of the assays, which should be strongly considered, especially in low-resources settings. INF-γ release assays are recommended for use as a confirmation tool when a patient with negative TST is suspected of having TB, or to exclude a positive TST result from BCG vaccination (Sun et al., 2010).

3.2.9 Interferon-gamma release assays and detection of TB in patients with immune-mediated inflammatory diseases

Studies involving immune-mediated inflammatory diseases (such as psoriasis, rheumatoid arthritis, etc.) indicated that INF-γ release assays are superior to the TST for detecting latent TB in both endemic and non-endemic areas (Ponce de Leon et al., 2005; Ponce de Leon et al., 2008; Sellam et al., 2007; Murakami et al., 2009; de Andrade et al., 2011).

Since most of the information on the performance of INF-γ release assays have been gathered from studies done in developed countries, it is important that further research on adults and children be done in developing countries where TB is endemic. These studies should include the presence of additional factors that have been reported to cause false negative results as high as 35.5 percent; these factors include HIV infection, malnutrition, impaired immune status, age, and the different ethnic backgrounds of patients (Pai et al., 2006; Menzies et al., 2007; Im et al., 1991; Landis & Koch, 1977; Legesse et al., 2010; Legesse et al., 2011 Apr 9;11:89).

Despite the progress that has been made in studying the use of INF-γ release assays, additional research is still required to study further the limitations of the assays and the ways to overcome them to improve the best utility of the tests in diagnosing and controlling TB (Lalvani & Pareek 2010; Mazurek et al., 2010).

4. Conclusions

Despite the continued research to identify the key Mtb antigens and biomarkers for developing the ideal diagnostic test, there is not yet a rapid, reliable, and economical method to diagnose both active and latent TB. The importance of diagnosing latent TB is often overshadowed in many parts of the world; however, it is key to controlling the spread of infection. In the last few years, new tests have been developed based on significant advances in understanding the genomic and immunology of Mtb. The new tests include the nucleic acid amplification test, QuantiFERON-TB and T-SPOT.TB, which have the advantages of higher specificity and sensitivity than the conventional tests—important for physicians so that they can avoid the inappropriate treatment of false-positive vaccinated individuals. Yet these new tests have disadvantages as well, including cost, training, and complexity. None of the available microbiological or immunological tests alone can accurately confirm the TB infection, while waiting for the culture results which can take weeks. Given the global burden of this disease, and its potential to spread rapidly, the importance of developing a novel assay or improving the existing methods for TB detection, active and latent, has never been greater.

5. References

Abebe F, Holm-Hansen C, Wiker HG, & Bjune G. (2007). Progress in serodiagnosis of M. tuberculosis infection. *Scand J Immuno*, 66: 176-191

Adams LV, Waddell RD, & Von Reyn CF. T-SPOT. (2008). TB Test(R) results in adults with Mycobacterium avium complex pulmonary disease. *Scand J Infect Dis,* 40(3): 196-203

Adetifa IM, Lugos MD, & Hammond A, et al. (2007). Comparison of two interferon gamma release assays in the diagnosis of Mycobacterium tuberculosis infection and disease in The Gambia. *BMC Infectious Diseases*, 7: 122

Akcay A, Erdem Y, & Altun B, et al. (2003). The booster phenomenon in 2-step tuberculin skin testing of patients receiving long-term hemodialysis. *Am J Infect Control,* 31(6): 371-374

Alonso V, Paul R, Barrera L, & Ritacco V. (2007). False diagnosis of tuberculosis by culture. *Medicina (B Aires),* 67(3): 287-294

Amdekar YK. (2010). How to optimize current (available) diagnostic tests. *Indian J Pediatr,* Mar; 78(3): 340-4

American Thoracic Society. (2000). Diagnostic standards and classification of tuberculosis in adults and children. *Am J Respir Crit Care Med*, 161: 1376-1395

Andersen P, Munk ME, Pollock JM, & Doherty TM. (2000). Specific immune-based diagnosis of tuberculosis. *Lancet*, 356: 1099-1104

Angeby KA, Hoffner SE, & Diwan VK. (2004). Should the 'bleach microscopy method' be recommended for improved case detection of tuberculosis? Literature review and key person analysis. *Int J Tuberc Lung Dis,* 8: 806–815

Anil P. (1995). Tuberculosis: a snap shot picture. *Health Millions*, 21(1): 8-9

Annam V, Karigoudar MH, & Yelikar BR. (2009). Indian J Pathol Microbiol. Improved microscopical detection of acid-fast bacilli by the modified bleach method in lymphnode aspirates. *Indian J Pathol Microbiol*, Jul-Sep; 52(3): 349-52

API Consensus Expert Committee. (2006). API TB Consensus Guidelines 2006: Management of pulmonary tuberculosis, extra-pulmonary tuberculosis, and tuberculosis in special situations. *J Assoc Physicians India,* 54: 219-234

Araujo Z, Waard JH, & Fernandez de Larrea C, et al. (2004). Study of the antibody response against Mycobacterium tuberculosis antigens in Warao Amerindian children in Venezuela. *Mem Inst Oswaldo Cruz*, 99: 517-524

Aris EA, Bakari M, Chonde TM, Kitinya J, Swai AB. (1999). Diagnosis of tuberculosis in sputum negative patients in Dar es Salaam. *East Afr Med J,* 76(11): 630-634

ATS MMWR Recommendations Report. (2000). Targeted tuberculin testing and treatment of latent tuberculosis infection. *MMWR,* 49 (PR6): 1-51

Attallah AM, Osman S, & Saad A, et al. (2005). Application of a circulating antigen detection immunoassay for laboratory diagnosis of extra-pulmonary and pulmonary tuberculosis. *Clin Chim Acta*, 356(1-2): 58-66

Baba K, Pathak S, & Sviland L, et al. (2008). Real-time quantitative PCR in the diagnosis of tuberculosis in formalin-fixed paraffin-embedded pleural tissue in patients from a high HIV endemic area. *Diagn Mol Pathol*, 17(2), 112-117

Babayiğit Hocaoğlu A, Olmez Erge D, Anal O, Makay B, Uzuner N, & Karaman O. (2011). Characteristics of children with positive tuberculin skin test. *Tuberk Toraks*, Jun; 59(2): 158-63

Bakir M, Millington KA, Soysal A, et al. (2008). Prognostic value of a T-cell-based, interferon-γ biomarker in children with tuberculosis contact. *Ann Intern Med*, 149 (11): 777- 87

Barnes PF, Lu S, Abrams JS, Wang E, Yamamura M, & Modlin RL. (1993). Cytokine production at the site of disease in human tuberculosis. *Infect Immun*, 61: 3482–9

Barnes PF, Mistry SD, Cooper CL, Pirmez C, Rea TH, & Modlin RL. (1989). Compartmentalization of a CD4+ T lymphocyte subpopulation in tuberculous pleuritis. *J Immunol*, 142: 1114–1119

Barnes PF. (1997). Rapid diagnostic tests for tuberculosis: progress but no gold standard. *Am J Respir Crit Care Med*, 155: 1497-8

Barrett-Connor E. (1979). The epidemiology of tuberculosis in physicians. *JAMA*, 241: 33–38

Bartu V, Havelkova M, & Kopecka E. (2008). QuantiFERON-TB Gold in the diagnosis of active tuberculosis. *J Int Med Res*, 36: 434–437

Behr MA, Wilson MA, & Gill WP, et al. (1999). Comparative genomic of BCG vaccines by whole-genome DNA microarrays. *Science*, 284: 1520-3

Bergamini BM, Losi M, Vaienti F, D'Amico R, Meccugni B, Meacci M, De Giovanni D, Rumpianesi F, Fabbri LM, Balli F, & Richeldi L. (2009). Performance of commercial blood tests for the diagnosis of latent tuberculosis infection in children and adolescents. *Pedatrics*, Mar; 123(3): e419-24

Biglino A, Crivelli P, Concialdi E, Bolla C, & Montrucchio G. (2008). Clinical usefulness of elispot assay on pericardial fluid in a case of suspected tuberculous pericarditis. *Infection*, 36:601–604

Bochme C, Molokova E, Minja F, Geis S, & Loscher T, et al. (2005). Detection of mycobacterial lipoarabinomannan with an antigen-capture ELISA in unprocessed urine of Tanzanian patients with suspected tuberculosis. *Trans R Soc Trop Med Hyg*, 99: 893–900

Boloursaz MR, Khalilzadeh S, Baghaie N, Khodayari AA, & Velayati AA. (2010). Radiologic manifestation of pulmonary tuberculosis in children admitted in pediatric ward-Massih Daneshvari Hospital: a 5-year retrospective study. *Acta Med Iran*, Jul-Aug; 48(4): 244-9

Bonnet M, Gagnidze L, Githui W, Guérin PJ, Bonte L, Varaine F, Ramsay A. (2011). Performance of LED-based fluorescence microscopy to diagnose tuberculosis in a peripheral health centre in Nairobi. *Int J Tuberc Lung Dis*, Jan; 15(1): 14-23

Bonnet M, Gagnidze L, Guerin PJ, Bonte L, Ramsay A, Githui W, & Varaine F. (2011). Evaluation of Combined LED-Fluorescence Microscopy and Bleach Sedimentation for Diagnosis of Tuberculosis at Peripheral Health Service Level. PLoS One. 2011;6(5):e20175. Epub 2011 May 31

Bonnet M, Ramsay A, Varaine F, Githui W, & Gagnidze L, et al. (2007). Reducing the number of sputa examined, and thresholds for positivity: an opportunity to optimize smear microscopy. *Int J Tuber Lung Dis,* 11: 953–958

Boom WH. (1996). The role of T-cell subsets in mycobacterium tuberculosis infection. *Infect Agents Dis,* 5(2): 73-81

Brock I, Ruhwald M, Lundgren B, Westh H, Mathiesen LR, & Ravn P. Latent tuberculosis in HIV positive, diagnosed by the M. tuberculosis specific interferon-gamma test. *Respir Res,* 7:56

Brodin P, de Jonge MI, & Majlessi L, et al. (2005). Functional analysis of early secreted antigenic target 6, the dominant T-cell antigen of M. tuberculosis, reveals key residues involved in secretion, complex formation, virulence and immunogenicity. *J Biol Chem,* 280(40): 33953-9

Brown TJ, Power EG, & French GL. (1999). Evaluation of three commercial detection systems for Mycobacterium tuberculosis where clinical diagnosis is difficult. *J Clin Pathol,* 52: 193-7

Bukhary ZA, & Alrajhi AA. (2004). Extrapulmonary tuberculosis, clinical presentation and outcome. *Saudi Med J,* 25: 881-885

Cağlayan V, Ak O, Dabak G, Damadoğlu E, Ketenci B, Ozdemir M, Ozer S, & Saygı A. (2011). Comparison of tuberculin skin testing and QuantiFERON-TB Gold-In Tube test in health care workers. *Tuberk Toraks,* 59(1): 43-7

Cambanis A, Ramsay A, Wirkom V, Tata E, & Cuevas LE. (2007). Investing time inmicroscopy: an opportunity to optimise smear-based case detection of tuberculosis. *Int J Tuberc Lung Dis,* 11: 40–45

Capelozzi VL, Faludi EP, Balthazar AB, Fernezlian SD, Filho JV, & Parra ER. (2011). Bronchoalveolar lavage improves diagnostic accuracy in patients with diffuse lung disease. *Diagn Cytopathol,* Jun 14; doi: 10.1002/dc.21743. [Epub ahead of print]

Cartuyvels R, de Ridder C, Jonckheere S, Verbist L, & van Eldere J. (1996). Prospective clinical evaluation of Amplicor Mycobacterium tuberculosis PCR test as a screening method in a low-prevalence population. *J Clin Microbiol,* 34: 2001-2003

Cashmore TJ, Peter JG, van Zyl-Smit RN, Semple PL, Maredza A, Meldau R, Zumla A, Nurse B, & Dheda K. (2010). Feasibility and diagnostic utility of antigen-specific interferon-gamma responses for rapid immunodiagnosis of tuberculosis using induced sputum. *PLoS One,* Apr 28; 5(4): e10389

Cattamanchi A, Huang L, Worodria W, den Boon S, Kalema N, Katagira W, Byanyima P, Yoo S, Matovu J, Hopewell PC, & Davis JL. (2011). Integrated strategies to optimize sputum smear microscopy: a prospective observational study. *Am J Respir Crit Care Med,* Feb 15; 183(4): 547-51. Epub 2010 Sep 17

Cattamanchi A, Smith R, Steingart KR, Metcalfe JZ, Date A, Coleman C, Marston BJ, Huang L, Hopewell PC, & Pai M. (2011). Interferon-gamma release assays for the diagnosis of latent tuberculosis infection in HIV-infected individuals: a systematic review and meta-analysis. *J Acquir Immune Defic Syndr,* Mar 1; 56(3): 230-8.

Caws M, Tho DQ, & Duy PM, et al. (2007). PCR-restriction fragment length polymorphism for rapid, low-cost identification of isoniazid-resistant Mycobacterium tuberculosis. *J Clin Microbiol*, 45(6): 1789-1793

Cengiz K, Seker A. (2006). Boosted tuberculin skin testing in hemodialysis patients. *Am J Infect Control*, 34(6): 383-387

Cesur S, Hoca NT, Tarhan G, Cimen F, Ceyhan I, Annakkaya AN, Aslan T, & Birengel S. (2010). Evaluation of Quantiferon-TB Gold and tuberculin skin test in patients with tuberculosis, close contact of patients, health care workers and tuberculosis laboratory personnel. *Mikrobiyol Bul*, Oct; 44(4):553-60

Chakravorty S, Sen MK, & Tyagi JS. (2005). Diagnosis of extrapulmonary tuberculosis by smear, culture, and PCR using universal sample processing technology. *J Clin Microbiol,* 43(9): 4357-62

Chang KC, Leung CC. (2010). Systematic review of interferon-gamma release assays in tuberculosis: focus on likelihood ratios. *Thorax*, Mar; 65(3): 271-6

Chaparas SD, Vandiviere HM, Melvin I, Koch G, & Becker C. (1985). Tuberculin test: Variability with the Mantoux procedure. *Am Rev Respir Dis*, 132: 175-177

Chaturvedi V, Gupta HP. (2001). Evaluation of integral membrane antigens of M. habana for serodiagnosis of extrapulmonary tuberculosis: association between levels of antibodies and M. tuberculosis antigens. *FEMS Immunol Med Microbiol*, 33: 1-7

Chedore P, Broukhanski G, Shainhouse Z, & Jamieson F. (2006). False-positive amplified Mycobacterium tuberculosis direct test results for samples containing Mycobacterium leprae. *J Clin Microbiol*, 44(2): 612-3

Chen J, Sun J, Zhang R, Liu L, Zheng Y, Shen Y, Wang Z, Sun F, Li L, & Lu H. (2011). T-SPOT.TB in the diagnosis of active tuberculosis among HIV-infected patients with advanced immunodeficiency. *AIDS Res Human Retroviruses,* Mar; 27(3): 289-94. Epub 2010 Oct 26).

Chiang IH, Suo J, & Bai KJ, et al. (1997). Serodiagnosis of tuberculosis. A study comparing three specific mycobacterial antigens. *Am J Respir Crit Care Med*, 156: 906-911

Chien HP, Yu MC, Wu MH, Lin TP, & Luh KT. (2000). Comparison of the BACTEC MGIT 960 with Lǫwenstein-Jensen medium for recovery of mycobacteia from clinical specimens. *Int J Tuberc Lung Dis*, 4: 866–870

Chihota VN, Grant AD, Fielding K, Ndibongo B, van Zyl A, Muirhead D, & Churchyard GJ. (2010). Liquid vs. solid culture for tuberculosis: performance and cost in a resource-constrained setting. *Int J Tuberc Lung Dis,* Aug; 14(8): 1024-31

Cho SN, Brennan PJ. (2007). Tuberculosis: diagnostics. *Tuberculosis (Edinb)*, 87(Suppl 1): S14-17

Clark SA, Martin SL, & Pozniak A, et al. (2007). Tuberculosis antigen-specific immune responses can be detected using enzyme-linked immunospot technology in human immunodeficiency virus (HIV)-1 patients with advanced disease. *Clin Exp Immunol,* 150(2): 238-44

Cohn DL. (2000). Treatment of Latent Tuberculosis Infection: Renewed Opportunity for Tuberculosis Control. *Clin Infect Dis*, 31(1): 120-124

Coll P, Garrigó M, Moreno C, & Martí N. (2003). Routine use of Gen-Probe Amplified Mycobacterium Tuberculosis Direct (MTD) test for detection of Mycobacterium tuberculosis with smear-positive and smear-negative specimens. *Int J Tuberc Lung Dis*, 7: 886-891

Comstock GW, Liveasy VT, & Woolpert SF. (1974). The Prognosis of a positive tuberculin reaction in childhood and adolescence. *Am J Epidemiol*, 99: 131-13

Corbett EL, Charalambous S, Moloi VM, Fielding K, Grant AD, Dye C, De Cock KM, Hayes RJ, Williams BG, & Churchyard GJ. (2004). Human immunodeficiency virus and the prevalence of undiagnosed tuberculosis in African gold miners. *Am J Respir Crit Care Med*, 170: 673–679

Corbett EL, Watt CJ, & Walker N, et al. (2003). The growing burden of tuberculosis: global trends and interactions with the HIV epidemic. *Arch Intern Med*, 163: 1009-21

Dacso CC. (1990). Skin Testing for Tuberculosis, In: *Clinical Methods: The history, PHISICAL, AND laboratory Examinations (3rd Edition),* Walker HK, Hail WD, & Hurst JW, editors. Boston: Butterworths

Daley P, Thomas S, & Pai M. (2007). Nucleic acid amplification tests for the diagnosis of tuberculous lymphadenitis: a systemic review. *Int J Tuberc Lung Dis*, 11(11): 1166-1176

Daniel TM, De Murillo GL, & Sawyer JA, et al. (1986). Field evaluation of enzyme-linked immunosorbent assay for the serodiagnosis of tuberculosis. *Am Rev Respir Dis*, 134: 662-5

Daniel TM. (1987). New approaches to the rapid diagnosis of tuberculosis meningitis. *J Infect Dis*, 155(4): 599-602

Daniel TM. (1990). The rapid diagnosis of tuberculosis: a selective review. *J Lab Clin Med*, 116:277-282

Davids V, HanekomWA, Mansoor N, Gamieldien H, & Gelderbloem SJ, et al. (2006) The effect of bacille Calmette-Guerin vaccine strain and route of administration on induced immune responses in vaccinated infants. *J Infect Dis*, 193: 531–536

Davis JL, Huang L, Worodria W, Masur H, Cattamanchi A, Huber C, Miller C, Conville PS, Murray P, & Kovacs JA. (2011). Nucleic acid amplification tests for diagnosis of smear-negative TB in a high HIV-prevalence setting: a prospective cohort study. *PLoS One*, Jan 27; 6(1): e1632

de Andrade Lima E, de Andrade Lima M, Barros de Lorena VM, de Miranda Gomes Y, Lupi O, & Benard G. (2011). Evaluation of an IFN-gamma Assay in the Diagnosis of Latent Tuberculosis in Patients with Psoriasis in a Highly Endemic Setting. Acta Derm Venereol. 2011 Jun 1. doi: 10.2340/00015555-1151.

Debord C, De Lauzanne A, Gourgouillon N, Guérin-El Khourouj V, Pédron B, Gaudelus J, Faye A, & Sterkers G. (2011). Interferon-gamma Release Assay Performance for Diagnosing Tuberculosis Disease in 0- to 5-year-old Children. *Pediatr Infect Dis J*, Jun 20

Demkow U, Filewska M, & Michalowska-Mitczuk D, et al. (2007). Heterogeneity of antibody response to myobacterial antigens in different clinical manifestations of pulmonary tuberculosis. *J Physiol Pharmacol*, 58(Suppl 5): S117-127

Dheda K, Davids V, Lenders L, Roberts T, Meldau R, Ling D, Brunet L, van Zyl Smit R, Peter J, Green C, Badri M, Sechi L, Sharma S, Hoelscher M, Dawson R, Whitelaw A, Blackburn J, Pai M, & Zumla A. (2010). Clinical utility of a commercial LAM-ELISA assay for TB diagnosis in HIV-infected patients using urine and sputum samples. *PLoS One*, Mar 24; 5(3): e9848

Dheda K, Smit RZ, Badri M, & Pai M. (2009). T-cell interferon-gamma release assays for the rapid immunodiagnosis of tuberculosis: clinical utility in high-burden vs. low-burden settings. *Curr Opin Pulm Med*, 15: 188–200

Dheda K, Van-Zyl Smit RN, Sechi LA, Badri M, & Meldau R, et al. Clinical diagnostic utility of IP-10 and LAM antigen levels for the diagnosis of tuberculous pleural effusions in a high burden setting. *PLoS One*, 4: e4689

Diacon AH, Maritz JS, Venter A, van Helden PD, Andries K, McNeeley DF, & Donald PR. (2010). Time to detection of the growth of Mycobacterium tuberculosis in MGIT 960 for determining the early bactericidal activity of antituberculosis agents. *Eur J Clin Microbiol Infect Dis*, Dec; 29(12): 1561-5. Epub 2010 Sep 4

Diel R, Loddenkemper R, Meywald-Walter K, Gottschalk R, & Nienhaus A. (2009). Comparative performance of tuberculin skin test, QuantiFERON-TB-Gold In Tube assay, and T-Spot.TB test in contact investigations for tuberculosis. *Chest*, 135(4): 1010–1018. doi: 10.1378/chest.08-2048)

Dinnes J, Deeks J, Kunst H, Gibson A, Cummins E, Waugh N, Drobniewski F, & Lalvani A. (2007). A systematic review of rapid diagnostic tests for the detection of tuberculosis. *Health Technol Assess*, 11(3): 1-196

Dogan E, Erkoc R, Sayarlioglu H, & Uzun K. (2005). Tuberculin skin test results and booster phenomenon in two-step tuberculin skin testing in hemodialysis patients. *Ren Fail*, 27(4): 425-8

Dominguez J, De Souza-Galvao M, Ruiz-Manzano J, Latorre I, Prat C, Lacoma A, Mila C, Jimenez MA, Blanco S, & Maldonado J, et al. (2009). T-cell responses to the mycobacterium tuberculosis-specific antigens in active tuberculosis patients at the beginning, during, and after antituberculosis treatment. *Diagn Microbiol Infect Dis*, 63:43–51

Dosanjh DP, Hinks TS, Innes JA, Deeks JJ, & Pasvol G, et al. (2008). Improved diagnostic evaluation of suspected tuberculosis. *Ann Intern Med*, 148:325–336

Dowdy DW, O'Brien MA, & Bishai D. (2008). Cost-effectiveness of novel diagnostic tools for the diagnosis of tuberculosis. *Int J Tuberc Lung Dis*, 12: 1021–1029

El-Masry S, El-Kady I, Zaghloul MH, Al-Badrawey MK. (2008). Rapid and simple detection of a mycobacterium circulating antigen in serum of pulmonary tuberculosis patients by using a monoclonal antibody and Fast-Dot-ELISA. *Clin Biochem*, 41(3): 145-151

Elliott AM, Halwiindi B, Hayes RJ, Luo N, & Tembo G, et al. (1993) The impact of human immunodeficiency virus on presentation and diagnosis of tuberculosis in a cohort study in Zambia. *J Trop Med Hyg*, 96: 1–113

Escamilla L, Mancilla R, Glender W, & López-Marín LM. (1996). Mycobacterium fortuitum glycolipids for the serodiagnosis of pulmonary tuberculosis. *Am J Respir Crit Care Med*, 154: 1864-1867

Ewer K, Deeks J, & Alvarez L, et al. (2003). A comparison of T-cell-based assay with tuberculin skin test for diagnosis of Mycobacterium tuberculosis infection in a school tuberculosis outbreak. *Lancet*, 361:1168-1173

Farhat M, Greenaway C, Pai M, & Menzies D. (2006). False-positive tuberculin skin tests: what is the absolute effect of BCG and non-tuberculous mycobacteria? *Int J Tuberc Lung Dis,* Nov;10(11):1192-204

FDA. 2005. Approval for the use of synthetic peptide antigens used in the QuantiFERON-TB Gold. P10033/S0006 www.fda.gov/cdrh/pma/pmadec04.html

Fine PEM. (1995). Variation in protection by BCG: implications of and for heterologous immunity. *Lancet,* 346: 1339-1345

Flynn JL, Chan J, Triebold KJ, Dalton DK, Stewart TA, & Bloom BR. (1993). An essential role for interferon-gamma resistance to mycobacterium tuberculosis infection. *J Exp Med,* 178: 2249-54

Franco-Álvarez de Luna F, Ruiz P, Gutiérrez J, & Casal M. (2006). Evaluation of the GenoType Mycobacteria Direct assay for detection of Mycobacterium tuberculosis complex and four atypical mycobacterial species in clinical samples. *J Clin Microbiol,* 44:3025-7

Frieden TR, Sterling TR, Munsiff SS, Watt CJ, & Dye C. Tuberculosis. Lancet. 2003;362(9387):887–899. doi: 10.1016/S0140-6736(03)14333-4) (Rapid diagnostic tests for tuberculosis: what is the appropriate use? American Thoracic Society Workshop. Am J Respir Crit Care Med. 1997;155(5):1804–1814),

Fukazawa K. (2007). Application and problems of QuantiFERON TB-2G for tuberculosis control programs: (1) Tuberculosis outbreak in a Cram school. *Kekkaku,* 82(1): 53-59

Gallegos AM, Pamer EG, & Glickman MS. (2008). Delayed protection by ESAT-6-specific effector CD4+ cells after airborne M. tuberculosis infection. *J Exp Med,* 205(10): 2359-2368

Gangane N, Anshu, & Singh R. (2008). Role of modified bleach method in staining of acid-fast bacilli in lymph node aspirates. *Acta Cytol,* May-Jun;52(3):325-8

Gebauer BS, Hricik DE, & Atallah A, et al. (2002). Evolution of the enzyme-linked immunosorbent spot assay for post-transplant alloreactivity as a potentially useful immune monitoring tool. *Am J Transplant,* 2, 857-866

Gérôme P, Fabre M, Soler CP, De Pina JJ, Simon F. (2009). Comparison of the mycobacteria growth indicator tube with solid culture for the detection of tuberculosis complex mycobacteria from blood. *Pathol Biol (Paris),* Feb; 57(1): 44-50. Epub 2008 Jun 30

Goessens WHF, de Man P, Koeleman GM, Luijendijk A, te Witt R, Endtz HP, van & Belkum A. (2005). Comparison of the COBAS AMPLICOR MTB and BDProbeTec ET assays for detection of Mycobacterium tuberculosis in respiratory specimens. *J Clin Microbiol,* 43:2563-6

Goletti D, Butera O, Bizzoni F, Casetti R, Girardi E, & Poccia F. (2006). Region of difference 1 antigen-specific CD4+ memory T cells correlate with a favorable outcome of tuberculosis. *J Infect Dis,* 194(7), 984-92

Gounder CR, Kufa T, Wada NI, Mngomezulu V, Charalambous S, Hanifa Y, Fielding K, Grant A, Dorman S, Chaisson RE, & Churchyard GJ. (2011). Diagnostic accuracy of a urine lipoarabinomannan enzyme-linked immunosorbent assay for screening ambulatory HIV-infected persons for TB. *J Acquir Immune Defic Syndr,* ePub ahead of print on Jul 13

Guerra RL, Hooper NM, Baker JF, Alborz R, Armstrong DT, Maltas G, Kiehlbauch JA, & Dorman SE. (2007).Use of the amplified mycobacterium tuberculosis direct test in a public health laboratory: test performance and impact on clinical care. *Chest,* 132:946-951

Haldar S, Chakravorty S, Bhalla M, De Majumdar S, & Tyagi JS. (2007). Simplified detection of Mycobacterium tuberculosis in sputum using smear microscopy and PCR with molecular beacons. *J Med Microbiol,* 56, 1356-62

Hamasur B, Bruchfeld J, Haile M, Pawlowski A, & Bjorvatn B, et al. (2001). Rapid diagnosis of tuberculosis by detection of mycobacterial lipoarabinomannan in urine. *J Microbiol Methods,* 45:41–52

Han M, Yue J, Lian YY, Zhao YL, Wang HX, & Liu LR. (2011). Relationship between single nucleotide polymorphism of interleukin-18 and susceptibility to pulmonary tuberculosis in the Chinese Han population. *Microbiol Immunol,* Jun; 55(6): 388-93

Han YM, Kim HS, Kim CH, Kang HJ, & Lee KM. Analysis of patients with positive acid-fast bacilli culture and negative T-SPOT.TB results. *Korean J Lab Med,* Aug; 30(4): 414-9

Hanna BA, Ebrahimzadeh A, & Elliott LB, et al. (1999). Multicenter evaluation of the BACTEC MGIT 960 system for recovery of mycobacteria. *J Clin Microbiol,* 37: 748–52

Harada N, Higuchi K, Yoshiyama T, Kawabe Y, & Fujita A, et al. (2008). Comparison of the sensitivity and specificity of two whole blood interferon-gamma assays for M. tuberculosis infection. *J Infect,* 56: 348–353

Harada N. (2006). Characteristics of a diagnostic method for tuberculosis infection based on whole blood interferon-gamma assay. *Kekkaku,* 81(11): 681-6

Harboe M, Oettinger T, Wiker HG, Rosenkrands I, & Andersen P. (1996). Evidence for occurrence of the ESAT-6 protein in Mycobacterium tuberculosis and virulent Mycobacterium bovis and for its absence in Mycobacterium bovis BCG. *Infect Immun,* 64: 16-22

Harries AD, Maher D, & Nunn P. (1997). Practical and affordable measures for the protection of health care workers from tuberculosisin low-income countries. *Bull World Health Organ,* 75: 477–89

Harris A. (2004). What is the additional yield from repeated sputum examinations by microscopy and culture? In: *Tuberculosis Case detection. Treatment and monitoring. 2nd ed.* Frieden TR (Ed.), 46-50, World Health Organization, Geneva.

Heeger PS, Greenspan NS, Kuhlenschmidt S, Dejelo C, Hricik DE, & Schulak JA. (2001). Pretransplant frequency of donor-specific, IFN-gamma-producing lymphocytes is a manifestation of immunologic memory and correlates with the risk of posttransplant rejection episodes. *J Immunol,* 163: 2267-75

Hill PC, Brookes RH, & Fox A, et al. (2004). Large-scale evaluation of enzyme-linked immunospot assay and skin test for diagnosis of Mycobacterium tuberculosis infection against a gradient of exposure in the Gambia. *Clin Infect Dis,* 38(7): 966-73

Hill PC, Fox A, Jeffries DJ, Jackson-Sillah D, Lugos MD, & Owiafe PK, et al. (2005). Quantitative T cell assay reflects infectious load of Mycobacterium tuberculosis in an endemic case contact model. *Clin Infect Dis,* Jan 15; 40(2): 273–8

Hobby GL, Holman AP, Iseman MD, & Jones JM. (1973). Enumeration of tubercle bacilli in sputum of patients with pulmonary tuberculosis. *Antimicrob Agents Chemother,* 4(2), 94-104

Hofmann-Thiel S, Turaev L, & Hoffmann H. 2010. Evaluation of the hyplex TBC PCR test for detection of Mycobacterium tuberculosis complex in clinical samples. *BMC Microbiol,* 2010 Mar 31;10:95

Honscha G, Von Groll A, & Valença M, et al. (2008). The laboratory as a tool to qualify tuberculosis diagnosis. *Int J Tuberc Lung Dis,* 12(2): 218-20

Hooja S, Pal N, Malhotra B, Goyal S, Kumar V, & Vyas L. (2011). Comparison of Ziehl Neelsen & Auramine O staining methods on direct and concentrated smears in clinical specimens. *Indian J Tuberc,* Apr; 58(2): 72-6

Hooper CE, Lee YC, & Maskell NA. (2009). Interferon-gammarelease assays for the diagnosis of TB pleural effusions: hype or real hope? *Curr Opin Pulm Med,* 15 (4): 358-65

Houghton RL, Lodes MJ, & Dillon DC, et al. (2002). Use of multiepitope polyproteins in serodiagnosis of active tuberculosis. *Clin Diagn Lab Immunol,* 9: 883-91

Huebner RE, Schein MF, Bass JB Jr. The tuberculin skin test. Clin Infect Dis. 17(6), 968-975 (1993).

Im JG, Webb WR, Han MC, & Park JH. (1991). Apical opacity associated with pulmonary tuberculosis: high-resolution CT findings. *Radiology,* 178(3): 727–31

Imaz MS, Comini MA, & Zerbini E, et al. (2001). Evaluation of the diagnostic value of measuring IgG, IgM and IgA antibodies to the recombinant 16-kilodalton antigen of M. tuberculosis in childhood tuberculosis. *Int J Tuberc Lung Dis,* 5,1036-43 (2001).

International Union Against Tuberculosis and Lung Disease. (1996). *Tuberculosis Guide for Low Income Countries, 4th ed.* International Union Against Tuberculosis and Lung Disease, Paris.

Jafari C, Ernst M, Kalsdorf B, Greinert U, Diel R, Kirsten D, Marienfeld K, Lalvani A, & Lange C. (2006). Rapid diagnosis of smear-negative tuberculosis by bronchoalveolar lavage enzyme-linked immunospot. *Am J Respir Crit Care,*174:1048–54

Jafari C, Thijsen S, Sotgiu G, Goletti D, Domínguez Benítez JA, Losi M, Eberhardt R, Kirsten D, Kalsdorf B, Bossink A, Latorre I, Migliori GB, Strassburg A, Winteroll S, Greinert U, Richeldi L, Ernst M, & Lange C. (2009). Tuberculosis Network European Trialsgroup. Bronchoalveolar lavage enzyme-linked immunospot for a rapid diagnosis of tuberculosis: a Tuberculosis Network European Trialsgroup study. *Am J Respir Crit Care,* Oct 1; 180(7): 666-73. Epub 2009 Jul 9

Jiang W, Shao L, Zhang Y, Zhang S, Meng C, Xu Y, Huang L, Wang Y, Wang Y, Weng X, & Zhang W. (2009). High-sensitive and rapid detection of Mycobacterium tuberculosis infection by IFN-gamma release assay among HIV-infected individuals in BCG-vaccinated area. *BMC Immunol,* 10: 31

Joh JS, Lee CH, & Lee JE, et al. (2007).The interval between initiation of anti-tuberculosis treatment in patients with culture-positive pulmonary tuberculosis and receipt of drug-susceptibility test results. *J Korean Med Sci,* 22(1): 26-29

Kabeer BSA, Raman B, Thomas A, Perumal V, & Raja A. Role of QuantiFERON-TB Gold, Interferon Gamma Inducible Protein-10 and Tuberculin Skin Test in Active Tuberculosis Diagnosis. PLoS ONE. 2010;5:9051–7) (Pia M, Zwerling A, Menzies D. Systematic review: T-cell-based assays for the diagnosis of latent tuberculosis infections; an update. Ann Intern Med. 2008;149:177–184)

Kabra SK, Lodha R, & Seth V. (2004). Some current concepts on childhood tuberculosis. *Indian J Med Res*, 120(4): 387-97

Kadival GV, D'Souza CD, Kolk AH, & Samuel AM. (1995). Polymerase chain reaction in the diagnosis of tuberculosis. Comparison of two target sequences for amplification. *Zentralbl Bakteriol*, 282(4): 353-61

Kampmann B, Hemingway C, Stephens A, Davidson R, & Goodsall A, et al. (2005). Acquired predisposition to mycobacterial disease due to autoantibodies to IFN-gamma. *J Clin Invest*, 115:2480–8

Kampmann B, Whittaker E, Williams A, Walters S, Gordon A, Martinez-Alier N, Williams B, Crook AM, Hutton AM, & Anderson ST. (2009). Interferon-gamma release assays do not identify more children with active tuberculosis than tuberculin skin test, *Eur Respir J*, 33 (6), 1250-3

Kang YA, Lee HW, & Yoon HI, et al. (2005). Discrepancy between the tuberculin skin test and the whole-blood interferon gamma assay for diagnosis of latent tuberculosis infection in an intermediate tuberculosis-burden country. *JAMA*, 293: 2756-61

Kang YA, Lee, HW, & Hwang SS, et al. (2007). Usefulness of whole-blood interferon-gamma assay and interferon-gamma enzyme-linked immunospot assay in the diagnosis of active pulmonary tuberculosis. *Chest*, 132(3): 959-65

Kanunfre KA, Leite OH, Lopes MI, Litvoc M, & Ferreira AW. (2008). Enhancement of diagnostic efficiency by a gamma interferon release assay for pulmonary tuberculosis. *Clin Vaccine Immunol*,15(6): 1028-30

Katsenos S, Nikolopoulou M, Gartzonika C, Manda-Stachouli C, Gogali A, Grypaiou C, Mavridis A, Constantopoulos SH, & Daskalopoulos G. (2011). Use of interferon-gamma release assay for latent tuberculosis infection screening in older adults exposed to tuberculosis in a nursing home. *J Am Geriatr Soc*, May; 59(5): 858-62

Kawabe Y. (2007). Application and problems of quantiFERON TB-2G for tuberculosis control programs--(2) clinical use of quantiFERON TB-2G. *Kakkaku*, 82(1): 61-66

Kehinde AO, Obaseki FA, Cadmus SI, & Bakare RA. (2005). Diagnosis of tuberculosis: urgent need to strengthen laboratory services. *J Natl Med Assoc*, Mar;97(3):394-6

Kent PT, Kubica GP. (1985). Public health mycobacteriology: a guide for the level III laboratory. Atlanta, GA, USA: Centers for Disease Control, 1985).

Khawcharoenporn T, Apisarnthanarak A, Sungkanuparph S, Woeltje KF, Fraser VJ. (2011). Tuberculin skin test and isoniazid prophylaxis among health care workers in high tuberculosis prevalence areas. *Int J Tuberc Lung Dis*, Jan; 15(1): 14-23

Kibiki GS, Mulder B, & van der Ven AJ, et al. (2007). Laboratory diagnosis of pulmonary tuberculosis in TB and HIV endemic settings and the contribution of real time PCR for M. tuberculosis in bronchoalveolar lavage fluid. *Trop Med Int Health*, 12(10): 1210-7

Kim HJ, Yoon HI, Park KU, Lee CT, & Lee JH. (2011). The impact of previous tuberculosis history on T-SPOT.TB interferon-gamma release assay results. *Int J Tuberc Lung Dis*, Apr; 15(4): 510-6

Kim HS, Kim CH, Hur M, Hyun IG, Park MJ, Song W, Park JY, Kang HJ, & Lee KM. (2010). Clinical usefulness of T-SPOT.TB test for the diagnosis of tuberculosis. *Korean J Lab Med*, Apr; 30(2): 171-7

Kim SH, Choi SJ, Kim HB, Kim NJ, Oh MD, & Choe KW. (2007). Diagnostic usefulness of a T-cell based assay for extrapulmonary tuberculosis. *Arch Intern Med,* 167(20): 2255-9

Kobashi Y, Mouri K, & Yagi S, et al. (2008). Usefulness of the QuantiFERON-TB 2G test for the differential diagnosis of pulmonary tuberculosis. *Intern Med,* 47(4): 237-43

Kobashi Y, Mouri K, Obase Y, Fukuda M, Miyashita N, & Oka M. (2007). Clinical evaluation of QuantiFERON TB-2G test for immunocompromised patients. *Eur Respir J,* 30(5): 945-50

Kobashi Y, Obase Y, Fakuda M, Yoshida K, Miyashita N, Oka M. (2006). Clinical revaluation of the QuantiFERON TB-2G test as a diagnostic methods for differentiating active tuberculosis from nontuberculous mycobacteriosis. Clin Infect Dis, 43: 1540-6

Kobashi Y, Sugiu T, Shimizu H, Ohue Y, Mouri K, Obase Y, Miyashita N, & Oka M. (2009). Clinical evaluation of the T-SPOT.TB test for patients with indeterminate results on the QuantiFERON TB-2G test. *Intern Med,* 48(3): 137-42. Epub 2009 Feb 2

Komiya K, Ariga H, Nagai H, Kurashima A, Shoji S, Ishii H, & Nakajima Y. (2011). Reversion rates of QuantiFERON-TB Gold are related to pre-treatment IFN-gamma levels. *J Infect,* Jul; 63(1): 48-53. Epub 2011 May 17

Kumar VG, Urs TA, & Ranganath RR. (2011). MPT 64 Antigen detection for Rapid confirmation of M.tuberculosis isolates. *BMC Res Notes,* Mar 24; 4: 79

Laal S, Samanich KM, & Sonnenberg MG, et al. (1997). Surrogate marker of preclinical tuberculosis in human immunodeficiency virus infection: antibodies to an 88-kDa secreted antigen of Mycobacterium tuberculosis. *J Infect Dis,* 176: 133-143

Lai CC, Tan CK, Lin SH, Liao CH, Huang YT, Wang CY, Wang JY, Lin HI, & Hsueh PR. (2010). Diagnostic value of an enzyme-linked immunospot assay for interferon-γ in genitourinary tuberculosis. *Diagn Microbiol Infect Dis,* Nov; 68(3): 247-50. Epub 2010 Sep 17).

Lai CC, Tan CK, Lin SH, Liu WL, Liao CH, Huang YT, & Hsueh PR. (2011). Diagnostic value of an enzyme-linked immunospot assay for interferon-γ in cutaneous tuberculosis. *Diagn Microbiol Infect Dis,* May; 70(1): 60-4

Lalvani A, Brookes R, & Wilkinson RJ, et al. (1998). Human cytolytic and interferon gamma-secreting CD8+ T lymphocytes specific for Mycobacterium tuberculosis. *Proc Natl Acad Sci USA,* 95: 270-5

Lalvani A, Hill AV. (1998). Cytotoxic T-lymphocytes against malaria and tuberculosis: from natural immunity to vaccine design. *Clin Sci (Lond),* 95, 531-8

Lalvani A, Nagvenkar P, & Udwadia Z, et al. (2001). Enumeration of T cells specific for RD1-encoded antigens suggests a high prevalence of latent Mycobacterium tuberculosis infection in healthy urban Indians. *J Infect Dis,* 183: 469-77

Lalvani A, Pareek M. (2010). Interferon gamma release assays: principles and practice. *Enferm Infect Microbiol Clin,* Apr;28(4):245-52. Epub 2009 Sep 24

Lalvani A, Pathan AA, & Durkan H, et al. (2001). Enhanced contact tracing and spatial tracing of M. tuberculosis infection by enumeration of antigen-specific T cells. *Lancet,* 357: 2017-21

Lalvani A, Pathan AA, & McShane H, et al. (2001). Rapid detection of M. tuberculosis infection by enumeration of antigen-specific T cells. *Am J Resir Crit Care Med,* 163, 824-8

Lalvani A. (2007). Diagnosing tuberculosis infection in the 21st century: new tools to tackle an old enemy. *Chest*, 131(6): 1898-1906

Landis JR, Koch GG. (1977). The measurement of observer agreement for categorical data. *Biometrics*, 33(1):159–174

Laszlo A, Gill P, Handzel V, Hodgkin MM, & Helbecque DM. (1983). Conventional and radiometric drug susceptibility testing of Mycobacterium tuberculosis complex. *J Clin Microbiol*, 18(6):1335–9

Latorre I, De Souza-Galvao M, Ruiz-Manzano J, Lacoma A, Prat C, Fuenzalida L, Altet N, Ausina V, & Dominguez J. (2009). Quantitative evaluation of T-cell response after specific antigen stimulation in active and latent tuberculosis infection in adults and children. *Diagn Microbiol Infect Dis*, 65:236–246

Latorre I, Martínez-Lacasa X, Font R, Lacoma A, Puig J, Tural C, Lite J, Prat C, Cuchi E, Ausina V, & Domínguez J. (2010). IFN-γ response on T-cell based assays in HIV-infected patients for detection of tuberculosis infection. *BMC Infect Dis*, Dec 10; 10: 348

Lawn SD, Edwards DJ, Kranzer K, Vogt M, Bekker LG, & Wood R. (2009). Urine lipoarabinomannan assay for tuberculosis screening before antiretroviral therapy diagnostic yield and association with immune reconstitution disease. *AIDS*, 2009 Sep 10; 23(14): 1875-80

Lee E, Holzman RS. (2002). Evolution and current use of the tuberculin test. *Clin Infect Dis*, 34: 365-370

Lee JE, Kim HJ, & Lee SW. (2011). The clinical utility of tuberculin skin test and interferon-γ release assay in the diagnosis of active tuberculosis among young adults: a prospective observational study. *BMC Infect Dis*, Apr 18; 11: 96

Lee JJ, Suo J, Lin CB, Wang JD, Lin TY, & Tsai YC. (2003). Comparative evaluation of the Bactec MGIT 960 system with solid medium for isolation of mycobacteria. *Int J Tuberc Lung Dis*, 7: 569–574

Lee JS, Jo EK, & Noh YK, et al. (2008). Diagnosis of pulmonary tuberculosis using MTB12 and 38-kDa antigens. *Respirology*, 13(3): 432-7

Lee SW, Jang YS, Park CM, Kang HY, Koh WJ, Yim JJ, & Jeon K. (2010). The role of chest CT scanning in TB outbreak investigation. *Chest*, May;137(5):1057-64

Legesse M, Ameni G, Mamo G, Medhin G, Bjune G, & Abebe F. (2010). Performance of QuantiFERON-TB Gold In-Tube (QFTGIT) for the diagnosis of Mycobacterium tuberculosis (Mtb) infection in Afar Pastoralists, Ethiopia. *BMC Infect Dis*, Dec 17; 10: 354

Legesse M, Ameni G, Mamo G, Medhin G, Bjune G, & Abebe F. (2011). Community-based cross-sectional survey of latent tuberculosis infection in Afar pastoralists, Ethiopia, using QuantiFERON-TB Gold In-Tube and tuberculin skin test. *BMC Infec Dis*, Apr 9;11:8

Lewinsohn DA, Gennaro ML, Scholvinck L, & Lewinsohn DM. (2004).Tuberculosis immunology in children: diagnostic and therapeutic challenges and opportunities. *Int J Tuberc Lung Dis*, 8(5): 658– 74

Leyten EM, Prins C, & Bossink AW, et al. (2007). Effect of tuberculin skin testing on a Mycobacterium tuberculosis 1212-6s-specific interferon-gamma assay. *Eur Respir J*, 29(6): 1212-6

Lighter-Fisher J, Peng CH, & Tse DB. (2010). Cytokine responses to QuantiFERON® peptides, purified protein derivative and recombinant ESAT-6 in children with tuberculosis. *Int J Tuberc Lung Dis,* Dec; 14(12): 1548-55

Ling DI, Flores LL, & Pai M. (2008). Commercial nucleic-acid amplification tests for diagnosis of pulmonary tuberculosis in respiratory specimens: meta-analysis and meta-regression. *PLoS One,* 3:e1536

Liu KT, Su WJ, & Perng RP. (2007). Clinical utility of polymerase chain reaction for diagnosis of smear-negative pleural tuberculosis. *J Clin Med Assoc,* 70(4): 146-151.

Lu D, Heeren B, & Dunne WM. (2002). Comparison of the Automated Mycobacteria Growth Indicator Tube System (BACTEC 960/MGIT) with Löwenstein-Jensen medium for recovery of mycobacteria from clinical specimens. *Am J Clin Pathol,* Oct;118(4): 542-5

Lyu J, Lee SG, Hwang S, Lee SO, Cho OH, Chae EJ, Lee SD, Kim WS, Kim DS, & Shim TS. (2011). Chest CT is more likely to show latent tuberculosis foci than simple chest radiography in liver transplantation candidates. *Liver Transpl,* Apr 19. doi: 10.1002/lt.22319. [Epub ahead of print

Mabaera B, Lauritsen JM, Katamba A, Laticevschi D, & Naranbat N, et al. (2007) Sputum smear positive tuberculosis: empiric evidence challenges the need for confirmatory smears. *Int J Tuber Lung Dis,* 11: 959–64

Madariaga MG, Jalali Z, & Swindells S. (2007). Clinical Utility of Interferon Gamma Assay in the Diagnosis of Tuberculosis. *J Am Board Fam Med,* 20:540–547. doi: 10.3122/jabfm.2007.06.070109)

Magana-Arachchi D, Perera J, Gamage S, & Chandrasekharan V. (2008). Low cost in-house PCR for the routine diagnosis of extra-pulmonary tuberculosis. *Int J Tuberc Lung Dis,* 12(3): 275-80

Mancuso JD, Tobler SK, Keep LW. (2008). Pseudoepidemics of TST conversions in the U.S. Army after recent deployments. *Am J Respir Crit Care Med.* 177(11):1285-9. (Epub Mar 20, 2008.)

Mandalakas AM, Hesseling AC, & Chegou NN, et al. High level of discordant IGRA results in HIV-infected adults and children. *Int J Tuberc Lung Di,* 12(4):417– 423

Manjunath N, Shankar P, Rajan L, Bhargava A, Saluja S, & Shriniwas. (1991). Evaluation of a polymerase chain reaction for the diagnosis of tuberculosis. *Tubercle,* 72: 21-27

Marais BJ, Pai M. (2007). Recent advances in the diagnosis of childhood tuberculosis. Arch Dis Child. 92(5): 446-452 (2007).

Mase SR, Ramsay A, Henry M, Ng V, & Hopewell PC, et al. (2007). The incremental yield of serial sputum smears in the diagnosis of tuberculosis: asystematic review. *Int J Tuber Lung Dis,* 11: 485–95

Mazurek GH, Jereb J, & Lobue P, et al. (2005). Guidelines for using the QuantiFERON-TB Gold test for detecting Mycobacterium tuberculosis infection, United States. *MMWR Recomm Rep,* 54(RR-15): 49-55

Mazurek GH, Jereb J, Vernon A, LoBue P, Goldberg S, Castro K; IGRA Expert Committee; Centers for Disease Control and Prevention (CDC). (2010). Updated guidelines for using Interferon Gamma Release Assays to detect Mycobacterium tuberculosis infection - United States, 2010. *MMWR Recomm Rep,* Jun 25; 59(RR-5): 1-25

Mazurek M, Jereb J, Vernon A, LoBue P, Goldberg S, & Castro K. Updated guidelines for using interferon gamma release assays to detect Mycobacterium tuberculosis infection—United States, 2010. *MMWR Recomm Rep*, 59(RR-5): 1–25

Menzies D, Pai M, & Comstock G. (2007). Meta-analysis: new tests for the diagnosis of latent tuberculosis infection: areas of uncertainty and recommendations for research. *Ann Intern Med*, 146(5), 340-54

Menzies D. (2000). What does tuberculin reactivity after bacille Calmette-Guerin vaccination tell us? *Clin Infect Dis*, 31 (Suppl 3): S71–74

Metchock BJ, Nolte FS, Wallace RJ Jr. (1999). Mycobacterium. In: *Manual of Clinical Microbiology*, Murray PR, Baron EJ, Pfaller MA, et al, eds. 7th ed. 399-437. ASM Press: Washington, DC.

Mfinanga GS, Ngadaya E, & Mtandu R, et al. The quality of sputum smear microscopy diagnosis of pulmonary tuberculosis in Dar es Salaam, Tanzania. *Tanzan Health Res Bull*, 9(3): 164-8

Middelkoop K, Bekker LG, Myer L, Dawson R, & Wood R. (2008). Rates of tuberculosis transmission to children and adolescents in a community with a high prevalence of HIV infection among adults. *Clin Infect Dis*, Aug 1; 47(3): 349-55

Minion J, Sohn H, & Pai M. (2009). Light-emitting diode technology for TB diagnosis: what is on the market? *Expert Rev Med Devices*,6: 341–5

Miorner H, Gebre N, & Karlsson U, et al. (1994). Diagnosis of pulmonary tuberculosis. *Lancet*, 344: 127

Miragliotta G, Antonetti R, Di Taranto A, Mosca A, & Del Prete R. (2005). Directdetection of Mycobacterium tuberculosis complex in pulmonary andextrapulmonary samples by BDProbeTec ET system. *New Microbiol*, 28: 67-73

Miret-Cuadras P, Pina-Gutierrez JM, & Juncosa S. (1996). Tuberculin reactivity in Bacillus Calmette-Guerin vaccinated subjects. *Tuber Lung Dis*, 77: 52–58

Mohan A, Pande JN, Sharma SK, Rattan A, Guleria R, & Khilnani GC. Bronchoalveolar lavage in pulmonary tuberculosis: a decision analysis approach. *QJM*, Apr;88(4):269-76

Morcillo N, Imperiale B, & Di Giulio B. (2010). Evaluation of MGIT 960 and the colorimetric-based method for tuberculosis drug susceptibility testing. *Int J Tuberc Lung Dis*, Sep; 14(9): 1169-75

Moreno S, Blazquez R, Novoa A, Carpena I, Menasalvas A, Ramirez C, & Guerrero C. (2001). The Effect of BCG Vaccination on Tuberculin Reactivity and the Booster Effect Among Hospital Employees. *Arch Intern Med*, 161:1760–1765. doi: 10.1001/archinte.161.14.1760).

Mori T, Sakatini M, & Yamagishi F, et al. (2004). Specific detection of tuberculosis infection: an interferon-gamma-based assay using new antigens. *Am J Respir Crit Care Med*, 170: 59-64

Munk ME, Arend SM, Brock I, Ottenhoff TH, & Andersen P. (2001). Use of ESAT-6 and CFP 10 antigens for diagnosis of extra-pulmonary tuberculosis. *J Infect Dis*, 183(1): 175-6

Murakami S, Takeno M, Kirino Y, Kobayashi M, Watanabe R, Kudo M, & Ihata A, et al. (2009). Screening of tuberculosis by interferon-gamma assay before biologic therapy for rheumatoid arthritis. *Tuberculosis*, 89: 139–41

Murray PR, Rosenthal KS, Kobayashi GS, et al. (1998). Mycobacterium. In: *Medical Microbiology*, Brown M, ed. 3rd ed. 319-330. Mosby: St Louis, MO

Muyoyeta M, de Haas PE, Mueller DH, van Helden PD, Mwenge L, Schaap A, Kruger C, van Pittius NC, Lawrence K, Beyers N, Godfrey-Faussett P, & Ayles H. (2010). Evaluation of the Capilia TB assay for culture confirmation of Mycobacterium tuberculosis infections in Zambia and South Africa. *J Clin Microbiol*, Oct; 48(10): 3773-5. Epub 2010 Aug 4

Nagi SS, Anand R, & Pasha ST, et al. (2007). Diagnostic potential of IS6110, 38kDa, 65kDa and 85B sequence-based polymerase chain reaction in the diagnosis of Mycobacterium tuberculosis in clinical samples. *Indian J Med Micobiol*, 25(1): 43-49

Nakanishi M, Demura Y, Ameshima S, Kosaka N, Chiba Y, Nishikawa S, Itoh H, & Ishizaki T. (2010). Utility of high-resolution computed tomography for predicting risk of sputum smear-negative pulmonary tuberculosis. *Eur J Radiol*, Mar: 545-50. Epub 2009 Jan 23

Newport MJ, Goetghebuer T, Weiss HA, Whittle H, & Siegrist CA, et al. (2004). Genetic regulation of immune responses to vaccines in early life. *Genes Immun*, 5: 122–129

Newton SM, Brent AJ, Anderson S, Whittaker E, & Kampmann B. (2008). Paediatric tuberculosis. *Lancet Infect Dis*, 8: 498–510

Ngamlert K, Sinthuwattanawibool C, McCarthy KD, Sohn H, Starks A, Kanjanamongkolsiri P, Anek-vorapong R, Tasaneeyapan T, Monkongdee P, Diem L, & Varma JK. (2009). Diagnostic performance and costs of Capilia TB for Mycobacterium tuberculosis complex identification from broth-based culture in Bangkok, Thailand. *Trop Med Int Health*, 2009 Jul;14(7):748-53. Epub 2009 Apr 23

Nicol M P, Davies M A, & Wood K, et al. (2009). Comparison of T-SPOT. TB assay and tuberculin skin test for the evaluation of young children at high risk for tuberculosis in a community setting. *Pediatrics*, 123: 38– 43

Nigussie M, Mamo G. (2010). Detection of acid fast bacilli (AFB) in tuberculous lymphadenitis among adult Ethiopians. *Ethiop Med J*, Oct; 48(4): 277-83

Nishimura T, Hasegawa N, & Mori M, et al. (2008). Accuracy of an interferon-gamma release assay to detect active pulmonary and extra-pulmonary tuberculosis. iInt J Tuberc Lung Dis, 12(3): 269-74

Noordhoek GT, Kaan JA, Mulder S, Wilke H, & Kolk AH. (1995). Routine application of the polymerase chain reaction for detection of Mycobacterium tuberculosis in clinical samples. *J Clin Pathol*, 48(9), 810-4

Oni T, Patel J, Gideon HP, Seldon R, Wood K, Hlombe Y, Wilkinson KA, Rangaka MX, Mendelson M, & Wilkinson RJ. (2010). Enhanced diagnosis of HIV-1-associated tuberculosis by relating T-SPOT.TB and CD4 counts. *Eur Respir J*, 2010 Sep;36(3):594-600. Epub 2010 Jan 14).

Ozekinci T, Ozbek E, & Celik Y. (2007). Comparison of tuberculin skin test and a specific T-cell-based test, T-Spot.TB, for the diagnosis of latent tuberculosis infection. *J Int Med Res*, Sep-Oct; 35(5): 696-703

Ozkutuk A, Kirdar S, Ozden S, & Esen N. (2006). Evaluation of Cobas Amplicor MTB test to detect Mycobacterium tuberculosis in pulmonary and extrapulmonary specimens. *New Microbiol*, 29:269-73

Oztürk N, Sürücüoğlu S, & Ozkütük N, et al. (2007). Comparison of interferon-gamma whole blood assay with tuberculin skin test for the diagnosis of tuberculosis infection in tuberculosis contacts. *Mikrobiyol Bul*, 41(2): 193-202

Pai M, Joshi R, Bandyopadhyay M, Narang P, Dogra S, Taksande B, & Kalantri S. (2007). Sensitivity of a whole-blood Interferon-gamma assay among patients with pulmonary Tuberculosis and variation in T-cell responses during anti-Tuberculosis treatment. *Infection*, 35(2): 98-108

Pai M, Kalantri S, & Dheda K. (2006). New tools and emerging technologies for the diagnosis of tuberculosis: part I. Latent tuberculosis. *Expert Rev Mol Diagn*, 6: 413–22

Pai M, Riley LW, & Colford JM Jr. (2004). Interferon-gamma assays in the immunodiagnosis of tuberculosis: a systemic review. *Lancet Infect Dis*, 4(12): 761-776

Pai M, Zwerling A, & Menzies D. (2008). Systematic review: T-cell-based assays for the diagnosis of latent tuberculosis infection: an update. *Ann Intern Med*, 149(3):177–184

Pai M. (2004). The accuracy and reliability of nucleic acid amplification tests in the diagnosis of tuberculosis. *Natl Med J India*,17(5): 233-236

Papay P, Eser A, Winkler S, Frantal S, Primas C, Miehsler W, Angelberger S, Novacek G, Mikulits A, Vogelsang H, & Reinisch W. (2011). Predictors of indeterminate IFN-γ release assay in screening for latent TB in inflammatory bowel diseases. *Eur J Clin Invest*, Mar 17

Park SY, Park YB, Choi JH, Lee JY, Kim JS, & Mo EK. (2009). The diagnostic value of interferon-γ assay in patients with active tuberculosis. *Tuberc Respir Dis*, 66:13–19

Patel VB, Bhigjee AI, Paruk HF, Singh R, Meldau R, et al. (2009). Utility of a novel lipoarabinomannan assay for the diagnosis of tuberculous meningitis in a resource-poor high-HIV prevalence setting. *Cerebrospinal Fluid Res*, 6:13

Patel VB, Singh R, Connolly C, Coovadia Y, Peer AK, Parag P, Kasprowicz V, Zumla A, Ndung'u T, & Dheda K. (2010). Cerebrospinal T-cell responses aid in the diagnosis of tuberculous meningitis in a human immunodeficiency virus- and tuberculosis-endemic population. *Am J Respir Crit Care Med.* Aug 15;182(4):569-77. Epub 2010 May 4)

Patil SA, Gourie-Devi M, & Anand AR, et al. (1996). Significance of mycobacterial immune-complex (IgG) in the diagnosis of tuberculin meningitis. *Tuber Lung Dis*, 77:164-7

Pavić I, Zrinski Topić R, Raos M, Aberle N, & Dodig S. (2011) May 12. Interferon- γ release assay for the diagnosis of latent tuberculosis in children younger than 5 years of age. *Pediatr Infect Dis J*, May 12 [Epub ahead of print]).

Pepper T, Joseph P, Mwenya C, et al. (2008). Normal chest radiography in pulmonary tuberculosis: implications for obtaining respiratory specimen cultures. *Int J Tuberc Lung Dis*, 12(4): 397-403

Perez-Stable EJ, Slutkin G. (1985). A demonstration of lack of variability among six tuberculin skin test readers. *Am J Public Health*, 75(11): 1341-3

Pérez-Then E, Shor-Posner G, Crandall L, & Wilkinson J. (2007). The relationship between nutritional and sociodemographic factors and the likelihood of children in th e Dominican Republic having a BCG scar. *Rev Panam Salud Publica*, Jun; 21(6): 365-72

Perkins MD. (2000). New diagnostic tools for tuberculosis. *Int J Tuberc Lung Dis*, 4(Suppl 2): S182-8

Pesanti EL. (1994). The negative tuberculin test. Tuberculin, HIV and anergy panels. *Am J Respir Crit Care Med*, 149:1699–709

Pfyffer GE. (1999). Nucleic acid amplification for mycobacterial diagnosis. *J Infect*, 39: 21-26

Piana F, Ruffo Codecasa L, Baldan R, Miotto P, Ferrarese M, & Cirillo DM. (2007). Use of T-SPOT.TB in latent tuberculosis infection diagnosis in general and immunosuppressed populations. *New Microbiol*, 30 (3), 286-90

Piersimoni C, Scarparo C, Piccoli P, Rigon A, Ruggiero G, Nista D, & Bornigia S. (2002). Performance assessment of two commercial amplification assays for direct detection of Mycobacterium tuberculosis complex from respiratory and extrapulmonary specimens. *J Clin Microbiol*, 40: 4138-42

Ponce de Leon D, Acevedo-Vasquez E, Alvizuri S, Gutierrez C, Cucho M, & Alfaro J, et al. (2008). Comparison of an interferon-gamma assay with tuberculin skin testing for detection of tuberculosis (TB) infection in patients with rheumatoid arthritis in a TB-endemic population. *J Rheumatol*, 35: 776–81

Ponce de Leon D, Acevedo-Vasquez E, Sanchez-Torres A, Cucho M, Alfaro J, & Perich R, et al. (2005). Attenuated response to purified protein derivative in patients with rheumatoid arthritis: study in a population with a high prevalence of tuberculosis. *Ann Rheum Dis*, 64: 1360–5

Pooran A, Booth H, Miller RF, Scott G, Badri M, Huggett JF, Rook G, Zumla A, & Dheda K. (2010). Different screening strategies (single or dual) for the diagnosis of suspected latent tuberculosis: a cost effectiveness analysis. *BMC Pulm Med*, Feb 22;10:7).

Powell RD 3rd, Whitworth WC, Bernardo J, Moonan PK, & Mazurek GH. (2011). Unusual interferon gamma measurements with QuantiFERON-TB Gold and QuantiFERON-TB Gold in-tube tests. *PLoS One*, 6(6):e20061. Epub 2011 Jun 8

Qiao D, Yang BY, Li L, Ma JJ, Zhang XL, Lao SH, & Wu CY. (2011). ESAT-6- and CFP-10-specific Th1, Th22 and Th17 cells in tuberculous pleurisy may contribute to the local immune response against Mycobacterium tuberculosis infection. *Scand J Immunol*, Apr; 73(4): 330-7

Raja A, Ranganathan UD, & Bethunaickan R. (2008). Improved diagnosis of pulmonary tuberculosis by detection of antibodies against multiple Mycobacterium tuberculosis antigens. *Diagn Microbiol Infect Dis*, 60(4), 361-8

Raja A, Uma Devi KR, Ramalingam B, & Brennan PJ. (2002). Immunoglobulin G, A and M responses in serum and circulating immune complexes elicited by the 16-kilodalton antigen of M. tuberculosis. *Clin Diag Lab Immunol*, 9(2), 308-12

Raja A, Uma Devi KR, Ramalingam B, & Brennan PJ. (2004). Improved diagnosis of pulmonary tuberculosis by detection of free and immune complex-bound ant -30 kDa antibodies. *Diagn Microbiol Infect Dis*, 50: 523-9

Ramalingam B, Uma DK, Swaminathan S, & Raja A. (2002). Isotype-specific antibody response in childhood tuberculosis against purified 38 kDa antigen of M. tuberculosis. *J Trop Pediatr*, 48: 188-9

Ramsay A, Bonnet M, Gagnidze L, Githui W, & Varaine F, et al. (2009). Sputum, sex and scanty smears: New case-definition may reduce sex disparities in smear-positive tuberculosis. *Int J Tuber Lung Dis*, 13: 613–9

Rangaka MX, Wilkinson KA, Seldon R, Van Cutsem G, Meintjes GA, Morroni C, Mouton P, Diwakar L, Connell TG, Maartens G, & Wilkinson RJ. (2007). Effect of HIV-1 infection on T-Cell-based and skin test detection of tuberculosis infection. *Am J Respir Crit Care Med*, 175: 514–20

Raviglione MC. (2003). The TB epidemic from 1992 to 2002. *Tuberculosis (Edinb)*, 83, 4-14

Ravn P, Demissie A, & Eguale T, et al. (1999). Human T cell responses to the ESAT-6 antigen from M. tuberculosis. *J Infect Dis*, 179(3): 637-45

Ravn P, Munk ME, & Andersen AB, et al. (2005). Prospective evaluation of a whole-blood test using Mycobacterium tuberculosis-specific antigens ESAT-6 and CFP-10 for diagnosis of active tuberculosis. *Clin Diagn Lab Immunol*, 12:491-6

Reischl U, Lehn N, Wolf H, & Naumann L. (1998). Clinical evaluation of automated COBAS AMPLICOR MTB assay for testing respiratory and nonrespiratory specimens. *J Clin Microbiol*, 36:2853-60

Ribeiro S, Dooley K, Hackman J, Loredo C, Efron A, & Chaisson RE, et al. (2009). T-SPOT.TB responses during treatment of pulmonary tuberculosis. *BMC Infect Dis*, 9: 23

Richeldi L, Ewer K, Losi M, et al. (2004). T-cell-based tracking of multidrug resistant tuberculosis infection after brief exposure. *Am J Respir Crit Care Med*, 170(3): 288-95

Richeldi L, Losi M, D'Amico R, Luppi M, Ferrari A, Mussini C, Codeluppi M, Cocchi S, Prati F, & Paci V, et al. (2009). Performance of tests for latent tuberculosis in different groups of immunocompromised patients. *Chest*,136: 198–204

Richeldi L. An update on the diagnosis of tuberculosis infection. (2006). *Am J Respir Crit Care Med*, n.d.: 736-47

Ritz N, Yau C, Connell TG, Tebruegge M, Leslie D, & Curtis N. (2011). Absence of interferon-gamma release assay conversion following tuberculin skin testing. *Int J Tuberc Lung Dis*, Jun;15(6): 767-9

Ruddy M, McHugh TD, & Dale JW, et al. (2002). Estimation of the rate of unrecognized cross-contamination with mycobacterium tuberculosis in London microbiology laboratories. *J Clin Microbiol*, 40(11): 4100-4

Runa F, Yasmin M, Hoq MM, Begum J, Rahman AS, Ahsan CR. (2011) Molecular versus conventional methods: clinical evaluation of different methods for the diagnosis of tuberculosis in Bangladesh. *J Microbiol Immunol Infect*, Apr; 44(2): 101-5. Epub 2011 Jan 14

Sahiratmadja E, Alisjahbana B, de Boer T, Adnan I, Maya A, Danusantoso H, Nelwan RH, Marzuki S, van der Meer JW, van Crevel R, van de Vosse E, & Ottenhoff TH. (2007). Dynamic changes in pro- and anti-inflammatory cytokine profiles and gamma interferon receptor signaling integrity correlate with tuberculosis disease activity and response to curative treatment. *Infect Immun*, Feb; 75(2): 820-9. Epub 2006 Dec 4

Salfinger M, Pfyffer GE. (1994). The new diagnostic Mycobacteriology laboratory. *Eur J Clin Microbiol Infect Dis*,13: 961-79

Santín Cerezales M, Benítez JD. (2011). Diagnosis of tuberculosis infection using interferon-γ-based assays. *Enferm Infecc Microbiol Clin*, Mar;29 Suppl 1:26-33

Sapkota BR, Ranjit C, & Macdonald M. (2007). Rapid differentiation of Mycobacterium tuberculosis and Mycobacterium leprae from sputum by polymerase chain reaction. *Nepal Med Coll J*, 9(1):12-16

Sauzullo I, Massetti AP, Mengoni F, Rossi R, Lichtner M, Ajassa C, Vullo V, & Mastroianni CM. (2011). Influence of previous tuberculin skin test on serial IFN-γ release assays. *Tuberculosis (Edinb)*, Jul; 91(4): 322-6. Epub 2011 Jun 12)

Schauf V, Rom WN, & Smith KA, et al. (1993). Cytokine gene activation and modified responsiveness to interleukin-2 in the blood of tuberculosis patients. *J Infect Dis*, 168: 1056–9

Sekiguchi J, Miyoshi-Akiyama T, & Augustynowicz-Kopeć E, et al. (2007). Detection of multidrug resistance in Mycobacterium tuberculosis. *J Clin Microbiol*, 45(1), 179-192

Sellam J, Hamdi H, Roy C, Baron G, Lemann M, & Puéchal X, et al. (2007). Comparison of in vitro-specific blood tests with tuberculin skin test for diagnosis of latent tuberculosis before anti-TNF therapy. *Ann Rheum Dis*, 66: 1610–5

Selwyn PA, Sckell BM, Alcabes P, Friedland GH, Klein RS, Schoenbaum EE. (1992). High risk of active tuberculosis in HIV-infected drug users with cutaneous anergy. *JAMA*, 268:504–9

Shams H, Weis SE, & Klucar P, et al. (2005). Enzyme-linked immunospot and tuberculin skin testing to detect latent tuberculosis infection. *Am J Respir Crit Care Med*, 172: 1161-8

Sinirtas M, Ozakin C, & Gedikoglu S. (2009). Evaluation of the fully automated BACTEC MGIT 960 system for testing susceptibility of Mycobacterium tuberculosis to front line antituberculosis drugs and comparison with the radiometric BACTEC 460 TB method. *Mikrobiyol Bul*, Jul;43(3):403-9.

Somoskovi A, Kodmon C, Lanstos A, Bártfai Z, Tamási L, & Füzy J, et al. (2000). Comparison of recoveries of Mycobacterium tuberculosis using the automated BACTEC MGIT 960 System, BACTEC 460 TB System and Lowenstein-Jensen Medium. *J Clin Microbiol*, 38:2395-7

Somoskvi A, Kidman C, & Lantos A, et al. (2000). Comparison of recoveries of Mycobacterium tuberculosis using the automated BACTEC MGIT 960 system, the BACTEC 460 TB system and Lǫwenstein-Jensen medium. *J Clin Microbiol*m 38: 2395–7

Somu N, Swaminathan S, Paramasivan CN, Vijayasekaran D, Chandrabhooshanam A, Vijayan VK, & Prabhakar R. (1995). Value of bronchoalveolar lavage and gastric lavage in the diagnosis of pulmonary tuberculosis in children. *Tuber Lung Dis*, Aug; 76(4): 295-9

Sørensen AL, Nagai S, Houen G, Andersen P, & Andersen AB. (1995). Purification and characterization of a low-molecular-mass T-cell antigen secreted by Mycobacterium tuberculosis. *Infect Immun*, 63: 1710-7

Soysal A, Torun T, Efe S, Gencer H, Tahaoglu K, & Bakir M. (2008). Evaluation of cut-off values of interferon -gamma-based assays in the diagnosis of M.tuberculosis infection. *Int J Tuberc Lung Dis*, 12: 50–6

Spyridis N, Chakraborty R, Sharland M, & Heath PT. (2007). Early diagnosis of tuberculosis using an INF-gamma assay in a child with HIV-1 infection and a very low CD4 count. *Scand J Infect Dis*, 39(10): 919-21

Starke J. (2009). Predictive values of blood tests to diagnose LTBI have not been established in children. *AAP News*, 30: 14

Stavri H, Ene L, Popa GL, Duiculescu D, Murgoci G, marica C, Ulea I, Cus G, & Popa MI. (2009). Comparison of tuberculin skin test with whole-blood interferon gamma assay and ELISA, in HIV positive children and adolescents with TB. *Roum Arch Microbiol Immunol*, 68(1), 14-19

Stefan DC, Dippenaar A, Detjen AK, Schaaf HS, Marais BJ, Kriel B, Loebenberg L, Walzl G, & Hesseling AC. (2010). Interferon-gamma release assays for the detection of Mycobacterium tuberculosis infection in children with cancer. *Int J Tuberc Lung Dis,* Jun; 14(6): 689-94

Stein CM, Zalwango S, Malone LL, Won S, Mayanja-Kizza H, Mugerwa RD, Leontiev DV, Thompson CL, Cartier KC, Elson RC, lyengar SK, Boom WH, & Whalen CC. (2008). Genome Scan of M. tuberculosis infection and Disease in Ugandans. *PloS ONE,* 3(12), e4094

Steingart K R, Ng V, & Henry M, et al. (2006). Sputum processing methods to improve the sensitivity of smear microscopy for tuberculosis: a systematic review. *Lancet Infect Dis,* 6: 664–74

Steingart KR, Henry M, Ng V, Hopewell PC, & Ramsay A, et al. (2006) .Fluorescence versus conventional sputum smear microscopy for tuberculosis: a systematic review. *Lancet Inf Dis,* 6: 570–81

Steingart KR, Ng V, & Henry M, et al. (2006). Sputum processing methods to improve the sensitivity of smear microscopy for tuberculosis: a systematic review. *Lancet Infect Dis,* 6(10): 664-74

Steingart KR, Ramsay A, & Pai M. (2007). Optimizing sputum smear microscopy for the diagnosis of pulmonary tuberculosis. *Expert Rev Anti Infect Ther,* 5: 327–31

Stephan C, Wolf T, Goetsch U, Bellinger O, Nisius G, Oremek G, Rakus Z, Gottschalk R, Stark S, Brodt HR, & Staszewski S. (2008). Comparing QuantiFERON-tuberculosis gold, T-SPOT tuberculosis and tuberculin skin test in HIV-infected individuals from a low prevalence tuberculosis country. *AIDS,* 22: 2471–9

Sun L, Yan HM, Hu YH, Jiao WW, Gu Y, Xiao J, Li HM, Jiao AX, Guo YJ, & Shen AD. (2010). IFN-γ release assay: a diagnostic assistance tool of tuberculin skin test in pediatric tuberculosis in China. *Chin Med J (Engl),* Oct; 123(20): 2786-91

Sutherland JS, de Jong BC, Jeffries DJ, Adetifa IM, & Ota MO. (2010). Production of TNF-alpha, IL-12(p40) and IL-17 can discriminate between active TB disease and latent infection in a West African cohort. *PLoS One,* Aug 24;5(8):e12365

Swaminathan S, Subbaraman R, & Venkatesan P, et al. (2008).Tuberculin skin test results in HIV-infected patients in India: implications for latent tuberculosis treatment. *Int J Tuberc Lung Dis,* 12(2):168-173

Syblo K. (1980). Recent advances in epidemiological research in tuberculosis. *Adv Tuberc Res,* 20: 1-63

Syed AKB, Sikhamani R, Swaminathan S, Perumal V, Paramasivam P, & Raja A. (2009). Role of Interferon Gamma Release Assay in Active TB Diagnosis among HIV Infected Individuals. *PLoS One,* 4(5): e5718

Takamatsu I. Study Group of QFT in Pediatrics. Multicenter study of QuantiFERON in child tuberculosis. Tokyo, Japan: Ministry of Health, Labour and Welfare, 2008);

Takashima T, Higuchi T. (2008). Mycobacterial tests. *Kekkaku,* 83(1), 43-59

Takayanagi K, Aoki M, Aman K, Mitarai S, Harada N, Higuchi K, Okumura M, Yoshiyama T, Ogata H, & Mori T. (2011). Analysis of an interferon-gamma release assay for monitoring the efficacy of anti-tuberculosis chemotherapy. *Jpn J Infect Dis,* 64(2): 133-8

Talati NJ, Seybold U, Humphrey B, Aina A, Tapia J, Weinfurter P, Albalak R, & Blumberg HM. (2009). Poor concordance between interferon-gamma release assays and tuberculin skin tests in diagnosis of latent tuberculosis infection among HIV-infected individuals. *BMC Infect Dis*, 9:15

Tessema TA, Hamasur B, Bjun G, Svenson S, & Bjorvatn B. (2001). Diagnostic evaluation of urinary lipoarabinomannan at an Ethiopian tuberculosis centre. *Scand J Infect Dis*, 33: 279–284.

Thomas MM, Hinks TS, Raghuraman S, Ramalingam N, Ernst M, Nau R, Lange C, Kosters K, Gnanamuthu C, & John GT, et al. (2008). Rapid diagnosis of mycobacterium tuberculosis meningitis by enumeration of cerebrospinal fluid antigen-specific T-cells. *Int J Tuberc Lung Dis*,12:651–7

Thornton CG, MacLellan KM, Brink TL, Passen S. (1998). In vitro comparison of NALC-NaOH, Tween 80 and C18-Carboxypropylbetaine for processing of specimens for recovery of mycobacteria. *J Clin Microbiol*, 36: 3558-66

Torres Costa J, Silva R, Ringshausen FC, Nienhaus A. (2011). Screening for tuberculosis and prediction of disease in Portuguese healthcare workers. *J Occup Med Toxicol*, Jun 9; 6: 19

Tortoli E, Cichero P, Piersonetti C, Simonetti MT, Gesu G, & Nista D. (1999). Use of BACTEC MGIT 960 for recovery of mycobacteria from clinical specimens: Multicenter study. *J Clin Microbiology*, 37: 3578-82

Toshiyama T, Harada N, Higuchi K, Sekiya Y, & Uchimura K. (2010). Use of the QuantiFERON-TB Gold Test for screening tuberculosis contacts and predicting active disease. *Int J Tuberc Lung Dis*, 14:819–27

Trusov A, Bumgarner R, & Valijev R, et al. (2009). Comparison of L umin™ LED fl uorescent attachment, fl uorescent microscopy and Ziehl-Neelsen for AFB diagnosis. *Int J Tuberc Lung Dis*, 13: 836–841

Tsiouris SJ, Austin J, & Toro P, et al. (2006). Results of a tuberculosis-specific IFN-gamma assay in children at high risk for tuberculosis infection. *Int J Tuberc Lung Dis*, 10 (8):939- 941

Tuberculosis Research Centre (ICMR), Chennai. (1999). Fifteen year follow up of trial of BCG vaccines in south India for tuberculosis prevention. *Indian J Med Res*, 110: 56-69

Tully G, Kortsik C, & Höhn H, et al. (2005). Highly focused T cell responses in latent human pulmonary M. tuberculosis infection. *J Immunol*, 174: 2174-84

Ulrichs T, Munk ME, & Mollenkopf H, et al. (1998). Differential T cell responses to M. tuberculosis ESAT-6 in tuberculosis patients and healthy donors. *Eur J Immunol*, 28: 3949-58

van Cleeff M, Kivihya-Ndugga L, Githui W, Ng'ang'a L, & Kibuga D, et al. (2005). Cost-effectiveness of polymerase chain reaction versus Ziehl-Neelsen smear microscopy for diagnosis of tuberculosis in Kenya. *Int J Tuberc Lung Dis*, 9: 877–883

van Cleeff MR, Kivihya-Ndugga LE, Meme H, Odhiambo JA, & Klatser PR. (2005). The role and performance of chest X-ray for the diagnosis of tuberculosis: a cost-effectiveness analysis in Nairobi, Kenya. *BMC Infect Dis*, 12(5), 111

Van Deun A, Aung KJ, Hamid Salim A, Gumusboga M, Nandi P, & Hossain MA. (2010). Methylene blue is a good background stain for tuberculosis light-emitting diode fluorescence microscopy. *Int J Tuberc Lung Dis*, Dec; 14(12): 1571-5

Van Deun A, Salim AH, Cooreman E, Daru P, & Das AP, et al. (2004). Scanty AFB smears: What's in a name? *Int J Tuber Lung Dis*, 8: 816–823

Van Deun, Chonde T M, Gumusboga M, & Rienthong S. (2008). Performance and acceptability of the FluoLED Easy module for tuberculosis fluorescence microscopy. *Int J Tuberc Lung Dis*, 12:1009–14

von Reyn CF, Horsburgh CR, Olivier KN, Barnes PF, Waddell R, Warren C, Tvaroha S, Jaeger AS, Lein AD, Alexander LN, Weber DJ, & Tosteson AN. (2001). Skin test reactions to Mycobacterium tuberculosis purified protein derivative and Mycobacterium avium sensitin among health care workers and medical students in the United States. *Int J Tuberc Lung Dis*, 2001; 5: 1122–8

Wang L, Turner MO, Elwood RK, Schulzer M, & FitzGerald JM. (2002). A meta-analysis of the effect of Bacille Calmette Guerin vaccination on tuberculin skin test measurements. *Thorax*, 57(9): 804–9

Weldingh K, Rosenkrands I, Okkels LM, Doherty TM, & Andersen P. (2005). Assessing the serodiagnostic potential of 35 Mycobacterium tuberculosis proteins and identification of four novel serological antigens. *J Clin Microbiol*, 43: 57-65

Whilley DM. Lambert SB, Bialasiewicz S, Goire N, Nissen MD, et al. (2008). False-negative results in nucleic acid amplification tests-do we need to routinely use two genetic targets in all assays to overcome problems caused by sequence variation? *Crit Rev Microbiol*, 34(2): 71-6

WHO. (2008). Global Tuberculosis Control: Surveillance, Planning and Financing. WHO, Geneva

WHO. (2006). Global Tuberculosis Control: Surveillance, Planning, and Financing. WHO, Geneva

WHO. (1994). The HIV/AIDS and tuberculosis epidemics: implications for TB control. WHO/TB/CARG (4)/94.4

WHO. (2009). New Diagnostic Working Group of the Stop TB Partnership. Pathways to better diagnostics for tuberculosis- A blueprint for the development of TB diagnostics. WHO, Geneva

WHO. (2010) Global TB control Report 2010. WHO, Geneva

WHO Tuberculosis Research office. (1995). Further studies of geographic variation in naturally acquired tuberculin sensitivity. Bull World Health Organization., 12,63-83

Wiker HG, Mustafa T, Bjune GA, & Harboe M. (2010). Evidence for waning of latency in a cohort study of tuberculosis. *BMC Infect Dis*,10:37

Wilkinson KA, Wilkinson RJ, Pathan A, Ewer K, Prakash M, Klenerman P, Maskell N, Davies R, Pasvol G, & Lalvani A. (2005). Ex vivo characterization of early secretory antigenic target 6-specific T cells at sites of active disease in pleural tuberculosis. *Clin Infect Dis*, 40:184–187

Wozniak TM, Saunders BM, Ryan AA, & Britton WJ. (2010). Mycobacterium bovis BCG-specific Th17 cells confer partial protection against Mycobacterium tuberculosis infection in the absence of gamma interferon. *Infect Immun*, Oct; 78(10): 4187-94. Epub 2010 Aug 2.

Yu CC, Liu YC, Chu CM, Chuang DY, Wu WC, & Wu HP. Factors associated with in vitro interferon-gamma production in tuberculosis. J Formos Med Assoc. 2011 Apr;110(4):239-46)

Zhang J, Chen Y, Nie XB, Wu WH, Zhang H, Zhang M, He XM, & Lu JX. (2011). Interleukin-10 polymorphisms and tuberculosis susceptibility: a meta-analysis. *Int J Tuberc Lung Dis,* May;15(5): 594-601

Zhao J, Wang Y, Wang H, Jiang C, Liu Z, Meng X, Song G, Cheng N, Graviss EA, & Ma X. (2011). Low agreement between the T-SPOT®.TB assay and the tuberculin skin test among college students in China. *Int J Tuberc Lung Dis,* Jan;15(1):134-6

Zheng YJ, Wang RH, Lin YZ, & Daniel TM. (1994). Clinical evaluation of the diagnostic value of measuring IgG antibody to 3 mycobacterial antigenic preparations in the capillary blood of children with tuberculosis and control subjects. *Tuber Lung Dis,* 75(5), 366-70

Zrinski Topić R, Zoričić-Letoja I, Pavić I, & Dodig S. (2011). Indeterminate results of QuantiFERON-TB Gold In-Tube assay in nonimmunosuppressed children. *Arch Med Res,* Feb;42(2):138-43

6

Diagnosis of Smear-Negative Pulmonary Tuberculosis in Low-Income Countries: Current Evidence in Sub-Saharan Africa with Special Focus on HIV Infection or AIDS

Claude Mambo Muvunyi[1,2] and Florence Masaisa[1,3]
[1]*Department of Clinical Chemistry, Microbiology and Immunology, Ghent University Hospital, De Pintelaan, Ghent,*
[2]*Department of Clinical Biology, Centre Hospitalier Universitaire-Butare, National University of Rwanda, Butare, Rwanda;*
[3]*Department of Internal Medicine, Centre Hospitalier Universitaire-Butare, National University of Rwanda, Butare,*
[1]*Belgium*
[2,3]*Rwanda*

1. Introduction

1.1 Background

Tuberculosis (TB) remains a major global public health problem and it persists as a major cause of human mortality and morbidity, affecting almost a third of the world's population [Sudre et al., 1992; WHO 2002]. There were 9.2 million new cases of tuberculosis worldwide in 2006, with the highest rates of disease in African countries. Despite efforts to control tuberculosis and reduce the rate of infections, the lack of accurate laboratory diagnosis hinders these efforts. The rapid spread of the human immunodeficiency virus (HIV) in sub-Saharan African countries has led to dramatic rises in incidence of TB cases and has been associated with worsening treatment outcomes, even in well functioning TB programmes [Raviglione et al., 1997]. The impact of the HIV epidemic on tuberculosis depends on the degree of overlap between the population infected with HIV and that infected with Mycobacterium tuberculosis. In sub-Saharan Africa the prevalence of both infections is high with considerable overlap between the infected populations, since the age distribution of both infections is concentrated in the 20-50-year age group. In 1994 there were an estimated 4.8 million people worldwide infected with both M. tuberculosis and HIV, of whom over 75% were reported to be living in sub-Saharan Africa (6). Worldwide estimates of the proportions of new tuberculosis cases attributable to HIV infection were 4% in 1990, 8% in 1995, projected to 14% by the year 2000 [WHO 2002]. HIV-related infection thus accounts for a relatively small but increasing proportion of the global tuberculosis burden. In sub-Saharan Africa, however, it accounts for a greater part of the burden: an estimated 30% or more of tuberculosis cases by the year 2000 [WHO 2002]. THE WORLD HEALTH

ORGANIZATION (WHO) estimated that both the number of cases of tuberculosis worldwide and the percentage attributable to coexisting HIV infection would increase substantially during the decade between 1990 and 2000 [WHO 2002]. Furthermore, most of this burden occurs among the low-income countries of the world, particularly those in sub-Saharan Africa, the region most heavily affected since the beginning of the HIV epidemic[Sudre et al., 1992].

Although both culture techniques and the introduction of nucleic acid-based tests can improve laboratory diagnosis [Perkins and Cunningham, 2007], these procedures are not widely available in most low-income countries. Instead, in most low income countries, the diagnosis of pulmonary tuberculosis (PT) still relies on the search for Acid-Fast Bacilli (AFB) in sputum smears, which has sensitivity between 50 and 80% in well-equipped laboratories [Aber et al., 1980]. In low-income countries, poor access to high-quality microscopy services contributes to even lower rates of AFB detection. Furthermore, in countries with high prevalence of both pulmonary tuberculosis and HIV infection, the detection rate is even lower owing to the paucibacillary nature of pulmonary tuberculosis in patients with HIV infection. In fact, HIV changes the presentation of smear-negative pulmonary tuberculosis from a slowly progressive disease with low bacterial load and reasonable prognosis, to one with reduced pulmonary cavity formation and sputum bacillary load, more frequent involvement of the lower lobes, and an exceptionally high mortality rate [Hopewell, 1992; Jones et al., 1993]. This means that there are many cases of PT that are not going to be diagnosed by this test, and they are denominated smear-negative pulmonary tuberculosis (SNPT). Therefore, it is often necessary to make a clinico-radiological diagnosis of smear-negative TB using an algorithm and to initiate empirical TB treatment while awaiting culture results. Therefore, early identification of persons who have TB, whether smear positive or smear negative, is desirable both to enable appropriate isolation procedures and to provide a basis for early institution of therapy. Conversely, correct prediction of persons who are unlikely to have TB is important as well to limit the expense and potential toxicity of empiric therapy. A clinical prediction rule (CPR) is defined as a "decision making tool for clinicians that includes three or more variables obtained from the history, or physical examination of the patient, or from simple diagnostic tests and that either provides the probability of an outcome or suggest a diagnostic or therapeutic course of action. Given the lack of resources to use sophisticated laboratory tests for this problem in most developing countries, we will try to develop a CPR to diagnose Smear-negative pulmonary tuberculosis.

The primary objective of this chapter will be to conduct a systematic review of the literature to gather data on evaluation of various criteria, algorithms, and clinical indicators used in low-income countries in the diagnosis of PT in people with suspected tuberculosis but repeated negative sputum smears with particular consideration of HIV infection or AIDS. This review will be of help therefore to develop it in the format of a score based on simple clinical variables for the diagnosis of Smear-negative pulmonary tuberculosis.

This article will describe the incidence, natural history and differential diagnoses of smear-negative pulmonary TB in HIV negative and HIV-positive patients. The various strategies that have attempted to address smear-negative TB will then be reviewed; highlighting plausible interventions for developing countries and areas for future research.

1.2 Definition of smear-negative pulmonary tuberculosis

Smear-negative tuberculosis is currently defined as symptomatic illness in a patient with at least two sputum smear examinations negative for AFB on different occasions in whom pulmonary tuberculosis is later confirmed by culture, biopsy, or other investigations[WHO 2007]. Guidelines from some developing countries like Malawi through their national Tuberculosis Program recommends that the diagnosis of smear negative TB be based on four criteria of (i) cough for more than 3 weeks, (ii) three sputum smears negative for AFB, (iii) no response to an antibiotic, and (iv) a chest x-ray compatible with TB[Hargreaves et al., 2000].

The following are suggested case definitions for use in HIV-prevalent settings[WHO 2007]

Smear-Positive Pulmonary Tuberculosis

- One sputum smear examination positive for AFB **and**
- Laboratory confirmation of HIV infection **or**
- Strong clinical evidence of HIV infection*

Smear-Negative Pulmonary Tuberculosis

- At least two sputum specimens negative for AFB **and**
- Radiographical abnormalities consistent with active tuberculosis **and**
- Laboratory confirmation of HIV infection **or**
- Strong clinical evidence of HIV infection* **and**
- Decision by a clinician to treat with a full course of antituberculosis chemotherapy

OR

- A patient with AFB smear-negative sputum which is culture-positive for *Mycobacterium tuberculosis*

1.3 Impact of HIV on TB infection

Persons with HIV-1 infection are at increased risk of active TB due to reactivation of latent TB and more rapid progression to disease after TB infection. It is well known that the risk of TB is greatly increased in HIV-infected persons, and some of the underlying mechanisms are being elucidated. Effective immunity to TB involves coordination of responses between the innate and adaptive immune systems, both of which are altered by HIV[Patel and Koziel, 2009]. The strongest risk factor for developing TB disease in HIV lies in helper T-cell type 1 (Th1) adaptive immunity, specifically the progressive decline in CD4 T-cell count associated with advanced HIV [Williams and Dye, 2003]. In patients with prior TB exposure as assessed by a positive Purified protein derivative (PPD) response, the incidence of TB is 2.6%/year for those with a CD4 T-cell count greater than 350/ml, 6.5%/year for those with aCD4 T-cell count from 200 to 350/ml, and 13.3%/year for those with a CD4 T-cell count less than 200/ml [Antonucci et al., 1995]. With decline of the CD4 T-cell count, there is also a higher risk of anergy to skin test reactions, suggesting dysfunction of delayed-type hypersensitivity dependent on Th1-type immunity [Markowitz et al., 1993]. There is also in vitro evidence for qualitative dysfunction of CD4 T cells in HIV. Compared with TB-infected patients without HIV infection, peripheral blood mononuclear cells from patients coinfected with HIV and TB have decreased proliferative T-cell responses and reduced IFN-g production to *Mycobacterium tuberculosis* in vitro, whereas anti-inflammatory IL-10 production is preserved [Zhang et al., 1994]. However, the observation that TB incidence increases shortly after HIV seroconversion, and before reduction in peripheral blood CD4 T-cell counts [Sonnenberg et al., 2005], suggests that HIV confers additional mechanisms of susceptibility to TB infection. Investigations into the progression of primary HIV infection to AIDS suggest that primary HIV infection is associated with a precipitous decrease in mucosal CD4 memory T cells [Brenchley et al., 2006a], which may set the stage for chronic immune activation and CD4 T-cell depletion through mucosal translocation of bacteria through the gut [Brenchley et al., 2006b]. Thus, mucosal CD4 memory T-cell depletion may provide a potential mechanism to account for disrupted T-cell function in early HIV infection, although whether similar events occur in the lung mucosa has not yet been established [Brenchley et al., 2008]. Indeed, primary HIV infection is associated with decreased PPD-specific IFN-secreting T cells [Sutherland et al., 2006; Geldmacher et al., 2008] and ESAT (early secreted antigenic target)-6–specific T cells [Geldmacher et al., 2008] in the blood, suggesting that early depletion of memory T cells may affect specific immunity to TB. Lung lavage enzymelinked immunospot (ELISPOT) studies also suggest decreased bacillus Calmette-Gue´rin (BCG)– or PPD-specific pulmonary CD4 T cells in asymptomatic HIV-infected persons compared with HIV-negative persons [Kalsdorf et al., 2009]. HIV–TB coinfection may also be associated with increased serum levels of IL-4, an anti-Th1 type cytokine that hinders immune response to MTb [Dheda et al., 2005]. Interestingly, alveolar lavage cells from coinfected individuals may have intact ability to secrete IFN-g in response to MTb antigens in vitro [Dheda et al., 2005], although this may not translate to equivalent cell function and cell numbers in vivo.

Independent of CD4 T-cell count, HIV also affects the function of innate immune cells, especially alveolar macrophages (AMs), which serve as the main reservoir for MTb infection [Russell, 2001; Dheda et al., 2009]. MTb has evolved to persist within macrophages in part through prevention of MTb phagosomal fusion with lysosomes, thus preventing intracellular killing of MTb [Brown et al., 1969; Mwandumba et al., 2004]. AMs can combat intracellular parasitization by releasing immune-activating cytokines or chemokines, and by programmed cell death or apoptosis [Oddo et al., 1998; Keane et al., 2000]. Apoptosis benefits the host by promoting intracellular killing of MTb [Oddo et al., 1998; Keane et al., 2000] and improving antigen presentation by additional phagocytes to activate adaptive immunity [Schaible et al., 2003; Winau et al., 2006]. Whereas asymptomatic HIV infection does not affect the intracellular growth of MTb [Day et al., 2004; Kalsdorf et al., 2009], AMs from asymptomatic HIV-infected subjects have increased phagocytosis of MTb [Day et al., 2004; Patel et al., 2007], decreased release of specific cytokines and chemokines [Saukkonen et al., 2002], and similarly impaired MTb phagosomal maturation [Mwandumba et al., 2004] compared with AMs from healthy subjects. AMs from HIV-infected subjects also have decreased apoptosis in response to MTb [Patel et al., 2007]; the mechanism may involve increased lung levels of IL-10 in HIV, which up-regulates BCL-3 (B-cell lymphoma 3–encoded protein), an apoptosis inhibitor [Patel et al., 2009]. HIV infection of macrophages also inhibits autophagy [Kyei et al., 2009], another cellular process that may be critical for macrophage intracellular killing of MTb [Gutierrez et al., 2004].

1.4 Rationale

The focus of this chapter is on sub-Saharan Africa (SSA). Countries in the developing world and especially in sub-Saharan Africa are the most affected by the TB epidemic. Worldwide, in 2008, the estimated global TB incidence rate was 139 cases per 100,000 population, which equates to 9.4 million (range, 8.9–9.9 million) incident TB cases. This represents an 11% increase in TB incidence rate and a 40% increase in the number of TB cases, compared with estimates from 1990[WHO 2009]. This global increase in rates was attributable to increases in the SSA and was mainly driven by the HIV epidemic. Particularly in SSA, mirroring the HIV epidemic, TB incidence and TB-associated death rates have doubled, and the number of TB cases and TB-related deaths has tripled in comparison with estimated figures from 1990[WHO 2009]. The HIV epidemic has fuelled the tuberculosis epidemic in the region. Of the 9.4 million incident cases in 2009, an estimated 1.0–1.2 million (11–13%) were HIV-positive, with a best estimate of 1.1 million (12%). Of these HIV-positive TB cases, approximately 80% were in the African Region (http://www.who.int/tb/publications/global_report/2010/). The relative risk of developing TB in HIV-positive individuals, compared with HIV-negative individuals, is 21 in high HIV prevalence countries and 37 in low HIV prevalence countries[WHO 2009]. Moreover, these co-infected people have at least a 30% lifetime risk of developing active tuberculosis, thus contributing to the increase in the number of tuberculosis cases in the region. In Africa, TB is often the first manifestation of HIV infection, and accounts for a disproportionate burden of morbidity and mortality in co-infected patients [Munyati et al., 2005].

As a consequence, HIV is the single most significant risk factor for the development of TB, and HIV patients are at increased risk for primary and reactivation disease, as well as exogenous reinfection [Sonnenberg et al., 2001]. The risk of death in co-infected patients is two to four times that of HIV individuals without TB, independent of CD4 count [Whalen et al., 1995; Connolly et al., 1999]. In addition, coinfected patients have a markedly greater risk of progression to AIDS compared with HIV patients without TB [Whalen et al., 1997]. The focus of this chapter is therefore sub-Saharan Africa, the region of the world most severely affected by the HIV/TB co-epidemic.

2. Search strategy

We used a combination of systematic review, document analysis, and global expert opinion to prepare this chapter. We identified relevant publications by searches of Medline, PubMed, Embase, HealthSTAR, and Web of Science with the keywords: "tuberculosis", "*Mycobacterium tuberculosis*", "sputum negative", "smear negative", AFB negative", "negative for AFB", "HIV" , "diagnosis" and "treatment" for papers published in English between 1990 and December, 2010. Studies were included in the review if they reported on tuberculous disease in people with HIV infection or AIDS in sub- Saharan Africa and if the disease had been stratified into smear-positive and smear-negative. We reviewed data for smear-negative pulmonary tuberculosis only for patients who were also HIV positive. All retrieved titles and abstracts were scrutinised for the relevance to the topic. Analytical studies that identified demographic, clinical, radiological, or simple laboratory based indicators facilitating the diagnosis of smear-negative tuberculosis were included. An assessment of methodological quality was undertaken for each paper.

We used the WHO definition of a case of smear-negative pulmonary tuberculosis: at least two sputum specimens negative for acid-fast bacilli, abnormalities on radiography consistent with active tuberculosis, no response to broad-spectrum antibiotics, and a decision by a clinician to treat with a full course of antituberculosis chemotherapy.

3. Frequency of smear-negative pulmonary tuberculosis

Given the immunopathological spectrum seen in HIV-infected TB patients, it would be expected that the proportion of patients with smear-negative PT should increase in areas where the prevalence of HIV is high. Initial impressions were that HIV infection in sub-Saharan Africa was associated with a large and predominant increase in smear-negative PT [Harries, 1990]. It is apparent from cross-sectional studies, however, that the majority of HIV-positive PT patients are smear positive, although the proportion of smear-negative patients is greater among those infected with HIV than among those who are HIV-negative [Elliott et al., 1990; Nunn et al., 1992]. Since the advent of HIV, the annual incidence of TB has more than doubled in some African countries [De Cock et al., 1992; Wilkinson and Davies, 1997], and there has been a disproportionate increase in the reported rate of smear-negative disease. A study in Zambia [Elliott et al., 1993] of over 100 patients with culture-positive PT found that 24% of those who were HIV-seronegative had a negative sputum smear, compared with 43% of those who were HIV-seropositive. With good routine reporting systems, the national tuberculosis programmes of countries such as Malawi and the United Republic of Tanzania have reported a larger increase in new cases of smear negative than of smear-positive PT in the last 10 years [Graf 1994].

Other studies showed that the proportion of cases of smear-negative pulmonary tuberculosis in HIV-positive tuberculosis patients ranged from 10% to 61% [Affolabi et al., ; Long et al., 1991; Elliott et al., 1993; Harries et al., 1997; Behr et al., 1999; Bruchfeld et al., 2002; Zachariah et al., 2003; Kang'ombe et al., 2004; Yassin et al., 2004; Chintu and Mwaba, 2005]. The apparent variation in the incidence of negative sputum smear between these studies may be due to differences in the study populations. Some studies were conducted among patients seen at specialist institution-based centres who may be more or less likely to be smear-positive depending on the referral procedure. The level of immunosuppression among the HIV-positive patients in the various studies may also have differed. Less severely immunocompromised HIV-positive patients tend to have classic cavitary TB which is smear-positive [De Cock et al., 1992; Desta et al., 2009]. As the level of immunocompromise increases with advancing HIV disease, atypical pulmonary features predominate and smear examinations prove less sensitive It is not clear at present whether these figures reflect the true pattern of PT or whether there is an over diagnosis or under diagnosis of smear-negative cases. Reports from national tuberculosis programmes of the pattern of PT are influenced by various factors such as the criteria used to diagnose smear-negative PT, the extent to which these criteria are followed in clinical practice, and the number of other respiratory diseases that can resemble and be misdiagnosed as PT. Moreover, access to health services and DOTS in most resource-constrained settings with high HIV infection rates is restricted and services reach only a fraction of the population. If the availability of these services were increased, we expect that a much higher frequency of disease would be seen. Negative smears could also be the result of poor quality smear microscopy from inadequate sputum collection, storage, and staining, reading errors, or poor laboratory services. In children, the diagnosis of pulmonary tuberculosis is especially difficult because the disease is paucibacillary and collection of sufficient sputum for smear microscopy and culture is difficult [Chintu and Mwaba, 2005]. HIV-positive patients with smear-negative tuberculosis are more likely to die during or before diagnosis than HIV-negative patients because of their immunosuppression, which leads to further under estimates of the magnitude of the problem.

4. Transmission of tuberculosis from smear negative patients

TB patients whose sputum smears are AFB negative are generally regarded as less infectious than those whose smears are positive. The relative TB transmission rate among patients with smear-negative, culture-positive pulmonary disease, compared with patients with smear-positive disease, was found to be 0.24 in cohort study in the Netherlands [Tostmann et al., 2008]. Overall, 17% of TB transmission events were attributable to source patients with sputum smear-negative, culture-positive disease [Tostmann et al., 2008]. These important findings are consistent with report from similar studies from San Francisco, California, and Vancouver, British Columbia [Behr et al., 1999; Hernandez-Garduno et al., 2004], collectively showing that in high-income countries, 10%-20% of TB transmission at the population level is attributable to source cases with smear-negative pulmonary TB. Tostmann and co-worker [Tostmann et al., 2008] speculated on the relevance of their data for countries in which HIV infection is endemic and rates of smear-negative TB disease are high. In these countries with a high incidence of TB, microscopic examination of sputum smear samples is often the only available diagnostic test for TB. As a result, patients with smear-negative TB do not receive a diagnosis in a timely manner; thus, disease may further develop, initiation of treatment may be delayed, and further TB transmission may occur [Siddiqi et al., 2003]. In view of these observations, one can conclude that transmission attributable to smear-negative pulmonary TB cases at the community level may be important in these regions.

Whether this is true for HIV-positive patients with pulmonary tuberculosis remains to be established. One study from Zambia concluded that patients with HIV-associated pulmonary tuberculosis were less infectious than seronegative patients [Elliott et al., 1993], whereas results from Zaire showed no difference in rates of infection among household contacts [Klausner et al., 1993]. Moreover, In sub-Saharan Africa, HIV infection has had a devastating impact on TB control [Lawn et al., 2006; WHO 2009]. In a study of a community in a township in Cape Town, South Africa, for example, the antenatal HIV seroprevalence rate is 30%, and the annual TB notification rate has increased to 11500 cases per 100,000 population [Lawn et al., 2006] almost 200-fold higher than TB rates in The Netherlands. This has been associated with a major and disproportionate increase in the rate of smear-negative disease among HIV-infected individuals [Lawn et al., 2006].

5. Diagnosis of smear negative TB in Sub-Saharan African

In the absence of rapid and simple tools to diagnose tuberculosis, health institutions should avail guidelines or algorithms to assist clinical decision-making in HIV-prevalent and resource-constrained settings, to expedite the diagnostic process and minimize incorrect diagnosis and mortality. As much as possible, patients should be correctly diagnosed and treated for smear-negative pulmonary tuberculosis; however, treatment of those without the disease should be avoided. The diagnosis of PT in adults in most African countries is based on simple techniques such as clinical assessment, sputum smear microscopy and chest radiography. Although specificity is high [Hargreaves et al., 2001; van Cleeff et al., 2003; Apers et al., 2004], major concerns include low sensitivity [Harries et al., 1997; Hargreaves et al., 2001] and delayed diagnosis of smear-negative disease [Harries et al., 1997; Colebunders and Bastian, 2000]. The accuracy of both microscopy and radiography is reduced by HIV, and so assessment of diagnostic approaches with existing methods and continuing research into new diagnostics are necessary [Colebunders and Bastian, 2000; Kivihya-Ndugga et al., 2003; Angeby et al., 2004].

Tuberculin skin testing in adults is not useful for individual diagnosis in populations with a high prevalence of M. tuberculosis infection. In addition, for HIV-infected individuals, there is the problem that cutaneous anergy increases as the CD4 lymphocyte count declines. In Zaire, over 50% of HIV-positive PT patients with a CD4 lymphocyte count <200/4l had a negative tuberculin skin test [Mukadi et al., 1993]. Techniques that are widely available in industrialized countries for obtaining pulmonary specimens (such as induced sputum and fibre-optic bronchoscopy with bronchoalveolar lavage) and for analysing them (such as culture, antigen detection and polymerase chain reaction) are beyond the resources of most hospitals in sub-Saharan Africa.

5.1 Criteria used to diagnose smear-negative TB

5.1.1 Clinical criteria

Smear-negative tuberculosis is found to be more common in older than younger patients in a country with low prevalence of HIV infection [Samb et al., 1999]. However, countries with high HIV prevalence have an even age distribution, probably because HIV affects younger age-groups [Parry, 1993]. HIV is also more common in patients with smear-negative tuberculosis than in those with smear-positive disease. As for clinical indicators, pulmonary TB remains the most frequent form of active TB in HIV-1 infected persons, even those with low CD4 counts. Although the clinical presentation of pulmonary TB is different to the presentation of pulmonary TB in HIV-1 uninfected patients, the most common symptoms remain cough, fever, night sweats and significant weight loss [Batungwanayo et al., 1992; Bruchfeld et al., 2002]. Relative to HIV-1 uninfected patients, weight loss and fever are more common, whereas haemoptysis is less common and some studies have reported a decreased proportion of patients with cough [Selwyn et al., 1998; Kassu et al., 2007]. Although HIV-infected persons with TB may have the classic symptoms of TB (eg, productive cough, chest pain, shortness of breath, hemoptysis, fever, night sweats, and/or weight loss), many such patients have few symptoms or have symptoms that are even less specific than those mentioned. Cough persisting for longer than 3 weeks warrants AFB microscopy, according to the current WHO guidance. However, one study, in an area of high HIV and tuberculosis prevalence, confirmed smear-negative tuberculosis in 35% of patients with cough unresponsive to antibiotics of only 1–3 weeks duration [Banda et al., 1998]. Most of these patients had atypical changes on chest radiography. That study suggests that pulmonary tuberculosis should be considered in patients with short duration of cough associated with weight loss and lack of response to antibiotics, particularly those who live in overcrowded places in areas with high prevalence of HIV infection and tuberculosis. It has been noted recently that a small proportion of HIV infected patients with TB are minimally symptomatic or asymptomatic, particularly in developing countries with a high burden of both HIV infection and TB [Bassett et al., 2009; Edwards et al., 2009].

A number of studies in Africa have tried to identify frequently occurring clinical features in smear-negative tuberculosis in areas with high prevalence of HIV infection and tuberculosis. A study, in Tanzania and Burundi, identified four clinical criteria for diagnosis of smear-negative tuberculosis [Samb et al., 1997]: presence of cough for longer than 21 days (odds ratio 5·43[1·95–15·1]); presence of chest pain for longer than 15 days (1·98 [0·77–5·12]); absence of expectoration (odds ratio for expectoration 0·42 [0·15–1·18]); and absence of shortness of breath (odds ratio for breathlessness 0·26 [0·01–0·66]). Diagnosis of smear negative tuberculosis by any two of these criteria exhibited high sensitivity but low specificity (sensitivity 85%, specificity 67%, positive predictive value 43%, and negative predictive value 94%). When three of the criteria were considered, the specificity improved while the sensitivity decreased (sensitivity 49%, specificity 86%, positive predictive value 50%, and negative predictive value 86%). The gold standard against which these clinical indicators were evaluated was Sputum culture, tissue histology, and positive clinical and radiological response to the antituberculosis therapy. However, patients with chronic lung disorders were excluded from the study, which limits the extent to which it can be generalised. The prevalence of HIV was high (71%) in both case and control groups.

In another hospital-based study in Ethiopia, the most frequent symptoms in patients with pulmonary tuberculosis (both smear positive and smear negative) than in those without pulmonary tuberculosis were loss of appetite, weight loss, fever, night sweats, chest pain, haemoptysis, and breathlessness were more common [Tessema et al., 2001]. However, patients with smear-negative tuberculosis had night sweats for a longer time. Smear-positive patients were more likely to have fever and weight loss than the smear negative group (odds ratios 4·1 [1·2–15·0] and 6·4 [2·3–17·8], respectively). The diagnosis by a group of tuberculosis physicians, which may have been due to lack of resources, although the authors do not clarify the reason in the paper, was used as the gold standard for diagnosis of pulmonary tuberculosis. However, in an area with low prevalence of HIV infection and high prevalence of tuberculosis, one study based in Senegal found no clinical features differentiating smear-negative from smear-positive tuberculosis other than the absence of cough (odds ratio 10·0 [1·96–50·0]) [Samb et al., 1997]. Limitations of this study were that it had a small sample size and that the diagnosis was confirmed by means of sputum culture in only 20% of cases. The overall prevalence of HIV in both case and control groups was 8·9%. Our search could only retrieve one study that included subjects from a population with low prevalence of both HIV infection and tuberculosis [Kanaya et al., 2001]. Cough with expectoration was considered as a negative predictor of smear-negative tuberculosis (odds ratio 0·3 [0·1–0·6]). This study could not identify any other differentiating clinical features, possibly owing to the small sample size.

5.1.2 Radiographic criteria

Although the classical radiographic hallmarks of PT are cavitation, apical distribution, bilateral distribution, pulmonary fibrosis, shrinkage and calcification, no pattern is absolutely diagnostic of tuberculosis. Interpretation of chest X-rays of individuals suspected to have PT is difficult. In the pre-HIV era, there was considerable inter- and intra-observer variation in chest X-ray interpretation by radiologists and chest physicians [Thoman 1979].

In sub-Saharan Africa with limited microbiological services, the problem is compounded because there are few trained radiologists or chest physicians, and in most district hospitals chest X-rays are interpreted by relatively inexperienced medical officers or paramedics., survey in Malawi showed that medical officers misdiagnosed a third of clinical vignettes, which described typical radiographic signs of tuberculosis [Nyirenda et al., 1999]. The nonspecific findings of pulmonary infiltrates, in the middle or lower lobes, in HIV positive PT patients adds to the difficulties of correct radiographic diagnosis. It is now well recognized in industrialized countries [Pedro-Botet et al., 1992; Greenberg et al., 1994] and countries in sub-Saharan Africa [Simooya et al., 1991; Abouya et al., 1995] that the chest X-ray can appear normal in HIV-positive PT patients.

Studies in sub-Saharan Africa revealed that tuberculous patients with HIV infection are more likely to have atypical chest radiographic appearances (pulmonary infiltrates with no cavities, lower-lobe involvement, intrathoracic lymphadenopathy, and even normal appearance) than tuberculous patients without HIV infection [Harries et al., 1998b; Banda et al., 2000]. In areas of high HIV and tuberculosis prevalence, 75% of patients with smear-negative tuberculosis are likely to have atypical chest radiographic findings [Tessema et al., 2001]. Patients with smear-negative tuberculosis are less likely to have cavities on the chest radiograph (odds ratio 2·56) than patients with smear positive tuberculosis [Samb et al., 1999]. In addition, smear-negative patients can also present with normal or only slightly abnormal chest radiographs [Harries et al., 1998a]. A study confirmed pulmonary tuberculosis by sputum culture in 21% of patients with suspected tuberculosis and negative smears and normal or slightly abnormal chest radiographs. 47% of such patients were found to have typical radiographic features after 3 months. A third of the culture-negative patients also developed typical radiographic signs of tuberculosis during follow-up. Authors from that study suggested that close monitoring of smear-negative patients with suspected tuberculosis and normal or slightly abnormal chest radiographs is useful in areas with high prevalence of HIV infection and tuberculosis.

5.1.3 Sputum smear microscopy

Microscopy for the detection of AFB is rapid, low cost, and detects the most infectious cases of tuberculosis, but needs maintenance of equipment, consistent supply of reagents, and proper training in interpretation of the slides [Foulds and O'Brien, 1998]. International guidelines recommend the microscopic examination of three serial sputum specimens for acid-fast bacilli (AFB) in the investigation of pulmonary TB suspects, and define a positive case as a case with at least two smear-positive results [WHO 2003]. Recent studies have shown that under routine conditions, evaluating TB suspects with two sputum smears is as effective as with three sputum smears and is accompanied with less laboratory work and thus reductions in the cost related to the TB workup [Ipuge et al., 1996; Gopi et al., 2004]. This strategy could leave more time for the examination of each slide, should the workload dictate a reduction in the number of examinations. For a smear to be positive, there must be at least 5000-10 000 acid-fast bacilli per mL sputum, but these bacilli could be released only intermittently from cavities [WHO 2004]. If the sensitivity of smear microscopy could be improved, it would be a valuable instrument for TB control [Angeby et al., 2004] and would improve the diagnosis of tuberculosis in both adults. Many investigators have suggested sputum liquefaction and concentration through centrifugation to improve detection of AFB in negative smears through direct microscopy. Liquefaction of sputum with sodium hypochlorite and concentration by either centrifugation or sedimentation is the most widely studied procedure [Angeby et al., 2004]. Studies carried out in developing countries have shown an increase of almost two fold in the sensitivity of AFB detection compared with direct microscopy [Gebre et al., 1995; Habeenzu et al., 1998]. A systematic review also showed that studies that used sputum processing with chemicals including bleach and centrifugation yielded a mean 18% increase in sensitivity and an incremental yield (positives with bleach minus positives with Ziehl-Neelsen stain only) of 9% [Steingart et al., 2006]. Specificity ranged from 96% to 100% with the bleach method alone and from 95% to 100% with the Ziehl-Neelsen method alone [Angeby et al., 2004]. In HIV-positive patients, sensitivity increased from 38·5% to 50·0% after concentration [Bruchfeld et al., 2000]. This improvement was less remarkable when compared with the sensitivity of direct microscopy supported by clinicians' judgment in diagnosing pulmonary tuberculosis. The main disadvantages of the bleach method are the additional processing time, the technique lacks standardisation, and its advantages over other sputum concentration methods are not clear [Colebunders and Bastian, 2000].

Fluorescence microscopy increases the probability of detecting AFB, especially if the sputum contains few bacteria, and hence improves the sensitivity of microscopy in HIV-positive patients. A systematic review of studies that used fluorescence microscopy showed that on average, in comparison with Ziehl-Neelsen microscopy, fluorescence microscopy showed a 10% increase in sensitivity and 9% incremental yield, and this improvement was not affected by HIV status [Kivihya-Ndugga et al., 2003; Steingart et al., 2006]. The methods had similar specificity, but fluorescence microscopy done on one or two specimens was more cost effective than the Ziehl-Neelsen method used on three sputum specimens [Kivihya-Ndugga et al., 2003].

6. Differential diagnosis of smear-negative TB

There have been a number of research studies in sub-Saharan Africa, using either induced sputum or fibre-optic bronchoscopy with bronchoalveolar lavage and transbronchial biopsy, to determine the range of pulmonary diseases found in patients with respiratory illness and negative AFB sputum smears. AFB microscopy lacks sensitivity compared with culture. In patients with culture-confirmed pulmonary TB, the sensitivity of AFB microscopy ranges from 22 to 80% [Kim et al., 1984]. In the setting of low income countries as elsewhere, there are a number of factors that influence the diagnosis of smear negative tuberculosis. These factors include the prevalence of tuberculosis in the population, the prevalence of HIV infection, and finally, the prevalence of other infections that may mimic tuberculosis. In under-resourced, over-worked TB control programmes, laboratories cannot cope with the influx of diagnostic and follow-up smear examinations, and smears may not be done at all. For example, in Botswana in 1992, 48% of patients reported with pulmonary tuberculosis had no smear examinations performed [De Cock and Wilkinson, 1995]. Alternatively, the sputum specimens collected may be inadequate in quality or number. Ipuge et al. [Ipuge et al., 1996] found that 83.4% of smear-positive cases were detected on the first specimen, 12.2% on the second, and 4.4% on the third, by Ziehl-Neelsen staining under routine programme conditions in Tanzania. Finally, the performance of the smears may be technically inadequate. Declining quality of smear examination is a particular problem in overburdened laboratories in HIV-endemic countries. When, as part of an epidemiological study of TB and HIV in Tanzania, Chum et al. [Chum et al., 1996] compared the sputum microscopy results obtained in local and reference laboratories, 29% of new smear-negative cases (on the basis of local microscopy) were found to be smear-positive by the reference laboratory. False-negative results can be due to inadequate staining, under- or over-decolourisation, or inspection of too few fields (i.e., a minimum of 100 fields of a Ziehl-Neelsen smear must be examined before reporting a negative result and this examination takes about 5–10 minutes) [WHO 1998].

Other diseases identified in patients suspected of having TB include bacterial pneumonia due to a wide range of pathogens, Pneumocystis carinii pneumonia (PCP), Kaposi's sarcoma, nocardiosis and fungal infections with Cryptococcus neoformans and Aspergillus fumigatus. Bacterial pneumonia is the main differential diagnosis in HIV-positive and HIV-negative individuals, while PCP, cryptococcosis, and nocardiosis are of increased importance in HIV-positive subjects. The reported rates of PCP in African HIV-positive patients with respiratory symptoms vary between 0 and 33%. [Abouya et al., 1992; Kamanfu et al., 1993; Batungwanayo et al., 1994; Greenberg et al., 1995; Malin et al., 1995; Daley et al., 1996; Grant et al., 1998].

This variation has not been fully explained, but has been attributed to differences in patient selection, the level of immunodeficiency of HIV-positive patients in Africa, the limited availability of specialized laboratory diagnostics, the failure to diagnose PCP in the presence of multiple other infections, and geographic differences in the prevalence of PCP [Batungwanayo et al., 1994; Malin et al., 1995]. HIV-associated nocardiosis may also be under diagnosed. Lucas et al. [Lucas et al., 1994] conducted an autopsy study of 247 HIV-positive cases in Abidjan, Ivory Coast, and found one case of nocardiosis for every nine TB cases. These medical conditions account for significant morbidity and mortality in patients presenting with 'smear-negative pulmonary disease' in HIV- and TB endemic developing countries. However, the pre-eminent position of TB as the major pathogen in these circumstances must be emphasised. Moreover, it is necessary to emphase the importance of appropriate diagnosis of smear negative tuberculosis, both in terms of public health to identify early infectious sources more rapidly, and in terms of individual health, to identify specific diseases that can be treated. "In areas of high prevalence of tuberculosis, the most common disease that occurs in someone with the clinical signs of tuberculosis but has a negative sputum smear is still tuberculosis

7. Conclusion and future perspective

Smear-negative pulmonary TB is an increasing clinical problem in developing countries affected by the dual HIV/TB epidemic. It is clear that in sub-Saharan Africa more information is required to help solve some of the problems surrounding the diagnosis of smear negative TB. Clear diagnostic criteria need to be developed and agreed upon, and these may vary from country to country according to the availability of diagnostic facilities. Management algorithms that have been validated by local studies should improve case detection. Where current WHO guidelines have been implemented, clinical audits have the potential to improve the quality of diagnosis of smear-negative tuberculosis. Wider use of sputum induction and evaluation of novel sputum processing techniques may also improve the investigation of these patients. Some authors have argued for the wider availability of

TB culture facilities in developing countries; however, these Utopian interventions will require increased financial and technical support from the international community. The contribution of false negative sputum smears to the overall burden of smear-negative TB and the deficiencies in the system that lead to false-negative results need to be addressed. Rates of misdiagnosis of smear-negative tuberculosis can be reduced by development of diagnostic tools, which incorporate the diagnosis of other non-tuberculosis pulmonary disorders. Extensive basic research to develop rapid, simple, and accurate tuberculosis diagnostic tools that can be used in laboratories and remote locations is essential. Increased political commitment, greater scientific interest, and massive investment are needed. At the same time, innovative means need to be sought to address the human resources issues in the diagnosis problem, such as strategic efforts to train adequate and efficient laboratory staff at all levels. New diagnostic techniques are required in addition to AFB microscopy for the identification of smear-negative tuberculosis. These need to be appropriate for use in low income countries. Research into development of more cost-effective microbiological and serological diagnostic solutions is under way. However, until such tests are widely available, diagnostic scoring systems and algorithms must be developed and validated to assist clinicians working in resource-poor settings. Research collaboration is required between countries with similar HIV prevalence to address these research needs and to develop joint management guidelines, which can be applied and evaluated in different situations.

8. References

Aber VR, Allen BW, Mitchison DA, Ayuma P, Edwards EA, Keyes AB: Quality control in tuberculosis bacteriology. 1. Laboratory studies on isolated positive cultures and the efficiency of direct smear examination. Tubercle 1980;61:123-133.

Abouya L, Coulibaly IM, Coulibaly D, Kassim S, Ackah A, Greenberg AE, Wiktor SZ, De Cock KM: Radiologic manifestations of pulmonary tuberculosis in hiv-1 and hiv-2-infected patients in abidjan, cote d'ivoire. Tuber Lung Dis 1995;76:436-440.

Abouya YL, Beaumel A, Lucas S, Dago-Akribi A, Coulibaly G, N'Dhatz M, Konan JB, Yapi A, De Cock KM: Pneumocystis carinii pneumonia. An uncommon cause of death in african patients with acquired immunodeficiency syndrome. Am Rev Respir Dis 1992;145:617-620

Affolabi D, Akpona R, Odoun M, Alidjinou K, Wachinou P, Anagonou S, Gninafon M, Trebucq A: Smear-negative, culture-positive pulmonary tuberculosis among patients with chronic cough in cotonou, benin. Int J Tuberc Lung Dis;15:67-70.

Angeby KA, Hoffner SE, Diwan VK: Should the 'bleach microscopy method' be recommended for improved case detection of tuberculosis? Literature review and key person analysis. Int J Tuberc Lung Dis 2004;8:806-815.

Antonucci G, Girardi E, Raviglione MC, Ippolito G: Risk factors for tuberculosis in hiv-infected persons. A prospective cohort study. The gruppo italiano di studio tubercolosi e aids (gista). JAMA 1995;274:143-148.

Apers L, Wijarajah C, Mutsvangwa J, Chigara N, Mason P, van der Stuyft P: Accuracy of routine diagnosis of pulmonary tuberculosis in an area of high hiv prevalence. Int J Tuberc Lung Dis 2004;8:945-951.

Banda H, Kang'ombe C, Harries AD, Nyangulu DS, Whitty CJ, Wirima JJ, Salaniponi FM, Maher D, Nunn P: Mortality rates and recurrent rates of tuberculosis in patients with smear-negative pulmonary tuberculosis and tuberculous pleural effusion who have completed treatment. Int J Tuberc Lung Dis 2000;4:968-974.

Banda HT, Harries AD, Welby S, Boeree MJ, Wirima JJ, Subramanyam VR, Maher D, Nunn PA: Prevalence of tuberculosis in tb suspects with short duration of cough. Trans R Soc Trop Med Hyg 1998;92:161-163.

Bassett I, Chetty S, Wang B, et al. Intensive TB screening for HIV infected patients ready to start ART in Durban, South Africa: limitations of WHO guidelines. In: Program and abstracts of the 16th Conference on Retroviruses and Opportunistic Infections (Montreal). 2009. Abstract 779.

Batungwanayo J, Taelman H, Dhote R, Bogaerts J, Allen S, Van de Perre P: Pulmonary tuberculosis in kigali, rwanda. Impact of human immunodeficiency virus infection on clinical and radiographic presentation. Am Rev Respir Dis 1992;146:53-56.

Batungwanayo J, Taelman H, Lucas S, Bogaerts J, Alard D, Kagame A, Blanche P, Clerinx J, van de Perre P, Allen S: Pulmonary disease associated with the human immunodeficiency virus in kigali, rwanda. A fiberoptic bronchoscopic study of 111 cases of undetermined etiology. Am J Respir Crit Care Med 1994;149:1591-1596.

Behr MA, Warren SA, Salamon H, Hopewell PC, Ponce de Leon A, Daley CL, Small PM: Transmission of mycobacterium tuberculosis from patients smear-negative for acid-fast bacilli. Lancet 1999;353:444-449.

Brenchley JM, Knox KS, Asher AI, Price DA, Kohli LM, Gostick E, Hill BJ, Hage CA, Brahmi Z, Khoruts A, Twigg HL, 3rd, Schacker TW, Douek DC: High frequencies of polyfunctional hiv-specific t cells are associated with preservation of mucosal cd4 t cells in bronchoalveolar lavage. Mucosal Immunol 2008;1:49-58.

Brenchley JM, Price DA, Douek DC: Hiv disease: Fallout from a mucosal catastrophe? Nat Immunol 2006a;7:235-239.

Brenchley JM, Price DA, Schacker TW, Asher TE, Silvestri G, Rao S, Kazzaz Z, Bornstein E, Lambotte O, Altmann D, Blazar BR, Rodriguez B, Teixeira-Johnson L, Landay A, Martin JN, Hecht FM, Picker LJ, Lederman MM, Deeks SG, Douek DC: Microbial translocation is a cause of systemic immune activation in chronic hiv infection. Nat Med 2006b;12:1365-1371.

Brown CA, Draper P, Hart PD: Mycobacteria and lysosomes: A paradox. Nature 1969;221:658-660.

Bruchfeld J, Aderaye G, Palme IB, Bjorvatn B, Britton S, Feleke Y, Kallenius G, Lindquist L: Evaluation of outpatients with suspected pulmonary tuberculosis in a high hiv prevalence setting in ethiopia: Clinical, diagnostic and epidemiological characteristics. Scand J Infect Dis 2002;34:331-337.

Bruchfeld J, Aderaye G, Palme IB, Bjorvatn B, Kallenius G, Lindquist L: Sputum concentration improves diagnosis of tuberculosis in a setting with a high prevalence of hiv. Trans R Soc Trop Med Hyg 2000;94:677-680.

Chintu C, Mwaba P: Tuberculosis in children with human immunodeficiency virus infection. Int J Tuberc Lung Dis 2005;9:477-484.

Chum HJ, O'Brien RJ, Chonde TM, Graf P, Rieder HL: An epidemiological study of tuberculosis and hiv infection in tanzania, 1991-1993. AIDS 1996;10:299-309.

Colebunders R, Bastian I: A review of the diagnosis and treatment of smear-negative pulmonary tuberculosis. Int J Tuberc Lung Dis 2000;4:97-107.

Connolly C, Reid A, Davies G, Sturm W, McAdam KP, Wilkinson D: Relapse and mortality among hiv-infected and uninfected patients with tuberculosis successfully treated with twice weekly directly observed therapy in rural south africa. AIDS 1999;13:1543-1547.

Daley CL, Mugusi F, Chen LL, Schmidt DM, Small PM, Bearer E, Aris E, Mtoni IM, Cegielski JP, Lallinger G, Mbaga I, Murray JF: Pulmonary complications of hiv infection in dar es salaam, tanzania. Role of bronchoscopy and bronchoalveolar lavage. Am J Respir Crit Care Med 1996;154:105-110.

Day RB, Wang Y, Knox KS, Pasula R, Martin WJ, 2nd, Twigg HL, 3rd: Alveolar macrophages from hiv-infected subjects are resistant to mycobacterium tuberculosis in vitro. Am J Respir Cell Mol Biol 2004;30:403-410.

De Cock KM, Soro B, Coulibaly IM, Lucas SB: Tuberculosis and hiv infection in sub-saharan africa. JAMA 1992;268:1581-1587.

De Cock KM, Wilkinson D: Tuberculosis control in resource-poor countries: Alternative approaches in the era of hiv. Lancet 1995;346:675-677.

Desta K, Asrat D, Lemma E, Gebeyehu M, Feleke B: Prevalence of smear negative pulmonary tuberculosis among patients visiting st. Peter's tuberculosis specialized hospital, addis ababa, ethiopia. Ethiop Med J 2009;47:17-24.

Dheda K, Chang JS, Breen RA, Haddock JA, Lipman MC, Kim LU, Huggett JF, Johnson MA, Rook GA, Zumla A: Expression of a novel cytokine, il-4delta2, in hiv and hiv-tuberculosis co-infection. AIDS 2005;19:1601-1606.

Dheda K, van Zyl-Smit RN, Meldau R, Meldau S, Symons G, Khalfey H, Govender N, Rosu V, Sechi LA, Maredza A, Semple P, Whitelaw A, Wainwright H, Badri M, Dawson R, Bateman ED, Zumla A: Quantitative lung t cell responses aid the rapid diagnosis of pulmonary tuberculosis. Thorax 2009;64:847-853.

Edwards D, Vogt M, Bangani N, et al. Baseline screening for TB among patients enrolling in an ART service in South Africa. In: Program and abstracts of the 16th Conference on Retroviruses and Opportunistic Infections (Montreal). 2009. Abstract 780.

Elliott AM, Luo N, Tembo G, Halwiindi B, Steenbergen G, Machiels L, Pobee J, Nunn P, Hayes RJ, McAdam KP: Impact of hiv on tuberculosis in zambia: A cross sectional study. BMJ 1990;301:412-415.

Elliott AM, Namaambo K, Allen BW, Luo N, Hayes RJ, Pobee JO, McAdam KP: Negative sputum smear results in hiv-positive patients with pulmonary tuberculosis in lusaka, zambia. Tuber Lung Dis 1993;74:191-194.

Foulds J, O'Brien R: New tools for the diagnosis of tuberculosis: The perspective of developing countries. Int J Tuberc Lung Dis 1998;2:778-783.

Gebre N, Karlsson U, Jonsson G, Macaden R, Wolde A, Asseta A, Mlorner H: Improved microscopical diagnosis of pulmonary tuberculosis in developing countries. Trans R Soc Trop Med Hyg 1995;89:191-193.

Geldmacher C, Schuetz A, Ngwenyama N, Casazza JP, Sanga E, Saathoff E, Boehme C, Geis S, Maboko L, Singh M, Minja F, Meyerhans A, Koup RA, Hoelscher M: Early depletion of mycobacterium tuberculosis-specific t helper 1 cell responses after hiv-1 infection. J Infect Dis 2008;198:1590-1598.

Gopi PG, Subramani R, Selvakumar N, Santha T, Eusuff SI, Narayanan PR: Smear examination of two specimens for diagnosis of pulmonary tuberculosis in tiruvallur district, south india. Int J Tuberc Lung Dis 2004;8:824-828.

Graf P. Tuberculosis control in high-prevalence countries. In: Davies PDO, ed. Clinical tuberculosis 1994. London, Chapman & Hall, 1994: 325-339.

Grant AD, Sidibe K, Domoua K, Bonard D, Sylla-Koko F, Dosso M, Yapi A, Maurice C, Whitaker JP, Lucas SB, Hayes RJ, Wiktor SZ, De Cock KM, Greenberg AE:

Spectrum of disease among hiv-infected adults hospitalised in a respiratory medicine unit in abidjan, cote d'ivoire. Int J Tuberc Lung Dis 1998;2:926-934.

Greenberg AE, Lucas S, Tossou O, Coulibaly IM, Coulibaly D, Kassim S, Ackah A, De Cock KM: Autopsy-proven causes of death in hiv-infected patients treated for tuberculosis in abidjan, cote d'ivoire. AIDS 1995;9:1251-1254.

Greenberg SD, Frager D, Suster B, Walker S, Stavropoulos C, Rothpearl A: Active pulmonary tuberculosis in patients with aids: Spectrum of radiographic findings (including a normal appearance). Radiology 1994;193:115-119.

Gutierrez MG, Master SS, Singh SB, Taylor GA, Colombo MI, Deretic V: Autophagy is a defense mechanism inhibiting bcg and mycobacterium tuberculosis survival in infected macrophages. Cell 2004;119:753-766.

Habeenzu C, Lubasi D, Fleming AF: 'improved sensitivity of direct microscopy for detection of acid-fast bacilli in sputum in developing countries. Trans R Soc Trop Med Hyg 1998;92:415-416.

Hargreaves NJ, Kadzakumanja O, Phiri S, Nyangulu DS, Salaniponi FM, Harries AD, Squire SB: What causes smear-negative pulmonary tuberculosis in malawi, an area of high hiv seroprevalence? Int J Tuberc Lung Dis 2001;5:113-122.

Hargreaves NJ, Phiri S, Kwanjana J, Nyangulu DS, Squire SB: Unrecognised mycobacterium tuberculosis. Lancet 2000;355:141; author reply 142-143.

Harries AD: Tuberculosis and human immunodeficiency virus infection in developing countries. Lancet 1990;335:387-390.

Harries AD, Banda HT, Boeree MJ, Welby S, Wirima JJ, Subramanyam VR, Maher D, Nunn P: Management of pulmonary tuberculosis suspects with negative sputum smears and normal or minimally abnormal chest radiographs in resource-poor settings. Int J Tuberc Lung Dis 1998a;2:999-1004.

Harries AD, Maher D, Nunn P: An approach to the problems of diagnosing and treating adult smear-negative pulmonary tuberculosis in high-hiv-prevalence settings in sub-saharan africa. Bull World Health Organ 1998b;76:651-662.

Harries AD, Nyangulu DS, Kangombe C, Ndalama D, Wirima JJ, Salaniponi FM, Liomba G, Maher D, Nunn P: The scourge of hiv-related tuberculosis: A cohort study in a district general hospital in malawi. Ann Trop Med Parasitol 1997;91:771-776.

Hernandez-Garduno E, Cook V, Kunimoto D, Elwood RK, Black WA, FitzGerald JM: Transmission of tuberculosis from smear negative patients: A molecular epidemiology study. Thorax 2004;59:286-290.

Hopewell PC: Impact of human immunodeficiency virus infection on the epidemiology, clinical features, management, and control of tuberculosis. Clin Infect Dis 1992;15:540-547.

Ipuge YA, Rieder HL, Enarson DA: The yield of acid-fast bacilli from serial smears in routine microscopy laboratories in rural tanzania. Trans R Soc Trop Med Hyg 1996;90:258-261.

Jones BE, Young SM, Antoniskis D, Davidson PT, Kramer F, Barnes PF: Relationship of the manifestations of tuberculosis to cd4 cell counts in patients with human immunodeficiency virus infection. Am Rev Respir Dis 1993;148:1292-1297.

Kalsdorf B, Scriba TJ, Wood K, Day CL, Dheda K, Dawson R, Hanekom WA, Lange C, Wilkinson RJ: Hiv-1 infection impairs the bronchoalveolar t-cell response to mycobacteria. Am J Respir Crit Care Med 2009;180:1262-1270.

Kamanfu G, Mlika-Cabanne N, Girard PM, Nimubona S, Mpfizi B, Cishako A, Roux P, Coulaud JP, Larouze B, Aubry P, et al.: Pulmonary complications of human immunodeficiency virus infection in bujumbura, burundi. Am Rev Respir Dis 1993;147:658-663.

Kanaya AM, Glidden DV, Chambers HF: Identifying pulmonary tuberculosis in patients with negative sputum smear results. Chest 2001;120:349-355.

Kang'ombe CT, Harries AD, Ito K, Clark T, Nyirenda TE, Aldis W, Nunn PP, Semba RD, Salaniponi FM: Long-term outcome in patients registered with tuberculosis in zomba, malawi: Mortality at 7 years according to initial hiv status and type of tb. Int J Tuberc Lung Dis 2004;8:829-836.

Kassu A, Mengistu G, Ayele B, Diro E, Mekonnen F, Ketema D, Moges F, Mesfin T, Getachew A, Ergicho B, Elias D, Aseffa A, Wondmikun Y, Ota F: Coinfection and clinical manifestations of tuberculosis in human immunodeficiency virus-infected and -uninfected adults at a teaching hospital, northwest ethiopia. J Microbiol Immunol Infect 2007;40:116-122.

Keane J, Remold HG, Kornfeld H: Virulent mycobacterium tuberculosis strains evade apoptosis of infected alveolar macrophages. J Immunol 2000;164:2016-2020.

Kim TC, Blackman RS, Heatwole KM, Kim T, Rochester DF: Acid-fast bacilli in sputum smears of patients with pulmonary tuberculosis. Prevalence and significance of negative smears pretreatment and positive smears post-treatment. Am Rev Respir Dis 1984;129:264-268.

Kivihya-Ndugga LE, van Cleeff MR, Githui WA, Nganga LW, Kibuga DK, Odhiambo JA, Klatser PR: A comprehensive comparison of ziehl-neelsen and fluorescence microscopy for the diagnosis of tuberculosis in a resource-poor urban setting. Int J Tuberc Lung Dis 2003;7:1163-1171.

Klausner JD, Ryder RW, Baende E, Lelo U, Williame JC, Ngamboli K, Perriens JH, Kaboto M, Prignot J: Mycobacterium tuberculosis in household contacts of human immunodeficiency virus type 1-seropositive patients with active pulmonary tuberculosis in kinshasa, zaire. J Infect Dis 1993;168:106-111.

Kyei GB, Dinkins C, Davis AS, Roberts E, Singh SB, Dong C, Wu L, Kominami E, Ueno T, Yamamoto A, Federico M, Panganiban A, Vergne I, Deretic V: Autophagy pathway intersects with hiv-1 biosynthesis and regulates viral yields in macrophages. J Cell Biol 2009;186:255-268.

Lawn SD, Bekker LG, Middelkoop K, Myer L, Wood R: Impact of hiv infection on the epidemiology of tuberculosis in a peri-urban community in south africa: The need for age-specific interventions. Clin Infect Dis 2006;42:1040-1047.

Long R, Scalcini M, Manfreda J, Jean-Baptiste M, Hershfield E: The impact of hiv on the usefulness of sputum smears for the diagnosis of tuberculosis. Am J Public Health 1991;81:1326-1328.

Lucas SB, Hounnou A, Peacock C, Beaumel A, Kadio A, De Cock KM: Nocardiosis in hiv-positive patients: An autopsy study in west africa. Tuber Lung Dis 1994;75:301-307.

Malin AS, Gwanzura LK, Klein S, Robertson VJ, Musvaire P, Mason PR: Pneumocystis carinii pneumonia in zimbabwe. Lancet 1995;346:1258-1261.

Markowitz N, Hansen NI, Wilcosky TC, Hopewell PC, Glassroth J, Kvale PA, Mangura BT, Osmond D, Wallace JM, Rosen MJ, Reichman LB: Tuberculin and anergy testing in hiv-seropositive and hiv-seronegative persons. Pulmonary complications of hiv infection study group. Ann Intern Med 1993;119:185-193.

Mukadi Y, Perriens JH, St Louis ME, Brown C, Prignot J, Willame JC, Pouthier F, Kaboto M, Ryder RW, Portaels F, et al.: Spectrum of immunodeficiency in hiv-1-infected patients with pulmonary tuberculosis in zaire. Lancet 1993;342:143-146.

Munyati SS, Dhoba T, Makanza ED, Mungofa S, Wellington M, Mutsvangwa J, Gwanzura L, Hakim J, Nyakabau M, Mason PR, Robertson V, Rusakaniko S, Butterworth AE, Corbett EL: Chronic cough in primary health care attendees, harare, zimbabwe: Diagnosis and impact of hiv infection. Clin Infect Dis 2005;40:1818-1827.

Mwandumba HC, Russell DG, Nyirenda MH, Anderson J, White SA, Molyneux ME, Squire SB: Mycobacterium tuberculosis resides in nonacidified vacuoles in endocytically competent alveolar macrophages from patients with tuberculosis and hiv infection. J Immunol 2004;172:4592-4598.

Nunn P, Gicheha C, Hayes R, Gathua S, Brindle R, Kibuga D, Mutie T, Kamunyi R, Omwega M, Were J, et al.: Cross-sectional survey of hiv infection among patients with tuberculosis in nairobi, kenya. Tuber Lung Dis 1992;73:45-51.

Nyirenda TE, Harries AD, Banerjee A, Salaniponi FM: Accuracy of chest radiograph diagnosis for smear-negative pulmonary tuberculosis suspects by hospital clinical staff in malawi. Trop Doct 1999;29:219-220.

Oddo M, Renno T, Attinger A, Bakker T, MacDonald HR, Meylan PR: Fas ligand-induced apoptosis of infected human macrophages reduces the viability of intracellular mycobacterium tuberculosis. J Immunol 1998;160:5448-5454.

Palomino JC, Cardoso S, Ritacco V (2007) Tuberculosis 2007: from basic science to patient care. Available: http://www.tuberculosistextbook.com/ tuberculosis2007.pdf. Accessed 2011 Jul 5.

Parry CM: Sputum smear negative pulmonary tuberculosis. Trop Doct 1993;23:145-146.

Patel NR, Koziel H. Lung defenses in the immunosuppressed patient. In: Agusti C, Torres A, editors. Pulmonary infection in the immunocompromised patient. Oxford: Wiley-Blackwell; 2009

Patel NR, Swan K, Li X, Tachado SD, Koziel H: Impaired m. Tuberculosis-mediated apoptosis in alveolar macrophages from hiv+ persons: Potential role of il-10 and bcl-3. J Leukoc Biol 2009;86:53-60.

Patel NR, Zhu J, Tachado SD, Zhang J, Wan Z, Saukkonen J, Koziel H: Hiv impairs tnf-alpha mediated macrophage apoptotic response to mycobacterium tuberculosis. J Immunol 2007;179:6973-6980.

Pedro-Botet J, Gutierrez J, Miralles R, Coll J, Rubies-Prat J: Pulmonary tuberculosis in hiv-infected patients with normal chest radiographs. AIDS 1992;6:91-93.

Perkins MD, Cunningham J: Facing the crisis: Improving the diagnosis of tuberculosis in the hiv era. J Infect Dis 2007;196 Suppl 1:S15-27.

Raviglione MC, Harries AD, Msiska R, Wilkinson D, Nunn P: Tuberculosis and hiv: Current status in africa. AIDS 1997;11 Suppl B:S115-123.

Russell DG: Mycobacterium tuberculosis: Here today, and here tomorrow. Nat Rev Mol Cell Biol 2001;2:569-577.

Samb B, Henzel D, Daley CL, Mugusi F, Niyongabo T, Mlika-Cabanne N, Kamanfu G, Aubry P, Mbaga I, Larouze B, Murray JF: Methods for diagnosing tuberculosis among in-patients in eastern africa whose sputum smears are negative. Int J Tuberc Lung Dis 1997;1:25-30.

Samb B, Sow PS, Kony S, Maynart-Badiane M, Diouf G, Cissokho S, Ba D, Sane M, Klotz F, Faye-Niang MA, Mboup S, Ndoye I, Delaporte E, Hane AA, Samb A, Coulaud JP, Coll-Seck AM, Larouze B, Murray JF: Risk factors for negative sputum acid-fast bacilli smears in pulmonary tuberculosis: Results from dakar, senegal, a city with low hiv seroprevalence. Int J Tuberc Lung Dis 1999;3:330-336.

Saukkonen JJ, Bazydlo B, Thomas M, Strieter RM, Keane J, Kornfeld H: Beta-chemokines are induced by mycobacterium tuberculosis and inhibit its growth. Infect Immun 2002;70:1684-1693.

Schaible UE, Winau F, Sieling PA, Fischer K, Collins HL, Hagens K, Modlin RL, Brinkmann V, Kaufmann SH: Apoptosis facilitates antigen presentation to t lymphocytes through mhc-i and cd1 in tuberculosis. Nat Med 2003;9:1039-1046.

Selwyn PA, Pumerantz AS, Durante A, Alcabes PG, Gourevitch MN, Boiselle PM, Elmore JG: Clinical predictors of pneumocystis carinii pneumonia, bacterial pneumonia and tuberculosis in hiv-infected patients. AIDS 1998;12:885-893.

Siddiqi K, Lambert ML, Walley J: Clinical diagnosis of smear-negative pulmonary tuberculosis in low-income countries: The current evidence. Lancet Infect Dis 2003;3:288-296.

Simooya OO, Maboshe MN, Kaoma RB, Chimfwembe EC, Thurairajah A, Mukunyandela M: Hiv infection in newly diagnosed tuberculosis patients in ndola, zambia. Cent Afr J Med 1991;37:4-7.

Sonnenberg P, Glynn JR, Fielding K, Murray J, Godfrey-Faussett P, Shearer S: How soon after infection with hiv does the risk of tuberculosis start to increase? A retrospective cohort study in south african gold miners. J Infect Dis 2005;191:150-158.

Sonnenberg P, Murray J, Glynn JR, Shearer S, Kambashi B, Godfrey-Faussett P: Hiv-1 and recurrence, relapse, and reinfection of tuberculosis after cure: A cohort study in south african mineworkers. Lancet 2001;358:1687-1693.

Steingart KR, Ng V, Henry M, Hopewell PC, Ramsay A, Cunningham J, Urbanczik R, Perkins MD, Aziz MA, Pai M: Sputum processing methods to improve the sensitivity of smear microscopy for tuberculosis: A systematic review. Lancet Infect Dis 2006;6:664-674.

Sudre P, ten Dam G, Kochi A: Tuberculosis: A global overview of the situation today. Bull World Health Organ 1992;70:149-159.

Sutherland R, Yang H, Scriba TJ, Ondondo B, Robinson N, Conlon C, Suttill A, McShane H, Fidler S, McMichael A, Dorrell L: Impaired ifn-gamma-secreting capacity in mycobacterial antigen-specific cd4 t cells during chronic hiv-1 infection despite long-term haart. AIDS 2006;20:821-829.

Tessema TA, Bjune G, Assefa G, Bjorvat B: An evaluation of the diagnostic value of clinical and radiological manifestations in patients attending the addis ababa tuberculosis centre. Scand J Infect Dis 2001;33:355-361.

Toman K. Tuberculosis case-finding and chemotherapy. Questions and answers. Geneva, World Health Organization, 1979.

Tostmann A, Kik SV, Kalisvaart NA, Sebek MM, Verver S, Boeree MJ, van Soolingen D: Tuberculosis transmission by patients with smear-negative pulmonary tuberculosis in a large cohort in the netherlands. Clin Infect Dis 2008;47:1135-1142.

van Cleeff MR, Kivihya-Ndugga L, Githui W, Nganga L, Odhiambo J, Klatser PR: A comprehensive study of the efficiency of the routine pulmonary tuberculosis diagnostic process in nairobi. Int J Tuberc Lung Dis 2003;7:186-189.

Whalen C, Horsburgh CR, Hom D, Lahart C, Simberkoff M, Ellner J: Accelerated course of human immunodeficiency virus infection after tuberculosis. Am J Respir Crit Care Med 1995;151:129-135.

Whalen C, Horsburgh CR, Jr., Hom D, Lahart C, Simberkoff M, Ellner J: Site of disease and opportunistic infection predict survival in hiv-associated tuberculosis. AIDS 1997;11:455-460.
Laboratory Services in Tuberculosis Control. Technical Series: Microscopy. WHO/TB/98.258. Geneva: World Health Organization, 1998.
Worl Health Organization (WHO): Global tuberculosis control, WHO report 2002 [http://www.who.int/gtb/publications] accessed 2011 Jul 13
World Health Organization. Treatment of tuberculosis. Guidelines for national programs. WHO/CDS/TB/2003.313. Geneva, Switzerland: WHO, 2003.
World Health Orgainization. Toman's Tuberculosis: Case detection, treatment and monitoring-questions and answers. WHO/HTM/TB/2004.334. Geneva: World Health Organization, 2004.
Worl Health Organization (WHO): Improving the diagnosis and treatment of smear-negative pulmonary and extra-pulmonary tuberculosis among adults and adolescents: recommendations for HIV-prevalent and resource-constrained settings. Geneva, World Health Organization, 2007. WHO/HTM/TB/2007.379 WHO/HIV/2007.01
World Health Organization. Global tuberculosis control: a short update to the 2009 report. December 2009. Geneva: World Health Organization, 2009.
World Health Organization. Global tuberculosis control: epidemiology, strategy, financing. WHO report 2009. Geneva, Switzerland: WHO; 2009
Wilkinson D, Davies GR: The increasing burden of tuberculosis in rural south africa--impact of the hiv epidemic. S Afr Med J 1997;87:447-450.
Williams BG, Dye C: Antiretroviral drugs for tuberculosis control in the era of hiv/aids. Science 2003;301:1535-1537.
Winau F, Weber S, Sad S, de Diego J, Hoops SL, Breiden B, Sandhoff K, Brinkmann V, Kaufmann SH, Schaible UE: Apoptotic vesicles crossprime cd8 t cells and protect against tuberculosis. Immunity 2006;24:105-117.
Yassin MA, Takele L, Gebresenbet S, Girma E, Lera M, Lendebo E, Cuevas LE: Hiv and tuberculosis coinfection in the southern region of ethiopia: A prospective epidemiological study. Scand J Infect Dis 2004;36:670-673.
Zachariah R, Spielmann MP, Harries AD, Salaniponi FL: Voluntary counselling, hiv testing and sexual behaviour among patients with tuberculosis in a rural district of malawi. Int J Tuberc Lung Dis 2003;7:65-71.
Zhang M, Gong J, Iyer DV, Jones BE, Modlin RL, Barnes PF: T cell cytokine responses in persons with tuberculosis and human immunodeficiency virus infection. J Clin Invest 1994;94:2435-2442.

7

Immunologic Diagnosis of Neurotuberculosis

Iacob Simona Alexandra[1], Banica Dorina[1], Iacob Diana Gabriela[2], Panaitescu Eugenia[2], Radu Irina[3] and Cojocaru Manole[4]
[1]*National Institute of Infectious Diseases "Matei Bals", Bucharest,*
[2]*The University of Medicine and Pharmacy "Carol Davila" Bucharest,*
[3]*The University of Bucharest,*
[4]*The "Titu Maiorescu" University*
Romania

1. Introduction

Tuberculosis (TB) is one of the most prevalent infectious diseases in the world, particularly in developing countries. The high incidence and mortality of TB in these countries mainly resides in the limited financial resources, the emergence of multiresistant strains and the spread of HIV infections. The key element for controlling TB is a rapid and early diagnosis which ensures the correct treatment and eradication of the infection source in the community. Current strategies for the development of a rapid and accurate diagnosis address 3 major objectives: improving the present diagnostic tools through better knowledge, developing new tests and increasing the accessibility to such diagnostic possibilities (Who Strategic Directions, 2006). The gold standard of diagnosis in TB is the identification of mycobacteria in the pathologic product using acid-fast smear microscopy and mycobacterial culture. Nevertheless the bacteriologic diagnosis is presently inefficient due to increasing number of smear-negative TB forms. This has led to the development of various complementary diagnostic methods such immunologic assays. The aim of the present chapter is to outline the literature data on the importance of the immunologic diagnosis in neurotuberculosis, a lethal localization of TB. It presents the current immunological assays and their practical value in the diagnosis of neurotuberculosis as complementary methods.

2. General data

Neurotuberculosis is represented by various central nervous system (CNS) tuberculous manifestations including : tuberculoma, tuberculous abscess, meningoencephalitis , spinal arachnoiditis and cerebral miliary tuberculosis. This diverse neurological frame mostly emerges as a result of the invasive potential as well as of the immune pathogeny of neurotuberculosis. The difficulty in the diagnosis of neurotuberculosis lies in the atypical clinical presentation and non-specific changes recorded by various diagnostic assays. The bacteriological exams of the cerebrospinal fluid (CSF) are still regarded as the sole diagnostic tools in the confirmation of neurotuberculosis. Nevertheless the bacteriological assay in neurological forms of TB has a low sensitivity and a considerable delay. As a rule, owing to the rapid evolution and increased mortality, the suspected neurotuberculosis patients frequently receive antituberculous treatment before bacteriological confirmation (Donald & Schoeman, 2004). A complete antituberculous treatment requires 6-12 months, during which serious adverse reactions could occur. On the other hand nontuberculous CNS infections with different treatment and high mortality could be overlooked. Therefore multiple research studies based on new diagnostic methods have been developed over the last 30 years aiming to improve the diagnostic efficiency in neurotuberculosis.

3. Diagnostic methods in neurotuberculosis

CSF analysis represents the basic element in the diagnosis of neurotuberculosis. The isolation and identification of mycobacteria in CSF are crucial for the diagnosis of neurotuberculosis. However as the CSF is a paucibacillar product, these methods often fail. All the same the CSF could present characteristic cytological and chemical changes which could be suggestive for the neurotuberculosis diagnosis in a specific clinical context. In several cases, especially in children and immunosupressed patients, the cytochemical changes of the CSF lack even these particular findings and the neurotuberculosis diagnosis is then ommited. During the past decades various complementary methods have been implemented to assist these difficulties. These currently include : nucleic acid amplification tests (NAATs), CSF adenosindeaminase (ADA) detection and immunologic assays.

3.1 Advantages and disadvantages of current diagnostic techniques in neurotuberculosis

Below are the main findings, advantages and disadvantages of each current diagnostic method in neurotuberculosis (Desai et al, 2006; Sonmeza et al, 2008; Nyendak et al, 2009; Davies & Pai 2008)

a. **CSF cytology.** *Main findings*: at the onset mixed pleocytosis with mainly lymphocytes(80-90%) and the presence of neutrophils (10-20%); in the later stages, only lymphocytes.

Advantages: rapid, inexpensive, sensitive method. *Disadvantages*: 1) Variable CSF cytology in the evolution of the disease, 2) Many atypical CSF aspects at the onset or throughout the evolution in immunodepressed hosts and children 3)Low specificity; 4)Normal CSF cytology cannot rule out localized forms of neurotuberculosis

b. **Biochemical CSF exam.** *Main findings*: high CSF protein level and low glucose.

Advantages: rapid, inexpensive. *Disadvantages*: 1) Very low specificity: many infections of the CNS share similar changes ; 2) CSF biochemical analysis is normal in localized forms of neurotuberculosis.

c. Bacteriologic CSF exam.

CSF smear. *Main findings*: the CSF smear detects mycobacteria using acid-fast bacilli stains (Ziehl-Neelsen or the Kinyoun method) as well as fluorescence staining.

Advantages: rapid, inexpensive, simple, specific, low technical demand. *Disadvantages*: 1) Very low sensitivity of 13-53%; nevertheless, fluorescence microscopy and certain processing methods have been developed to improve the sensitivity; 2) The CSF smear cannot distinguish between different species of mycobacteria ; moreover, it is difficult to detect nontuberculous mycobacteria; 3) The procesessing is prone to contamination with environmental or water-borne saprophitic mycobacteria; 4) Results depend on the CSF volume (a positive result requires >6ml of CSF) and on the number of samples (repeated analysis of lumbar punctures increases diagnostic yield); 5) False negative smear results in localized forms of cerebral TB.

CSF culture. *Main findings*: isolation and identification of mycobacteria on selective media (solid or liquid media).

Advantages: 1) Represents the definitive proof of active TB (gold standard). 2) Enables the performance of an antibiogram; 3) better sensitivity, than the CSF smear. *Disadvantages*: 1) Sensitivity depends on the number of samples, CSF volume and mycobacteria loading (CSF enrichment techniques could be used); 2) Large differences between media on efficiency and price; 3) Adequate laboratory infrastructure and trained personnel are necessary; 4) Detection requires minimum 14 days even on selective media; 5) Negative CSF culture in localized neurotuberculosis.

d. **Nucleic acid amplification tests (NAATs).** *Main findings*: detect mycobacteria nucleic acid in serum and CSF using the *PCR* assay.

Advantages: *NAAT*s exhibits a high specificity (88%-100%), good positive predictive value and rapid processing. Due to its specificity it could be used for treatment monitoring. *Disadvantages*: 1) *NAAT*s have a highly variable sensitivity and low negative predictive value, especially in smear-negative and extrapulmonary TB; the sensitivity of the *PCR* method (33% to 90%) is highly dependent on the mycobacteria loading and variable for each *PCR* technique; 2) *PCR* becomes rapidly negative after treatment; 3) In-house *NAAT*s produces highly variable results compared to commercial, standardized *NAAT*s. Nevertheless, commercial *NAATs* show a potential role in confirming the diagnosis of TB meningitis, although their overall low sensitivity precludes the use of these tests to rule out the diagnosis with certainty; 4) The high price makes them prohibitive in poor countries with the highest prevalence of TB.

e. **The adenosine deaminase (ADA) detection**

Advantages: rapid; inexpensive; high diagnostic accuracy. *Disadvantages:* 1) Low specificity: it cannot rule out bacterial meningitis. 2) Not standardized.

f. **Histologic exam.** *Main findings*: reveals tissue mycobacteria and characteristic granulomatous aspects.

Advantages: 1) Very high specificity. 2) The main diagnosis method for localised cerebral TB. *Disadvantages:* 1) Invasive method; 2) Histology does not distinguish between mycobacteria or different granulomatous diseases; 4)Belated result (requires one or two days)

g. **Imaging methods.** *Main findings:* indicates complications of neurotuberculosis (hydrocephalus, vasculitis) and localized forms of neurotuberculosis. *Advantages*: improves the differential diagnosis and treatment evaluation. *Disadvantages*: 1) Images are not pathognomonic for TB; 2) High exposure to radiation; 3) Very expensive.

Conclusion: None of the current methods meets the criteria required by an efficient diagnostic test: rapid, accurate and readily applicable. Treatment in neurotuberculosis is therefore implemented according to the association of epidemiological, clinical criteria, bacteriologic CSF examination and different complementary laboratory methods dependent on the technical level of each laboratory. The decision on which tests to use should consider country-level technical facilities and other relevant factors, such as cost and availability. The lack of standardisation in the use of these methods renders their comparison more difficult.

3.2 Reason for the development of immunologic assays in neurotuberculosis

Unlike latent TB, neurotuberculosis is characterized by active CNS lesions accompanied by an intense cellular and humoral immune response. Both T cells and B cells are active during mycobacteria replication suggesting the potential use of immune markers in cerebral TB. Immune diagnostic tools also assessed antigens released by *M.tbc* in the CSF or specific antibodies. Beginning with 1990, numerous antigens and antibodies were screened for the diagnosis of neurotuberculosis in endemic areas. Studies on these methods proved a good specificity and simple, inexpensive and rapid results. Nevertheless the low sensitivity and the development of molecular techniques decreased the importance of these methods in neurotuberculosis diagnosis. The immunological diagnosis continues to be considered in TB endemic areas due to the increasing number of immunological biomarkers detection (Walzl et al, 2011). Over the past years, T cell-based IFNg release assays (IGRAs) performed on T cell isolated from the CSF, were found senzitive and specific for TB meningitis. IGRAs restored the interest in the immunological methods for TB diagnosis even in countries with high financial support. (Thomas et al, 2008).

3.3 The advantages and disadvantages of immunologic diagnostic methods in the diagnosis of neurotuberculosis

a. Determination of mycobacterial antigens or antimycobacterial antibodies in serum and CSF fluid. (Thomas et al, 2008; Patel et al, 2010)

Advantages: 1) Rapid , inexpensive, simple technique, minimal training requirements compared to molecular methods. 2) Specific detection of the intrathecal synthesis of antimycobacterial antibodies and of mycobacterial antigens in the CSF.

Disadvantages: 1) Highly inconsistent estimates of sensitivity and specificity correlated with the method used, detected type of antigen or antibody and mycobacteria load; however combinations of select antigens provide higher sensitivity compared to single antigens. 2) False negative results particularly in immunodepressed hosts; 3) Specificity can be affected by cross reactions between different mycobacteria or other bacterial species (*Nocardia, Leishmania*); 4) Some methods (*ELISA*) require specific equipment, skilled technicians and refrigerated reagents.

b. **IFN-γ release assays (IGRAs)** The two methods presently used are *QuantiFERON-Gold (QFT-G)* method and *T-SPOT.TB* method. Both can substitute the tuberculin skin test (*TST*) in routine clinical practice, especially where *BCG* vaccination is prevalent.

Avantages: rapid and specific. 2) Applied in few studies of neurotuberculosis with a sensitivity of 90% and specificity of 100% in cases of negative bacteriological TB meningitis.

Disadvantages: 1) Requires appropiate lab-facility; 2) Expensive; 3) T cell lymphopenia and anergy resulting from disseminated TB or advanced HIV infection, lead to the lack of *ELISPOT* responses. 4) False negative results in patients with atypical CSF (few lymphocytes). 5) False positive results in the case of blood contamination during puncture.

Conclusion. The immunological diagnosis in neurotuberculosis reflects the present knowledge related to the immune pathogenesis of TB. Addition of new immunologic data and a more complex interpretation of the results could improve the diagnostic value of these methods.

4. Imunologic response in NTB

TB is primarily a pulmonary disease. The protective immunity in infections with *M.tbc* is ensured by the macrophageal activity, CD4T cell response and Th1 cytokines. Consequently, the immune response frequently leads to the formation of granuloma, an organized and efficient form of defence. The granulomas include mycobacteria with a modified metabolism and potential of active replication which increases in case of immunodepression. The granulomas adjacent to the meninges or cerebral vessels increase the risk of CSF mycobacteria invasion. Mycobacteria reaching the subarachnoidial space release antigens and induce an intense inflammatory response. Since 1990, these antigens have been acknowledged as potential markers for the diagnosis of TB meningitis.

4.1 Mycobacterial antigens (general data, classification, role)

M.tbc encodes about 4000 proteins. As mycobacteria are extremely dynamic they release a variable number of antigens according to the clinical form of TB, the duration of the infection and the host immune response. The recognition of relevant mycobacterial antigens by T cell subsets is an essential step in triggering the protective immunity in TB. A functional classification of these antigens is presently unavailable, nor is the selection of antigens for the development of efficient serological diagnostic tools. Sequencing of the M.tbc genome in 1998 and the knowledge in proteogenomics led to the identification of numerous immunogenic antigens specific for *M. tbc* and *M .bovis*. These specific antigens differ from environmental mycobacterias or BCG vaccine strains and could be used in the immunologic TB diagnosis. However no specific antigen or set of antigens has been yet recognized in TB and no set of antigens has been established for diagnosis with confidence. The release of a certain antigen is induced by a large number of factors such as the type of infection (active or inactive), the host immune status (imunocompetent or immunodeppressed), local immune metabolism or ph conditions, mycobacteria viability (viable mycobacteria release other antigens than dormant bacilli), mycobacteria virulence and the infection site. The immunogenicity of these antigens also differs: only a small number of the antigens released in the culture media (25%) induced the synthesis of specific antibodies. (Samanich et al, 2000). The variability of released antigens under different conditions and their immunogenicity hinders an accurate selection and represents a serious obstacle in the immunodiagnostic development of TB. A cocktail combining a large number of antigens (10 to 12 recombinant antigens or poly-proteins) appears to be a reasonable choice for increasing both the sensitivity and the specificity of immunologic diagnostic methods (Raja et al, 2008). The classification and nomenclature of mycobacteria antigens is not unitary. There are more names and classifications for one antigen depending on localization (cellular wall, cellular membrane and cytoplasm antigens) and structure (lipids, proteins, polysaccharides and their complexes). Proteic antigens are secreted in active lesions and have proved a great potential in the serological diagnosis, either alone or in poly-protein complexes (Houghton et al, 2002) , while glycolipidic antigens are released in immunodepressed hosts especially. A detailed presentation of mycobacteria antigens belongs to Young (Yang et al, 1992). Several of these proteic antigens have already been included in diagnostic tests for neurotuberculosis: antigens of 38 kDa, 16 kDa, 88 kDa, MPT51, CFP-10, antigen 85B (associated to the protein 30-31 kDa), lipoarabinomannan (LAM), antigen A60, antigen 5, cord factor. The roles assigned to mycobacteria antigens are often contradictory and not fully understood. The documented activity of mycobacteria antigens is diverse: enhancing the immune response (antigen 85, P320, A60) , triggering the delayed-type hypersensitivity (proteic antigens), interfering with the adhesion of mycobacteria on host cells, promoting phagosome-lysososme fusion. Certain antigens (LAM, 30kDa antigen, antigen 6) also induce cellular immunodepression by inhibiting various functions of the macrophages, or T Lymphocytes and assisting in the formation of granulomas.

4.2 Antimycobacterial antibodies (general data, relevance, dynamics)

M. tbc is resistant to antimycobacterial antibodies. Stimulation of the humoral immunity using polysaccharide conjugated vaccines has not been efficient and antimycobacterial antibodies are not considered protective (Glatman-Freedman et al, 2000). Nevertheless their presence could influence the immune response. Thus the presence of B lymphocytes surrounding granulomas suggests the involvement of humoral immunity in latent forms of TB .The appearance of plasmocytes in the CSF also suggests a potential role of specific antibodies in TB meningitis. Numerous studies have attempted to identify specific antibodies in active TB but the present data is incomplete. The antigenic variability of mycobacteria is mirrored by the heterogenity of the released antibiodies. The repertoir of released antibodies appears to be diverse and correlated to many factors (the lesion's evolution and localization, the immune status etc) (Davidow et al, 2005). As in the case of antigens, the type of the released antibodies in different hosts and different forms of TB is unpredictable. Thus anti 38kDa are elevated in pulmonary TB while LAM antibodies and anti 16 kda increase in the CSF of patients with TB meningitis; anti 38 kDa have been associated with a poor outcome, while anti 19kda suggested a good prognosis. Anti38kDa are released in the presence of cavitary lesions and have not been found in patients who do not present such lesions such as immunodeppresed hosts. Anti 85 complex are present in large quantities in disease forms confirmed by positive smear as well as in severe forms. By comparison, lower amounts were found in forms with negative smears or minimal lesions. (Wiker & Harboe, 1992). Antibody responses are correlated with the bacillary load. Under these circumstances the level of IgG was regarded by some authors as an index for the antigenic load with possible implications in treatment follow-up (Fadda et al, 1992). The present knowledge on the role of antimycobacterial antibodies is the result of numerous immunologic diagnostic studies but their implication in the TB pathogenesis is still little known. IgM antibodies were found in different groups of patients with TB including vaccinated patients and are frequently found in HIV patients. Their presence marks the colonization with mycobacteria or the risk of TB relapse. IgA antibodies are rarely found.

They are detected in the CSF, pericardial and pleural liquid. They could appear in a state of anergy or in the absence of IgG antibodies, sometimes indicating an aberrant immune response Th2 like. Immune complexes are frequently correlated with IgA antibodies and severe disease. A protective effect of IgA of short duration has been observed in the early stages of TB. IgG antibodies appear during chronic disease; high titres are maintained even during treatment. These are the main type of antibodies observed in neurotuberculosis (Maes, 1991).

The dynamic synthesis of antimycobacterial antibodies

Different stimuli were documented to trigger the antimycobacterial antibodies in the primary versus post primary infection or active versus inactive TB. The hummoral immune response following BCG vaccination indicates that IgM anti PPD increase progressively until the third month, followed by an increase of IgG. The antibody dynamics in TB infection could be similar (Maes et al, 1989), but it also depends on the clinical form and treatment starting. IgA serum antibodies appear immediately after IgM and precede IgG, but the CSF dynamics could vary. IgG antibodies are prevalent in both active and inactive cases (Kaplan & Chase, 1980). During treatment for primary tuberculosis antimycobacteria antibodies are present in low titres, exhibit a slow increase and are directed against a low number of antigens. (Kaplan & Chase, 1980). Only 11-46% of patients display an initial titre of antibodies, but the number of cases subsequently increases to 60%. In relapse forms of TB the serum reacts with a larger number of antigens, the IgG titre is higher and rapidly increases under treatment. A detectable IgG titre is initially recorded in 66% of patients but reaches 75-100% of patients in the later stages. Similar conclusions were published in other studies in which TB relapse forms produced a positive serology in 100% of patients compared to 11% in primary TB (Julian et al, 1997). Seroconversion under treatment in patients with TB exceeds 3-8 weeks in patients with a negative titre at the onset, while in those with positive onset titres the antibody increase is rapid and immediate. The titre of antimycobacterial antibodies in the serum and CSF is higher in treated compared to untreated patients (Kaplan & Chase 1980). Some authors consider that in primary TB the maximum titre could emerge after 3 months of treatment. The presence of antimycobacterial antibodies in large quantities in relapse as well as in the treated forms is a significant advantage in the serodiagnosis of neurotuberculosis (as the latter frequently occurs as a relapse). The main disadvantage is related to the slow antibody dynamics in primary infections.

4.3 The intrathecal synthesis of antimycobacterial antibodies in NTB

CNS dissemination of mycobacteria is assisted by alveolar macrophages and their interaction with epithelial cells. Although the hematomeningeal barrier ensures the CNS protection from systemic immune reactions, the nevrax is still the site of intense inflammatory reactions. The intracerebral immune reactions are supported by the phagocytic cells of CNS, such as astrocytes and endothelial cells. (de Micco & Toga, 1988) The complex of astrocytes and endothelial cells is also connected to microglial cells, oligodendrocytes and hematopoetic stem cells. All these cells could activate lymphocytes and release inflammatory cytokines. Moreover, the lymphocytes crossing the hematomeningeal barrier synthesize intrathecal immunoglobulins (Ig). The intrathecal synthesis of specific antibodies was first observed in neurotuberculosis by Kinman. He showed that the stimulation of CSF lymphocytes by PPD leads to their intense proliferation

(Kinnman et al, 1981). Subsequent studies revealed a local production of antimycobacterial antibodies anti PPD in the CSF (Kalish et al, 1983). In 1990, Sindic proved the presence of IgG in the CSF against the antigen of *M. tbc* H37Ra and A60 (Sindic et al, 1990) In this study antimycobacterial antibodies appeared in the subarachnoid space as early as 15 days after clinical onset and persisted up to 69 months. The delayed immune response after the disappearance of the antigenic stimulus could persist as a result of immune disorders of active B cells clones. A similar response was also observed in other nontuberculous meningoencephalitis even 8 years later. IgG generally dominate the CNS humoral immune response, but in some cases IgA are also present (Felgenhauer & Schädlich, 1987). The antimycobacterial antibodies synthesis could be detected and quantified in the CSF, resulting in titres that could be higher in the CSF compared to the serum. Furthermore the increase of the Ig index in the CSF is a proof of the local synthesis of antimycobacterial antibodies (Kinman et al, 1981). The intrathecal synthesis of antimycobacterial antibodies released in the CSF is specific for cerebral TB and thus represents a solid argument in favor of the neurotuberculosis diagnosis.

5. Immunologic methods used in the diagnosis of neurotuberculosis

Immunological assays are rapid and easy to process but their use in TB is disputed due to contradictory results on sensitivity. Nevertheless, immunologic methods could be considered as complementary diagnostic tools especially in poor areas and smear-negative CSF neurotuberculosis. The most commonly used serological assay in neurotuberculosis is enzyme-linked immunosorbent assay (ELISA). Rapid methods (such as immunodot) are only seldom used. ELISA is automated and able to simultaneously analyse a high number of samples and different antibodies (Ig G, IgM or IgA). The evaluation of serological assays requires the accuracy of the following parameters: the sensitivity (probability of a positive test in people with neurotuberculosis), the specificity (probability of a negative test in uninfected people), the positive predictive value (probability that the person is infected when the test is positive) and the negative predictive value (probability that the person is uninfected when the test is negative).

5.1 The enzyme-immuno-assay (ELISA) technique

ELISA technique was first introduced in the serological diagnosis of TB in 1976. It detectes the antigen/antibody-enzyme linked complexes, with the antigen affixed to a solid adsorbent surface. Despite its highly variable sensitivity and specificity, studies on pulmonary TB proved that it is rapid and simple to process, suggesting its use in the extrapulmonary TB diagnosis. There are several comercial ELISA kits (Anda Biological using antigen A60, Omerga Pathozyme TB using antigen 38 kDa, Pathozyme TB complex with antigen 38 kDa and antigen 16 kDa, Pathozyme Myco with antigen 38 kDa and lypopolissaharidic antigen), and various in-house antibody-ELISA detection tests. Numerous ELISA studies were performed for the detection of different antigens and antibodies released in the pulmonary and extrapulmonary TB. Daniel and Debanne published a reference study in 1987 (Daniel & Debanne, 1987) analysing ELISA results in different forms of TB. They concluded that ELISA sensitivity of 25-100% and specificity of 76-100% were highly variable depending on the used antigen. A subsequent systematic revue on ELISA studies also revealed an extremely variable sensitivity of 0-100% and specificity of 59-100% in pulmonary TB and modest results in TB meningitis (sensitivity of 48% and specificity of 82%) (Steingart et al, 2007).

5.2 Interferon-γ-release assays (IGRAs)

There are currently 2 methods measuring the IFN-γ released by sensitized T cells: QuantiFERON-Gold *In Tube* (Cellestis Ltd) which measures IFN-γ-released in whole blood following *ex vivo* stimulation with ESAT-6, CFP-10 and TB 7.7 antigens and the T-SPOT.TB method (Oxford Immunotec Ltd) which measures IFN-γ-released by peripheral blood mononuclear cells following *ex vivo* stimulation with ESAT-6 and CFP-10. These 2 methods were initially approved for the diagnosis of latent TB, displaying a higher efficiency compared to tuberculin skin tests (TST). Their use was later extended for the diagnosis of active TB including HIV-infected patients. Recent studies on TB meningitis using both methods revealed only modest results. (Thomas et al, 2008, Patel et al, 2010). Thus the specificity in the diagnosis of active TB was generally low (59-79%) while the sensitivity was between 79% (non HIV patients) and 64% (HIV patients) (Sester et al, 2011). Nevertheless more optimistic results in TB meningitis were also reported (Murakami et al, 2008).

5.3 Other techniques used in the immune diagnosis of neurotuberculosis

The immunoblot technique is based on the electrophoretic separation of proteins (antigens or antibodies from serum or CSF), blotting for separate fractions on nitrocelulosis and identification of each proteic fraction with a specific anti-serum conjugated with a complex of streptavidin-biotin preoxidase (calitative reaction). The immunoblot technique was previously used by several authors in the diagnosis of mycobacterial infections. Most antigens recorded in these studies weighted between 30-45 kDa. However, only a part of the serum antigens identified in pulmonary TB were also recorded in the CSF in TB meningitis. In a study by Mathai the patients with TB meningitis presented 27 kDa, 30kDa, 45 kDa and 5kDa *M.tbc* antigens (Mathai et al, 1994). The latter was found in another study in 70% of patients with TB meningitis (Mathai et al, 1991). Patil also identified 30-40kDa antigens in the CSF but lower amounts of 14kDa and 18-25kDa antigens (Patil et al, 1996). Katti identified mostly 30-32kDa and 71kDa antigens in the CSF of patients with TB meningitis (Katti, 2001). Literature data also reveals the predominance of 30kDa antigen in the CSF. Research proved that 30 kDa protein is also a member of the Ag 85 complex (Ag 85 A and Ag 85 B), an antigen frequently detected in TB meningitis. This emphasizes the importance of 30 kDa antigen as a CSF marker in various forms of TB meningitis. **ImmunoDOT** is an rapid-test format, dipstick ELISA that allows patients to be tested for multiple parameters simultaneously. Up to five or six different tests may be completed simultaneously on a single sample, making it ideal for users who require fast, and reliable diagnostic tests in a single patient format. ImmunoDot or other rapid techniques are suitable for low CSF volumes and limited resources laboratories. **Haemagglutination assays** such as reverse passive haemagglutination (RPHA) using polyclonal or monoclonal antibodies, could be used in the serum and CSF, with a variable sensitivity in the diagnosis of TB meningitis. (Venkatesh et al, 2007). The use of a polyclonal serum generally proved more efficient. The main limitation of this method was connected to the variable sensitivity (50-94%) and to the short shelf-life of red-cell labelled antibodies; both listed drawbacks could be amended (Katti, 2001). The method is interesting from the perspective of using a single sample for the detection of both antibodies and antigens in biologic products and for measuring antigens and antibody dilutions needed in treatment monitoring. **Radioimmunoassay (RIA)** has been used for the TB diagnosis since 1987, with variable results. The method could follow the antigens level in the CSF during treatment which enables its use in treatment monitoring (Kadival et al, 1987). In conclusion, neurotuberculosis presently employs a wide range ofimmunologic diagnostic techniques. Their results however are not influenced by the method as much as by the detected antigens or antibodies. Presented below is the diagnostic value of the main antigens and antibodies detected in the serum and CSF in patients with neurotuberculosis.

6. Diagnostic value of immunological assays in studies of adults with neurotuberculosis

6.1 Mycobacterial antigens detection in neurotuberculosis

The mycobacterial antigens detection in CSF samples evidence active meningeal infection and could hold a diagnostic value. Hence, several *M.tbc* antigens have been analyzed as potential markers for the TB menigitis diagnosis. Moreover, quantitative determination of antigens could be useful for treatment monitoring. Attempts to detect mycobacterial antigens in neurotuberculosis have been made since 1984 employing mostly agglutination tests, *ELISA* with different variants or other methods (Venkatesh et al, 2007; Sumi et al, 2002; Radhacrishnan et al, 1990; Katti, 2001; Kashyap et al, 2009). Numerous antigens were evaluated: 55-kDa antigen, 14 kDa, PPD, 62 kDa, ag 85 complex , 30-32 kDa protein, LAM, Ag Mtbc, *M. tbc* H37Rv. The main conclusions of these studies are listed below.

a. **Method efficiency.** The specificity of methods: 69-100%. The sensitivity variation depended on the diagnosis criteria: in bacteriologically confirmed TB meningitis 79-100%; 67-92% in unconfirmed cases and 50-100% in both confirmed and unconfirmed cases.
b. **Comments**. The evaluated antigens were extremely different for each study. The sensitivity of methods was highly variable too. No method or specific antigen rendered a higher efficiency, although more studies have confirmed the presence of 30Kda antigen (ag 85 complex) in the CSF and simultaneous use of more antigens improved the methods sensitivity. The highly variable results could derive from the reduced level of antigen in the CSF, as well as from the lack of complete information connected with the precise type of antigens released in the CSF in TB meningitis.

6.2 Antimycobacterial antibodies detection in neurotuberculosis

Irrespective of localisation, antigentic stimulation in mycobacteria infections induces the synthesis of specific antibodies in the serum. In neurological localizations however, antibodies also appear in the CSF as a result of intratechal synthesis (Sindic et al, 1990; Kinmann et al, 1981; Kalish et al, 1983) and active secretion by choroidal plexuses. False positive antibodies in the CSF are possible in areas endemic for TB, where healthy persons or patients with pulmonary TB present high serum levels of antimycobacterial antibodies able to difusse from the serum to the CSF. The assesment of the intratechal synthesis of antimycobacterial antibodies could help ascertain such false positive reactions. Most studies analyzing the presence of the antimycobacterial antibodies in CSF were performed in imunocompetent adults with TB meningitis. The detected antibodies involved more antigens either isolated or simultaneous (LAM, PPD, A60, M.tbc, Ag 5, 14kDa, 19 kDa, 27 kDa, 30 kDa, 35 kDa, 40 kDa, Ag H37Ra, LAM, 30 kDa, 65 kDa heat shock protein, ESAT-6 antigen). In addition, most authors focused on the detection of IgG type antibodies using ELISA. Below are the main findings of these studies (Thakur & Mandal, 1996; Maheshwari et al, 2000; Patil1et al, 1996; Kashyap et al 2009; Mudaliar et al, 2006).

a. **Method's efficiency**. The specificity of antimycobacterial antibodies detection ranged between 92-100% but the positive predictive value was high. False positive results were recorded in patients who also presented pulmonary TB or as a result of cross-reactivity; 65 antigen kDa belonging to stress proteins was most frequently involved in cross reactions with other bacteria. The sensitivity of methods was highly variable: 30-100% in the studies with a single tested antigen and 61-100% when testing multiple antigens Chandramuki et al, 1989; Mathai et al, 1990a). The sensitivity was correlated with diagnosis criteria as follows: 80-90% sensitivity in bacteriologically confirmed tuberculous meningitis, 30-62% sensitivity in unconfirmed cases, 58% sensitivity in histologically confirmed tuberculomas and 70-87% sensitivity in clinically TB meningitis. Large differences between studies were also noticed depending on antibodies detection (for *LAM*, the sensitivity varied between 58-85% and for A60, the sensitivity ranged from 38 to 100%).
b. **Comments.** Almost all studies were perfomed in patients with TB meningitis. Nevertheless, a study on tuberculoma revealed A60 antibodies in these patients too. This indicates the potential use of the serodiagnosis in localized forms of neurotuberculosis, in which noninvasive diagnotic tools are presently unavailable. The variability of the recorded results was connected with more factors: 1) the use of different antigens (several studies indicate *LAM* antigen as immunodominant in the CSF; 2) the use of different dilutions: higher dilutions of the CSF decreased the sensitivity; 3) the immune status of different patients: low antibody detection in immunodepressed patients (only 10%) compared to immunocompetent hosts (50%); 4) almost all studies analyzed IgG antibodies, while only few also considered IgM or IgA. The antigens which induced IgM antimycobacterial antibodies were different from those responsible for IgG. IgG antibodies were mostly directed against *LAM* or 14 kDa antigen (74% of the total patients), suggesting that using these antigens could raise the efficiency. 5) some studies disclosed that simultaneous detection of serum and CSF antimycobacterial antibodies improved the CSF results compared to serum detection only. (Srivastava et al, 1994); however other studies reported inferior CSF sensitivity compared to the serum sensitivity.(Ghoshal et al, 2003). 6) the sensitivity of antibodies detection increased during treatment with 18% for both IgG and IgA detection.

Conclusion. There is a large number of serological studies dedicated to neurotuberculosis, with extremely different results. They are hard to compare as a result of using different study protocols and different antibodies detection. Despite the unconfindence which these studies arose, serologic diagnosis is widely used in poor countries. The standardisation of the methods in what regards the recommended antigens (type, concentration) and the immunological assay, could help improve the immunological diagnosis. One advantage of this method is the CSF specificity of antigens and intrathecal antimycobacterial antibodies synthesis and also the increased antibody level during antituberculous treatment, which renders this method useful for a retrospective diagnosis.

6.3 Intrathecal synthesis of antimycobacterial antibodies in neurotuberculosis

TB meningitis prompts a vigorous humoral local response proved by CSF intrathecal synthesis of antimycobacterial antibodies. Sindic proved that most antibodies synthesized intrathecally are directed against antigen A60 (Sindic et al, 1990). He also revealed the presence of Ig in the subarahnoidian space after 14-27 days of disease and their persistence after several years. A higher Ig G index is presently regarded as a strong argument in favor of the humoral local response induced by mycobacteria. All the same not all Ig detected in the CSF belong to antimycobacterial antibodies. Unspecific IgG were also found in other diseases affecting the CNS as a results of an immunosuppresive abberation. This immune impairment allows B cell multiplication and antibody persistence accounting for false positive results. Fals positive CSF results could also be found after passive transfer of antimycobacterial antibodies from the serum in the subarachnoid space. The mathematical evaluation of the intrathecal synthesis takes into account the presence of antibodies and IgG level in serum and CSF could highlight these false positive results.

6.4 Personal contribution. The intrathecal synthesis of antimycobacterial antibodies in patients with TB meningitis

The sole presence of antimycobacterial antibodies in the CSF cannot define the local inflammatory response since any form of TB accompanied by high titres of antibodies could promote their passive transfer in the CSF. The intrathecal synthesis was instead acknowledged as a typical finding in neurotuberculosis and an alternative for improving the specificity and positive predictive value of diagnosis in TB meningitis.The aim of our study was to evaluate the presence of antimycobacterial antibodies released as a result of the intrathecal synthesis in TB meningitis and to differentiate them from unspecific Ig.

Subjects. The study was performed on 21 adult patients with TB meningitis. A total of 34 CSF samples were collected, all having proved positive for antimycobacterial antibodies. The samples were collected after starting the antituberculous treatment, between 3 and 140 days after the clinical onset of the disease. Diagnosis criteria of TB meningitis were based on clinical characteristic features, CSF characteristic features (CSF lymphocytosis, increased protein and decreased sugar), evidence of pulmonary or extrapulmonary TB and positivity of CSF Lowenstein culture (for 3 patients only). Antimycobacterial antibodies were detected through ELISA using glycolipidic (GL) antigens and A60antigen.

Methods. Two types of comparative antigens were used for ELISA: GL antigen (0,1 ml sol of 10micrograms/ml of purified glycolipid in hexan obtained from Cantacuzino laboratories, Romania) and A60 (Andaelisa mycobacteria IgG, IgM, IgA kits, from Anda Biologicals, Strasbourg, France).

a. Elisa anti GL antigen detection method steps: 0,1 ml of ½ diluted CSF and 0,1 ml of conjugate (protein A-peroxidase) were distributed in microplates at 37^0 C for 1 hour; 0,1 ml *OPD* (peroxide and ortophenylendiamine) substrate in citric acid-sodium citrate buffer, 0,1 M, pH =5, was used. The reaction was prolonged for 30 minutes, at 37^0C, at dark. The optical densities (OD) were read with a Multiscan MCC Reader, at 450 nm. Serum Ig isolated from immunised rabbits with *Mtbc* suspension were used as positive controls. Cut off was established at two standard deviations above the level considered normal. The level of antibodies was expressed in international units (UI). The baseline serounit for the CSF fluid was 0 UI.

b. Elisa antiA60 detection steps: the CSF fluid was diluted 1/10 according to the kit instructions; anti-human IgG, IgA, IgM were conjugated to peroxidase (one hour at $37^{0}C$). The baseline serounits were: 125 for IgG, 200 for IgA serounits and 0.8 for IgM antibodies. Supplementary analysis in all subjects included: serum and CSF albumin expressed in mg/ml) (Ortodiagnosis) and serum and CSF Ig (radial passive immunodifussion). Albumin index, IgG index and IgG intratechal synthesis were calculated using the following mathematical formula (Tibbling 1977):

1. **Albumin index** (mg/ml)= CSF albumin/ serum albumin ratio. The normal value of CSF albumin was considered < 35mg% and between 3500-5000 mg% for serum albumin. The normal value of the *albumin index* is < $7x10^{-3}$ (0.007). Higher values suggest the permeability of the hematomeningeal barrier and the possibility of a passive transfer of antimycobacterial antibodies from the blood to the CSF.
2. **IgG index** (mg/ml)= (CSF IgG/serum IgG) / (CSF albumin /serum albumin) ratio.The normal value of the IgG index is ≤0.7. Higher values indicate increased IgG synthesis.
3. **IgG intratechal synthesis** of antimycobacterial antibodies was acquired using the formula: (CSF antimycobacterial antibodies of IgG type/CSF IgG) / (serum antimycobacterial antibodies of IgG type/serum IgG) ratio. Antimycobacterial antibodies of IgG type were measured in *ELISA* units. Serum and CSF IgG were quantified in mg/ml. The normal value of the intratechal synthesis calculated using this formula is < 1.

Results. The intrathecal synthesis was present 3 days after clinical onset and persisted up to 140 days after onset. The intrathecal synthesis against GL antigen was assessed in 31 samples while anti A60 antibodies were assessed only in 19 samples, out of the total of 34 CSF samples. 19 CSF samples were studied comparatively for the intrathecal synthesis of anti GL antibodies and antiA60: anti GL antibodies were detected in 7 samples only (22,58%) and anti A60 in 15 patients (78,94%).Eighteen from the 19 CSF samples (94,73%) presented the intrathecal synthesis of either anti GL antibodies or anti A60.Results are displayed in table 1.

Antimycobacterial antibodies of IgG type	Total CSF samples	CSF samples positive for the intrathecal antibody synthesis	CSF samples positive for a high albumin index	CSF samples positive for **a high** IgG index
GL-IgG antibodies	31	7 from 31 samples (22,58%)	33 from 34 samples (97,05%)	24 from 34 samples (70,58%)
A60-IgG antibodies	19	15 from 19 (78,94%)		
GL and A60 IgG antibodies	19	18 from 19 (94,73%)		

Table 1. Results of the albumin index, IgG index and the intrathecal synthesis of antimycobacterial anti GL and A60 in patients with TB meningitis

Observations. High values of the IgG index were recorded in 70, 58% cases and high values of the albumin index suggesting an increased permeability of the hematomeningeal barrier were noticed in 97,05% of patients. Only a part of the patients positive for CSF anti GL or A60 antibodies also exhibited an intrathecal synthesis. This finding confirms the transfer of antibodies from the serum into the CSF, through the hematomenigeal barrier. We also observed a significantly lower anti GL intrathecal synthesis compared to anti A60. In our study the simultaneous detection of intrathecal synthesis increased the CSF detection of antimycobacterial antibodies.

Conclusions. This study recorded the intrathecal synthesis of at least one type of antimycobacterial antibodies (GL or A60) in 94,73% of the TB meningitis patients even after specific treatment starting. The current study is also one of the few confirming the intrathecal synthesis of antimycobacterial antibodies in TB meningitis. Our findings support the value of the immunologic diagnosis, be it retrospective, after specific treatment starting.

7. Diagnostic value of immunological assays in children with neurotuberculosis

TB meningitis in children develops after hematogenic dissemination from the pulmonary infection site. Thus it manifests as a progressive primary disease, while in adults it commonly arises as a relapsing form of TB. The neurologic signs and symptoms become obvious 2 weeks after the onset. CSF changes are frequently unspecific and cases with a normal CSF examination have also been described in TB encephalopathy. The first obstacle in the diagnosis lies in obtaining adequate CSF and sputum samples. Moreover the bacteriological diagnosis in TB meningitis is disappointing: acid fast bacilli stain is positive in only 15% of cases and culture in only 30% of cases. The prognosis is poor and a rapid diagnosis is imperious. Most treatment regimens in children TB meningitis are initiated based on clinical, epidemiological data and pulmonary radiological features, without a bacteriological confirmation. The most adequate methods in the neurotuberculosis diagnosis in children are the molecular techniques (Lawn & Zumla, 2011). These are rapid and specific, but the high cost prevents their use on a wider scale in poor countries. At the same time, some countries are reluctant to employ molecular techniques in the TB diagnosis in children (Consensus Statement on Childhood Tuberculosis, 2010). Therefore the serological methods could be an alternative, but there are few studies on children and their efficiency is variable. The lack of knowledge related to the type of antigen released in this age group causes highly unspecific results. The serologic diagnosis is based on antigens randomly chosen, considered as immunodominant in adult TB (Raja et al, 2001). However certain results yielded by serologic techniques deserve credit for having revealed additional information on the immune pathogenesis of TB in children. According to these the titre of antimycobacterial antibodies and TST in children under 2 years are influenced by BCG vaccination which prompts persistent titres of antimycobacterial antibodies. Children between 0-4 years display a decreased humoral immune response despite a strong cellular immune response. (Seth et al, 1993). Subsequently the titre of antimycobacterial antibodies increases with age (Delacourt et al, 1993). Children with primary lesions of TB or calcified lesions also present increased titres of serum antibodies. As a result there is a high risk of false positive reactions in TB endemic areas. Thus the serologic diagnosis of active TB is not regarded as a plausible alternative for diagnosis in children. In addition, the serologic results in children with pulmonary and extrapulmonary TB exhibit an extremely varied sensitivity (20.7%-85%) (Rosen, 1990, Alde et al, 1989). Results with a better sensitivity were retrieved for A60, antigen 85 complex, 30 kDa or combinations of multiple antigens (Delacourt et al, 1993, Dayal et al, 2008, Raja et al, 2001). The specificity depends on the antigen used or the type of detected antibodies (Raja, 2001, Delacourt et al, 1993). There are also studies suggesting a correlation between the titre of antibodies and the antituberculous treatment. This implies the monitoring of antibodies titre in the pediatric management of TB. (Sireci et al, 2007). However the above mentioned results are considered of little practical value and irrelevant for the current diagnostic methods in TB. Other immunologic assays such as IGRAs although unrelated to the BCG vaccination and with a high specificity appear not to be advantageous in all cases of active TB in children. (Kampmann et al, 2009). There are few serologic studies in children with TB meningitis which displayed a high variable sensitivity. A comparative analysis on these studies is hindered by the diverse antigens used and discordant results (Dole et al, 1989; Srivastava et al, 1998) (table 9). Serious errors of interpretation are important for the above mentioned reasons.

The efficiency of serologic techniques in children with neurotuberculosis is low: sensitivity of 30%-100% and specificity of 62-96%. The sensitivity was influenced by the CSF dilution, the type of detected antibody and the chosen antigen. The sensitivity was similar for the serum and CSF.

Comments. ELISA was the technique most commonly used. Best results involved antimycobacterial antibodies A60, 30 Kda and *M. bovis* BCG towards Ag 5 and LAM. Some studies considered the detection of IgM more relevant than IgG. The detection of antigens in the CSF proved more useful compared to the finding of antibodies in TB meningitis.

8. Diagnostic value of immunological assays in studies of HIV patients with neurotuberculosis

The neurotuberculosis diagnosis in HIV infected patients is probably overevaluated. The TB patients with HIV often present miliaria forms, extrapulmonary localisations of TB and extensive vasculisis, accompanied by specific HIV manifestations. The difficulty to recognize the neurologic forms of TB increases with the advancing immunodepression. The low inflammatory response in HIV patients generates an atypical CSF aspect and repeated confusions with meningitis of other aetiology. At the same time, the TB aetiology should always be included in the differential diagnosis due to its frequency in the evolution of the HIV infection. TB meningitis usually appears as a relapse and only rarely during primary infection. Bacteriological confirmation is delayed and its sensitivity is under dispute: some authors recorded a higher number of false negative smear sample results while others maintained that the sensitivity is similar in both HIV and non-HIV infected patients. Therefore in order to raise the cases diagnosed one should consider the addition of invasive investigations and high cost molecular techniques. The immunologic methods of diagnosis in immunodepressed hosts have been little evaluated. HIV patients display a decreasing Th1 count, sustaining the Th2 stimulation of B cells and the synthesis of antimycobacterial antibodies. Specific tests of cell immunity (IGRAs, TST) are disappointing (Pai & Lewinsohn, 2005) but the humoral immune response appears to persist for a long time. An advantage of the serologic diagnosis is that of the high titres of antimycobacterial antibodies in relapse forms which comprise the majority of TB forms in HIV patients. Certain authors observed an increased IgG in the serum of HIV patients with pulmonary TB compared to controls (Van Vooren et al,1994). No difference has been observed between pulmonary TB and extrapulmonary TB in what regards humoral immunity (Daleine et al, 1995). The essential difference resides in the released antigens. A serologic study in HIV patients with TB infection concluded that only 14 antigens induced the antibody synthesis in these patients. Interestingly, most antigens between 32-45KDa (except for 38 Kda) failed to elicit a humoral reponse (Zhou et al, 1996). The best results involved glycolipidic antigens , especially LOS, LAM, DAT, PGL (Patel et al, 2009) and high molecular weight proteic antigens (ag 85Kda, 88Kda) (Laal et al, 1997). LAM positivity has been associated with HIV co-infection and low CD4 T cell count. Below are the conclusions of ten studies performed in patients with HIV and TB infection using Elisa and numerous antigens (LOS, LAM , 88kDa , PPD , 38 kDa, 88 kDa, A60 or antigen combinations such as PPD and DAT, PPD and SLIV or PPD and LAM.

Main findings. Various studies revealed an extremely variable sensitivity (0-95%), not only for different antigens included in the same study, but also for the same antigen in different studies (such as the high variable sensitivity for LAM in different studies: 35-95%). Only the selection of LOS antigen has led to concordant results between studies. Despite the dysfunctional cellular immune responses in HIV patients, several investigators have reported the presence of antibodies against *M. tbc,* TB16.3, TB9.7, MPT 51, MTB 81 and 88 kDa antigens (Laal et al, 1997). Comparative studies also revealed that the sensitivity for certain antigens (PPD, *M.tbc*) doubles in patients who are HIV negative compared to HIV positive. Moreover the sensitivity is higher in HIV patients compared to AIDS patients. However the level of anti A60 IgG remains elevated in patients with AIDS or with a negative TST result. Despite the low sensitivity the specificity of the Mycodot test was high.

Comments. Secondary TB elicits a stronger serologic response than primary TB and could account for the differences between the different groups of patients (Maes, 1991). However none of the mentioned studies classified the patients as primary or secondary TB. On the other hand an attempt to classify according to the bacteriological confirmation revealed a higher detection sensitivity for antimycobacterial antibodies in patients with confirmed TB (57%) than in patients with unconfirmed TB (30%) (Kameswaran et al, 2002). Antimycobacterial antibodies could predict tuberculosis in HIV patients in some studies. A study by Amicosante proved the appearance of antimycobacterial antibodies one year before the clinical onset of tuberculosis in 67% of HIV infected patients. (Amicosante et al, 1994). The early prediction and diagnosis of neurotuberculosis rendered by antibodies are extremely important for an early starting of antituberculous chemotherapy. Unfortunately only few HIV patients with neurotuberculosis are recorded in the evaluation of extrapulmonary TB and it is difficult to estimate the real value of serologic methods.

9. Diagnostic value of immunological assays in patients with neurologic nonmycobacterial infections

Nontuberculous mycobacteria infections with neurologic or systemic localizations exhibit a low titre of IgG (Oliver et al, 2001). In addition the presence of corresponding antibodies in HIV patients suggests colonization (usually involving the digestive tract) rather than infection (Maes 1991). Thus studies on patients with AIDS and disseminated infection with

M.avium failed to detect any IgG antimycobacterial antibodies in the serum, unlike patients with AIDS and pulmonary infection with *M.avium* (Daniel et al, 1990). A study on the IgG, IgM, IgA released against antigen LAM has triggered no immune response in mycobacteria infections other than TB (Demkow et al, 2006). There are also studies upholding the possibility of a serologic diagnosis in HIV patients with nontuberculous mycobacteria infection using antigens extracted from PPD-B /M. intracellulare, PPD-Y/M. kansasii, PPD-F/M. fortuitum) Nevertheless the serologic diagnosis is presently impractical in the case of nontuberculous mycobacteria infections and there are no available studies regarding HIV patients with neurotuberculosis.

10. The interpretation of serologic results in the diagnosis of neurotuberculosis. Reasons for false positive and negative results

Immunoenzymatic techniques are the most frequently used techniques for the detection of antimycobacterial antibodies in the CSF. The detection of CSF and serum antimycobacterial antibodies through such methods is specific, inexpensive, rapid, but displays a moderate sensitivity and requires a correct interpretation of the data.

Reasons for false negative results. Most false negative results are related to the low level of antimycobacterial antibodies in the serum or CSF, along with inadequate technical parameters. The low titre of antibodies could be the consequence of: a) decreased antigenic stimulation induced by reduced metabolism of mycobacteria; b) reduced antibodies synthesis as a result of a congenital or acquired immunodeficiency; c) antigen fixation in the immune complexes; d) early detection. The use of inadequate technical parameters correlates with: a) a cut off too highly set; b) too high dilutions (the current CSF dilutions of 1/10 appear to exceed the titre of antibodies); c) belated CSF processing; d) improper storing conditions.

Reasons for false positive results in the CSF: a) excessive amount of serum antibodies able to cross the blood barier (a finding usually related to pulmonary TB); b) cross reaction with other infections (Nocardia, Corynebacterium) , the rheumatoid factor, or other diseases (sarcoidosis, pulmonary neoplasm, autoimmune diseases); c) immune hiperreactivity unable to suppress the antibody synthesis after the disappearance of the stimulus; f) insufficient purification of the antigens; g) high prevalence of TB and a low cut-off.

11. Improvement possibilities of serologic techniques in neurotuberculosis

The improvement of immunologic results in neurotuberculosis diagnosis is first related to the knowledge advance of TB immunopathology. The current improvement strategies focus on the following: a) The discovery of highly specific antigens; b) Polyproteins or multiple antigens concurrent detection; c) Cut-off value adapted to the geographic area TB endemicity and to the CSF sample (the predicted cut off value for the CSF is of 40 serounits of IgG instead of 200 serounits required by pulmonary TB); d) The removal of immune complexes; e) Repeated serologic detection after onset and during treatment; f) Simultaneous screening for antibodies IgM, IgG, IgA; g) Simultaneous detection of antibodies and antigenes using rapid techniques; h)The use of low dilutions for the immunosuppressed patients); i) Intrathecal synthesis detection; j) Correlation with immunologic markers (the CD4 level, immunogram) for a correct interpretation of the immune status.

12. Conclusions

a. The value and limits of the immunologic diagnosis in NTB

The detection of mycobacteria antigens and antimycobacterial antibodies in the CSF, as well as in the serum of patients with neurotuberculosis could augment the diagnosis suspicion and ensure a rapid treatment. Increasing the efficiency of the immunologic diagnosis in neurotuberculosis requires antigens that are specific for neurological localizations as well as standardized and sensitive methods. Immunoserological studies on neurotuberculosis generally involve methods with a good specificity and acceptable senzitivity. The rapidity and increased specificity are the main advantages of these methods. Still, these diagnostic methods cannot replace the bacteriological exam and are presently unstandardised, which hinders the results comparison. In addition, the correct interpretation requires complex data (not always available) related to the onset, treatment, medical history, other localizations of tuberculosis and the immunologic status. In the absence of these data, the results obtained through serological methods cannot be relevant.

b. The possibilities of performing the immunologic diagnosis in NTB

Despite the numerous diagnostic tools presently available, the neurologic forms of TB often remain undetected and lead to an increased mortality. Neurologic localizations are mostly smear negative and require a rapid diagnosis. The only rapid diagnosis method employs molecular techniques which are too expensive for developing countries. Moreover, starting antituberculous treatment before the collection of specific pathological products decreases the sensitivity of both bacteriological and molecular methods. The immunologic methods are inexpensive and could also be used after treatment starting. The rapid methods (Dot) do not even require trained personnel, the results are available without delay and the reagents are easy to store. As long as the interpretation of the results is correct, the serological methods deliver significant information and a rapid orientation in the diagnosis at a low cost.

c. The practical value of the immunologic diagnosis as a complementary method in developing countries with a high prevalence of TB

The immunologic methods studied in neurotuberculosis hold a practical value once their results are included in an internationally accepted algorithm for diagnosis. However, the use of these diagnostic methods and reports on cost-efficiency are regarded with reluctance. Literature data published between 2004-2008 on TB case definitions includes only 1 study which considers ELISA IgM detection useful in TB meningitis (Kalita et al, 2007).Three other studies consider that a positive TST test could exhibit only a potential utility in the diagnosis of TB. (Marais et al, 2010) There is also insufficient experience in order to appreciate the efficiency of IGRAs assays in the diagnosis of neurotuberculosis. Therefore the immunologic diagnosis in neurotuberculosis is not currently accepted in the international guidelines as a complementary diagnosis for the confirmation of the diagnosis of neurotuberculosis. Nevertheless serologic diagnostic methods are in use in developing countries and provide rapid orientative data in TB meningitis. However each assay should be validated using controls from that specific area and a part of the technical criteria are also to be adapted to that area in terms of cut off value and used antigens. Standardised diagnostic criteria for TB meningitis as well as standardised immunologic methods could render correct forthcoming comparisons between immunologic studies. It could also establish the real value of these methods especially in poor countries with a high prevalence for tuberculosis and reduced possibilities of diagnosis.

13. Acnowledgments

This work was supported by CNCSIS-Grant project 1165/2508/2008

14. References

Alde, S., Piñasco, H., Pelosi F., Budani H., Palma-Beltran O. & Gonzalez-Montaner LJ. (1989). Evaluation of an enzyme-linked immunosorbent assay (ELISA) using an IgG antibody to Mycobacterium tuberculosis antigen 5 in the diagnosis of active tuberculosis in children. *Am Rev Respir Dis.*, Vol.139, No.3, (Mar 1989), pp. 748-751.

Amicosante, M., Richeldi, L., Monno, L., Cuboni, A., Tartoni, P., Angarano, G., Orefici, G. & Saltini C. (1997). Serological markers predicting tuberculosis in human immunodeficiency virus-infected patients. *Int J Tuberc Lung Dis.* No 5 (Oct 1997), pp 435-440.

Chandramuki, A., Bothamley, G., Brennan, P.& Ivanyi J. (1989). Levels of antibody to defined antigens of Mycobacterium tuberculosis in tuberculous meningitis. *J Clin Microbiol.* Vol. 27, No. 5, (May 1989), pp. 821-825.

Cho, T., Park, S., Cho, S., Lee, H., Kim, S., Kim, S.& Lee, B.(1995). Intrathecal synthesis of immunoglobulin G and Mycobacterium tuberculosis-specific humoral immune response in tuberculous meningitis. *Clin Diagn Lab Immunol.* Vol.2, No.3, (May 1995), pp. 361-364.

Consensus Statement on Childhood Tuberculosis Working group on Tuberculosis, Indian Academy of Pediatrics (IAP), (2010). *Indian Pediatrics,* Vol. 47 (Jan 17, 2010), pp. 41-55.

Daleine, G.& Lagrange, P. (1995). Preliminary evaluation of a Mycobacterium tuberculosis lipooligosaccharide (LOS) antigen in the serological diagnosis of tuberculosis in HIV seropositive and seronegative patients. *Tuber Lung Dis.*, Vol.76, No.3, (Jun 1995), pp. 234-239.

Daniel, P., Kataaha, P.& Eriki, P.(1990). AIDS patiens with coexisting tuberculosis can be diagnosic serologicaly while thouse wih M. avium disease cannot, *ARRD* 141, Vol.141, No.4 (Feb 1990), A264.

Daniel, T.& Debanne, S. (1987). The serodiagnosis of tuberculosis and other mycobacterial diseases by enzyme-linked immunosorbent assay. *Am Rev Respir Dis.* Vol.135, No.5, (1987 May), pp.1137-1151.

Davidow, A., Kanaujia, G., Shi, L., Kaviar, J., Guo, X., Sung, N.& Kaplan, G.(2005). Menzies D, Gennaro ML. Antibody profiles characteristic of Mycobacterium tuberculosis infection state. *Infect Immun.* , Vol.73, No.10 (Oct 2005), pp. 6846-6851.

Davies, P., Pai, M.,(2008). The diagnosis and misdiagnosis of tuberculosis. *Int J Tuberc Lung Dis.*Vol 12, No 11, (Nov 2008), pp. 1226-1234Dayal, R., Singh, A., Katoch, V., Joshi,

B., Chauhan, D., Singh, P., Kumar, G.& Sharma V. (2008).Serological diagnosis of tuberculosis. *Indian J Pediatr.* Vol.75, No.12, (Dec 2008), pp. 1219-21.

Dayal, R., Singh, A., Katoch, V., Joshi, B., Chauhan, D., Singh, P., Kumar, G.& Sharma V. (2008).Serological diagnosis of tuberculosis. *Indian J Pediatr.* Vol.75, No.12, (Dec 2008), pp. 1219-21.

de Micco C.& Toga, M. (1988). The immune status of the central nervous system. *Rev Neurol (Paris), Vol.* 144, No.12, (1988) pp.776-788.

Delacourt C, Gobin J, Gaillard JL, de Blic J, Veron M, Scheinmann P.Value of ELISA using antigen 60 for the diagnosis of tuberculosis in children. *Chest.*,Vol. 104, No.2, (Aug 1993) ,pp. 393-398.

Demkow, U., Białas-Chromiec, B., Filewska, M., Zielonka, T., Michałowska-Mitczuk, D., Kuś, J., Broniarek-Samson, B., Augustynowicz-Kopeć, E., Zwolska, Z.& Rowińska-Zakrzewska, E. (2006). Humoral immune response against mycobacterial antigens in patients with tuberculosis and mycobacterial infections other than tuberculosis. *Pneumonol Alergol Pol.* Vol.74, No. 2, (2006), pp. 203-208

Desai, D., Nataraj, G., Kulkarni, S., Bichile, L., Mehta, P., Baveja, S., Rajan, R., Raut, A.& Shenoy, A. (2006). Utility of the polymerase chain reaction in the diagnosis of tuberculous meningitis. *Res Microbiol.* Vol. 157, No.10, (Dec 2006), pp. 967-70.

Dole, M., Maniar, P., Lahiri, K.& Shah, M. (1989). Enzyme-linked immuno-assay for the detection of mycobacterium tuberculosis specific IgG antibody in the cerebrospinal fluid in cases of tuberculous meningitis. *J Trop Pediatr.* Vol. 35, No.5, (Oct 1989), pp. 218-220.

Donald, P. & Schoeman, J. (2004). Tuberculous meningitis. *N Engl J Med* Vol. 351 (Oct 21, 2004), pp. 1719-1720

Fadda, G., Grillo, R., Ginesu, F., Santoru, L., Zanetti, S.& Dettori, G. (1992). Serodiagnosis and follow up of patients with pulmonary tuberculosis by enzyme-linked immunosorbent assay. *Eur J Epidemiol.* Vol.8, No.1, (Jan 1992), pp. 81-87.

Felgenhauer, K. & Schädlich, H. (1987). The compartmental IgM and IgA response within the central nervous system. *J Neurol Sci.* Vol.77, No 2-3, (Feb 1987), pp.125-135.

Ghoshal, U., Kishore, J., Kumar, B.& Ayyagari, A. (2003). Serodiagnosis of smear and culture-negative neurotuberculosis with enzyme linked immunosorbent assay for anti A-60 immunoglobulins. *Indian J Pathol Microbiol.* Vol.46, No.3, (Jul 2003), pp. 530-534.

Glatman-Freedman, A., Casadevall, A., Dai, Z., Jacobs, WR Jr., Li, A., Morris, S., Navoa, J, Piperdi, S., Robbins, J., Schneerson, R., Schwebach, .&J Shapiro, M. (2004). Antigenic Evidence of Prevalence and Diversity of Mycobacterium tuberculosis Arabinomannan , *J Clin Microbiol.* Vol. 42, No 7, (Jul 2004), pp. 3225-3231.

Houghton, R., Lodes, M., Dillon, D., Reynolds, L., Day, C., McNeill, P., Hendrickson, R., Skeiky, Y., Sampaio, D., Badaro, R, Lyashchenko, K.& Reed, S.(2002). Use of multiepitope polyproteins in serodiagnosis of active tuberculosis. *Clin Diagn Lab Immunol.*Vol.9, No. 4, (Jul 2002), pp. 883-891

Julián, E., Matas, L., Ausina, V.& Luquin, M. (1997). Detection of lipoarabinomannan antibodies in patients with newly acquired tuberculosis and patients with relapse tuberculosis. *J Clin Microbiol.*, Vol.35, No.10, (Oct 1997), pp. 2663-2664.

Kadival, G., Samuel, A., Mazarelo, T. & Chaparas, S. (1987). Radioimmunoassay for detecting Mycobacterium tuberculosis antigen in cerebrospinal fluids of patients with tuberculous meningitis. *J Infect Dis.*, Vol.155, No. 4, (Apr 1987), pp. 608-611Kalish, S., Radin, R., Levitz, D., Zeiss, C.& Phair, J. (1983). The enzyme-linked immunosorbent assay method for IgG antibody to purified protein derivative in cerebrospinal fluid of patients with tuberculous meningitis. *Ann Intern Med.*, Vol.99, No.5, (Nov 1983), pp. 630-633.

Kalita, J., Misra, U.& Ranjan, P. (2007). Predictors of long-term neurological sequelae of tuberculous meningitis: a multivariate analysis. *Eur J Neurol.*Vol.14, No.1, (Jan 2007), pp 33-37.

Kameswaran, M., Shetty, K., Ray, M., Jaleel, M.& Kadival, G.. (2002). Evaluation of an in-house-developed radioassay kit for antibody detection in cases of pulmonary tuberculosis and tuberculous meningitis. *Clin Diagn Lab Immunol.*, Vol.9, No. 5, (Sep 2002), pp. 987-993.

Kaplan, M.& Chase, M. (1980). Antibodies to mycobacteria in human tuberculosis. I. Development of antibodies before and after antimicrobial therapy. *J Infect Dis.*, Vol.142, No.6, (Dec 1980), pp. 825-834.

Kashyap, R., Ramteke, S., Morey, S., Purohit, H., & Daginawala, H.(2009). Diagnostic value of early secreted antigenic target-6 for the diagnosis of tuberculous meningitis patients. *Infection.* Vol.37, No.6, (Dec 2009), pp. 508-513.

Kampmann, B., Whittaker, E., Williams, A., Walters, S., Gordon, A., Martínez-Alier N, et al.(2009). Interferon-gamma release assays do not identify more children with active TB than TST. *Eur Respir J.*, Vol.33, (2009), pp. 1374-1378

Katti, M. (2001). Immunodiagnosis of tuberculous meningitis: rapid detection of mycobacterial antigens in cerebrospinal fluid by reverse passive hemagglutination assay and their characterization by Western blotting. *FEMS Immunol Med Microbiol.*,Vol.31, No.1, (Jul 2001), pp. 59-64.

Kinnman, J., Link, H. & Frydén, A. (1981). Characterization of antibody activity in oligoclonal immunoglobulin G synthesized within the central nervous system in a patient with tuberculous meningitis. *J Clin Microbiol.* , Vol.13, No 1, (Jan 1981), pp. 30-35.

Laal, S.,Samanich, K., Sonnenberg,M., Zolla-Pazner, S., Phadtare J.& Belisle J. (1997). Human humoral responses to antigens of Mycobacterium tuberculosis: immunodominance of high-molecular-mass antigens. *Clin Diagn Lab Immunol.*, Vol.4, No.1, (Jan 1997), pp. 49–56.

Lawn, S.& Zumla, A. (2011). Tuberculosis. *Lancet.* Vol 2, No 378(9785), (Jul 2011), pp. 57-72.

Maes, R., Homasson, J., Kubin, M.& Bayer M.(1989). Development of an enzyme immunoassay for the serodiagnostic of tuberculosis and mycobacterioses. *Med Microbiol Immunol.*, Vol.178, No.6, (1989), pp. 323-335.

Maes, R. (1991). Clinical usefulness of serological measurements obtained by antigen 60 in mycobacterial infections: development of a new concept. *Klin Wochenschr.*, Vol. 69, No.15, (Oct 1991), pp. 696-709.

Maheshwari, A., Gupta, H., Gupta, S., Bhatia, R.& Datta, K.(2000). Diagnostic utility of estimation of mycobacterial antigen A60 specific immunoglobulins in serum and CSF in adult neurotuberculosis. *J Commun Dis.*,Vol.32, No. 1, (Mar 2000), pp. 54-60.

Marais, S., Thwaites, G., Schoeman, J., Török, M., Misra, U., Prasad, K., Donald, P., Wilkinson, R.& Marais, B. (2010). Tuberculous meningitis: a uniform case definition for use in clinical research. *Lancet Infect Dis.*, Vol.10, No.11, (Nov 2010), pp. 803-12.

Mathai, A., Radhakrishnan, V.& Shobha S.Diagnosis of tuberculous meningitis confirmed by means of an immunoblot method. *J Infect.*, Vol.29, No.1, (Jul 1994), pp. 33-39.

Mathai, A., Radhakrishnan, V.& Thomas, M. (1991). Rapid diagnosis of tuberculous meningitis with a dot enzyme immunoassay to detect antibody in cerebrospinal fluid. *Eur J Clin Microbiol Infect Dis.*, Vol.10, No.5, (May 1991), pp. 440-443.

Mudaliar, A., Kashyap, R., Purohit, H., Taori, G.& Daginawala, H. (2006).Detection of 65 kD heat shock protein in cerebrospinal fluid of tuberculous meningitis patients. *BMC Neurol.*, Vol. 15, No.6, (Sep 2006), pp.34-36.

Murakami, S., Takeno, M., Oka, H., Ueda, A., Kurokawa, T., Kuroiwa, Y.& Ishigatsubo Y. (2008). Diagnosis of tuberculous meningitis due to detection of ESAT-6-specific gamma interferon production in cerebrospinal fluid enzyme-linked immunospot assay. *Clin Vaccine Immunol.*, Vol.15, No. 5, (May 2008), pp. 897-899.

Nyendak, M., Lewinsohn, D.& Lewinsohn, D. (2009). New diagnostic methods for tuberculosis. *Current Opinion in Infectious Diseases*, Vol.22, No 2, (April 2009), pp. 174-182

Oliver, A., Maiz, L., Cantón, R., Escobar, H., Baquero, F.& Gómez-Mampaso, E. (2001). Nontuberculous mycobacteria in patients with cystic fibrosis. *Clin Infect Dis.*, Vol.1, No 32(9), (May 2001), pp. 1298-303.

Park, S., Lee, B., Cho, S., Kim, W., Lee, B. & Kim, J. (1993). Diagnosis of tuberculous meningitis by detection of immunoglobulin G antibodies to purified protein derivative and lipoarabinomannan antigen in cerebrospinal fluid. *Tuber Lung Dis.*,Vol.74, No.5, (Oct 1993), pp. 317-322.

Patel, V., Bhigjee, A., Paruk, H., Singh, R., Meldau, R., Connolly, C.& Dheda, K. (2009). Utility of a novel lipoarabinomannan assay for the diagnosis of tuberculous meningitis in a resource-poor high-HIV prevalence setting. *Cerebrospinal Fluid Res.*, Vol.6, (Nov 2, 2009), pp.13-18.

Patel, V., Singh, R., Connolly, C., Kasprowicz, V., Zumla, A. & Dheda K. (2010). Comparison of a clinical prediction rule and a LAM antigen-detection assay for the rapid diagnosis of TBM in a high HIV prevalence setting. *PLoS One*, Vol.5, No. 12, (Dec 22, 2010) : e15664.Patil, S., Gourie-Devi, M., Chaudhuri, J.& Chandramuki, A. (1996). Identification of antibody responses to Mycobacterium tuberculosis antigens in the CSF of tuberculous meningitis patients by Western blotting. *Clin Immunol Immunopathol.*, Vol.81, No.1, (Oct 1996), pp. 35-40.

Radhakrishnan, V., Annamma, M.& Shobha S. (1990). Correlation between culture of Mycobacterium tuberculosis and IgG antibody to Mycobacterium tuberculosis antigen-5 in the cerebrospinal fluid of patients with tuberculous meningitis. *J Infect.*, Vol.21, No.3, (Nov 1990), pp. 271-277.

Raja, A., Ranganathan, U.& Bethunaickan, R. (2008). Improved diagnosis of pulmonary tuberculosis by detection of antibodies against multiple Mycobacterium tuberculosis antigens., *Diagn Microbiol Infect Dis.* ,Vol.60, No.4, (Apr 2008), pp. 361-368.

Rosen E. (1990). The diagnostic value of an enzyme-linked immune sorbent assay using adsorbed mycobacterial sonicates in children. *Tubercle*, Vol.71, No.2, (Jun 1990), pp. 127-130.

Samanich, K., Keen, M., Vissa, V., Harder, J., Spencer, J., Belisle, J., Zolla-Pazner, S.& Laal S. (2000). Serodiagnostic potential of culture filtrate antigens of Mycobacterium tuberculosis. *Clin Diagn Lab Immunol.* ,Vol.7, No.4, (Jul 2000), pp. 662-668.

Sester, M., Sotgiu, G., Lange, C., Giehl, C., Girardi, E., Migliori, G., Bossink, A., Dheda, K., Diel, R., Dominguez, J., & Manissero D. (2010). Interferon-γ release assays for the diagnosis of active tuberculosis: a systematic review and meta-analysis. *Eur Respir J.*,Vol.37, No.1, (Jan 2011), pp 100-111.

Seth, V., Kabra, S., Beotra, A. & Semwal OP. (1993).Tuberculous meningitis in children: manifestation of an immune compromised state. *Indian Pediatr.* Vol.30, No.10, (Oct 1993), pp. 1181-1186.

Sindic, C., Boucquey, D., Van Antwerpen, M., Baelden, M., Laterre, C.& Cocito C. (1990). Intrathecal synthesis of anti-mycobacterial antibodies in patients with tuberculous meningitis. An immunoblotting study. *J Neurol Neurosurg Psychiatry.*, Vol.53, No.8, (Aug 1990), pp. 662-666.

Sireci, G., Dieli, F., Di Liberto, D., Buccheri, S., La Manna, M., Scarpa, F., Macaluso, P., Romano, A., Titone, L., Di Carlo, P., Singh, M., Ivanyi, J.& Salerno A. (2007). Anti-16-kilodalton mycobacterial protein immunoglobulin m levels in healthy but purified protein derivative-reactive children decrease after chemoprophylaxis. *Clin Vaccine Immunol.*, Vol.14, No.9, (Sep 2007), pp. 1231-1234.

Sonmeza, G., Ersin Ozturka, E., Sildiroglua, O., Mutlua, H., Cucea, F.,M. Senolb, G., Kutluc, A., Basekima, C.& Kizilkaya E. (2008). MRI findings of intracranial tuberculomas, *Clinical Imaging,* Vol. 32, No. 2, (March 2008), pp. 88-92

Srivastava, K., Bansal, M., Gupta, S., Srivastava, R., Kapoor, R., Wakhlu, I.& Srivastava BS. (1998). Diagnosis of tuberculous meningitis by detection of antigen and antibodies in CSF and sera. *Indian Pediatr.*, Vol.35, No.9, (Sep1998), pp. 841-850.

Srivastava, L., Prasanna, S.& Srivastava, V.(1994). Diagnosis of tuberculous meningitis by ELISA test. *Indian J Med Res.*, Vol.99, (Jan 1994), pp. 8-12.

Steingart, K., Ramsay, A.& Pai, M. (2007). Commercial serological tests for the diagnosis of tuberculosis: do they work? *Future Microbiol.*, Vol.2, No.4, (Aug 2007), pp. 355-359.

Sumi, M., Mathai, A., Reuben, S,. Sarada, C., Radhakrishnan, V., Indulakshmi, R., Sathish, M., Ajaykumar, R.& Manju, Y. (2002). A comparative evaluation of dot immunobinding assay (Dot-Iba) and polymerase chain reaction (PCR) for the laboratory diagnosis of tuberculous meningitis. *Diagn Microbiol Infect Dis.*, Vol. 42, No.1, (Jan 2002), pp. 35-38.

Thakur, A.& Mandal, A. (19960. Usefulness of ELISA using antigen A60 in serodiagnosis of neurotuberculosis. *J Commun Dis.*,Vol.28, No.1, (Mar 1996), pp. 8-14.

Thomas, M., Hinks, T., Raghuraman, S., Ramalingam, N., Ernst, M., Nau R., Lange C., Kösters K., John, G., Marshall, B.& Lalvani A. (20087). Rapid diagnosis of Mycobacterium tuberculosis meningitis by enumeration of cerebrospinal fluid antigen-specific T-cells. *Int J Tuberc Lung Dis.* Vol.12, No.6, (Jun 2008), pp. 651-657

Tibbling, I. (1977). Establishment of reference values. Scand. J. Clin.G., H. Link, and S. Ohman. Principles of albumin and IgG analyses in neurological disorders. *Lab. Invest.*, No. 37, (1977), pp. 385-390.

Van Vooren, J., Launois, P., Huygen, K., Leguenno, B.& Drowart A. (1994). Detection of anti-85A and anti-85B IgG antibodies in HIV-infected patients with active pulmonary tuberculosis. *Eur J Clin Microbiol Infect Dis.*, Vol.13, No.5, (May 1994), pp. 444-446.

Venkatesh, K., Parija, S., Mahadevan, S.& Negi, V. (2007). Reverse passive haemagglutination (RPHA) test for detection of mycobacterial antigen in the cerebrospinal fluid for diagnosis of tubercular meningitis. *Indian J Tuberc.*, Vol.54, No.1, (Jan 2007),pp. 41-48.

Young, D., Kaufmann, S., Hermans, P. & Thole, J. (1992). Mycobacterial protein antigens: a compilation. *Mol Microbiol.*, Vol.6, No.2, (Jan 1992), pp. 133-145.

Walzl, G., Ronacher, K., Hanekom, W., Scriba, T.& Zumla,A. (2011). Immunological biomarkers of tuberculosis, *Nature Reviews Immunology*, Vol.11, No.5, (May 2011), pp.343-354.

Wiker & Harboe M, (1992). The antigen 85 complex: a major secretion product of Mycobacterium tuberculosis. *Microbiol Rev.*, Vol.56, No.4,(Dec 1992), pp. 648–661.

8

Diagnostic Methods for *Mycobacterium tuberculosis* and Challenges in Its Detection in India

Shamsher S. Kanwar
Department of Biotechnology
Himachal Pradesh University, Summer Hill, Shimla
India

1. Introduction

Tuberculosis (TB) is one of the world's oldest and most important disseminating infectious diseases that still accounts for a high morbidity and mortality among adults. Despite high prevalence, case detection rates are low, posing major hurdles for TB control in developed and developing countries. Traditional diagnosis of TB bacilli depends upon smear positivity in sputum samples, culture and chest radiography. All these tests have known limitations. Conventional tests for detection of drug resistance are slow, tedious and difficult to perform in field conditions. For rapid diagnosis, new methods include newer versions of nucleic acid amplification tests, immune-based assays, skin patch test and rapid culture systems. For drug resistance analysis line-probe assays, bacteriophage-based assays, molecular beacons and microscopic observation drug susceptibility assay are available. An ideal test for TB is still not available and fast emergence of drug resistant tubercle strains aided by the ever-increasing HIV AIDS-epidemic in third-world countries has stressed the need of rapid diagnostic test(s) to show the presence of mycobateria in the clinical samples. Microscopy and culture are still the major backbone for laboratory diagnosis of tuberculosis; new methods including molecular diagnostic tests have evolved over a period of time. The majority of molecular tests have been focused on: (i) detection of nucleic acids both DNA and RNA, which are specific to *Mycobacterium tuberculosis*, by amplification techniques such as polymerase chain reaction (PCR) focusing on detection and molecular epidemiology of *M. tuberculosis*; and (ii) detection of mutations in the genes which are associated with resistance to anti-tuberculosis drugs by sequencing or nucleic acid hybridization. The development and use of rapid diagnostic tools become increasingly important in addressing the emergence and treatment of multi-drug resistant (MDR) and extreme-drug (XDR) resistant *M. tuberculosis* strains.

Tuberculosis remains one of the most challenging bacterial diseases in spite of development of a realm of antibiotics and diagnostic molecular biology techniques. The tubercle bacillus was discovered more than two hundred years ago and substantial advancements have been made in our knowledge about the development of tuberculosis in human. The organism seems to evolve over a period of time in terms of its ability to survive the action of front line anti mycobacterial antibiotics by developing appropriate antibiotic resistant mechanisms. The estimated mortality by World Health Organization reports over 1.7 million deaths in 2006 and 9 million new cases of tuberculosis [WHO 2008]. The economic burden of management of disease in patients in the prime of their age is enormous because of prolonged antibiotic treatment. In spite of availability of anti mycobacterial drugs, tuberculosis remains one of the major health problems facing mankind particularly in developing countries. Presently, about one third of word's population is infected with *Mycobacterium tuberculosis*. Currently, the number of people dying of tuberculosis is more than any other infectious diseases. Death from tuberculosis comprises 25% of all avoidable deaths in developing countries [Ramachandran and Parmasivan 2003]. Nearly 95% of all tuberculosis cases and 98% of deaths due to tuberculosis are in developing countries and 75% of tuberculosis cases are in the economically productive age group. Currently, more people die of tuberculosis than from any other infectious disease. In India, out of a total population of more than 1 billion, approximately 2 million develop active disease and up to half a million die of tuberculosis. It also imparts a financial burden on the economy in terms of out-put losses because of premature deaths and ill health. To add to the existing cost burden, the cumulative effect is seen because of ever increasing number of new TB cases associated with HIV patients and about 1.8 million of these are co-infected with TB [Ramachandran and Paramasivan 2003].

2. Traditional methods of tuberculosis detection, management and limitations

Robert Koch discovered the tubercle bacillus in 1882, and there after methods of staining these microorganisms were developed to assist the diagnosis of the disease. Early diagnosis of the tuberculosis in the patients is a challenging task especially in the pauci-bacillary and extra-pulmonary forms. The conventional methods that are still the mainstay of the diagnosis of TB like Tuberculin test/ Montoux test, radiological examination and other imaging methods and sputum smear microscopy have their own limitations. Sputum smear microscopy requires 10,000 to 1,00,000 organisms/ ml and acid fast bacilli could be any pathogenic or saprophytic mycobacteria. Although smear microscopy may be made more convenient by using various fluorochromes (auramine, rhodamine, FITC etc.) but the scarce presence of tuber bacilli in the sputum has its own disadvantage. The smear positivity has to be supplemented with the culture positivity that has its own limitations because of failure of bacilli to grow or often become contaminated with other microbes. The slow growth of the tubercle bacilli on medium lingers on the confirmation of the causative organism. Histopathology is characteristic but there could be problems to get representative specimen, and non-specific features. Immunoassay based approaches are doubtful as the antibodies and the antigens may persist for some time after control of the clinical or sub-clinical disease. Thus Acid Fast Bacilli (AFB) staining of clinical material followed by smear microscopy remains the most cost effective, frequently used microbiological test for detection of TB. The major drawback of sputum smear microscopy is its poor sensitivity, especially to be ~70% in a recent review [Steingart et al., 2006]. Although the AFB staining is easy to perform in the field settings especially in the poor third world countries as well in the developing countries but the sensitivity of sputum smear microscopy is clearly less in many settings and may be sometimes as low as ~35% in some situations with high rates of TB and HIV co-infection [Khatri and Frieden 2002]. Compounding the poor test sensitivity is in adequate or absent test quality assurance in some recourse-constrained settings, further cut down the over all yield of the microscopy, driving up the laboratory workload as more sputum tests per patient are performed in an effort to reach a diagnosis, and increasing delay in diagnosis and patient's compliance to repeated follow-up [Dorman 2010]. Moreover drug-susceptibility status cannot be determined from the smear microscopy.

Unfortunately, the world's largest democracy India has over 1.2 billion people and this overpopulated country also has the highest burden of tuberculosis in the world. India accounts for about 20% incidence of tuberculosis besides a high incidence of global occurrence of multi drug resistant (MDR) tuberculosis. The poor sanitation conditions, thickly populated urban and rural area, scanty medical services in villages and rural area, malnourishment, insensitivity of private sector towards quick diagnosis, treatment and management of TB positive patients and higher cost of non-standard methods of diagnosis of TB are some of the important reasons of concern. It is obvious that any global effort towards control and eradication of TB and fast emerging MDR-TB is invariably dependent upon success of concerted efforts to contain the spread of this contagious disease. In India, the National TB Programme (NTP) was initiated in 1962. However, the poor infrastructure, inadequate funding, administrative lack-luster approach, irregular drug supply, non-standard and multiple anti-tuberculosis drug therapy, irregularity or non-compliance of patients to the clinician and a long treatment period had little effect on containing the spread of TB and controlling the emerging MRD-TB strains. The management and control of TB was further compounded and complicated with low rates of TB case detection, compliance of treatment regimen (30%), high rate of default (40-60%) and continuing high mortality (1: 2000) the NTP programme had little success rate. To overcome the deficiencies of NTP a Revised National Tuberculosis Control Programme (RNTCP) was launched by the Government of India in 1997, based on the global DOTS (Directly Observed Treatment, Short Course) approach that was used to exert an epidemiological impact by achieving 70% case detection and 85% cure rate. It was an encouraging sign that by 2002, 100% of the Indian population was covered by the India's own drug-delivery model - the DOTS programme, making this extended coverage as India's most significant public health accomplishment. The RNTCP thus achieved a pronounced success in cure rates (>80% in new infectious cases), substantial decline in mortality with low rate (<10%) of default [Khatri and Frieden 2002; TB India 2009; Bhargava et al., 2011].

3. Tuberculosis and HIV epidemic

In spite of improvement in public health system, participation of private sector in TB detection and management still the sputum smear microscopy test is most commonly used in public health settings to detect pulmonary TB. This method has roughly 50% chance of detection. Unfortunately, a significant number of people outside the public health sector, where the most common test is the serological (various types of ELISA for detection of *M. tuberculosis* antigens; or anti-*M. tuberculosis* IgG or IgM antibodies) that are expensive and means nothing. The global impact of converging dual epidemics of tuberculosis and human immunodeficiency virus (HIV) is one of the major challenges of the present time. In India, there are 2.5 million people living with HIV and AIDS at the end of 2007 while the incidence of TB was `1.8 million cases per year [WHO 2008, WHO Global Tuberculosis Program 1992].

In a survey carried out among new TB patients by RNTCP in 2007, HIV sero-prevalence varied widely and ranged from 1-13.8% across the 15 districts [Swaminathan and Narendran 2008]. Pulmonary involvement occurs in about 75% of all HIV-infected patients with TB [Devivanayagam et al., 2001; Ahmad and Shameen 2005]. Moreover, the interaction between HIV and TB in persons co-infected with HIV and TB is bi-directional and synergistic. As HIV progresses, there is cutaneous anergy as well as impaired tissue containment of mycobacteria leading to widespread dissemination of mycobacteria. While TB can develop at any CD4 count, extra-pulmonary and disseminated forms of the diseases are more common as immunodeficiency increases. Thus HIV infection is associated not only with an increased incidence of TB but also with altered clinical manifestations especially in the advanced stages of the disease. The cost management of anti-HIV and anti-TB therapy in the patients becomes a daunting task that compromises the success rate of containment and spread of TB from HIV infected patients. Current guidelines recommend that irrespective of HIV status, TB management require a minimum of 6 months of treatment with four drugs (including rifampin) in the intensive phase and two drugs in the continuation phase. In India, under the RNTCP, patients with newly diagnosed TB receive a 6-month thrice-weekly regimen 9cat I - $2EHRZ_3/4RH_3$) while those with relapse, default or failure receive an 8-months regimen (cat II - $2SEHRZ_3/1SEHRZ_3/5EHR_3$). The lifetime risk of TB in immuno-competent persons is 5% to 10%, but HIV positive individuals; there is a 5% to 15% annual risk of developing active TB diseases [Swaminathan et al., 2000]. WHO estimated 9.2 million new cases of TB globally in 2006 (139 per 100,000); of whom 7,09,000 (7.7%) were HIV positive (WHO 2008). India, China, Indonesia, South Africa and Nigeria rank 1st to 5th in terms of incident TB cases.

The first and foremost step in the diagnosis of TB is its accurate and early detection. To achieve this objective a number of methods have been developed and reported (Table 1) that achieve early growth of *M. tuberculosis* [Katoch and Sharma 1997; Katoch 2004].

4. Anti-TB drug resistance

The overall pattern of drug resistance to first line anti TB therapy is similar in HIV positive and negative patients; however, MDR-TB is marginally higher (3-4%) in HIV positive patients with newly diagnosed tuberculosis status [Swaminathan 2005]. Rifampicin mono-resistance is more common in HIV infected patients and arises independently from mutations in drug susceptible strains. Treatment of MDR-TB should employ at least 3-4 new drugs. The regimen should include an aminoglycoside and be given under direct observation. Extensively drug resistant (XDR) TB strains have emerged and have been reported from India [Singh et al., 2007; Thomas et al., 2007]. Such strains appeared to be as an outcome of the mismanagement of TB. It seems that XDR-TB is practically untreatable and thus an attempt may be made to limit its spread by strengthening the TB control programme. Presently, there is no national policy regarding TB preventive therapy for HIV positive patients in India [Swaminathan and Narendran 2008]. A clinical trial conducted at the Tuberculosis Research Center, Chennai investigated two different regimens; a 6-month regimen of ethambutol and isoniazid vs. a 3-year regimen of isoniazid alone, in order to establish ideal duration of therapy. In a TB-endemic country like India, consideration shall be given to provide preventive therapy to HIV-infected persons. Line probe assays, a family

S. No.	Method	Concept	Reference(s)
1	BACTEC system	Generation and detection of radioactive CO_2 from substrate palmitic acid. Used world-over, detection of growth in 5-7 d. Inclusion of (NAP: beta nitro alpha acetylamine beta hydroxy propiophenone) distinguishes *M. tuberculosis* [inhibition] from other mycobacteria.	Venkataram et al., 1998; Bemer et al., 2002
2	Mycobacteria growth indicator tube (MGIT)	Developed by Becton Dickinson, growth detection by non-radioactive fluorochrome detection; useful in drug screening, early detection of mycobacterium growth in 7-12 d.	Bemer et al., 2002; Tortoli et al., 1999
3	MB/BacT system	Developed by Organon Technika; colorimetric detection of bacterial growth in, cultures; also useful for drug susceptibility testing	Brunello and Fontana 2000
4	TK Medium	Developed by Salubris, Inc., MA, USA is a novel colorimetric system that indicates growth of mycobacteria by changing its color, also discriminates between mycobacteria and contamination, and enables drug susceptibility testing. Test is low cost and simple. Sensitivity of TK medium is comparable to the LJ-medium.	Kocagoz et al., 2004; Salubris, Inc.
5	Septi-Check	Bi-phase system developed by Roche. Consists of enriched selective broth and a slide having non-selective Middlebrook agar on one side and two sections on other side: one with NAP + egg-containing agar, and second with chocolate agar for detection of contaminating microbes.	Isenberg et al., 1991

S. No.	Method	Concept	Reference(s)
6	Reporter phages/ Bronx box	Use of mycobacterium-specific phage(s) and a reporter gene (luciferase) for detection of growth and drug-susceptibility to anti-TB drugs. Viability detection by either emission of light from microbe due to activation of luciferase gene or production of plaque on an indicator strain of mycobacteria; results availability in 2 d.	Riska et al., 1999; Wilson et al., 1997; Krishnamurthy et al., 2002
7	E-test	Use of gradient of drug on a paper-strip; useful for drug susceptibility testing of *M. tuberculosis*.	Kirk et al., 1998
8	Flow cytometry	Use of FACS for drug susceptibility testing, high cost of equipment and trained operator are the drawbacks.	Kakkar et al., 2000
9	Line-probe assay	A novel DNA strip-based test that uses PCR and reverse hybridization methods for rapid detection of mutations associated with drug resistance. Designed to identify *M. tuberculosis* complex and simultaneous detection of mutations associated with drug resistance.	Morgan et al., 2005

Table 1. Methods of early detection of *M. tuberculosis*.

of novel DNA strip-based tests use PCR and reverse hybridization methods for the rapid detection of mutations associated with drug resistance. These kits [INNO-LiPA Rif TB kit, Innogenetics NV, Gent, Belgium; GenoType MTBDR assay; Hain Life-science GmbH, Nehren, Germany] are not currently FDA approved for use in USA. Line-probe assays are designed to identify *M. tuberculosis* complex and simultaneously detect mutations associated with drug resistance. In June 2008, WHO announced a new policy statement endorsing the use of line probe assays for rapid screening of patients at risk of MRD-TB (http://www.who.int/tb/en/). However, the line probe assays are not recommended as a complete replacement for conventional culture and drug susceptibility testing. Culture is still required for smear-negative specimens and conventional drug susceptibility testing is still necessary to confirm XDR-TB.

5. Ineffective TB diagnostics in India

Ineffective TB diagnostics are a lucrative market in India. Patients seeking TB care in the private medical institutes are commonly subjected to diagnostic tests i.e. the anti-body-based blood tests, including ELISA that are completely ineffective at detecting TB. This is because a large number of the world's population has anti-TB antibodies, though only 10% of them do develop the active form of the disease. Obviously if patients who do not have TB are misdiagnosed, they could undergo 6-months of nasty toxic anti-TB chemotherapy. If patients have active TB and the test missies it, the disease may worsen and they may continue to spread the disease in their community. According to a preliminary analysis of over 80 labs in India, it is estimated that patients undergo more than 1.5 million useless TB antibody tests each year (WHO recommends against inaccurate tuberculosis tests by Kelly Morris; www.thelancet.com vol 377 Jan 8, 2011). The absence of any regulatory mechanisms results in the import of these dubious diagnostics from France, UK, USA and other countries, where these tests are not approved for TB diagnosis. These tests generate at least US $ 15 million. In a country that has ~100,000 labs this is probably a fraction of the enormous total market. Accurate diagnose is critical to the control of tuberculosis in India, particularly in view of the fact that India has set new targets as a part of RNTCP, which includes early detection of 90% of all TB cases by year 2015.

6. Molecular diagnosis of TB in Indian context

In India various institutes working on TB have sufficient technical expertise and financial affordability to use molecular diagnostic methods for detection of tubercle bacilli in the samples. For a laboratory with good sample load and which is using rapid methods for early growth detection the additional cost of sample analysis shall not be significant. If 10-25 isolates/ growths are assessed for identity simultaneously, additional cost for each isolate using a non-radioactive detection system like digoxigenin (DIG) should not be more than 200-250 rupees (~US $ 4-5). Similarly for a PCR system using primers, which are not patented, cost should be in similar range as prices of primers and reagents have considerably been reduced during the last couple of years [Katoch 2004]. The nucleic acid amplification tests (NAATs) are designed to amplify nucleic acid regions specific to the *Mycobacterium tuberculosis* complex. Such tests may be used directly on clinical samples/ sputum samples. Nucleic acid amplification test (NAAT) commercial kits are available under various brands like Amplified *M. tuberculosis* Direct Test (MTD; Gen-Probe Inc., CA, USA), the Amplicor *M. tuberculosis* (MTB) tests (Roche Molecular Diagnostics, CA, USA and the BD ProbeTec ET assay (BD Biosciences, MD, USA. Besides in-house lab developed PCR assays vary widely in their protocols and vary from lab to lab. In-house NAAT are cheap and are often used in research in developing countries where commercial NAATs are quite expensive to test large number of samples and thus in-house PCR technique/ protocol(s) provide a cheap option (Pai 2004). However, all the detection methods including the conventional AFB-staining, skin tuberculin test and new generation NAAT tests have some advantages as well as limitations (Table 2).

Method	Use	Intended use	Advantages	Limitations
AFB smear microscopy	Rapid tubercle bacilli detection	Community	Needs moderate training, microscope and low investment	Low sensitivity
Culture on solid media	Mycobacterial growth and drug susceptibility assay	Referral lab	Good sensitivity; gold standard	Long time to detect growth of bacteria
Chest radiography	Pulmonary TB detection	Referral by clinician	Indications and use not restricted to TB	Low specificity & sensitivity, trained clinician needed
Tuberculin skin test	Detection of *M. tuberculosis*	Community	Extensive clinical and published experience	Sensitivity decreases in immuno-comprised persons, positive reaction in BCG vaccinees
γ-Interferon release assay	Detection of *M. tuberculosis* infection	Referral to reference lab	Highly specific for *M. tuberculosis*	Trained manpower, poor sensitivity especially in immunocompro mised hosts
Automated, non-integrated NAAT	Pulmonary TB detection	Reference lab	High sensitivity, rapidity and detection of mutations in MDR-TB strains.	Moderately trained personnel and equipment, laborious and possible cross-contamination among specimens
Culture in liquid media [MGIT; BacT/ Alert and others]	TB detection and as a prerequisite to drug-susceptibility testing	Referral lab	High sensitivity (more sensitivity than liquid media)	Long time for detection; less than solid medium but high contamination rate in some settings

Method	Use	Intended use	Advantages	Limitations
Line probe assay	TB detection and drug susceptibility testing	Reference lab	Poor sensitivity in smear-negative samples, short analysis time	Labor intensive, potential for cross-contamination, requires extensive training
Strip-based Mycobacterium species identification	Species identification i.e. TB versus non-TB in cultures positive for mycobacterial growth	Referral lab	Accurate, requires minimal-training/ equipment/ consumables	Moderate training in handling of pathogenic microbes

Adapted from references: Pai et al., 2006; Perkins and Cunningham 2007; Nyendak et al., 2009; WHO and Stop TB Partnership 2009; Dorman 2010.

Table 2. Tuberculosis diagnostic methods in use, recently endorsed by WHO and under development.

7. Challenges in the TB care and control

At present a vigorous approach is needed to proactively detect the TB cases under RNTCP. The DOT service providers may be actively involved in identifying fresh potential TB patients in their community and getting them diagnosed for TB. Another possibility is contact tracing of both adults and children diagnosed to have TB. Such approach is currently being followed in HIV programs and could be considered to improve upon the case detection rate. Further prevalence studies in different parts of India may be conducted systematically to determine the existing burden of TB. The district level data will be quite helpful in achieving a realistic figure of TB cases.

Lab strengthening: In most cases among the poorest strata of people living in slums or rural areas the sputum transportation is difficult to reach populations is a major consideration and TB is quite commonly said to be poor man's disease. Thus inadequate number of microscopic centers/ labs put the burden on existing microscopic centers that causes a delay in the reporting of the results of the sputum samples. Most labs conduct AFB testing and are ill equipped to perform culture of tubercle bacilli.

Migrant populations: Presently, there is no national level strategy and guidelines for tuberculosis care and control for the migrant population in India who move from one state or place to another one as a part of their jobs or in search of jobs. Millions of migrants are currently working in unorganized job sectors with no health facilities, insurance facilities and work place policy for disease care and control like TB, HIV etc. Such workers are solely dependent on the relatively expensive private health sector for their healthcare. Accessing those migrants at their residences and working places with the key messages of TB, DOTS and RNTCP is extremely challenging because of the geographically scattered areas and huge number of migrants. Also women engaged in unorganized job sectors are particularly prone to tuberculosis due to continuous exploitation by the employers. The migrant workers should be mapped in the urban and peri-urban areas (construction sites, street dwellers, illegal residents along the railway tracts, brick kilns etc.) and should be provided RNTCP services (like sensitization on TB, identification of suspected TB cases, referral and tracking) through community-based programs as part of the extended TB monitoring and care program and activities. Moreover, the TB component may be introduced into the existing HIV programs for migrant workers after collaboration with National AIDS Control Programs (NACO).

New TB testing tools: For 100% detection of the TB cases new technologies and techniques shall be establishes that are reasonably cheap, rapid and easily available. Recently a new PCR based diagnostic kit has been developed through a partnership between Cepheid and Foundation for Innovative New diagnostics, the University of Medicine and Density of New Jersey, the Bill and Melinda Gates Foundation and national Institute of Health (U.S.). The study demonstrated high sensitivity and specificity, identifying 98% of patients with TB and correctly identified 98% of bacteria resistant to rifampin.

Besides PCR, some novel tests involving use of beacons for the rapid detection of mutations associated with drug resistance have been reported [Varma-Basil et al., 2004]. Employing Xpert/RIF kit 1,700 patients were screened at five sites across the world including Mumbai, and using this PCR 98% of patients with TB and resistant to rifampin were correctly identified. This PCR needed about 100 minutes compared to current tests that may take up to 3 months to have results. Unfortunately, the PCR NAATs are performed in a few national labs and specialized private hospitals only. Facilities for culture and drug susceptibility testing of TB cultures in India are grossly inadequate [Bhargava 2011]. As of 2008, only 17 accredited facilities were doing culture and drug-susceptibility testing (~0.1 facility/ 10 million residents against 1/ 10 million). Efforts are underway to enhance the number of labs/ facilities to 43 to perform drug-susceptibility testing. The RNTCP has started to include rapid diagnostic methods to perform culture and drug-susceptibility testing so as to prevent delay in management of MDR-TB patients.

8. Conclusion

TB one of the most communicable diseases is still evading accurate diagnosis because of lack and development of cheap, less labor/ equipment intensive, highly specific and sensitive methods. Culture positivity in sputum positive samples is still considered to be a gold standard as this method provides a further lead in accessing the drug susceptibility of the grown mycobacterial cultures. Currently, most of the tools/ techniques in demonstration or late-stage validation are sputum based and thus are likely to result in incremental gains in rate of TB detection. Still there is an urgent need to develop and validate a mycobacterial culture based or NAAT-based technique that is close to 100% specificity and sensitivity. The need to fast develop such techniques is urgent because of development of MDR mycobacterial strains in third-world countries as these countries are also experiencing an increased burden of HIV-positive patients. The previous decade has shown how despite '100% coverage' and impressive case detection and cure rates, TB continues to be an epidemic of magnanimous magnitude in India. Thus in India a staunch collaboration between RNTCP, NACO and private partners is the need of the hour to contain the fast spread of MRD *M. tuberculosis* strains.

9. References

Ahmad Z and Shameem M (2005). Manifestations of tuberculosis in HIV infected patients. JIACM 6: 302-305.

Bemer P, Palicova F, Rusch-Gerdes S, Dugeon HB and Pfyffer GE (2002). Multicentre evaluation of fully automatic BACTEC mycobacteria growth indicator tube 960 system for susceptibility testing of *Mycobacterium tuberculosis*. J Clin Microbiol 40: 150-154.

Bhargava A, Pinto l and Pai M (2011). Mismanagement of tuberculosis in India: causes, consequences and the way forward. Hypothesis 9: 1-13.

Brunello F and Fontana R (2000). Reliability of the MB-BactT system for testing susceptibility of *Mycobacterium tuberculosis* complex strains to anti-tuberculous drugs. J Clin Microbiol 38: 872-873.

Deivanayagam CN, Rajasekaran S, Senthilnathan V, Krishnarajasekhar R, Raja K, Chandrasekar C, Palanisamy S, Samuel DA, Jothivel G and Elango SV (2001). Clinico-radiological spectrum of tuberculosia among HIV-sero-positives - a Tambaram study. Indian J Tuberc 49: 123-127.

Dorman SE (2010). New diagnostic tests for tuberculosis: Bench, bedside and beyond. Clin Infect Dis 50: S173-S177.

Isenberg HD, D'Amate RF, Heifets L, Murray PR, Scardamaglia M, Jacob MC et al., (1991). Collaborative feasibility study of a biphasic system (Roche Septi-Chek AFB) for rapid detection and isolation of mycobacteria. J Clin Microbiol 29: 1713-1722.

Kakkar N, Sharma M, Ray P, Seth S and Kumar S (2000). Evaluation of E-test for susceptibility testing of mycobacteria to primary antitubercular drugs. Indian J Med Res 111: 168-171.

Katoch VM (2004). Newer diagnostic techniques for tuberculosis. Indian J Med Res 120: 418-428.

Katoch VM and Sharma VD (1997).Advances in the diagnosis of mycobacterial diseases. Indian J Med Microbiol 15: 49-55.

Khatri GR and Frieden T (2002). Controlling tuberculosis in India. N Engl J Med 347: 1420-1425.

Kirk SM, Schell RF, Moore AV, Callister SM and Mazurek GH (1998). Flow cytometric testing of susceptibilities of *Mycobacterium tuberculosis* isolates to ethambutol, isoniazid and rifampicin in 24 hours. J Clin Microbiol 36: 1568-1571.

Kocagoz T, O'Brien R and Perkins M (2004). A new colorimetric culture system for the diagnosis of tuberculosis. Int J Tuberc Lung Dis 8: 1512-1513.

Krishnamurthy A, Rodrigues C and Mehta AP (2002). Rapid detection of rifampicin resistance in *Mycobacterium tuberculosis* by phage assay. Indian J Med Microbiol 20: 211-214.

Morgan M, Kalantri S, Flores L and Pai M (2005). A commercial line probe assay for the rapid detection of rifampicin resistance in Mycobacterium tuberculosis. A systemic review and meta-analysis. BMC Infect Dis 5: 62.

Nyendak MR, Lewinsohn DA and Lewinsohn DM (2009). New diagnostic methods for tuberculosis. Curr Opin Infect Dis 22: 174-182.

Pai M (2004). The accuracy and reliability of nucleic acid amplification tests in the diagnosis of tuberculosis. Natl Med J India 17: 233-236.

Pai M, Kalantri S and Dheda K (2006). New tools and emerging technologies for the diagnosis of tuberculosis: Part II. Active tuberculosis and drug resistance. Expert Rev Mol Diagn 6: 423-432.

Perkin MD and Cunningham J (2007). Facing the crisis: Improving the diagnosis of tuberculosis in the HIV era. J Infect Dis 196(Suppl 1): S15-S27.

Ramachandran R and Parmasivan CN (2003). What is new in the diagnosis of tuberculosis? Part I: Techniques for diagnosis of tuberculosis. Indian J Tuberculosis 50: 133-141.

Riska PF, Su Y, Bardarov S, Freundlish L, Sarkis G, Hatfull G et al., (1999). Rapid film-based determination of antibiotic susceptibility of *Mycobacterium tuberculosis* strains by using a luciferase reporter phage and the Bronx box. J Clin Microbiol 37: 1144-1149.

Singh S, Sankar MM and Gopinath K (2007). High rate of extensively drug-resistant tuberculosis in Indian AIDS patients. AIDS 21: 2345-2347.

Steingart KR, Henry M, Ng V et al., (2006). Fluorescence versus conventional smear microscopy for tuberculosis: A systemic review. Lancet Infect Dis 6: 570-581.

Swaminathan S and Narendran G (2008). HIV and tuberculosis in India. J Biosci 33: 527-537.

Swaminathan S, Paramasivan CN, Ponnuraja C, Iliayas S, Rajasekaran S and naryanan PR (2005). Anti-tuberculosis drug resistance tuberculosis in South India. Int J Tuberc Lung Dis 9: 896-900.

Swaminathan S, Ramachandran R, Baskaran G and Paramsivan CN (2000). Risk of development of tuberculosis in HIV infectd patients. Int J Tuberc Lung Dis 4: 839-844.

TB India (2009). RNTCP status report.

Thomas BE, Ramachandran R, Anitha S and Swaminathan S (2007). Feasibility of routine HIV testing among TB patients through a voluntary, counseling and testing center VCTC). Int J Tuberc Lung Dis 11: 1296-1301.

Tortoli E, Cichero P, Piersimoni C, Simonetii T, Gesu G and Nistta D (1999). Use of BACTEC MGIT for recovery of mycobacteria from clinical specimens: multicentric study. J Clin Microbiol 37: 3578-3582.

Varma-Basil M, El-Hajj H, Colangeli R et al., (2004). Rapid detection of rifampin resistance in *Mycobacterium tuberculosis* isolates from India and Mexico by a molecular beacon assay. J Clin Microbiol 42: 5512-5516.

Venkataraman P, Herbert D and Paramasivan CN (1998). Evaluation of BACTEC radiometric method in the early diagnosis of tuberculosis. Indian J Med Res 108: 120127.

WHO (2008). Global tuberculosis control: surveillance, planning, financing. WHO report 2008. WHO/HTM/TB/2008.393. Geneva.

WHO Global Tuberculosis Program (1992). Tuberculosis programme review, India, September 1992.

Wilson S, Al-Suwaidi A, McNerny R, porter J and Drobniewski F (1997). Evaluation of a new rapid bacteriophage based method for the drug susceptibility testing of *Mycobacterium tuberculosis*. Nature Med 3: 415-418.

World Health Organization (1997). Prevalence and incidence of tuberculosis in India. A comprehensive review. WHO/TB/97, 231.

World Health Organization Stop TB partnership (2009). New laboratory diagnosis tools for tuberculosis control. http://www.apps.who.int/tdr.

9

Management of TB in HIV Subjects, the Experience in Thailand

Attapon Cheepsattayakorn
Thai Board of Preventive Medicine (Public Health Science)
10th Zonal Tuberculosis and Chest Disease Centre, Chiang Mai,
10th Office of Disease Prevention and Control,
Department of Disease Control,
Ministry of Public Health,
Thailand

1. Introduction

Currently, tuberculosis (TB) remains a major public health threats of humankind. It has been occurred since antiquity and is the second communicable-disease cause of death after the human immunodeficiency virus (HIV)/ acquired immunodeficiency syndrome (AIDS). Of the mycobacterial diseases, TB is by far the most important because of its most virulence. Most of the disease and nearly all of the deaths occurs in the developing countries. Co-infection with HIV/AIDS and TB represents a public health crisis worldwide. An estimated 2 billion people worldwide carry latent infection and more than 8 million persons develop active TB each year. Approximately, 3 million people per year die from TB (WHO, 2010). Various comorbidities, especially the immunocompromised statuses will accelerate the TB sickness and deaths. The prevalence of primary drug- (Jiang et al., 2011) and multidrug-resistant (MDR) (Wells, 2010) pulmonary TB among the immunocompromised populations is globally increased. In Thailand, total-estimated TB cases is more than 140,000, now ranking 18 of the 22 high-burden countries of the world (WHO, 2010). The clinical features of active TB are very highly variable, depend on the immune status of the host and the site and extent of disease. New diagnostic, therapeutic, preventive and control strategies for TB are heavily investigated throughout the world. How we can rapidly diagnose TB within few hours and how we can shorten the treatment regimens to weeks or days. World elimination of TB is expected to occur in 2050 when the incidence is 1 patient per 1 million populations per year (WHO, 2010).

2. Epidemiology

While HIV/AIDS has continued to pose greater threats to the public health system worldwide which is a major risk of double increasing within the first year after *Mycobacterium tuberculosis* exposure and 10% per year for developing TB (Barnes et al., 1991, as cited in Silva et al., 2010 & Sonnenberg et al., 2001, as cited in Nachega & Maartens, 2009). Now it is clear that non-communicable comorbidities such as diabetes mellitus, especially type 2 (Goldhaber-Fiebert et al., 2011), malignancies, chronic renal failure, immunosuppressive drug uses as well as biological modifiers such as rituximab and infliximab are undoubtedly adding to the multiple burdens the people suffer. A previous study in The Philippines demonstrated 37.4% of central nervous system TB among patients with systemic lupus erythematosus (SLE) (Vargas et al., 2009). Multiple immune system abnormalities contribute to high prevalence of TB with SLE (Prabu & Agrawal, 2010). Fatal tuberculous myositis at the left thigh was also reported in a 55-old-male patient with primary Sjögren's syndrome (Huang et al., 2010). TB patients with diabetes type 2 have lower antimicrobial peptides gene expression that contribute to enhance the TB-reactivation risk (Gonzalez-Curiel et al., 2011). A recent study conducted in India showed the ranks of risk factors for developing of TB disease as the following: diabetes (30.9%), smoking (16.9%), alcoholism (12.6%), HIV/AIDS (10.6%), malignancies (5.8%), chronic hepatic diseases (3.9%), history of TB contact (3.4%), chronic corticosteroid therapy (2.9%), chronic renal diseases and malnourishment (1.5%) (Gupta et al., 2011). No evidence was found that TB increases the risk of diabetes (Young et al., 2010). There has been a recent evidence of increased risk of lung malignancies among pulmonary TB patients and may increase further with coexisting chronic obstructive pulmonary disease (COPD) (Yu et al., 2011). A annual TB report of the fiscal year 2009 demonstrated that TB patients in northern Thailand who had COPD, HIV/AIDS, hypertension and diabetes mellitus ranked 1 to 4 of the specific causes of death (10th Zonal Tuberculosis and Chest Disease Centre, Chiang Mai, Thailand and the 10th Office of Disease Prevention and Control, Chiang Mai, Thailand, 2009 Tuberculosis annual report). A study in Brazil revealed that among the non-HIV-infected immunocompromised patients with TB, the only factor statistically related to mortality was the need for mechanical ventilation (Silva et al., 2010). In 2009, a total of 300,000 HIV-positive TB patients were enrolled on co-trimoxazole preventive therapy, and almost 140,000 were enrolled on antiretroviral therapy. In 2006 northern Thailand survey, only 69.6% and 63.1% of the HIV- infected/AIDS patients received co-trimoxazole prophylaxis therapy and antiretroviral therapy, respectively (10th Zonal Tuberculosis and Chest Disease Centre, Chiang Mai, Thailand and the 10th Office of Disease Prevention and Control, Chiang Mai, Thailand, 2006 Tuberculosis annual report). Almost 80,000 persons living with HIV were provided with isoniazid preventive therapy. This represents less than 1% of estimated number of HIV- infected persons worldwide. The 2015 targets are HIV testing of 100% of TB patients, enrolment of 100% of HIV-infected TB patients on antiretroviral therapy and co-trimoxazole preventive therapy while in 2009 revealed only 26%, 75% and 37%, respectively (WHO, 2010).

In northern Thailand, TB is the most common opportunistic infection among HIV-infected/AIDS individuals (38.9%) (Cheepsattayakorn et al., 2009). The highest prevalence of TB co-infected with HIV/AIDS in northern Thailand appeared in 1999 which was 48.8% of the total registered TB cases in the same year compared to 12.2% of the country (10th Zonal Tuberculosis and Chest Disease Centre, Chiang Mai, Thailand and the 10th Office of Disease Prevention and Control, Chiang Mai, Thailand, 2005 Tuberculosis annual report, Figure 1). In 2004 northern Thailand survey revealed that the extrapulmonary site of TB among HIV-infected/AIDS cases was accounted for 18.7% of the total TB cases, especially TB of the jugular lymph nodes (Cheepsattayakorn & Cheepsattayakorn, 2009). A recent study of extrapulmonary TB in a Caucasian population demonstrated that the proportion of extrapulmaonry TB has been increased while the overall incidence of TB has been reduced (Garcia-Rodriguez et al., 2011). This could be explained by an increase of life expectancy. There is no statistically significant difference between the development of pulmonary and extrapulmonary TB among diabetic persons (Young et al,. 2010). A recent study in the United States and Mexico revealed high diabetes prevalence among newly-diagnosed TB cases which was 39% in Texas and 36% in Mexico, respectively (Restrepo et al., 2011). A recent study on TB among end-stage renal disease (ESRD) patients in Taiwan showed that the independent risk factors for TB infection in ESRD are male gender, old age, chronic obstructive pulmonary disease (COPD), and silicosis (Li et al., 2011). A survey between 2001-2007 in northern Thailand showed the highest incidence of TB among the populations with more than 64 years of age (10th Zonal Tuberculosis and Chest Disease Centre, Chiang Mai, Thailand and the 10th Office of Disease Prevention and Control, Chiang Mai, Thailand, 2007 Tuberculosis annual report, Figure 2).

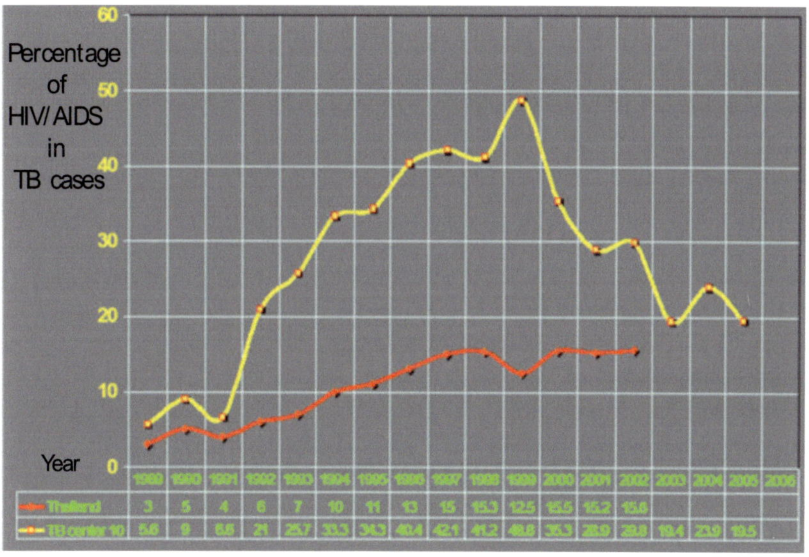

Fig. 1. TB/HIV/AIDS sentinel surveillance in northern Thailand between 1989-2005.

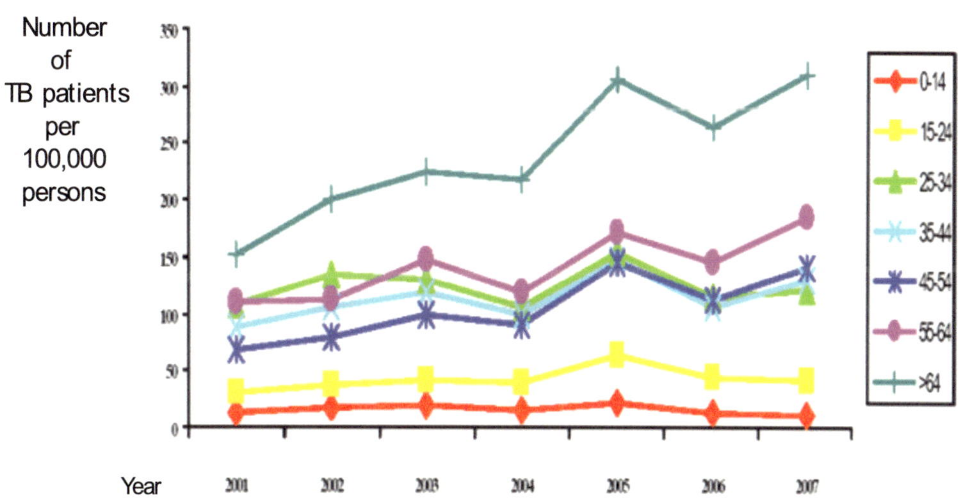

Fig. 2. Incidence of TB patients by ages in northern Thailand between 2001-2007.

3.Tuberculosis investigations in immunocompromised patients

3.1 Acid-Fast Bacilli (AFB) smear and culture

The finding of AFB on stained specimens is the only reliable and affordable rapid diagnostic method of TB which has lower yield (40%-70%) compared to the mycobacterial culture (75-90%) (Nachega & Maartens, 2009).

3.2 Interferon-gamma release assays

Since 2001, development of interferon-gamma release assays (IGRAs) for the detection of TB infection has been initiated in addition to the tuberculin skin test (TST). It detects sensitization to *Mycobacterium tuberculosis* by measuring interferon-gamma release in response to *Mycobacterium tuberculosis* complex antigens (Converse et al., 1997, Rothel et al., 1990 & Streeton et al., 1998, as cited in Mazulek et al., 2010 & Walsh et al., 2011). QuantiFERON-TB test (QFT) (Cellestis Limited, Carnegie, Victoria, Australia) was the first assay approved by the Food and Drug Administration (FDA) in 2001 (FDA, 2010 & Mazurek & Villarino, 2003, as cited in Mazulek et al., 2010). The QuantiFERON-TB Gold test (GFT-G) (Cellestis Limited, Carnegie, Victoria, Australia) was the second IGRA approved by FDA in 2005 (FDA, 2010 & Mazulek et al., 2005, as cited in Mazulek et al., 2010). The United States Centers for Disease Control and Prevention (CDC) published guidelines for using QFT and QFT-G in 2003 and 2005, respectively (Mazurek & Villarino, 2003, Mazulek et al., 2005, as cited in Mazulek et al., 2010). The CDC recommended that a positive interferon-gamma release test should be confirmed with a TST (Mazurek & Villarino, 2003, as cited in Hopewell, 2005). A recent study compared the sensitivity of QFT- G to enzyme-linked immunospot (ELISPOT) among pulmonary TB including HIV - negative immunocompromised patients and demonstrated the superiority of ELISPOT over QFT-G at the low lymphocyte count conditions, not depending on gender, age, and nutritional status (Komiya et al., 2010).

Many studies have been shown that these new assays are useful for diagnosis of active TB in both immunocompromised patients and immunocompetent ones such as HIV/AIDS, diabetes mellitus, systemic immunosuppressant administration, malignant diseases and chronic renal failure (Ito et al., 2011, Nachega & Maartens, 2009, Tan et al., 2010 & Walsh et al., 2011). The sensitivity of the interferon-gamma release assays are not compromised by serum glucose levels in TB patients with diabetes (Walsh et al., 2011) including other immunocompromised TB patients (Ito et al., 2011). A study demonstrated that, unlike the tuberculin skin test, the sensitivity of these assays are less interfered by moderately advanced HIV status (Rangaka et al., 2007, as cited in Nachega & Maartens, 2009). The QFT-G assay has higher detection rate of the latent TB infection than the TST. It may has lower sensitivity among the immunocompromised persons but requires shorter turnaround time than the TST (Baboolal et al., 2010). A previous study of QuantiFERON-TB Gold In-Tube (QFT-GIT) showed 33.4% of indeterminate results among HIV-infected/AIDS patients with CD4-T cell count below 200 cells/μL and the TST has higher degree of agreement than QFT-GIT in patients with immune-mediated inflammatory diseases. This study results indicated that the performance of QFT-GIT varied between different types of immunocompromised patients (Sauzullo et al., 2010). The CDC do not recommend the blood interferon-gamma release assay for pregnant women, individuals with HIV/AIDS, individuals with increased risk of TB, screening children younger than 17 years old, contacts with an infectious case of TB, or individuals being evaluated for suspected TB (Mazurek & Villarino, 2003, as cited in Hopewell, 2005).

3.3 Imaging

Several chest roengenographic pictures plays a critical role in the diagnosis of TB in HIV-infected/AIDS patients, however, the degree of immunosuppression is a core determinant of the roentgenographic appearance. Most notably the presence of bilateral hilar lymphadenopathy is highly suggestive of TB, but is not diagnostic (Nachega & Maartens, 2009, Figure 3). When a CD4+ T-cell count is higher than 200 cells/µL, the pulmonary infiltrates are characteristic adult picture with cavitation and upper lobe predominance. But when a CD4+ T-cell count is below 200 cells/µL, the pulmonary infiltrates shift toward atypical patterns for adults: hilar or mediastinal adenopathy, and mid- ,lower-zone or military infiltrates (Nachega & Maartens, 2009, Figure 4). Pleural effusion can occur with any CD4+ T-cell count (Havlir & Barnes, 1999, as cited in Nachega & Maartens, 2009, Post et al., 1995, Long et al., 1991, as cited in Nachega & Maartens, 2009, Perlman et al., 1997, Wendel & Sterling, 2002, as cited in Nachega & Maartens, 2009, Figure 5). There is no statistically significant pulmonary shadowing among old patients with TB (Toure' et al., 2010).

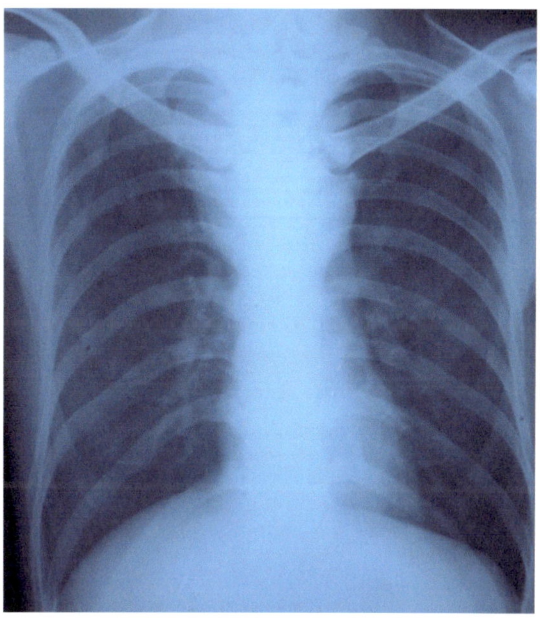

Fig. 3. Chest roentgenogram from the initial presentation of a 34-year-old Thai male with HIV-infection/AIDS who attended the tenth Zonal Tuberculosis and Chest Disease Centre, Chiang Mai, Thailand showing bilateral hilar adenopathy. The sputum smears for AFB and cultures revealed positive results. Diagnosis of pulmonary TB was made.

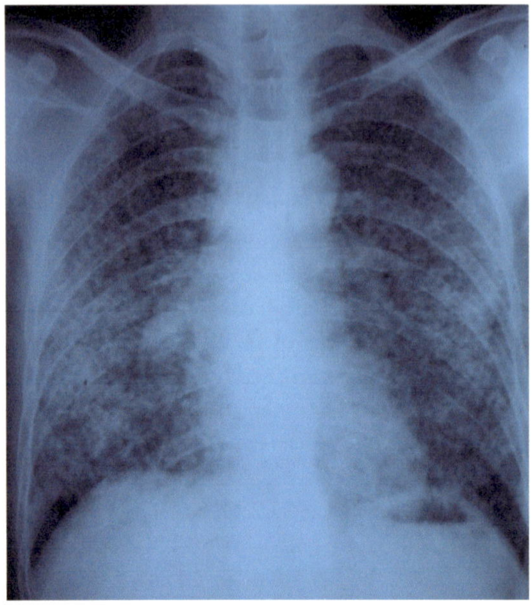

Fig. 4. Chest roentgenogram from initial presentation of a 44-year-old Thai female with chronic smoking who attended the tenth Zonal Tuberculosis and Chest Disease Centre, Chiang Mai, Thailand showing military infiltrates. Her three consecutive sputum smears for AFB and cultures revealed negative results. After completeness of anti-TB chemotherapy her chest roentgenogram completely resoluted.

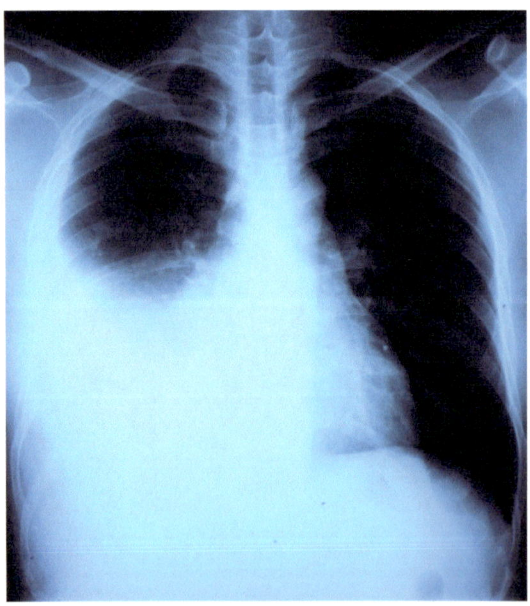

Fig. 5. Chest roentgenogram from initial presentation of another 34-year-old Thai male with HIV-infection/AIDS who attended the tenth Zonal Tuberculosis and Chest Disease Centre, Chiang Mai, Thailand showing a right massive pleural effusion. His pleural biopsy revealed tuberculous pleurisy.

A recent study of TB patients with diabetes conducted in India revealed that lower lung field involvement was predominant (84%) as compared to upper lung field. Cavitation was predominantly confined to the lower lung field (80%) while nodular lesions were found in 36% and exudative lesions were found in 22% (Patel et al.,2011). A previous report in 2000 also demonstrated a higher lower-lung field involvement (Perez-Guzman et al., 2000, as cited in Patel et al.,2011). Some investigators have demonstrated no major differences of the roentgenographic pictures (Bacakoglu et al., 2001, as cited in Patel et al.,2011) while other previous studies have reported more common multiple cavities among diabetic patients (Sen et al., 2009, as cited in Patel et al.,2011). There are not clear reasons for atypical images in TB patients with diabetes.

Alveolar infiltration which indicates tuberculous pneumonia mostly occurs in the upper lung fields is frequently found in HIV-infected/AIDS (20%) and diabetes (15%) patients (Moreira et al., 2011).

Other imaging techniques may be helpful depending on localization of the clinical manifestations. Magnetic resonance imaging (MRI) or computed tomography (CT) scans are specifically detection of TB of the central nervous system (Figure 6 A & B) while ultrasonography can detect intraperitoneal TB such as splenic microabscesses, mesenteric lymphadenopathy and hepatic tuberculous granulomas. CT of the chest is superior to chest roentgenogram to demonstrate latent TB infiltrate in patient with hepatic transplantation (Lyu et al., 2011).

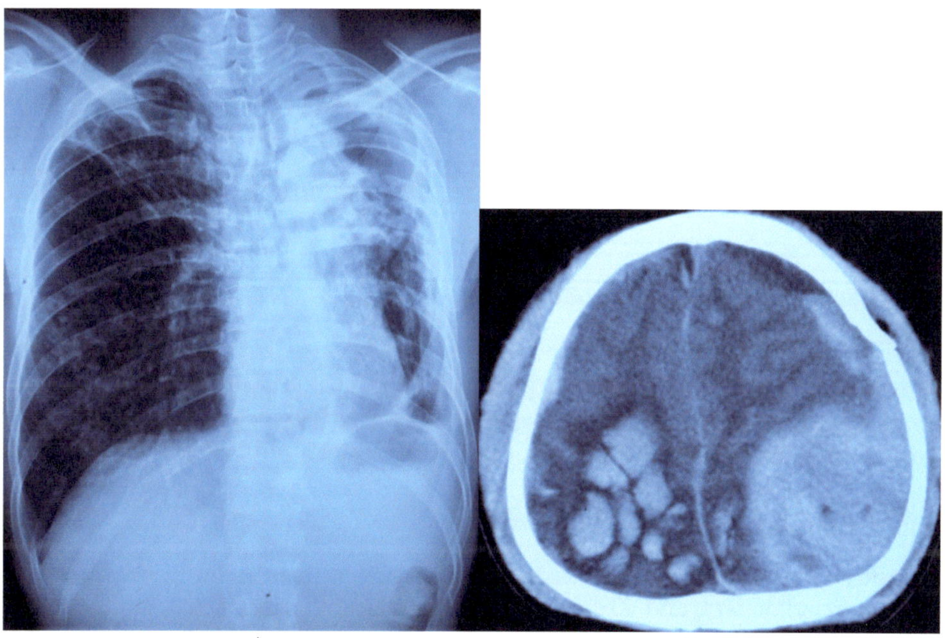

A B

Fig. 6. A: Chest roentgenogram from initial presentation of a 46-year-old Thai male with HIV-infection/AIDS who attended the tenth Zonal Tuberculosis and Chest Disease Centre, Chiang Mai, Thailand showing bilaterally diffuse reticulo-nodular infiltrates with left pleural effusion. His three consecutive sputum smears for AFB and cultures revealed positive results. B: Computed tomography of the brain from initial presentation of the same patient in Figure 6 A showing multiple tuberculous granulomas with various sizes throughout both parietal lobes.

3.4 Tuberculin skin test

The tuberculin skin test is now the standard technique to detect the latent TB infection. The sensitivity and specificity of the TST in immunocompromised persons with TB infection are very low. A study on latent TB infection during renal replacement therapy in India demonstrated that TST was insensitive and nonspecific to detect latent TB infection (Bhowmik et al., 2010). The TST in HIV-infected/AIDS patients is more likely to be negative due to the declines of the CD4+ T-cell count (Markowitz et al., 1993, as cited in Nachega & Maartens, 2009). More than 5 mm. induration on the Mantoux test in HIV-infected/AIDS patients is a positive result but this has been challenged by a previous study with sensitivity of 64.3% at a cutoff value of 10 mm. and of 71.2% at a cutoff value of 5 mm. and after adjustment for tuberculosis-specific anergy, the sensitivity was 67.6% and 74.5%, respectively (Cobelens et al., 2006, as cited in Nachega & Maartens, 2009). The sensitivity and specificity of TST for diagnosis of latent TB infection in patients on renal replacement therapy were only 20% and 9%, respectively, showed in a previous study (Agarwal et al., 2010). The only benefit and effectiveness of the positive-result TST is TB preventive therapy (Woldehanna & Volmink, 2004, as cited in Nachega & Maartens, 2009).

3.5 Tissue aspiration, excision and biopsy

Aspiration of lymph node with macroscopic tuberculous caseation demonstrates positive results 40.8% of cases (Bem et al., 1993, as cited in Nachega & Maartens, 2009, Pithie & Chicksen, 1992, as cited in Nachega & Maartens, 2009). Patients with negative-result aspiration should be performed needle-core biopsy or excisional biopsy. First needle-core biopsy made a definite diagnosis in 85% of cases (Wilson et al., 2005, as cited in Nachega & Maartens, 2009).

3.6 Mycobacterial molecular identification modalities

3.6.1 Amplicor Polymerase Chain Reaction (PCR)

A previous study in Kenya showed that the sensitivity and specificity of this technique were 93% and 94%, respectively and did not affected by the HIV status (Kivihya-Ndugga et al., 2004, as cited in Cheepsattayakorn & Cheepsattayakorn, 2006).

3.6.2 IS6110-PCR

The sensitivity of this technique was 100% in smear-positive, 81.8% in smear- negative, 66.7% in extrapulmonary, and 42.9% in blood specimens of HIV-infected/AIDS patients as demonstrated in a study (Schijman et al., 2004, as cited in Cheepsattayakorn & Cheepsattayakorn, 2006).

3.6.3 Nested PCR

This technique was studied in urine specimens of the HIV-infected/AIDS participants and revealed the sensitivity of 40.5% in smear-positive, 66.7% in smear-negative, and 57.1% in extrapulmonary cases. The overall specificity was 98.2%. This study results were different in the non-HIV-infected/AIDS and HIV-infected/AIDS patients (Torrea et al., 2005, as cited in Cheepsattayakorn & Cheepsattayakorn, 2006).

3.6.4 GeneXpert MTB/RIF test

This test is based on nucleic acid amplification and detection of an *Mycobacterium tuberculosis*-specific region of the *rpoB* gene, use real-time PCR with molecular beacons. It also detects mutation associated with rifampicin resistance. It is fully automated system which integrates sputum processing, deoxy-ribonucleic acid extraction, and amplification to diagnose TB. Its results are available within 90 minutes. It is minimized biosafety and contamination because of its closed system (Lockman, 2011). A clinical study conducted in Azerbaijan, India, Peru and South Africa showed the sensitivity of this test for only one sputum specimen examination was 92.2% for all positive-culture, 98.2% for positive AFB smear and positive culture, and 72.5% for negative AFB smear and positive culture cases with a specificity of 99.2%. When 3 specimens were tested the sensitivity was 97.6%, 99.8%, and 90.2% with a specificity of 98.1%, respectively (Boehme et al., 2010, as cited in Lockman, 2011). This test would increase case finding by 30% (replacing or adding to the conventional sputum AFB smear) and MDR case finding by 3-fold (replacing sputum culture and conventional drug-susceptibility testing) (Boehme et al., 2011, as cited in Lockman, 2011). The WHO stated in 2010 that this test should be used as the initial diagnostic test in persons suspected of being HIV/AIDS-associated TB or MDR-TB and it may be used as a follow-on test in smear-negative specimens where HIV/AIDS and/or MDR are of lesser concern (WHO, 2010, as cited in Lockman, 2011). Thailand will soon start using 4 GeneXpert MTB/RIF units in collaboration with the United States CDC.

4. Diagnosis of pulmonary tuberculosis (Sociedade Brasileira de Pneumologia e Tisiologia, 2004 & WHO, 2010)

The diagnosis of pulmonary TB is based on meeting one or more the following criteria: 3.1 detection by two positive sputum smear examinations 3.2 detection by one positive sputum smear examination and positive sputum culture 3.3 detection by one positive sputum smear examination and roentgenographic pictures consistent TB positive sputum culture or 3.4 clinical manifestations, epidemiological findings and roentgenographic pictures consistent TB, together with a favorable response to anti-TB drugs.

5. Antituberculous chemotherapy

There have been substantial studies from both prospective and retrospective demonstrated that standard 6-month rifampicin and isoniazid-contained regimens supplemented by pyrazinamide and ethambutol are effective for cure in treating HIV-seropositive patients with TB (Hopewell & Chaisson, 2000). The WHO recommends standard regimen (2HRZE/4HR, H=isoniazid, R=rifampicin, Z=pyrazinamide, E=ethambutol) for new TB patients with seropositive-HIV and all TB patients living in HIV-prevalent settings should receive daily antituberculous therapy at least during the intensive phase (Khan et al., 2010, as cited in WHO, 2010). Co-trimoxazole preventive therapy should be started as soon as possible and prescribed throughout antituberculous therapy (International Standards for

Tuberculosis Care (ISTC), 2009, as cited in WHO, 2010) which substantially reduces mortality among these patients (Harries et al., 2009, as cited in WHO, 2010 & WHO, 2006). The standard 6-month regimen is currently recommended for treating TB of any site, excepts of the central nervous system, which is recommended 2HRZE/7HR or 2HRZE/10HR (Nachega & Maartens, 2009). Recurrent rates of pulmonary TB among patients with and without HIV/AIDS have varied among various studies, mostly of 5% or less (Kassim et al., 1995, as cited in Nachega & Maartens, 2009, Chaisson et al., 1996, as cited in Nachega & Maartens, 2009, el-Sadr et al.,1998, as cited in Nachega & Maartens, 2009, Connolly et al.,1999, as cited in Nachega & Maartens, 2009 & Sterling et al., 1999, as cited in Nachega & Maartens, 2009). The recurrent rates of TB among HIV-infected/AIDS patients were associated with the duration of rifampicin-based regimens which rifampicin durations of 2-3, 5-6, and more than 7 months were associated with rates of 4, 2, and 1.4 cases per 100 person-years, respectively (Korenromp et al., 2003, as cited in Nachega & Maartens, 2009). WHO and the International Union Against Tuberculosis and Lung Disease (IUATLD) recommends a standardized 6-month rifampicin-based regimen with directly observed treatment for highly TB/HIV-endemic, low- income countries for at least the first 2 months for all positive-sputum smear cases (Korenromp et al., 2003, as cited in Nachega & Maartens, 2009). The IUATLD recommends an 8-month regimen (2HRZE/6HE) for negative-smear HIV-infected/AIDS cases but this regimen is related to high relapse rates (Korenromp et al., 2003, as cited in Nachega & Maartens, 2009). A study in Zaire among HIV-infected/AIDS-related TB patients demonstrated that additional 3 months in the continuation phase (2HRZE/7HR) of the standardized 6- month short-course regimen (2HRZE/4HR) resulted in 1% versus 8% of relapse rates, respectively but the survival rates were no different in patients given extended regimen (Perriens et al., 1995, as cited in Hopewell & Chaisson, 2000). Other studies revealed relapse rates of TB with various treatment regimens among HIV-infected/AIDS patients between 2%-7% (Kassim et al., 1995, as cited in Hopewell & Chaisson, 2000, Chaisson et al., 1996, as cited in Hopewell & Chaisson, 2000, el-Sadr et al., 1998, as cited in Hopewell & Chaisson, 2000). The United States CDC , the American Thoracic Society (ATS) and the Infectious Disease Society of America (IDSA) recommend the extension of the continuation phase from 6 to 9 months of the standardized 6-month rifampicin-based regimen for patients with positive cultures and cavitary TB, regardless of the HIV status (Chaisson & Nachega, 2010). Acquired- rifampicin resistance has been occurred among HIV-infected with advanced immune suppression treated with twice weekly rifampicin-based or rifabutin-based regimens (Chaisson & Nachega, 2010). The continuation phase of isoniazid plus rifapentine once weekly is contraindicated in HIV-infected/AIDS patients because of acquired resistance to rifamycins and unacceptably high rate of relapse (Chaisson & Nachega, 2010). Patients with CD4-T cell count < 100 cells/μL should receive daily or three-times weekly regimens (Chaisson & Nachega, 2010). WHO recommends the same regimens for extrapulmonary and pulmonary TB excepts longer treatment for TB of bone or joint and TB of meninges (WHO, 2010). Progress against TB is being made on several fronts. Several new drugs are being studied for TB therapy, including nitroimidazopyrans (e.g., PA-824), quinolone (moxifloxacin & gatifloxacin), oxazolidinones (e.g., PNU-100480, linezolid), macrolides (e.g., clarithromycin, azithromycin), ring-substituted imidazoles, and diamines (e.g., SQ109). Finally, new TB vaccines is being directed toward developing and should be ready for human testing within a few years.

6. Empirical antituberculous therapy

Empirical therapy will often initiated pending culture results in areas where mycobacterial culture is available, especially in areas of high proportion of sputum smear-negative cases and relatively rapid disease progression of HIV-related TB. Three consecutive-negative smear results, a compatible chest roentgenogram, and no response to a 2-week trial of antibiotics for pneumonitis is the common case definition for negative-smear pulmonary TB used in resource-poor settings (WHO, 2010, Figure 7). This case definition has been modified by WHO to include consideration of acutely-ill patients (especially with Pneumocystis pneumonia). If there has been a clinical response with negative-culture results, the empirical therapy should be continued. A previous study of case definitions in South Africa demonstrated high positive predictive value for a modified case definition of negative-smear pulmonary TB and case definitions of extrapulmonary TB and found that improvement of symptoms, Karnosky performance score, and serum C-reactive protein level were very sensitive to evaluation of the empirical therapy, excepted improvement of body weight and hemoglobin level (Wilson et al., 2006, as cited in Nachega & Maartens, 2009). The specificity of case definitions cannot be 100% so patients who have no response to empirical therapy within 2-8 weeks need to be investigated for alternative diagnoses discontinuation of their empirical therapy (Nachega & Maartens, 2009). In developing countries, the national TB control programs and the international agencies discourage the clinical trials of antituberculous therapy.

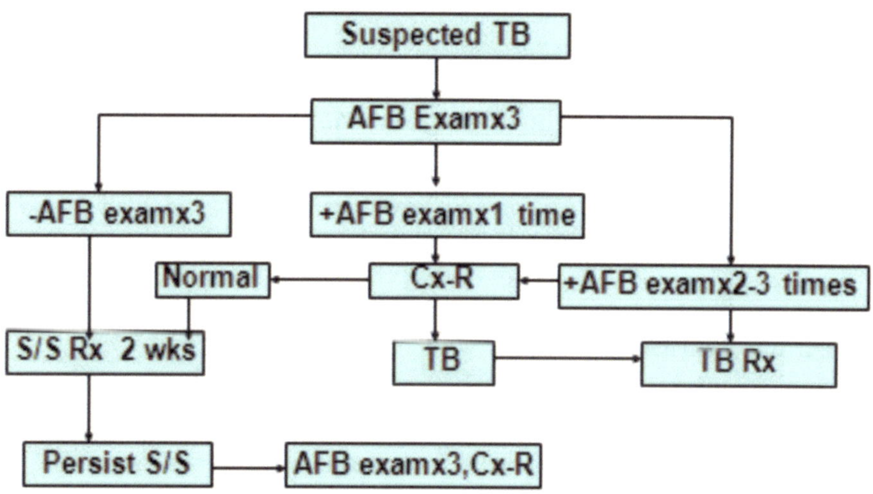

Fig. 7. TB case management (WHO, 2010)

7. Antiretroviral therapy

TB patients with advanced HIV disease/AIDS indicates antiretroviral therapy (ART) which improves survival (Harries et al., 2009, as cited in WHO, 2010), reduces TB disease rates by 60% at a population level, by up to 90% at personal level and reduces TB recurrence rates by 50% (Lawn & Churchyard, 2009, as cited in WHO, 2010 & Golub et al., 2008, as cited in WHO, 2010). Patients co-administered ART and antituberculous therapy may increase risk of adverse drug reactions, especially hepatitis (McIlleron et al., 2007, as cited in Nachega & Maartens, 2009). Around 25%-40% of these patients develop the so-called immune reconstitute inflammatory syndrome (IRIS) which paradoxically deteriorate TB disease (Lawn et al., 2005, as cited in Nachega & Maartens, 2009). Factors related to an increased risk of TB-IRIS include rapidly decreasing viral loads, lower CD4+ T-cell count and more shorter intervals between starting of antituberculous therapy and ART (Lawn et al., 2005, as cited in Nachega & Maartens, 2009). These worsening clinical manifestations should be excluded notably poor compliance to antituberculous therapy, systemic drug hypersensitivity reactions, MDR-TB, and new opportunistic infections. The most common manifestation of TB-IRIS is enlarging lymphadenopathy with caseous necrosis. The optimal timing of starting ART in relation to starting antituberculous therapy is unclear but TB treatment should always be initiated first, and waits at least until the patient is tolerating the antituberculous therapy before initiating ART as soon as possible and within the first 8 weeks of initiating antituberculous therapy (Nachega & Maartens, 2009 & WHO, 2010). All active-TB patients living with HIV should be initiated ART irrespective of CD4+ T-cell count (WHO, 2009, as cited in WHO, 2010). In 2010 Thailand's guidelines, starting ART when CD4 T-cell count is below 350 cells/µL. Patients who are already receiving an ART regimen, ART should be continued (Nachega & Maartens, 2009). WHO recommends the first-line ART regimens contain two nucleoside reverse transcriptase inhibitors (NRTIs-zidovudine (AZT) or tenofovir disproxil fumarate (TDF) plus lamivudine (3TC) or emtricitabine (FTC)) plus one non-nucleoside reverse transcriptase inhibitors (NNRTI-efavirenz (EFV) or nevirapine (NVP)) (WHO, 2010). In Thailand, the available regimens are stavudine plus lamivudine plus efavifenz or stavudine plus lamivudine plus nevirapine or stavudine plus lamivudine plus indinavir or ritonavir (Cheepsattayakorn & Cheepsattayakorn, 2009).

8. Adjunctive glucocorticoids in TB patients with HIV-infection/AIDS

There is lacking of evidence base for adjunctive glucocorticoids among these patients. There is likely to be a mortality benefit when used in HIV-infected/AIDS patients with tuberculous meningitis and pericarditis, but more larger studies are needed (Nachega & Maartens, 2009).

9. Adjuvant immunotherapy

A previous study demonstrated that immunization with killed *Mycobacterium vaccae* had ability to modify immune response to TB, but failed to showed clinical benefit in HIV-infected/AIDS patients (Mwinga et al., 2002, as cited in Nachega & Maartens, 2009).

10. Monitoring during antituberculous therapy

Sputum-smear examinations at the completion of the intensive phase of treatment course is a conditional, rather than a strong WHO recommendation (WHO, 2010). The evidence of a positive smear at this stage has a very poor ability to predict relapse or pretreatment isoniazid resistance (WHO, 2010). A positive-sputum smear at the end of the intensive phase among new patients should trigger sputum-smear examinations at the end of the third month and if it is positive, sputum culture and antituberculous-drug susceptibility testing should be done (WHO, 2010). There is no longer recommends to extend the intensive phase for patients have a positive-sputum smear at the end of the second month of treatment course (WHO, 2010).

11. Antituberculous therapy in non-HIV-infected immunocompromised patients

Regimens used in these patients are the same as used in HIV-infected/AIDS patients except regimens used in military TB, TB of bone or joint, and meninges which are more longer than 6 months, usually at least 8 months (WHO, 2010).

12. Treatment of latent TB infection

The IUATLD conducted a study in Eastern Europe and revealed that 3 months of isoniazid therapy reduced the TB incidence by 20%, 66% for 6 months, and 75% for 12 months (Chaisson & Nachega, 2010). This study also resulted in 92% reduction in TB risk for patients completing 12 months of isoniazid compared to 69% decrease for patients completing the standard-6 month regimen. A recent study in Alaskan populations revealed that the optimal duration of isoniazid therapy was 9 months therefore, the new ATS/CDC recommendation is 9 months of isoniazid as the preferred regimen, and the alternative regimen is 6 months (Chaisson & Nachega, 2010). A previous study in northern Thailand showed that 78% of HIV-infected/AIDS patients did not have TB disease at the end of 24 months after completion of 9 months of isoniazid therapy (Cheepsattayakorn, 1998, as cited in Cheepsattayakorn & Cheepsattayakorn, 2009).

13. Bacille Calmette-Gue'rin (BCG) vaccination

The protective benefit of BCG for active TB disease and death is about 50% (Chaisson & Nachega, 2010). It decrease hematogenous dissemination of primary TB infection and so reduces the incidence of military TB and childhood tuberculous meningitis (Chaisson & Nachega, 2010). BCG should not be given to immunocompromised individuals, including those with HIV-infection/AIDS, or to pregnant women (Hopewell, 2005).

14. Further research areas

It demonstrates that the WHO's DOTS strategy for case finding and effectively treating cases is not sufficient to eliminate TB, particularly in countries with HIV epidemics. Neither combination ART nor treatment of latent TB infection has a significant impact on community TB incidence. The most effective measures are reduced HIV incidence and improved TB case finding and treatment success rates. A better understanding of natural immunity to TB and its pathogenesis may contribute to the development of a new more effective vaccine. The genome sequencing of *Mycobacterium tuberculosis* promises to produce a new generation of TB control research.

15. References

Agarwal SK, Gupta S, Bhow D & Mahajan S. (2010). Tuberculin skin test for the diagnosis of latent tuberculosis during renal replacement therapy in an endemic area: a single center study. *Indian J Nephrol,* Vol. 20, No. 3, (July 2010), pp. 132-136, ISSN: 0971-4065.

Baboolal S, Ramoutar D & Akpaka PE. (2010). Comparison of the QuantiFERON®-TB assay and tuberculin skin test to detect latent tuberculosis infection among target groups in Trinidad & Tabago. *Rev Panam Salud Publica,* Vol. 28, No. 1, (July 2010), ISSN: 1020-4989, doi: 10.1590/S1020- 4982010000700006

Bacakoglu F, Basoglu OK, Cok G, Sayiner A & Ates M. (2001). Pulmonary tuberculosis in patients with diabetes mellitus. *Respiration,* Vol. 68, No. 6 , (November-December 2001), pp. 595-600, ISSN: 0993-9490.

Barnes PF, Bloch AB, Davidson PT & Snider DE Jr. (1991). Tuberculosis in patients with human immunodeficiency virus infection. *N Eng J Med,* Vol. 324, No. 23, (June 1991), pp. 1644- 1650, ISSN: 0028-4793.

Bem C, Patil PS, Elliot AM, Namaambo KM, Bharucha H & Porter JD. (2010). The value of wide-needle aspiration in diagnosis of tuberculous lymphadenitis in Africa. *AIDS,* Vol. 7, No. 9, (September 2010), pp. 1221-1225, ISSN: 0269-9370.

Bhowmik D, Agarwal SK, Gupta S & Mahajan S. (2010). Tuberculin skin test for diagnosis of latent tuberculosis during renal replacement therapy in an endemic area: a single center study. *Indian J Nephrol,* Vol. 20, No. 3, (October 2010), pp. 132-136, ISSN: 0971-4065.

Boehme CC, Nabeta P, Hillemann D, Nicol MP, Shenai S, Krapp F, Allen J, Tahirli R, Blakemore R, Rustomjee R, Milovic A, Jones M, O'Brien SM, Persing DH, Ruesch-Gerdes S, Gotuzzo E, Rodrigues C, Alland D & Perkins MD. (2010). Rapid molecular detection of tuberculosis and rifampicin resistance. *N Eng J Med,* Vol. 363, No. 11, (September 2010), pp. 1005-1015, ISSN: 0028- 4793.

Boehme CC, Nicol MP, Nabeta P, Michael JS, Gotuzzo E, Tahirli R, Gler MT, Blakemore R, Worodria W, Gray C, Huang L, Caceres T, Mehdiyey R, Raymond L, Whitelaw A, Sagadevan K, Alexander H, Albert H, Cobelens F, Cox H, Alland D & Perkins MD. (2011). Feasibility, diagnostic accuracy, and effectiveness of decentralized use of the xpert MTB/RIF test for diagnosis of tuberculosis and multidrug resistance: a multicentric implementation study. *Lancet,* Vol. 377, No. 9776, (April 2011), pp. 1495-1505, ISSN: 0099-5355.

Chaisson RE, Clermont HC, Holt E, Holt EA, Cantave M, Johnson MP, Atkinson J, David H, Boulos R, Quinn TC & Halsey NA. (1996). Six-month supervised intermittent tuberculosis therapy in Haitian patients with and without HIV infection. *Am J Respir Crit Care Med,* Vol. 154, No. 4 Pt 1 (October 1996), pp. 1034-1038, ISSN: 1073-449X.

Chaisson RE & Nachega JB. (2010). Tuberculosis. In: *Oxford textbook of Medicine.* Warrell DA, Cox TM, Firth JD & Ogg GS., pp. (810-831), Oxford University Press, 978-0-1992-0485-4, Oxford.

Cheepsattayakorn A. (1998). Isoniazid prophylactic therapy in HIV-infected individuals. *Thai Journal of Tuberculosis and Chest Diseases,* Vol. 19, No. 3, (July-September 1998), pp. 149-157, ISSN: 0125-5029.

Cheepsattayakorn A & Cheepsattayakorn R. (2006). Rapid diagnosis of pulmonary tuberculosis by polymerase chain reaction and other advanced molecular diagnostic technologies in comparison to conventional bacteriological methods. *Thai Journal of Tuberculosis Chest Diseases and Critical Care,* Vol. 27, No. 3, (July-September 2006), pp. 191- 216, ISSN: 0125-5029.

Cheepsattayakorn A & Cheepsattayakorn R. (2009). The outcome of tuberculosis control in special high-risk populations in northern Thailand: an observational study. *Journal of Health Systems Research*, Vol. 3, No. 4, (October-December 2009), pp. 558-566, ISSN: 0858-9437.

Cobelens FG, Egwaga SM, van Ginkel T, Muwinge H, Matee MI & Borgdorff MW. (2006). Tuberculin skin testing in patients with HIV infection: limited benefit of reduced cutoff values. *Clin Infect Dis*, Vol. 43, No. 5, (September 2006), pp. 634-639, ISSN: 1058-4838.

Connolly C, Reid A, Davies G, Sturm W, McAdam KP & Wilkinson D. (1999). Relapse and mortality among HIV-infected and uninfected patients with tuberculosis successfully treated with twice weekly directly observed therapy in rural South Africa. *AIDS*, Vol. 13, No. 12, (August 1999), pp. 1543-1547, ISSN: 0269-9370.

Converse PJ, Jones SL, Astemborski J, Vlahov D & Graham NM. (1997). Comparison of a Tuberculin-interferon-gamma assay with the tuberculin skin test in high-risk adults: effect of human immunodeficiency virus infection. *J Infect Dis*, Vol. 176, No. 1, (July 1997), pp. 144- 150, ISSN: 0022-1899.

el-Sadr WM, Perlman DC, Matts JP, Nelson ET, Cohn DL, Salomon N, Olibrice M, Medard F, Chirgwin KD, Mildvan D, Jones BE, Telzak EE, Klein O, Heifets L & Hafner R. (1998). Evaluation of an intensive intermittent-induction regimen and duration of short-course treatment for human immunodeficiency virus-related pulmonary tuberculosis. Terry Beirn Community Programs for Clinical Research on AIDS (CPCRA) and AIDS Clinical Trials Group (ACTG). *Clin Infect Dis*, Vol. 26, No. 5, (May 1998), pp. 1148-1158, ISSN: 1058-4838.

Food and Drug Administration. (2010). QuantiFERON-TB-P010033. June 16, 2010, Available from: http://www.fda.gov/MedicalDevices/ProductandMedicalProcedures/DeviceApprovals- ApprovedDevices/ucmo84025.htm

Food and Drug Administration. (2010). QuantiFERON-TB Gold-P010033/S006. June 16, 2010, Available from: http://www.fda.gov/MedicalDevices/ProductandMedicalProcedures/DeviceApprovals- ApprovedDevices/ucmo84025.htm

Garcia-Rodriguez JF, Alvarez-Diaz H, Lorenzo-Garcia MV, Marino-Callejo A, Ferna'ndez-Rial A & Sesma-Sa'nchez P. (2011). Extrapulmonary tuberculosis: epidemiology and risk factors. *Enferm Infecc Microbiol Clin*, (May 2011), ISSN: 0213-005X, [Epub ahead of print].

Goldhaber-Fiebert JD, Jeon CY, Cohen T & Murray MB. (2011). Diabetes mellitus and tuberculosis in countries with high tuberculosis burdens: individual risk and social determinants. *Int J Epidemiol*, Vol. 40, No. 2, (April 2011), pp. 417-428, ISSN: 0300-5771.

Golub JE, Astemborski J, Ahmed M, Cronin W, Mehta SH, Kirk GD, Vlahov D & Chaisson RE. (2008). Long-term effectiveness of diagnosing and treating latent tuberculosis infection in a cohort of HIV-infected and at risk injection drug users. *J Acquir Immune Defic Syndr*, Vol. 49, No. 5, (December 2008), pp. 532-537, ISSN: 1525-4135.

Gonzalez-Curiel I, Castaneda-Delgado J, Lopez-Lopez N, Araujo Z, Hernandez-Pando R, Gandara- Jasso B, Macias-Segura N, Enciso-Moreno A & Rivas-Santiago B. (2011). Differential expression of antimicrobial peptides in active and latent tuberculosis and its relationship with diabetes mellitus. *Hum Immunol*, Vol. 72, No. 8, (August 2011), pp. 656-662, ISSN: 0198-8859.

Gupta S, Shenoy VP, Mukhopadhyay C, Bairy I & Muralidharan S. (2011). Role of risk factors and socio-economic status in pulmonary tuberculosis: a search for the root cause in patients in a tertiary care hospital, South India. *Trop Med Int Health*, Vol. 16, No. 1, (January 2011), pp. 74-78, ISSN: 1360-2276.

Harries AD, Zachariah R, Lawn SD. (2009). Providing HIV care for co-infected tuberculosis patients: a perspective from sub-Saharan Africa. *Int J Tuberc Lung Dis*, Vol. 13, No. 1, (January 2009), pp. 6-16, ISSN: 1027-3719.

Havlir DV & Barnes PF. (1999). Tuberculosis in patients with human immunodeficiency virus infection. *N Eng J Med,* Vol. 340, (February 1999), pp. 367-373, ISSN: 0028-4793.

Hopewell PC. (2005). Tuberculosis and other mycobacterial diseases. In: *Murray and Nadel's textbook of respiratory medicine*, Mason RJ, Murray JF, Broaddus VC & Nadel JA, pp. 979-1043, Elsevier Saunders, Inc, ISSN: 0-7216-0327-0, Philadelphia.

Hopewell PC & Chaisson RE. (2000). Tuberculosis and human immunodeficiency virus infection. In: *Tuberculosis: a comprehensive international approach*, Reichman LB & Hershfield ES, pp. 525-552, Marcel Dekker, Inc, ISSN: 0-8247-8121-X, New York.

Huang CC, Liu MF, Lee NY, Chang CM, Lee HC, Wu CJ & Ko WC. (2010). Fatal tuberculous myositis in a immunocompromised adult with primary Sjögren's syndrome. *J Formos Med Assoc*, Vol. 109, No. 9, (September 2010), pp. 680-683, ISSN: 0929-6646.

International Standards for Tuberculosis Care (ISTC). (2009). *The Hague, Tuberculosis Coalition for Technical Assistance (2nd ed)*, World Health Organization, Geneva.

Ito I, Tada K, Ootera H, Sakurai T & Iwasaki H. (2011). Analysis of usefulness of a whole blood interferon-gamma assay (QuantiFERON TB-2G) for diagnosing active tuberculosis in immunocompromised patients. *Kekkaku*, Vol. 86, No. 2, (February 2011), pp. 45-50, ISSN: 0022-9776.

Jiang JR, Yen SY & Wang JY. (2011). Increased prevalence of primary drug-resistant pulmonary tuberculosis in immunocompromised patients. *Respirology*, Vol. 16, No. 2, (February 2011), pp. 308-313, ISSN: 1323-7799.

Kassim S, Sassan-Morokro M, Ackah A, Abouya LY, Digbeu H, Yesso G, Coulibaly IM, Coulibaly D, Whitaker PJ & Doorly R. (1995). Two year follow-up of persons with HIV-1-associated and HIV-2-associated pulmonary tuberculosis treated with short-course chemotherapy in West Africa. *AIDS*, Vol. 9, No. 10, (October 1995), pp. 1185-1191, ISSN: 0269-9370.

Khan FA, Minion J, Pai M, Royce S, Burman W, Harries AD & Menzies D. (2010). Treatment of active tuberculosis in HIV co-infected patients: a systematic review and meta-analysis. *Clin Infect Dis*, Vol. 50, No. 9, (May 2010), pp. 1288-1299, ISSN: 1058-4838.

Kivihya-Ndugga L, van Cleeff M, Juma E, Kimwomi J, Githui W, Oskam L, Schuitema A, van Soolinger D, Nganga L, Kibuga D, Odhiambo J & Klatser P. (2004). Comparison of PCR with the routine procedure for diagnosis of tuberculosis in a population with high prevalence of tuberculosis and human immunodeficiency virus. *J Clin Microbiol*, Vol. 42, No. 3, (March 2004), pp. 1012-1015, ISSN: 0095-1137.

Komiya K, Ariga H, Nagai H, Teramoto S, Kurashima A, Shoji S & Nakajima Y. (2010). Impact of peripheral lymphocyte count on the sensitivity of 2 interferon-gamma release assays, QFT- G and ELISPOT, in patients with pulmonary tuberculosis. *Intern Med*, Vol. 49, No. 17, (September 2010), pp. 1849-1855, ISSN: 0918-2918, doi: 10.2169/internalmedicine.49.3659

Korenromp EL, Scano F, Williams BG, Dye C & Nunn P. (2003). Effects of human immunodeficiency virus infection on recurrence of tuberculosis after rifampicin-based treatment: an analytical review. *Clin Infect Dis*, Vol. 37, No. 1, (July 2003), pp. 101-112, ISSN: 1058- 4838.

Lawn SD, Bekker L-G & Miller RF. (2005). Immune reconstitution disease associated with Mycobacterial infections in HIV-infected individuals receiving antiretrovirals. *Lancet Infect Dis*, Vol. 5, No. 6, (June 2005), pp. 361-373, ISSN: 1473-3099.

Lawn SD & Churchyard G. (2009). Epidemiology of HIV-associated tuberculosis. *Curr Opin HIV AIDS*, Vol. 4, No. 4, (July 2009), pp. 325-333, ISSN: 1746-630X.

Li SY, Chen TJ, Chung KW, Tsai LW, Yang WC, Chen JY & Chen TW. (2011). Mycobacterium tuberculosis infection of end-stage renal disease patients in Taiwan: a national longitudinal study. *Clin Microbiol Infect*, (January 2011), 1469-0691, Jan 24. doi: 10.1111/j.1469- 0691.2011.03473.x [Epub ahead of print].

Lockman S. (June 6, 2011). A new era: molecular tuberculosis diagnosis. Title, In: *Search Medscape News*, June 29, 2011, Available from: http://www.medscape.com/viewarticle/745030?src=nl_topic

Long R, Scalcini M, ManfredaJ, Carre' G, Philippe E, Hershfield E, Sekla L & Stackiw W. (1991). Impact of human immunodeficiency virus type 1 on tuberculosis in rural Haiti. *Am Rev Respir Dis*, Vol. 143, No. 1, (January 1991), pp. 69-73, ISSN: 1073-449X.

Lyu J, Lee SG, Hwang S, Lee SO, Cho OH, Chae EJ, Lee SD, Kim WS, Kim DS & Shim TS. (2011). Chest CT is more likely to show latent tuberculosis foci than simple chest radiography in liver transplantation candidates. *Liver Transpl*, Vol. 17, No. 8, (August 2011), pp. 963-968, ISSN: 1527- 6465, doi: 10.1002/lt.22319

Markowitz N, Hansen NI, Wilcosky TC, Hopewell PC, Glassroth J, Kvale PA, Mangura BT, Osmond D, Wallace JM, Rosen MJ & Reichman LB. (1993). Tuberculin and anergy testing in HIV-seropositive and HIV-seronegative persons. Pulmonary Complications of HIV Infection Study Group. *Ann Intern Med*, Vol. 119, No. 3, (August 1993), pp. 185-193, ISSN: 0003-4819.

Mazulek GH, Jereb J, LoBue P, Iademarco MF, Metchock B & Vernon A. (2005). Guidelines for using the QuantiFERON-TB Gold test for detecting Mycobacterium tuberculosis infection, United States. *MMWR*, Vol. 54, No. RR15, (December 2005), pp. 49-55, ISSN: 1057-5987.

Mazulek GH, Jereb J, Vernon A, LoBue P, Goldberg S & Castro K. (2010). Updated guidelines for using interferon-gamma release assays to detect Mycobacterium tuberculosis infection--- United States, 2010. *MMWR*, Vol. 59, No. RR05, (June 2010), pp. 1-25, ISSN: 1057-5987.

Mazurek GH & Villarino ME. (2003). Guidelines for using the QuantiFERON-TB test for diagnosing latent Mycobacterium tuberculosis infection. *MMWR*, Vol. 52, No. RR02, (January 2003), pp. 15-18, ISSN: 1057-5987.

McIlleron H, Meintjes G, Burman WJ & Maartens G. (2007). Complications of antiretroviral therapy in patients with tuberculosis-drug interactions, toxicity and immune reconstitute inflammatory syndrome. *J Infect* Dis, Vol. 196 (Suppl 1), (August 2007), pp. S63-75, ISSN: 0022- 1899.

Moreira J, Fochesatto JB, Moreira AL, Pereira M, Porto N & Hochhegger B. (2011). Tuberculous pneumonia: a study of 59 microbiologically confirmed cases. *J Bras Pneumol*, Vol. 37, No. 2, (April 2011), pp. 232-237, ISSN: 1806-3713.

Mwinga A, Nunn A, Ngwira B, Chintu C, Warndorff D, Fine P, Darbyshire J & Zumla AI; LUSKAR collaboration. (2002). Mycobacterium vaccae (SRL 172) immunotherapy as an adjunct to Standard antituberculosis treatment in HIV-infected adults with pulmonary tuberculosis: a randomized placebo-controlled trials. *Lancet*, Vol. 360, No. 9339, (October 2002), pp. 1050-1055, ISSN: 0099-5355.

Nachega JB & Maartens G. (2009). Clinical aspects of tuberculosis in HIV-infected adults, In: *Tuberculosis: a comprehensive clinical reference*, Schaaf HS & Zumla AI, pp. 524-531, Suanders Elsevier, ISSN: 978-1-4160-3988-4, London.

Patel AK, Rami KC & Ghanchi FD. (2011). Radiological presentation of patients of pulmonary tuberculosis with diabetes mellitus. *Lung India*, Vol. 28, No. 1, (January-March 2011), pp. 70, ISSN: 0970-2113.

Perez-Guzman C, Torres-Cruz A, Villarreal-Velarde H & Vargas MH. (2000). Progressive age- related changes in pulmonary tuberculosis images and the effect of diabetes. *Am J Respir Crit Care Med*, Vol. 162, No. 5, (November 2000), pp. 1738-1740, ISSN: 1073-449X.

Perlman DC, el-Sadr W, Nelson ET, Matts JP, Telzak EE, Salomon N, Chirgwin K & Hafner R. (1997). Variation of radiographic patterns in pulmonary tuberculosis by degree of human immunodeficiency virus-related immunosuppression. The Terry Beirn Community Programs for Clinical Research on AIDS (CPCRA). The AIDS Clinical Trials Group (ACTG). *Clin Infect Dis*, Vol. 25, No. 2, (August 1997), pp. 242-246, ISSN: 1058-4838.

Perriens JH, St. Louis ME, Mukadi YB, Brown C, Prignot J, Pouthier F, Portaels F, Willame JC, Mandala JK, Kaboto M, Ryder RW, Roscigno G & Piot P. (1995). Pulmonary tuberculosis in HIV-infected patients in Zaire: a controlled trial of treatment for either 6 or 12 months. *N Eng J Med*, Vol. 332, No. 12, (March 1995), pp. 779-784, ISSN: 0028-4793.

Pithie AD & Chicksen B. (1992). Fine-needle extrathoracic lymph-node aspiration in HIV-associated sputum-negative tuberculosis. *Lancet*, Vol. 340, No. 8834-8835, (n.d. 1992), pp. 1504- 1505, ISSN: 0099-5355.

Post FA, Wood R & Pillay GP. (1995). Pulmonary tuberculosis in HIV infection: radiographic appearance is related to CD4+ T-lymphocyte count. *Tuber Lung Dis*, Vol. 76, No. 6, (December 1995), pp. 518-521, ISSN: 0962-8479.

Prabu VNN & Agrawal S. (2010). Systemic lupus erythematosus and tuberculosis: a review of complex interactions of complicated diseases. *J Postgrad Med*, Vol. 56, No. 3, (August 2010), pp. 244-250, ISSN: 0022-3859, doi: 10.4103/0022-3859.68653

Rangaka MX, Wilkinson KA, Seldon R, Van Cutsem G, Meintjes GA, Morroni C, Mouton P, Diwakar L, Connell TG, Maartens G & Wilkinson RJ. (2007). Effect of HIV-1 infection on T cell based and skin test detection of tuberculosis infection. *Am J Respir Crit Care Med*, Vol. 175, No. 5, (March 2007), pp. 514-520, ISSN: 1073-449X.

Restrepo BI, Camerlin AJ, Rahbar MH, Wang W, Restrepo MA, Zarate I, Mora-Guzma'n F, Crespo-Solis JG, Briggs J, McCormick JB & Fisher-Hoch SP. (2011). Cross-sectional assessment reveals high diabetes prevalence among newly-diagnosed tuberculosis cases. *Bull World Health Organ*, Vol. 89, No. 5, (May 2011), pp. 352-359, ISSN: 0042-9686.

Rothel JS, Jones SL, Corner LA, Cox JC & Wood PR. (1990). A sandwich enzyme immunoassay for bovine interferon-gamma and its use for detection of tuberculosis in cattle. *Aust Vet J*, Vol. 67, No. 4, (April 1990), pp. 134-137, ISSN: 0005-0423.

Sauzullo I, Mengoni F, Scrivo R, Valesini G, Potenza C, Skroza N, Marocco R, Lichtner M, Vullo V & Mastroianni CM. (2010). Evaluation of QuantiFERON-TB Gold In-Tube in human immunodeficiency virus infection and in patients candidates for anti-tumor necrosis factor- alpha treatment. *Int J Tuberc Lung Dis*, Vol. 14, No. 7, (July 2010), pp. 834-840, ISSN: 1027-3719.

Schijman AG, Losso MH, Montoto M, Saez CB, Smayevsky J & Benetucci JA. (2004). Prospective evaluation of in-house polymerase chain reaction for diagnosis of mycobacterial diseases in patients with HIV infection and lung infiltrates. *Int J Tuberc Lung Dis*, Vol. 8, No. 1, (January 2004), pp. 106-113, ISSN: 1027-3719.

Sen T, Joshi SR & Udwadia ZF. (2009). Tuberculosis and diabetes mellitus: Merging epidemics. *J Assoc Physicians India*, Vol. 57, (May 2009), pp. 399-404, 0004-5772.

Silva DR, Menegotto DM, Schulz LF, Gazzana MB & Dalcin PdeTR. (2010). Clinical characteristics and evolution of non-HIV-infected immunicompromised patients with an in- hospital diagnosis of tuberculosis. *J Bras Pneumol*, Vol. 36, No. 4, (August 2010), pp. 475-484, ISSN: 1806-3713.

Sociedade Brasileira de Pneumologia e Tisiologia. (2004). 11 Consenso Brasileiro de Tuberculose-Diretrizes Brasileiras para Tuberculose. *J Bras Pneumol*, Vol. 30 (Puppl 1), (n.d. 2004), pp. S4-S56, ISSN: 1806-3713.

Sonnelberg P, Murray J, Glynn JR, Shearer S, Kambashi B & Godfrey-Faussett P. (2001). HIV-1 and recurrence, relapse, and reinfection of tuberculosis after cure: a cohort study in South African mineworkers. *Lancet*, Vol. 358, No. 9294, (November 2001), pp. 1687-1693, ISSN: 0099-5355.

Sterling TR, Alwood K, Gachuhi R, Coggin W, Blazes D, Bishai WR & Chaisson RE. (1999). Relapse rates after short-course (6-month) treatment of tuberculosis in HIV-infected and uninfected persons. *AIDS*, Vol. 13, No. 14, (October 1999), pp. 1899-1904, ISSN: 0269-9370.

Streeton JA, Desem N & Jones SL. (1998). Sensitivity and specificity of a gamma-interferon blood test for tuberculosis infection. *Int J Tuberc Lung Dis*, Vol. 2, No. 6, (June 1998), pp. 443-450, ISSN: 1027-3719.

Tan CK, Lai CC, Chen HW, Liao CH, Chou CH, Huang YT, Yang WS, Yu CJ & Hsueh PR. (2010). Enzyme-Linked immunospot assay for interferon-gamma to support the diagnosis of tuberculosis in diabetic patients. *Scand J Infect Dis*, Vol. 42, No. 10, (October 2010), pp. 752- 756, ISSN: 0036-5548.

Tenth Zonal Tuberculosis and Chest Disease Centre, Tenth Office of Disease Prevention and Control, Chiang Mai, Thailand. (2005). *Tuberculosis annual report*, Tenth Zonal Tuberculosis and Chest Disease Centre, Tenth Office of Disease Prevention and Control, Chiang Mai, Thailand.

Tenth Zonal Tuberculosis and Chest Disease Centre, Tenth Office of Disease Prevention and Control, Chiang Mai, Thailand. (2006). *Tuberculosis annual report*, Tenth Zonal Tuberculosis and Chest Disease Centre, Tenth Office of Disease Prevention and Control, Chiang Mai, Thailand.

Tenth Zonal Tuberculosis and Chest Disease Centre, Tenth Office of Disease Prevention and Control, Chiang Mai, Thailand. (2007). *Tuberculosis annual report*, Tenth Zonal Tuberculosis and Chest Disease Centre, Tenth Office of Disease Prevention and Control, Chiang Mai, Thailand.

Tenth Zonal Tuberculosis and Chest Disease Centre, Tenth Office of Disease Prevention and Control, Chiang Mai, Thailand. (2009). *Tuberculosis annual report*, Tenth Zonal Tuberculosis and Chest Disease Centre, Tenth Office of Disease Prevention and Control, Chiang Mai, Thailand. Toure' NO, Dia Kane Y, Diatta A, Ba Diop S, Niang A, Ndiaye EM, Thiam K, Mbaye FB, Badiane M & Hane AA. (2010). Tuberculosis in elderly persons. *Rev Mal Respir*, Vol. 27, No. 9, (November 2010), pp. 1062-1068, ISSN: 0761-8425.

Torrea G, Van de Perre P, Ouedraogo M, Zougba A, Sawadogo A, Dingtoumda B, Diallo B, Defer MC, Sombie' I, Zanetti S & Sechi LA. (2005). PCR-based detection of the Mycobacterium tuberculosis complex in urine of HIV-infected and uninfected pulmonary and extrapulmonary tuberculosis patients in Burkina Faso. *J Med Microbiol*, Vol. 54, No. Pt 1, (January 2005), pp. 39-44, ISSN: 0022-2615.

Vargas PJ, King G & Navarra SV. (2009). Central nervous system infections in Filipino patients with systemic lupus erythematosus. *Int J Rheum Dis*, Vol. 12, No. 3, (September 2009), pp. 234-238, ISSN: 1756-1841.

Walsh MC, Camerlin AJ, Miles R, Pino P, Martinez P, Mora-Guzma'n F, Crespo-Solis JG, Fisher- Hoch SP, McCormick JB & Restrepo BI. (2011). The sensitivity of interferon-gamma release assays is not compromised in tuberculosis patients with diabetes. *Int J Tuberc Lung Dis*, Vol. 15, No. 2, (February 2011), pp. 179-184, ISSN: 1027-3719.

Wells CD. (2010). Global impact of multidrug-resistant pulmonary tuberculosis among HIV-infected and other immunocompromised hosts: epidemiology, diagnosis, and strategies for management. *Curr Infect Dis Rep*, Vol. 12, No. 3, (May 2010), pp. 192-197, ISSN: 1523-3847.

Wendel KA & Sterling TR. (2002). Tuberculosis and HIV. *AIDS Clin Care*, Vol. 14, No. 2, (February 2002), pp. 9-15, ISSN: 1043-1543.

Wilson D, Nachega J, Chaisson R & Maartens G. (2005). Diagnostic yield of peripheral lymph node needle-core biopsies in HIV-infected adults with suspected smear-negative tuberculosis. *Int J Tuberc Lung Dis*, Vol. 9, No. 2, (February 2005), pp. 220-222, ISSN: 1027-3719.

Wilson D, Nachega J, Morroni C, Chaisson RE & Maartens G. (2006). Diagnosing smear-negative tuberculosis using case definitions and treatment response in HIV-infected adults. *Int J Tuberc Lung Dis*, Vol. 10, No. 1, (January 2006), pp. 31-38, ISSN: 1027-3719.

Woldehanna S & Volmink J. (2004). Treatment of latent tuberculosis infection in HIV infected persons. *Cochrane Database Syst Rev*, No. 1, (n.d. 2004): CD000171, ISSN: 1469-493X.

World Health Organization. (2010). *Global tuberculosis control: WHO report 2010*, World Health Organization, ISSN: 978 92 4 156406 9, Geneva.

World Health Organization. (2006). *Guidelines on co-trimoxazole prophylaxis for HIV-related infections among children, adolescents and adults in resource-limited settings: recommendations for a public health* approach, ISSN: 97892 4 159470 7, Geneva.

World Health Organization. (2009). Key recommendations, In : *Rapid advice for antiretroviral therapy for HIV infection in adults and adolescents*, June 6, 2011, Available from: http://www.who.int/hiv/pub/arv/rapid_advice_art.pdf

World Health Organization. (2010). About WHO expert group and STAG-TB recommendations, In: *Roadmap for rolling out Xpert MTB/RIF for rapid diagnosis of tuberculosis and MDR-TB*, June 6, 2011, Available from: http://www.who.int/tb/laboratory/roadmap_xpert_mtb-rif.pdf

World Health Organization. (2010). *Treatment of tuberculosis: guidelines* (4th ed), World Health Organization, ISSN: 978 92 4 154783 3, Geneva.

Young F, Wotton CJ, Critchley JA, Unwin NC & Goldacre MJ. (2010). Increased risk of tuberculosis disease in people with diabetes mellitus: record-linkage study in a UK population. *J Epidemiol Community Health*, (November 2010), ISSN: 0143-005X, Nov 24. [Epub ahead of print].

Yu YH, Liao CC, Hsu WH, Chen HJ, Liao WC, Muo CH, Sung FC & Chen CY. (2011). Increased lung cancer risk among patients with pulmonary tuberculosis: a population cohort study. *J Thorac Oncol*, Vol. 6, No. 1, (January 2011), pp. 32-37, ISSN: 1556-0864.

10

Mycobacterium tuberculosis: Biorisk, Biosafety and Biocontainment

Wellman Ribón
Universidad Industrial de Santander, Bucaramanga
Colombia

1. Introduction

1.1 Biorisk, biosafety and biocontainment: A life or death process

Safety at workplaces, occupational diseases, pandemics, international travel, public transportation, day care centers, nursing homes, and jails, among others, are situations we are frequently involved in and whose impact and risks we are not aware of but could change the course of our lives. When we travel abroad on business or vacation usually our expectations are high, but we have no information on the process undertaken to secure passengers health, as well as community and environmental safety. When we share a closed space such as an airplane, we should be aware of some diseases, especially air borne diseases, to be able to assess exposure risk and minimize it by adopting biosafety measures (individual, collective or both), and have the proper infrastructure to contain or isolate such risk.

Based on this multifactor approach, scientists and experts on *Mycobacterium tuberculosis* biology, on chemical agents, personal protective equipment (PPE), industrial air purifiers, building design, laboratory equipment and different transportation means join their efforts to harmonize the life of communities around the planet.

Every community should make an effort to acquire a culture aimed at preserving their physical integrity and environmental quality because this process is not restricted to expert laboratories. Anti-pandemic plans presently emphasize that communities are the main pillar to contain these devastating events and such a perspective must transcend the usual scenarios such as hospitals, laboratories, universities, public transportation, supermarkets, movie theaters, etc.

The debate today is heated, and there is an extensive and sometimes emphatic documentation. Many of the aspects involved are described separately, but we must remember that they should be integrated so as to avoid implementing isolated components that may have been successful elsewhere but are not reproducible in our own settings. The present chapter is no exception: we collected the minimum information required to develop the safety data sheet and start the risk assessment; we describe the basic, most general biosafety measures adopted internationally, and we offer a guide on essential biocontainment measures (some of which are described in the section dedicated to biosafety). Such a structure responds solely to academic purposes, but we have to remember that in reality they are inclusive, inseparable processes aimed at the same results. They are the starting point to strengthen the process in any institution, and, therefore, risk assessment should be done together with experts from different disciplines and based on updated knowledge, as well as on the identification of protection elements that may be included in the process and adapted to specific infrastructures and resources. This is the only way to develop a practical and reliable process. Besides, contingency plans should be designed to respond to unexpected catastrophic events such as bioterrorist attacks (Wheelis 2002) and natural disasters.

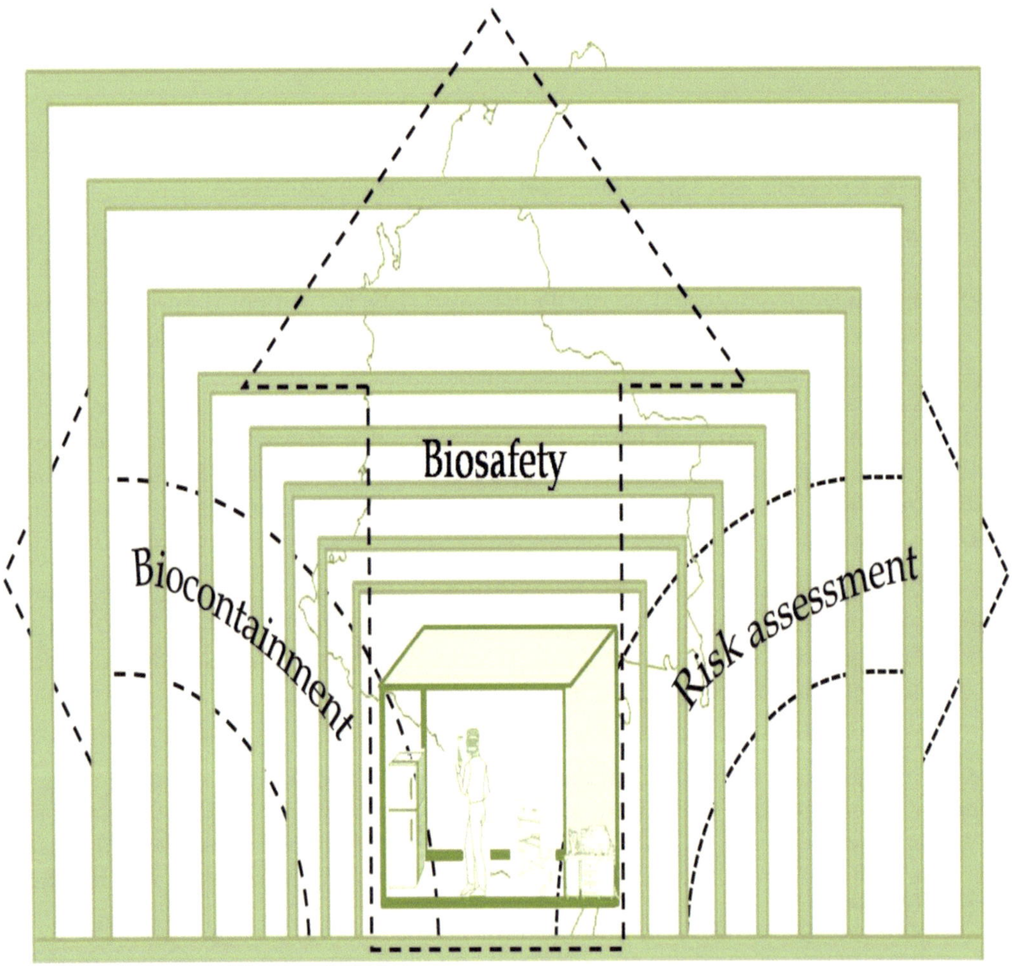

Fig. 1. Calculating risk levels and negative and positive impact according to the safety procedures.

Finally, as this is a complex and dynamic process, you should determine a specific, known and daily situation and then identify exposure risks, the PPE presently in use and consider and assess if you can contain the risk and prevent it from having greater magnitude. Figure 1 will help you in calculating risk levels and negative and positive impact according to your present procedures. Remember human fragility and the fact that probably many of the elements mentioned are no at your disposal, but you can resort to those available in your day-to-day scenario. Human beings are not disposable or reusable, but they are biodegradable or incinerable depending on the circumstances, and that is why the process described in this chapter must be seen as conducive to a better quality of life or to death.

2. Biorisk

The following is a description of various characteristics of the microorganism which are useful in understanding biorisk, biosafety, and biocontainment. *M. tuberculosis* is a pathogen that has been extensively studied; the majority of information required for risk-evaluation of each procedure or work situation can be easily consulted in publications of such renowned international organizations as: The World Health Organization (WHO); The Centers for Disease Control and Prevention (CDC); the National Institutes of Health (NIH); Sandia National Laboratories; American Biological Safety Association (ABSA); Asociación Mexica de Bioseguridad (AMEXBIO), and in the domestic regulations of each country. The updated versions of this information can be accessed through the systematic review of professional scientific publications. Each institutional biosafety committee is responsible for implementing, and ensuring compliance with, the relevant guidelines and regulations. The *M. tuberculosis* safety data sheet should be prepared in each laboratory, posted in a conspicuous location, and accessible to all personnel who work in the area. Staff should be diligent in the risk assessment of their tasks and procedures, request the required PPE, and comply with containment measures in order to guarantee their safety and that of their colleagues and the environment.

2.1 Safety date sheet

2.1.1 Identification of the microorganism, (Riley 1961, Kunz 1982, Wayne 1984 and Grange 1990)

Agent name: *Mycobacterium tuberculosis*

Taxonomy

Domain: Bacteria

Phylum: Actinobacteria

Class: Actinomycetes

Order: Actinomycetales

Family: Mycobacteriaceae

Genus: *Mycobacterium*

Specie: *tuberculosis*

2.1.2 Biological characteristics

Condition: bacteria aerobic

Grow: slow-growing

Motility: non-motile

Spore: non-endospore forming* (aspect in discussion by Ghosh 2009 and Traag 2010)

Acid-Fast Bacillus (AFB)

Allergenic: no

Cancerous: no

Abortive: no

Toxins forming: no

Immunosupressor: no

Capable of mutating in the host: yes

Recommended pictogram:

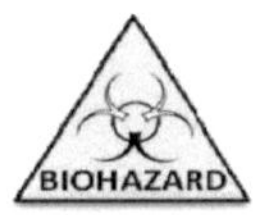

2.1.3 Mode of transmission

Usually airborne human to human (inhalation of infectious aerosols or infected droplets) or dermal inoculation and possible ingestion, it is not transmitted through sexual contact, and there has been no documentation of vertical transmission. (Wells 1955 and Verhagen 2011)

Disease:

Tuberculosis (TB) (second leading cause of death worldwide)

Latent TB infection

Multidrug resistant TB (MDR TB)

Extensively drug resistant TB (XDR TB)

Host:

Humans, nonhuman primates, and commonly used laboratory animals: pigs, cats, dogs, sheep, cattle, rodents and seals. Some domestic animals, in contact with people suffering from TB, are able to develop TB and become themselves a source of infection. (Grange 1990, National Research Council. 1997 and 2003, Hankenson 2003, Krauss 2003, and Cousins 2003)

Infectious dose for humans: is very low (ID_{50} 1-10 bacilli by inhalation route), a sputum of an infected patient can contain several millions of bacilli per milliliter.(Riley, 1957 and 1961 and CDC 1999)

Communicability: high, human to human with symptoms.

Incubation period: long (years), may progress to pulmonary or disseminated disease.

Vectors: none

Zoonosis: by inhalation or direct contact with infected animal or tissues from infected animal.

Survival on inanimate surfaces at different relative humidities: *M. tuberculosis* can survive for several days on inanimate surfaces; 70 days on carpet, 45 days on clothing, 105 days on paper, 90 to 120 days on dust, 6 to 8 months in sputum in a cool and dark room, 45 days in manure, and 49 days in guinea pig tissue.(Kunz 1982, and Rubin 1991)

Geographical localization: worldwide

2.1.4 Detection

Latent TB infection has been traditionally identified by the tuberculin skin test (TST, Mantoux or PPD); currently the new generation of test entails interferon gamma (IFN-γ) release assays (IGRAs: Quantiferon and T-SPOT.TB).

Diagnosis of TB: acid fast stain of sputum samples, culture, phenotypic and genotypic identification of *M. tuberculosis*, DNA fingerprinting (Rozo 2010) and drug susceptibility testing and tissue exams.

Possibility of viewing the bacillus in clinical specimens: yes, through examination of clinical sample for acid-fast bacilli (AFB), fluorescence microscopy and light-emitting diode (LED)

Growth in culture media: yes, frequently in Lowenstein-Jensen (LJ), Ogawa Kudoh (OK) or liquid culture as modified Middlebrook 7H9 broth, the *M. tuberculosis* is of slow growth, between 4 to 8 weeks, from clinical samples. (Welch 1993)

Rapid identification of *M. tuberculosis*: through the employment of methods such as nucleic acid hybridization methods, lateral flow assays, line probe assays, and DNA sequencing.

2.1.5 Epidemiology

Risk population: it is relatively more prevalent in immigrants, minorities, the elderly, persons with acquired immunodeficiency syndrome (AIDS) and among healthcare workers, and laboratory personnel who are occupationally exposed.

Mortality and morbidity: mortality for TB, depending on the country, MDR TB 50% to 70% of the patients not treated within a period of two years. Mortality is higher in patients with TB/AIDS. The morbidity in TB is high.

Perception of malicious use: low

2.1.6 Surveys of laboratory-acquired infection and prophylaxis

Laboratory personnel should undergo an annual PPD or IGRAs, and workers with a positive test should be evaluated for active TB; in accidental exposure the laboratory personnel should be tested 3 to 6 months after the event and should be offered prophylaxis if is required in TB, but the referenced isoniazid (INH) prophylaxis is not applicable in MDR TB.

Vaccine: Bacille Calmette Guerin (BCG), attenuate live vaccine, with limited protection. (Lietman 1999)

Treatment: therapy with multiple drugs

First line: INH, rifampin (RIF), pyrazinamide (PZA), ethambutol (EMB), streptomycin (SM).

Second line: Amikacin, capreomycin, ciprofloxacin, ethionamide, kanamycin, levofloxicin. Ofloxacin and *para*-aminosalicylic acid for MDR TB and XDR TB.

2.1.7 Prevention and control

Exposure control-personal protection: PPE such as respiratory protection (fit-tested respirators with N-95 rating) (Occupational Safety and Health Administration -OSHA- 2003 and 2004), hand protection, eye protection, skin and body protection, and hygiene measures.

Containment:

Objective: to prevent aerosol exposure or dermal inoculation.

Biosafety level (BSL) 2 can be used for low-risk procedures, such as making smear and diagnosis activities including primary culture of clinical specimens potentially infected by bacilli of *M. tuberculosis* s with PPE. (Welch 1993)(American Thoracic Society 1993)

BSL-3 can be used for high-risk procedures, such as handling solid and liquid positive culture, secondary cultures for diagnostic or research activities, DNA or RNA extraction (only in the initial stages of the procedure)(Castro 2009, Warren 2006, and NIH 2002), biochemical test, centrifugations, pipetting, mechanical homogenizing, sonication, heating or boiling, work with bacteriological loops, preparation and manipulation of frozen sections, animal studies, infected clinical specimens and others with PPE. (CDC. 1999 and 2006, and Hankenson 2003)

2.1.8 Disinfection, inactivation and sterilization of *M. tuberculosis*

Efficient disinfectants are:

0.4-5 phenol during 10 minutes

5% formaldehyde during at least 10 minutes

1-2% Glutaraldehyde during 30 minutes

0.2-5% Sodium hypochlorite for one minute

70-96% Ethyl alcohol during 2 minutes

3-10% Hydrogen peroxide during 5 minutes

2-10%, 75ppm Iodophore

Mix of iodine + iodophores or ethyl alcohol

Mix of paraformaldehyde + glutaraldehyde or formalin

Susceptible to moist heat sterilization at 121°C for 15 minutes at 121 pounds of pressure in autoclave.

Note: quaternary ammoniums inhibit tubercle bacilli but do not kill them. Please check the efficacy of each disinfectant in your own laboratory conditions.

Ultraviolet dosage required: 10.000 μW-s/cm^2 at 254 nanometer for 99.9% destruction of bacillus.

2.1.9 Transport information

WHO classification of infective microorganisms by risk groups (RG):

RG 3 (high individual risk, low community risk): a pathogen that usually causes serious human or animal disease but does not ordinarily spread from one infected individual to another. Effective treatment and preventive measures are available (WHO 2004).

Cultures positives for *M. tuberculosis* require packing measures, and labeled as "Infectious substance". The triple packaging should be utilized according to the International Air Transport Association (IATA) and Dangerous Goods regulation and WHO recommendations. *M. tuberculosis* (cultures only) is included in Category A, UN 2814 (Infectious Substances, affecting humans) see table 1. (IATA 2006)

Infections substance	**Class**	**Division**	**Category**	**Proper shipping name**	**UN Number**	**Packing instruction (PI)**
M. tuberculosis cultures only	6	6.2	A	Infections substance	2814	602

Table 1. General information of *M. tuberculosis* for international shipping.

2.1.10 Biosafety functions officer

Mistakes and accidents, which result in over-exposure to infectious materials, should be immediately reported and corrective measures should be taken to avoid a repetition of the event.

Mandatory: personnel concerned with mycobacteria activity should be experienced and under the supervision of the head of the laboratory.

2.2 Epidemiology of hospital and laboratory acquired TB

The epidemiology is defined as the study of the distribution and determinants of diseases and injuries in human populations. Inherent in the definition of epidemiology is the necessity of measuring the amount of disease in a population by relating the number of cases to a population base. One of the unfortunate consequences of working with infectious materials is the potential for acquiring an infection. The laboratory acquired infections (LAI) due to a wide variety of viruses, bacteria, parasites and fungi have been described. In the absence of precise data on LAIs, epidemiological methods provide the necessary tools to evaluate the extent and nature of personnel exposures. Although the precise risk of infection after an exposure remains poorly defined, surveys of LAIs suggested that *Brucella* species, *Shigella* species, *Salmonella* species, *M. tuberculosis* and *Neisseria meningitidis* are the most common causes. Early surveys of laboratory acquired TB found an incidence of TB among laboratory personnel 3-9 times greater than that in the general population (Harrintong 1976 and Reid 1957). The *M. tuberculosis*, the causative organism of TB, has distinction of repeatedly being ranked within the top five most commonly LAI (Pike 1976, 1978, and 1979). The OSHA in 1996, 1997, 2003 and 2004, promulgated withdrawal of the 1997 proposed standard on occupational exposure to TB. Along with the withdrawal of the 1997 standard, the respirator-specific standard, 29 CFR 1910.139, was also withdraw. The effect of withdrawing these standards is the application of the general industry respiratory protection standard, 29 CFR 1910.134, for all occupations, to those workplaces that provide respiratory protection from TB.

According to WHO, TB remains the second leading cause of death worldwide, killing 2 million people each year. In many developed countries, TB is considered a disease of the past. However, the impact of this disease can be devastating even today specially in poor countries. An estimated 9.4 million new cases of TB globally, with most cases occurring in resource limited or resource poor countries. In addition to that, much of deadliness of TB epidemic has to do with the virulent synergy between Human Immunodeficiency Virus (HIV) and TB. Recently, MDR-TB and XDR TB have had devastating effects on populations of HIV infected individuals in developing countries.

2.3 Risk assessment

Risk assessment was defined by Boa (Boa 2000), as "the use of factual information to define the health effects of exposure to individuals or populations to hazardous materials and situations"

The CDC and the NIH provided the basic definition for risk in their *Biosafety in Microbiological and Biomedical Laboratories*: -"Risk" implies the probability that harm, injury, or disease will occur. In the environment of the research, microbiological, teaching, and biomedical laboratories, the assessment of risk focuses first and foremost on the prevention of laboratory associated infections and the likelihood that the agent can be used as a weapon and the consequences of bioattack with the agent. The risk assessment helps to assign the BSL, PPE required, laboratory and facilities design, equipment that can be used, procedures and practices that can be implemented and that reduce, to a minimum, the personnel and the environmental risk of exposure to an agent. The risk evaluation should be made by the person with the best knowledge of the microorganism (*M. tuberculosis*) and the available containment measures. The risk assessment can be quantitative in the presence of known hazards or qualitative when the data will be incomplete or unknown.

The CDC and NIH recommend that the laboratory director or principal investigator, in close collaboration with the institutional biosafety committee, be responsible for assessing risk in order to set the BSL for the work.

The risk assessments should be conducted periodically and the analysis should include: new variables; updated information and procedures related to *M. tuberculosis*; management of the TB; MDR TB or XDR TB, and new international regulations applicable to the malicious use of the bacillus or bacillus-infected substances.

The CDC and NIH include the following important factors in a risk assessment:

1. The pathogenicity of the infectious or suspected infectious agent, in this case *M. tuberculosis*, including disease incidence and severity (morbidity and mortality). **Remark**: The more severe the potentially acquired disease, the higher the risk. With respect to *M. tuberculosis*, one has to consider the types of resistance (TB, MDR TB, and XDR TB).
2. The route of transmission (parenteral, airborne or ingestion). **Remark:** The greater the aerosol potential, the higher the risk (for *M. tuberculosis* the mode of transmission **is** usually airborne).
3. Agent stability: aerosol infectivity and the agent´s ability to survive over time in the environment. Factors such as desiccation, exposure to sunlight or ultraviolet light, or exposure to chemical disinfectants must be considered.
4. The infectious dose of *M. tuberculosis*.
5. The concentration (number of infectious organisms per unit volume).
6. The origin of the potentially infectious materials.
7. The availability of data from animal studies, in the absence of human data.
8. The established availability of an effective prophylaxis or therapeutic interventions.
9. Medical surveillance.
10. Evaluation of the experience and skill level of at-risk personnel.

Sandia National Laboratories International Biological Threat Reduction department worked with biosafety, infectious disease, and risk experts to develop a systematic and standardized methodology for biological safety risk assessments. This standardized methodology will enhance biosafety risk assessments by allowing them to be both repeatable and quantifiable. This methodology is not intended as an all-hazards assessment, but is focused on the risks associated with biological materials being handled in a laboratory setting. Sandia National Laboratories defined criteria related to:

- Agent factors which impact the biosafety risk to humans,
- Agent factors which impact the biosafety risk to animals,
- Procedures used for the activity being assessed, procedures and processes involving animals used for the procedure being assessed.

A "scoring system" was developed for each criterion, with zero defined as the absence of the element defined by the criterion and four defined as the highest possible value for the element (for some elements the highest possible value is the worst case and for others the highest possible value is the best case). For example:

Is this agent known to cause infection via inhalation in humans (to cause infection via droplets or droplet nuclei that have entered the upper or lower respiratory tract) in a laboratory setting?

4=Preferred route

2= A possible route

1=Unknown

0=Not a route

Taking the via inhalation in humans scenario for an agent which cannot cause infection via inhalation the score will be zero; for an agent which via inhalation as *M. tuberculosis* is the preferred route of infection the score will be four.

The biosafety risk assessment model has been coded into a software package which runs on Microsoft'sc .Net Framework. The software, titled "BioRAMSoftware.exe" (Version 1.0 dated September 2010), was planned to be released open source and discussions have started to freely license the software to organizations. The BioRAMSoftware allows visitors to provide the scores for all the criteria in a simple tool by answering a set of questions. The BioRAMSoftware calculates the risk scores using the algorithms and weights defined in the model and methodology. The BioRAMSoftware also allows visitors to modify the wording of questions and the definitions of the scoring scales to better reflect a unique laboratory situation or language differences. The software then produces a numeric and graphical document with the relative risk rankings for the visitors and a chart identifying the impact each question had on the final results. This feature is useful in understanding and communicating the risks, as well as providing guidance on risk management or mitigation efforts. Also, visitors can view and, if needed, modify the weights. The methodology outlined is consistent with internationally accepted risk assessment schemes and also parallels international biosafety risk assessment guidance.

Biosafety RAM includes generalized definitions of how to conduct a biosafety risk assessment:

Evaluate the biological agents that exist at the facility.

Evaluate the facility processes and procedures.

Evaluate the existing biorisk mitigation measures.

You can establish the procedures and concrete situations based upon your institution's particular environment, geographical conditions, and risk assessment. The BioRAMSoftw is available on: http://www.sandia.gov/

The selection should include all situations and procedures that represent a risk for employees, the community, the natural environment, and animals. Biosafety and biocontainment measures should then be implemented based upon each institution's particular situation. A risk assessment should be initiated that defines the specific problem. The method of risk assessment should be simple; easy to apply and interpret; and should permit a quantitative classification of risk on a scale ranging from very low, low, moderate, high, and very high risk.

A risk assessment should include the characteristics of *M. tuberculosis* that are described in the safety data sheet. The intrinsic properties and the laboratory techniques that are likely to generate infectious aerosols should be evaluated based upon each particular situation. For example, in a research laboratory one should establish the difference between the characteristics of bacteria's under study; the H37Ra (ATCC 25177) used in some experiments is classified as a RG 2 pathogen, while the H37Rv (ATCC 2618) strain is designated as RG 3 pathogen. The information collected in the risk assessment may confirm changes in the pathogenicity of the specific microorganism and, therefore, the risk assessment may be altered enough to require an increase in the BSL and PPE for its containment. For example, bacteria which have developed resistance to multiple therapeutic drugs, such as *M. tuberculosis* MDR or XDR are considered to be a higher risk due to the lack of treatment alternatives and are to be handled with more stringent precautions. This bacteria is RG 3, but the extra precautions required for safe work with *M. tuberculosis* MDR would not be expected to take it to a higher containment level than BSL 3.

The laboratory diagnosis of TB should determine the percentage of positivity of pathogenic mycobacteria of clinical specimens submitted for the *M. tuberculosis* test; reported studies estimate that only 1% is positive; however, this data will obviously vary according to region and the number of samples that each laboratory processes. Additionally, the following factors are of crucial relevance in the risk assessment:

- *M. tuberculosis* can be isolated from virtually any type of human or animal specimens.
- The infectious dose in humans is very low and some samples processed in a diagnostic laboratory, such as the sputum of an infected patient, can contain several millions of bacilli per milliliter.
- The infection predominantly occurs by inhalation of airborne bacilli and the manipulation of liquid clinical specimens that likely involves generation of infectious aerosols, although percutaneous injury or infection by secondary transmission through the use of contaminated PPE or laboratory surfaces may also result in infection (Miller 1987, and Muller 1988).

Studies of air transmission of TB conducted during the first half of the last century by Wells (Wells 1955), led to the framing of the concept of the "droplet nucleus." The great majority of laboratory technicians generate droplets of liquid or aerosols and each droplet may contain one or more bacillus. The aerosols that are produced can be classified according their size:

Droplet nuclei: with a size ranging from 1 to 10 μm in diameter and a velocity of propagation of 0.2 to 18 cm/minute or 0.1 to 1 μm in diameter and a velocity of propagation of 0.005 to 0.2 cm/minute.

Dust: with a size ranging from 10 to 100 μm in diameter and a velocity of propagation of 18 to 1800 cm/minute.

Droplet: with a size ranging from 100 to 400 μm in diameter and a velocity of propagation of 1800 to 15200 cm/minute. These particles containing *M. tuberculosis* can remain airborne from minutes to hours.

Larger droplets would not dry and could rapidly contaminate laboratory equipment and surfaces, and fingers or gloves, resulting in a secondary contamination of mouth and nasal cavities. The droplets settle very slowly and dry, and they are transformed into droplet nuclei. These droplet nuclei float in the air of a room and are spread by very small air currents; when inhaled they can settle in alveolar spaces and infect the employee.

Remark: among the laboratory techniques used for the identification and characterization of *M. tuberculosis,* the following ones are likely to increase the risk of contamination or to generate infectious aerosols producing droplet nuclei, such as: centrifugations, pipetting, mechanical homogenizing, sonication, heating, boiling, work with bacteriological loops, preparation and manipulation of frozen sections, handling of containers with clinical specimens, acid-fast staining, manipulation of solid and liquid cultures, flow cytometry, and animal studies.

The risk assessment should also be conducted in hospitals, healthcare units, respiratory isolation areas, ambulatory assistance spaces, and for the TB or non- TB patients transiting through the institution.

3. Biosafety

Biosafety currently involves a large, interdisciplinary group of professionals gathered with the unique objective of guaranteeing that the risk of contracting infection for employees of the institution, and animals, is reduced to a minimum, and that the environment is protected. Currently, however, many of the decisions implemented to reduce biorisk, and contain infectious agents, are also employed by the community-at-large as part of anti-pandemic programs. These activities are dynamic and are strengthened by recent scientific and industrial advances. Changes in the biological characteristics of microorganisms, and the pace of modern life, have generated host-parasite relations that facilitate the transmission of illnesses that are devastating for humanity. Thanks to the groups engaged in interdisciplinary, scientific work, many of these unusual relationships have been disclosed. General and basic recommendations, of a compulsory nature, to ensure biosecurity in the manipulation and containment of *M. tuberculosis*, are discussed below.

WHO classifies microorganisms within four RGs according to infectious characteristics, availability of treatment, preventive measures, and the possibility of containing dissemination (WHO 2004):

RG 1: no or low individual and community risk

RG 2: moderate individual risk, low community risk

RG 3: high individual risk, low community risk

RG 4: high individual and community risk

Current classifications, similar to those created by WHO, have been developed by other institutions, such as: Standars Australia/New Zealand 2002, Canadian Laboratory Biosafety Guidelines (Laboratory Centre for Disease Control 1996), European Economic Community Directive (Comission of the European Communities 2000), NIH Recombinant DNA guidelines, and CDC/NIH guidelines (NIH 2002).

M. tuberculosis is located within these classifications as a microorganism RG3; therefore, its management requires the implementation of PPE consistent with its biological characteristics; a level of security in facilities and laboratory equipment that will minimize the risk of infection and maximize the capability of containment; and measures focused on preventing the intentional, malicious use of this microorganism by the institution's staff or outside parties.

The WHO's *Laboratory Biosafety Manual*, 3rd ed., 2004, which addresses the general principles of biosecurity, establishes the recommended BSLs for the management of microorganisms according to their RG, offers examples of laboratory practices that should be frequently conducted, and the requisite safety equipment. The BSL designations are based on a combination of the containment facilities; design features, equipment, construction, practices and operational procedures required for working with agents belonging to the various RGs. The laboratory facilities are designated as:

- BSL 1 – basic laboratory: for microorganisms in RG 1; an example of a facility would be a basic teaching laboratory; requirements include a good microbiological technique, open bench work, and an autoclave for sterilization of material. The use of PPE is recommended in all procedures; however, safety equipment such as a biological safety cabinet (BSC) is not required.
- BSL 2 - basic laboratory: for microorganisms in RG 2; examples of laboratories are primary health services, primary level hospitals, diagnostic, teaching and public health. Require an implementation of good microbiological technique plus PPE in all procedures; biohazard signs, open benches or ventilation (inward air flow or mechanical via building system) plus BSC for the potential aerosols and autoclave. Various procedures related to the identification of *M. tuberculosis* through clinical samples are conducted at this BSL; therefore, specific PPE measures are obligatory in order to minimize the risk of infection. The following are some accepted procedures for the identification of *M. tuberculosis* through clinical samples:
- Making smear microscopy and diagnostic activities including primary culture of clinical specimens potentially infected by bacilli of *M. tuberculosis.* (Welch 1993)
- Extraction of DNA, RNA, proteins, cell compounds, and molecular methodologies, following the inactivation, death, and lysis of the microorganism; and, having previously determined that the experimental protocol for the extraction and separation of the bacterial components is completely secure in the particular laboratory conditions in which it is conducted (Burgos 2004, Castro 2009 and Warren 2006).
- BSL 3 – laboratory with containment conditions for microorganisms in RG3; examples of laboratories are special diagnostic, production facilities, national tuberculosis reference laboratory and research laboratories; all of the conditions that apply for BSL 2 are included, plus specific PPE, controlled access with double-door entry, isolation laboratory, room sealable for decontamination, directional air flow, ventilation (inward air flow, mechanical via building system and filtered air exhaust), safety equipment as BSC class II or III and autoclave, preferably double –ended. Positive, viable samples of *M. tuberculosis, M. tuberculosis* MDR, and *M. tuberculosis* XDR should be handled at this BSL (Sessler 1983), including the following activities:
- Handling solid and liquid positive culture
- Secondary cultures for diagnostic or research activities
- DNA or RNA extraction (initial step of each protocol)
- Biochemical test for *M. tuberculosis* identification
- Bacterial suspension preparation
- Detection drugs resistance
- Centrifugations
- Pipetting
- Mechanical homogenizing

- Sonication, heating or boiling
- Work with bacteriological loops
- Preparation and manipulation of frozen sections (biopsies)
- Animal studies
- Infected clinical specimens and others

BSL 4 - laboratory with maximum containment: for microorganisms in RG 4; this is the maximum containment-BSL and includes all of the requirements of BSL 3 plus airlock entry, airlock with shower, effluent treatment, BSC class III, shower exit, and special waste disposal.

Remark: although some of the precautions may appear to be unnecessary for some organisms, and no clinical or hospital laboratory has complete control over the specimens it receives, the staff may occasionally and unexpectedly be exposed to organisms in higher RGs; therefore, each employee is responsible for his/her own safety; this implies the obligatory and continuous use of PPE, and biosecurity and biocontainment measures, equipment and facilities while in areas of biological risk.

General considerations to guarantee biosecurity in each of the established levels are provided in the recommendations issued by WHO, CDC, NIH (American Thoracic Society 1983, Kent 1985, and CDC 1999 WHO 2004). Compliance with these measures should be part of a culture of biosecurity and professional responsibility. We consider it important to stress some of the following, specific measures for the handling of potentially contaminated material, or material infected with *M. tuberculosis*, in accordance with the requisite level of biosecurity:

BSL 2:

- The international biohazard sign should be displayed on the doors of rooms where the clinical specimens for the search of *M. tuberculosis* are being processed.
- The laboratory personnel have specific training in handling agents such as *M. tuberculosis* and are directed by a competent scientist.
- Access to the laboratory is limited when work is being conducted.
- Extreme precautions are taken with contaminated sharp items.
- The procedure in which infectious aerosols or splashes may be created are conducted in CBS (remember that the risk of aerosols possibly infected with *M. tuberculosis* in a clinical sample such as sputum, or a biopsy, vary according to the number of cases in a region and the number of samples processed by a laboratory; therefore, procedures including making smear microscopy should be conducted in a color booth with biological containment and specific filters for the retention of chemical vapors emitted during the coloration process) and additionally, films and smears for microscopy should be handled with forceps, stored appropriately, and sterilized before disposal.
- Persons wash their hands after they handle viable materials, after removing gloves, and before leaving the laboratory.
- Eating, drinking, smoking, handling contact lenses, and applying cosmetics are not permitted in the work areas.
- All procedures are performed carefully to minimize the creation of splashes or aerosols.

- The work surfaces are decontaminated on completion of work or at the end of the day and after any spill or splash of viable material with disinfectants that are effective against *M. tuberculosis*.
- The wastes are decontaminated before disposal by an approved decontamination against *M. tuberculosis*.
- An insect and rodent control program is in effect.

Recommendations for special procedures:

- Access to the laboratory is restricted by the laboratory director when the work with *M. tuberculosis* includes possibly infectious substances. **Remark:** persons who are at increased risk of acquiring infection, or for whom infection may have serious consequences, are not permitted in the laboratory. Every person, upon initiating employment, should have a medical exam and laboratory tests in order to confirm that he/she is not at risk. Each institution should establish requirements to guarantee that all staff members are clinically suited for this type of work; this process should be conducted in coordination with occupational health professionals, health insurers, and experts in risk assessment and biosafety. In some countries, such as Colombia, vaccination with BCG is indicated; in those nations that have imposed this requirement, the employer should request the appropriate certificate to document the vaccination.
- A degree of precaution must always be taken with any contaminated sharp items, including needles and syringes, slides, pipettes, capillary tubes and scalpels. These items should be used only when absolutely necessary and should be discarded in appropriate containers for subsequent decontamination, thereby preventing the formation of aerosols.
- Spills and accidents that result in over-exposure to substances possibly infected with *M. tuberculosis* are immediately reported to the chief. Medical evaluation and surveillance, and prophylaxis or treatment, should be provided based upon the severity of the accident and estimated risk of the procedure that was being conducted. Each institution should implement protocols for biorisk containment in order to maintain biosecurity; all personnel (housekeeping, professional, administrative, students, and others authorized to enter work areas) should be familiar with these policies. All laboratory areas should include a containment kit that facilitates the rapid implementation of corrective measures following an accident, including an appropriate disinfectant for laboratory surfaces and equipment, PPE, absorbent paper, tweezers for removal of glass particles, and signs to restrict access to the area where the accident occurred. The accident response should conclude with an analysis of causes and implementation of corrective measures.

BSL 3:

All general guidelines governing standard microbiological practices are applicable, in addition to the measures included in BSLs 1 and 2.

- The two person rule should apply, whereby no individual ever works alone in the laboratory.
- All procedures involving the *M. tuberculosis* manipulation are conducted within BSC.

- The laboratory has special engineering design features; however, in the case of those laboratories that do not possess all of these features, good ventilation, illumination, and disinfection of surfaces should be employed in order to guarantee good biosafety. Access to the laboratory is restricted, utilize standard microbiological practices. The decision to implement this modification of BSL 3 recommendations should be made only by the laboratory director.
- The laboratory doors are kept closed when experiments are in progress.
- The laboratory personnel receive the appropriate immunizations with BCG Vaccine or test for the infection surveillance with *M. tuberculosis,* TST or IGRAs.
- The biosafety manual specific to the laboratory is prepared or adopted by the laboratory director and biosafety precautions are incorporated into standard operating procedures.
- The laboratory and support personnel receive specific training about the potential hazards associated with *M. tuberculosis*.
- The laboratory director is responsible for ensuring that before working with *M. tuberculosis*, all workers demonstrate proficiency in standard microbiological practices and experience in handling *M. tuberculosis*.

The CDC and NIH, besides providing orientation about standard microbiological practices and special practices for each BSL, also describe the safety equipment or primary barriers and the laboratory facilities or secondary barriers (CDC 2000). In the following section we reproduce some of these recommendations and include information pertaining to the handling of *M. tuberculosis*:

Safety equipment or primary barriers for BSL 2

- All procedures should be conducted in BSC class II; the selection of BSC should be based upon the actual conditions of each laboratory as reflected in the risk assessment; all BSC's should include at least one HEPA (high efficiency particulated air) filter with at least 99.97% efficiency in retaining particles of 0.3 micrometers, protecting both the operator and the environment; various types may also provide greater protection for the product.

BSC class II type A1:

- Re-circulates 70% and removes 30% to the interior of the laboratory
- Minimum inflow 75 fpm
- Gas jets, volatile toxic chemicals, and radionucleotides cannot be used
- Includes a front aperture and guillotine-type window

BSC class II type A2:

- Re-circulates 70% and removes 30% to the interior of the laboratory
- Minimum inflow 100 fpm
- Gas jets, volatile toxic chemicals, and radionucleotides cannot be used
- Includes a front aperture and guillotine-type window
- Installation of a tube can allow 30% of the air to be ventilated to the exterior of the lab; traces of radionucleotides and small quantities of volatile, toxic liquids can be used

The two types of BSC class II can be used in BSLs 1, 2, and 3 (National Sanitation Foundation International -NSF- 2002).

- The centrifugation of specimens should be done in closed containers, i.e., centrifuge safety cups; these containers are opened only in BSC class II.
- Protective elements such as goggles, mask, and face shield, should be used in order to prevent splashes or sprays of material possibly contaminated with *M. tuberculosis* or other infectious substances. These measures should be used continuously while working, preferably when BSC protection is not available.
- Clothing appropriate for the laboratory should be used, such as impermeable uniforms, gowns that close at the back, caps, shoe protectors, and other items that the institution may consider to be necessary. Laboratory clothing should be used only in the laboratory and is not permitted in other areas such as cafeterias, bathrooms, libraries, on public transportation, offices, etc.

Remark: "all protective clothing is either disposed of in the laboratory or laundered by the institution; it should never be taken home by personnel."

- When working with contaminated material, on contaminated surfaces or equipment, it is recommended that two pairs of gloves be used. Every laboratory should establish a protocol for the disinfection of gloves and hand washing upon completing work.

The laboratory facilities or secondary barriers for BSL 2:

- Laboratory installations should be isolated from public areas, when possible
- Hand-washing and eyewash should be available
- Laboratory facilities, furniture and chairs, should be easy to clean and disinfect; avoid the use of carpets and rugs.
- The laboratory should not be accessible to unauthorized persons.

Safety equipment or primary barriers for BSL 3

- All PPE specific for the manipulation of *M. tuberculosis* should be used, including: caps, shoe protectors, impermeable clothing, and gowns that close in the back. These elements should be disinfected prior to leaving BSL 3 for the laundry or to be discarded.
- Frequent change of gloves and hand washing is recommended. Disposable gloves are not reused. Respiratory and face protection are used when handling or monitoring infected animals.
- In the case of *M. tuberculosis*, infected material is handled in BSC class II; the possibility of using BSC class II type B should be considered based upon the characteristics and risk assessment of each laboratory.

BSC class II type B1:

Re-circulates 40% and removes 60% to the exterior of the laboratory
Minimum inflow 100 fpm
Permits traces of radionucleotides and small quantities of volatile, toxic chemicals; the use of gas burners is not recommended.

BSC class II type B2:

Re-circulates 0% and removes 100% to the exterior of the laboratory

Minimum inflow 100 fpm

Recommended for the handling of radionucleotides and volatile, toxic chemicals; the use of gas burners is not recommended.

Remark: each laboratory should develop its own protocols for the use and disinfection of BSC, according to the instructions of the manufacturer, frequency of use, and risk assessment. The decision to use a BSC class III should be based upon the risk assessment of each laboratory.

Some PPE serve an important function, especially given the current, particular situation concerning *M. tuberculosis*. The short-term prospects of obtaining a vaccine or new, alternative methods of treatment are remote, and the evolving strain of *M. tuberculosis* that is resistant to various, contemporary therapies dictate effective methods of personal protection. Presently, individual respiratory protection is the most recommended measure, and not only for laboratory staff; these devices should also be used by hospital personnel (physicians, nurses, respiratory therapists, and administrative personnel who attend patients, among others); additionally, it is necessary to remark upon the differences between respirators and surgical masks (American National Standard Institute 1992, CDC 1994). The surgical masks provide protection against pathogens present in droplets emitted by coughing; protection is limited to the nose and mouth as the mask does not completely cover the face; therefore, masks do not provide protection against infection contained in droplet nuclei. These masks are now recommended for use by TB patients as they move throughout the hospital or when they are within confined spaces. Respirators, on the other hand, are designed to provide protection against pathogenic microorganisms contained in droplet nuclei; these can include respirators for the retention of particulates or the purification of air. Respirators that purify air function with batteries that power a ventilator providing filtered air to the user; this protective item can be disinfected, allows the change of HEPA filters, and guarantees a level of 100% purification of air. A particulate respirator can be reusable and employ filters that are easily replaced; the equipment can be disinfected and permits installation of a new filter. These respirators do not prevent transmission when used by infected persons. Disposable face respirators are made of filtered material that impedes the passage of large and small particles contained in the air; some include a valve for expelling air. The National Institute of Occupational Safety and Health -NIOSH- 2003 and 2004) has approved nine types of respirators for the retention of particulates. Differences include capacity to filter air, and resistance of the filter to oil (partially or strongly resistant). See table 2. Any of these can be used when handling *M. tuberculosis*.

General characteristics of respirators			
Class of respirators		**Resistance to oils**	**% of retention**
R	95	Resistant	95
	99	Resistant	99
	100	Resistant	99.97
P	95	Partial	95
	99	Partial	99
	100	Partial	99.97
N	95	No	95
	99	No	99
	100	No	99.97

Table 2. General characteristics of respirator.

Correct training in the use and care of these items is indispensable in order to guarantee their protective function; the respirators should be properly adjusted to the face; the perception of odors or the presence of air leaks is an indication that the respirator is not functioning properly. **Remark:** These elements are for individual use and should be discarded when alterations, stains, porosity, or humidity are present.

The laboratory facilities or secondary barriers for BSL 3:

- All doors and windows should remain closed.
- A double-door system should be in place that does not allow both doors to be open at the same time (an alarm should sound if this occurs).
- A special ventilation system with HEPA filters and negative pressure should be installed.
- All procedures should be conducted in BSC.
- Autoclaves, preferably double-ended, should be on-site, in the laboratory room.
- A constant supply of electricity, water, disposal, and gas should be guaranteed; filters and other necessary items should be available in order to ensure the containment of *M. tuberculosis* and other pathogens.
- All necessary equipment should be available in order to conduct all processes and avoid the entrance and exit of material that should be contained.
- All procedures that occur at this BLS should be documented and approved by the laboratory director and the institution's biosafety committee, who should then monitor compliance with the policies.
- Illumination should be adequate and should avoid reflections on cabinet windows and on other materials that would impair the vision of the operator.
- Installations and integrated systems at this BSL should be monitored and inspected periodically.
- Work areas should include decontamination systems and an adequate waste-disposal program (a company should be employed that specializes in this area).
- Equipment should be located in such a manner that facilitates disinfection below and between the items.
- Equipment and work surfaces should be resistant to the action of disinfectants.
- Professionals are now available who specialize in the planning, construction, and maintenance of laboratories at BSL 3; they should be consulted and evaluated by the biosafety committee of each institution.

3.1 Biosafety and hospital control

Hospital patient care areas, waiting rooms, healthcare units, respiratory isolation areas, and TB patients transiting through the institution, are just some examples of areas that require PPE for workers personnel and the requisite BSL in order to minimize the risk of exposure (CDC 1996). The implementation of biosafety and biocontainment measures in the hospital should begin with the creation of a TB control committee responsible for risk assessment (CDC 2003). The committee should be responsible for the following functions:

- Comprised of professionals who are expert in the area of biological changes of *M. tuberculosis* and its forms of resistance.

- The risk area should be identified
- Provide preventive measures and guidelines for patient isolation; identify, intervene and monitor the transmission risk areas
- Develop protocols for the management of patients, accidents in areas of risk, anti-pandemic plans, and for other situations that may arise
- supervise the compliance with protocols and guidelines

The areas that comprise the greatest risk of transmission in a hospital, and over which the TB control committee should focus its attention, are: ambulatory waiting rooms; radiology room; broncoscopy and sputum induction rooms; respiratory isolation rooms; ventilator assistance areas; emergency room; autopsy room; and microbiology or micobacteria laboratories. A detailed analysis indicates that these areas comprise almost 70% of the services provided by a general hospital; therefore, the activities of the TB control committee should be continuous and rigorous.

One of the effective measures used to diminish the transmission of MDR TB and XDR TB in the community is the placement of the patient in a respiratory isolation room; the room should have HEPA filters for the recirculation of air with a minimum replacement of six air changes per hour. The room should have negative pressure, guarantee the privacy of the patient, permit effective disinfection measures, and preferably contain an anteroom in order to minimize escape risk.

The TB control committee should delegate authority to a designated professional to decide which ambulatory or hospitalized patients should be located within the isolation area. The patient should receive clear instructions regarding behavior while in the respiratory isolation area (Garner 1996). For example, the patient should cover his/her mouth and nose when coughing in the room; upon leaving the room, the patient should cover his/her mouth and nose with a surgical mask. Healthcare personnel should avoid, to the maximum extent possible, entering the isolation area (Chen 1994). A small number of professionals should care for the patient and, when doing so, utilize a special mask such as N95, or respirators.

Remark: the TB control committee should monitor areas where patients gather, and should prepare guidelines to ensure that patients with suspected respiratory illness, pediatric patients, infectious persons, and geriatric patients are not in the same waiting room.

The TB control committee should also develop guidelines for ambulatory care areas that provide for adequate ventilation, illumination, and periodic disinfection with effective chemical agents against the pathogens most frequently encountered in this area. Air conditioners and ventilators are permitted only when used in conjunction with HEPA air filtration systems (American Institute of Architects 2001). The assistance room should include a ventilator that maintains a barrier between the physician and patient. Air flow should be directed toward the air that enters through doors and windows. See figure 2.

3.2 Biosafety in the teaching laboratory

The teaching laboratories are usually found in academic institutions to provide a venue for instructing students on how sciences are conducted and for training in specific applications. This laboratory in all discipline is unique in at least one important aspect. As a general rule and particularly at introductory levels, teaching laboratories tend to be densely populated

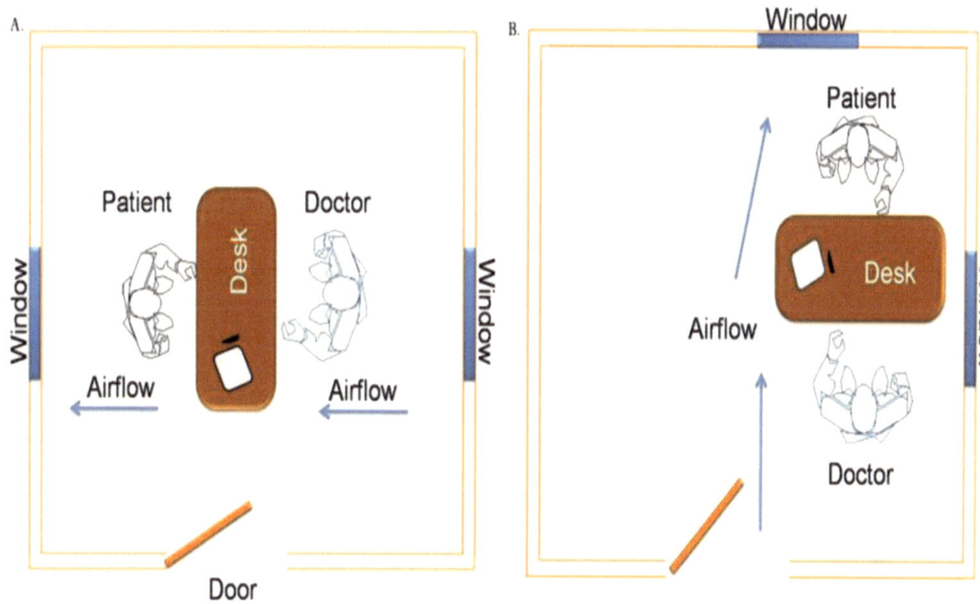

Fig. 2. Basic biosafety recommendations at the healthcare units.
On http://www.who.int/docstore/gtb/publications/healthcare/index.htm the WHO has proposed practical and low cost interventions to reduce nosocomial transmission.

with large numbers of individuals with limited experience in hazard of a science laboratory and certain number of then may be immunocompromised. Please answer the question ¿Are teaching laboratories less safe than others laboratories? The correct answer is no, because in this space de student must to learn the specific topics for risk assessment, biosafety and biocontainment. Is a responsibility of educational institutions to teach about of biosafety with the international and national guidelines and the use of PPE. (WHO 1992, CDC 1999, 2002, and 2005, Food and Drug Administration 2004).

3.3 Biosafety in the pharmaceutical industry

The microorganisms used in pharmaceutical companies are extremely diverse, encompassing bacteria, viruses, fungi, helminthes and protozoa. The pharmaceutical companies that use pathogenic microorganisms to produce or testing drugs, and vaccine must establish a broad range of biosafety practice to ensure the safety of their workers and their product. During the scale up, the biosafety practices employed should be in harmony with the international guidelines to ensure that the manufacturing process and product may be used and sold internationally. The biosafety in the pharmaceutical encompasses both laboratory scale practices and requires a well organized and implemented program of risk assessment, risk management, program evaluation and modification (Advisory Committee on Dangerous Pathogens 1998). More information: CDC 1997 and http://pharmacos.eudra.org/F2/eudralex/vol-4/pdfs-en/anx02en200408.pdf

4. Biocontainment

The biocontainment measures are very important, they arise from an adequate handling that an institution must do of their risk assessment, biological level, procedures, biosecurity measures, PPE, standards and protocols in order to prevent malicious use. The implementation and strict adherence of standard microbiological practices, it is currently considered the best measure of biocontainment for *M. tuberculosis* and other infectious substances is. The adoption of a biosafety culture together with a good laboratory practice and facilities design is a guarantee to preserve the environment and control risk.

The design of laboratories, as well as the supportive health and engineering staff faces great challenges like: to guarantee the maintenance of long-term infrastructure, to build efficiently at a reasonable cost and conscious planning of energy and water, localization of these laboratories (If the possibility is offered, this should be discussed with the regional development plans in each region). The biocontainment culture in an institution should anticipate the management of unexpected situations and for this; the institution must have contingency plans and emergency procedures.

4.1 The contingency plan must include

Operative procedures for the risk assessment, identification of high risk areas, to identify as much specific as possible to the population at risk and their characteristics, emergency transportation for the personnel exposed and prioritize this work when an incident occur, inventory of resources, suppliers commitment with availability of treatments, availability of PPE and properly trained personnel in the proper use and final disposal. Precise actions and simulations to verify the effectiveness of the evacuation plan and estimate the possibility of natural disaster like earthquakes powerful, storms and flooding, depending on the geographic region. (Lindell 1996 and, Young 2004)

Emergency procedures should include practical protocols, effective and achievable depending on the resources of the institution, these biocontainment protocols should include all possible events or accidents according with common activities like: ingestion or inhalation of potentially infectious material, broken containers and infectious spilled substances, breakage of tubes in centrifuges, puncture wounds, cuts and abrasions.

The police and fire departments should be involved in the development of emergency and contingency plans for fire or natural disasters, but they need to take a special training. Since, it is impossible to prevent all incidents of this nature, some precautions must be followed. These are some examples of what can be done to minimize the possibility of releasing pathogenic organism into the environment as the result of a natural disaster: post notices on all incubators, refrigerators, freezers and other storage facilities and contents listing persons to be notified in case of incident, secure store in culture collections, damage resistant cabinets or containers, cabinets or shelving provide for storing books, equipment, chemicals and others that close securely with doors, do not store heavy boxes and equipment above bench level.

5. Disinfection and sterilization

Understanding the importance of decontamination, cleaning, sterilization and disinfection is vital for implementing a laboratory biosafety plan. The descending order of resistance to

Disinfection					
Reagent	**Concentration**	**Time exposure**	**Action**	**Funtion**	**Dificulties**
Phenol	0.4 - 5%	10 minutes	Protein denaturation	Efficient disinfectants	Irritant, toxic, corrosive
Formal-dehyde	5%	10 minutes	Protein alkylation	Efficient disinfectants	Cutaneous irritant, respiratory irritant, eye irritant
Glutaral-dehyde	1 - 2%	20 - 30 minutes	Membrane disruption	Efficient disinfectants, or decontaminating surfaces	Toxic, cutaneous irritant, eye irritant
Sodium hypochlorite	0.2 - 5%, 5000 ppm, 1g/L	1 - 2 minutes	Enzymatic inhactivation	Efficient disinfectants	Toxic, corrosive, cutaneous irritant, respiratory irritant, eye irritant
Ethyl alcohol	70%, 96%	2 minutes	Protein action, membrane disruption	Surface disinfectant, mycobacterial disinfectants	Eye irritant
Hydrogen peroxide	3 - 10%	5 minutes	Free radicals, lipid and proteins action	Disinfectants	Corrosive, respiratory irritant
Iodophore	2 - 10 %, 75 ppm		Iodination and oxidation of proteins	Disinfectants	Cutaneous irritant, respiratory irritant, eye irritant, corrosive
Mix 1 : Iodine + ionophores, or ethyl alcohol	variable	variable	Iodination and oxidation of proteins	Efficient disinfectants	Cutaneous irritant, respiratory irritant, eye irritant, corrosive
Mix 2: paraformal dehyde + glutaraldeh yde or formalin solutions.	2- 5%	10 - 30 minutes	Protein alkylation, membrane disruption	Inactivation	Toxic, cutaneous irritant, respiratory irritant, eye irritant

Table 3. Summarizes the properties of some liquid germicides that are recommended again *M. tuberculosis*.

germicidal chemicals is: bacterial spores, Mycobacteria (especially *M. tuberculosis*), small viruses (Non lipid), fungi, vegetative bacteria, and medium size viruses (lipid) (Favero 1998, and 2001, and CDC 2003). Each laboratory must evaluate the efficacy of germicides. See table 3 (Kunz 1982, Best 1988, 1990, Rubin 1991, Rutala 1991, Sattar 1995, Schwebach 2001, and Blackwood 2005). Is essential that manufacturer's recommended use dilutions are followed.

Sterilization: susceptible to moist heat sterilization at 121°C for 15 minutes at 121 pounds of pressure.

6. Packing and shipping biological materials

The care and responsibility that one assumes when transporting infected material that contains live *M. tuberculosis* serve to guarantee the biosecurity of this important process. The transportation of infected material can occur within the same hospital (from the patient's room to the laboratory) or to an outside location (other institutions, cities, or countries). The transport of material infected with *M. tuberculosis* to areas within a hospital or laboratory should be made using resistant containers that can be easily disinfected; the container should have a hermetic seal capable of containing infectious substances during accidents, or until such time as the substances can be handled in a BSC. Currently, various organizations have prepared guidelines that should be used in order to reduce the risk of infection to personnel and the environment.

Current regulations governing the transport of hazardous items include obligatory actions that apply to the three parties involved in the process: the recipient (should receive import authorization and provide the appropriate documentation); the transporter or operator (should use a verification list, accept or reject the items to be transported, provide training, adequate documentation and instructions) and the shipper who should comply with packaging norms (should classify, identify and package the infected material, place markings and labels, document and have emergency plans in place).

The majority of the guidelines established for the transport of hazardous materials have been issued by the following agencies:

- International Civil Aviation Organization (ICAO), a specialized United Nations (UN) agency with the regulations entitled "Safe Transport of Dangerous Goods by Air"
- The IATA with regulations entitled "IATA Dangerous Goods Regulations
- The U.S. Department of Transportation (DOT) with regulations entitled "United States Hazardous Material Uniform Safety Act."

These regulations are similar with respect to the following guidelines: classification and naming of diagnostic specimens and infectious substances; marking and labeling packaging material; training and certification of personnel; practical suggestions for classifying diagnostic specimens and infectious substances; resources for additional information and documentation; and instructions for completing a shipper's declaration for dangerous goods. This can change significantly as a result of investigations or sudden pandemics which may necessitate new measures and regulations.

IATA requirements and DOT regulations provide minimum requirements for packing and shipping diagnostic specimens and infectious substances. These provisions include:

- Classification and naming of the substances to be shipped: select the appropriate IATA packing instructions; in the case of category A material, submit the necessary information to complete the shipper's declaration. The substance or material should be classified in one of the nine IATA specified classes (1-explosivos, 2- gases, 3- flammable liquids, 4- flammable solids, 5- oxidizing substances and organic peroxides, 6- toxic and infectious substances, division 6.1: toxic substances, division 6.2 infectious substances, 7- radioactive materials, 8- corrosives and 9-miscellaneous dangerous goods) (IATA 2006).
- The classification 6.2 must be divided into one of nine IATA specific groups such as: -category A infectious substances, -category B infectious substances, –exempt human or animal specimens, -exempt substances, -patient specimens, -genetically modified organisms, -biological products, - infected animals, -medical waste.

The category A substances are specifically designated as pathogens which can be dangerous to both individual and public health. Category A pathogens and substances likely to contain category A pathogens must be assigned UN number UN2814 for infectious substances that affect humans or UN2900 for infectious substances affecting animals.

- The selection of package and packing the shipment correctly: after having classified the infectious substance, the shipper must officially name the Category A or B material; the substances must then be assigned one of the more than 3,000 IATA specified, and internationally recognized, UN numbers accompanied by the proper shipping name as provided by IATA regulations. This list provides information about 14 items, identified in alphabetical order from A to N, for each of the proper shipping names; this data is required in order to complete the shipper's declaration.

The PI describes the minimum standards for the safe transport of various biological materials. Shippers are legally obligated to comply with the regulations. Materials must be packaged properly in order to ensure the safety of all personnel who handle the package before, during, and after shipment. Clinical laboratories transporting category A infectious substances should use PI 602; for category B infectious materials, PI 650 should be used.

The PI 602 used for the packaging of infectious material should comply with the following requirements: leakproof and pressure-resistant for the first and second containers; absorbent between the first and second containers; list of contents between the second container and outer package; rigid outer packaging; positively sealed first container; name, address, and telephone number of responsible person on outer package or air waybill; shipper declaration for dangerous goods; outer packaging marking and labels; and strict manufacturing specifications. See table 4:

- The outer package should include appropriate markings and labels: labeling is the act of placing informational labels or stickers onto the surface of an outer package. The shipper is responsible for the proper marking and labeling of the outer shipping container. The labels and markings include:

Column	Information		
A	United Nations number of the proper shipping name/description	**2814**	
B	Proper shipping name/description	Infectious Substance, Affecting Humans (Liquid)	Infectious Substance, Affecting Humans (Solid)
C	Class or division of dangerous good	6.2	6.2
D	NA		
E	Hazard label required on the outer package	Infectious substance	Infectious substance
F	NA		
G	NA		
H	NA		
I	PI to use for passenger and cargo aircraft	602	602
J	Maximum allowable amounts to be shipped in passenger and cargo aircraft	50 ml	50 g
K	PI to use for cargo aircraft only	602	602
L	Maximum allowable amounts to be shipped in cargo aircraft only	4 liters	4 kg
M	Applicable special provisions and exceptions	A81 A140	A81 A140
N	Emergency response code	11Y	11Y

Table 4. Shipping requirements for infection substances (*M. tuberculosis*).

- Name and direction of the shipper, name, address and telephone number of the responsible party, as provided by IATA regulations. The diamond-shaped infectious substances label should be used when shipping contaminated material, accompanied by a label which shows the proper shipping name, UN number, and quantity of the substances; the package orientation label must also be included and placed on opposite sides of the entire package. Additional markings may be included as required. The "cargo aircraft only" label indicates that the package may be shipped only in cargo, and not on passenger, aircraft; this label is used if the infectious substance is over 50 ml but less than 4 liters per the outer package being shipped. The "overpack" markings indicate that an overpack is used and that inner packages comply with the regulations. Packaging that meets UN specifications is marked by a "UN" inside of a circle and a series of letters and numbers which indicate the type of package, class of goods the package is designed to carry, the manufacturer, authorizing agency, and manufacturing date. The designation "Class 6.2" indicates that the container is approved for shipping infectious substances.(see figure 3)

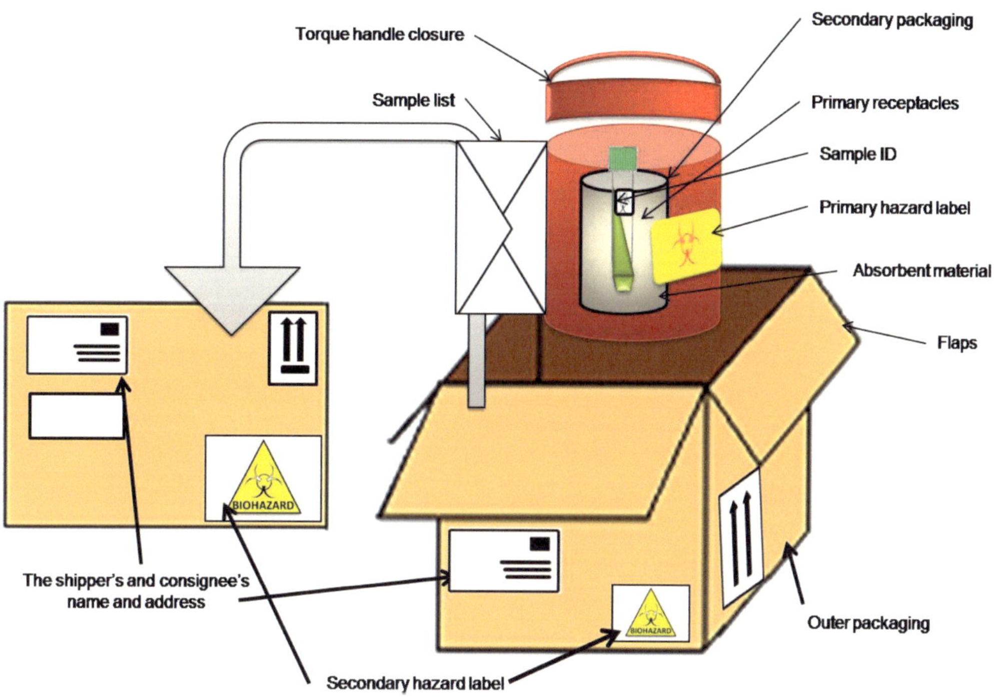

Fig. 3. Biomedical packaging for infectious substances, marking and labeling packages established by agencies governing transportation of dangerous goods.

- The relevant document: the preparation and delivery of a shipper's declaration is necessary in order to formalize a legal contract; this document is required for category A substances; however, it is not required for category B material. These documents should be completed in their entirety.
- Training for personnel: competent authorities such as the CDC offer training in the transport of infectious substances to laboratory personnel, members of biosecurity committees, and professionals in different areas.(IATA 2006, U.S. Department of Transportation 2004, and 2006, and WHO 2004, and 2005) Additional information concerning these regulations is available at http://www.iata.org or http://www.who.int/crs/resourceces/publications/biosafety/WWHO_CDS-EPR-2007_2/en/index.html

7. Conclusion

Is buying biosafety and biocontainment the best option?

The growing number of professionals infected by *M. tuberculosis*, many of whom have died due to this without knowing for certain the source of infection or exposure (whether the community or their workplace), and the dramatic figures of deaths caused by TB around the world among people infected or not with HIV confront us with a question to which we have no answer: Did the person get infected in a hospital waiting room, in an international flight? When did it happen? We don't know, and that is why it is so important to enhance community awareness on these issues.

Risk assessment and the adoption of biosecurity and biocontainment measures with the participation of academic institutions, scientists, designers and community at large represent paying the right price and obtaining the expected impact.

8. Self evaluation

Self evaluation:

1. What is *M. tuberculosis*?
   a. Fungi
   b. Bacteria
   c. Virus
   d. Other
2. Which is *M. tuberculosis* mode of transmission?
   a. Airborne
   b. Sexual contact
   c. Vertical transmission.
3. How is *M. tuberculosis* spread person to person?
   a. Inhalation of infectious aerosol or infected droplets
   b. Water
   c. Foods
   d. Clothes
4. What is a N95?
   a. Respirator
   b. Surgical mask
   c. HEPA filter
5. Is the infectious dose of *M. tuberculosis* less than 1000 bacilli by inhalation route in humans?
   a. Yes
   b. No
   c. Is unknown
6. What are the tests for TB infection?
   a. PPD or IGRAs
   b. BCG
   c. PPE

7. What is the meaning of microorganisms RG 3
   a. no or low individual and community risk
   b. high individual and community risk
   c. high individual risk, low community risk
   d. moderate individual risk, low community risk
8. What IATA category is *M. tuberculosis*?
   a. Category A
   b. Category B
   c. Category PI
9. The sterilization conditions for *M. tuberculosis* included?
   a. 121°C for 15 minutes at 121 pounds of pressure
   b. 121°C for 90 minutes at 140 pounds of pressure
   c. 15°C for 15 minutes at 121 pounds of pressure
   d. Unknown

9. References

Advisory Committee on Dangerous Pathogens. 1998. The Large Scale Contained Use of Biological Agents. Her Majesty's Stationery Office, London, England.

American Institute of Architects, Committee on Architecture for Health.2001. Guidelines for Construction and Equipment of Hospital and Medical Facilities. American Institute of Architects Press, Washington, D.C.

American National Standard Institute. 1992. American National Standard for Respirator Protection (ANSI Z88.2). American National Standards Institute, New York, N.Y.

American Thoracic Society. 1983. Levels of laboratory services for mycobacteria diseases. Am. Rev. Dis. 128:213.

Best M, Sattar S.A., Springthorpe V.S., Kennedy M.E. 1988. Comparative mycobactericidal efficacy of chemical disinfectans in suspension and carrier test. Appl Environ Microbiol. 54:2856-8.

Best M, Sattar S.A., Springthorpe V.S., Kennedy M.E. 1990. Efficacies of selected disinfectants against *Mycobacterium tuberculosis*. J Clin Microbiol 28:2234-9.

Blackwood K.s., Burdz T.V., Turenne C.Y., Sharma M.K., Kabani A.M. Wolfe J.N. 2005. Viability testing of material derived from *Mycobacterium tuberculosis* prior to removal from a containment Level-III Laboratory as part of a laboratory risk Assessment program. *BMC Infectious Diseases,* 5, (4): 1-7.

Boa, E., J. Lynch, and D.R. Liliquist. 2000. Risk Assessment Resource. American Industrial Hygiene Association, Fairfax, Va.

Burgos M.V., Mendez J.C., Ribón W. 2004. Molecular epidemiology of tuberculosis: methodology and applications. Biomédica. 24(Supl.):188-201

Castro C., González., Rozo J., Puerto G., Ribón W. 2009. Biosafety evaluation of the DNA extraction protocol for *Mycobacterium tuberculosis* complex species, as implemented at the Instituto Nacional de Salud, Colombia. Biomédica. 29:561-6

Centers for Disease Control and Prevention and National Institutes of Health. 1999. Biosafety in Microbiological and Biomedical laboratories, 4th ed. U.S. Government Printing Office, Washington, D.C. Centers for Disease Control and Prevention and

National Institutes of Health. 2006. Biosafety in Microbiology and Biomedical laboratories, 5th ed. U.S. Government Printing Office, Washington, D.C.

Centers for Disease Control and Prevention and the Healthcare Infection Control Advisory Committee. 2003. Guidelines for environmental infection control in health care facilities: recommendation of CDC and the Healthcare Infection Control Advisory Committee.

Centers for disease Control and Prevention. 1994. Guidelines for preventing the transmission of *Mycobacterium tuberculosis* in health-care facilities, 1994. Mor. Mortal. Wkly. Rep. 43(RR-13):1-132.

Centers for Disease Control and Prevention. 1996. Guideline for isolation precautions in hospitals. Am. J. Infect. Control 42:24-45.

Centers for Disease Control and Prevention. 1997. Goals Working safely with *Mycobacterium tuberculosis* in clinical, public health, and research laboratories.

Centers for Disease Control and Prevention. 2002. Guideline for hand hygiene in health-care settings. Morb. Mortal. Wkly. Rep. 51(RR-16):1-44.

Centers for Disease Control and Prevention. 2005. Possession, Use, and Transfer of Select Agents and Toxins. 42 CFR parts 72 and 73. U.S. Department of Health and Human Services. Fed. Regist. 70:13293-13325.

Centers for Diseases Control and Prevention and National Institutes of Health. 2000. Primary Containment for Biohazards: Selection, Installation and Use of Biological Safety Cabinets, 2nd ed. J. R. Richmond and R.W. McKinney (ed.) U.S. Government Printing Office, Washington, D.C.

Chen, S.-K., D. Vesley, L.M. Brosseau, and J.H. Vincent. 1994. Evaluation of single-use mask and respirators for protection of health care workers against mycobacterial aerosols. Am. J. Infect. Control. 22:65-74.

Commission of the European Communities. 2000. Directive 2000/54/EC of the European Parliament and of the Council of 18 September 2000 on the protection of workers from risks related to exposure to biological agents at work (seventhindividual directive within the meaning of Article 16 (1) of Directive 89/391/EEC). Official journal of the European Communities, L262/21-45,17.10.2000.

Cousins D.V., Bastida R., Cataldi A., Redrobe S., Dow s., Duignan P., Murray A., Dupont C., Ahmed N., Collins d. M. butler W.R., Dawson D., Rodriguez D., Loureiro J., Romano M.I., Alito A., Zumarraga M., Bernardelli A. 2003. Tuberculosis in seals caused by a novel member of the *Mycobacterium tuberculosis* complex: *Mycobacterium pinnipeddi* sp. Nov. Int Syst Evol Microbiol, 53,1305-1314.

Favero, M. 1998. Developing indicators for sterilization, p.119-132. In W.A. Rutala (ed.), Disinfection, Sterilization and Antisepsis in Health Cara. Association for Professionals in Infection Control and Epidemiology, Inc., Champlain, N.Y.

Favero, M. 2001. Sterility assurance: concepts for patient safety, p.110-119. In W.A. Rutala (ed.), Disinfection, Sterilization and antisepsis: Principles and Practices in Healthcare Facilities. Association for Professionals in Infection Control and Epidemiology, Inc., Washintong, D.C.

Favero, M., and W. Bond. 2001. Chemical disinfection of medical surgical material, p. 881-917.In S.S. Block (ed.) Disinfection, Sterilization, and Preservation, 5th ed. Lippincott, Williams and Wilkins, Philadelphia, Pa.

Food and Drug Administration. 2004. 21 CFR Part 211. Current Good Manufacturing Practices for finished pharmaceuticals. U.S. Code of Federal Regulations.

Garner, J.S., and the Hospital Infection Control Practices Advisory Committee. 1996. CDC guideline for isolation precautions in hospitals. Am. J. Infect. Control 24:24-52.

Garner, J.S., and the Hospital Infection Control Practices Advisory Committee. 1996. CDC guideline for isolation precautions in hospitals. Am. J. Infect. Control 24:24-52.

Ghosh J., Larsson P., Singh B., Pettersson B., Islam N., Sarkar S., Dasgupta S., and Kirsebom L. 2009. Sporulation in mycobacteria. PNAS 106: 10781–10.

Grange J.M. Tuberculosis. In: Topley and Wilson Principles of Bacteriology, Virology and Immunology, 9th ed. Year book, 1990. vol.3,p.94-121.

Hankenson, F. C., N.A. Johnson, B.J. Weigler, and R.F. Di Giacomo.2003.Overview: Zoonoses of occupational health importance in contemporary laboratory animal research. Comp. Med. 53:570-601.

Harrintong J.M., Shannon H.S. Incidence of tuberculosis, hepatitis, brucellosis and shigellosis in British Medical Laboratory workers. Br Med J 1976;1:759-62.

International Air Transport Association. 2006. IATA Dangerous Goods Regulations, 47th ed. International Air Transport Association, Montreal, Canada.

International Air Transport Association. 2006. Infectious Substances Shipping Guidelines, 7th ed. Ref. N°9052-07. International Air Transport Association, Montreal, Quebec, Canada.

Kent, P. T., and G. P. Kubica. 1985. Public Health Mycobacteriology. A guide for the level III Laboratory. Centers for Disease Control, Atlanta, Ga.

Krauss, H., A. Weber, M. Appel, B. Enders, H.D. Isenberg, H.G. Schiefer, W. Slenczka, A. von Graevenitz, and Zahner. 2003. Zoonoses: Infectious Diseases Transmissible from Animals to humans, 3rd ed. ASM Press, Washintong, D.C.

Kunz R., Gunderman KC. The survival of *Mycobacterium tuberculosis* on surfaces at different relative humidities. Zent Bakt Hyg 1982; 176. 105-115.

Laboratory Center for Diseases Control, Health Protection Branch, Health Canada. 1996. Laboratory Biosafety guidelines, 2nd ed. Ministry of Supply and Services, Ottawa, Ontario, Canada.

Lietman, T., and S. Blower.1999. Tuberculosis vaccines. Science 286:1300-1301.

Lindell, M. K., and R. W. Perry. 1996. Addressing gaps in environmental emergency planning hazardous materials releases during earthquakes. J. Environ. Planning Manag. 39:529-545.

Miller C.D. Songer J.R., Sullivan J.F. 1987. A twenty-five year review of laboratory acquired human infections at the National Animal Disease Center. Am Ind hyg assoc J, 48,271-275.

Muller H.E. 1988 Laboratory-acquired mycobacterial infection. Lancet, 2:331.

National Institute of Health. 2002. NIH guidelines for research involving recombinant DNA molecules (NIH guidelines). Fed. Regist. 59:34496 (July 5, 1994) as amended. (http:www4.od.nih.gov/oba/rac/guidelines/guidelines_html).

National Institutes of Health. 2002. NIH Guidelines for Research Involving Recombinant DNA Molecules (NIH Guidelines), 59 FR 34496 (July 5, 1994), as amended.

National Researgh Council. 1997. Occupational Health and Safety in the Care and Use of Research Animals. National Academy Press, Washintong, D.C.

National Researgh Council. 2003. Occupational Health and Safety in the Care and Use of Nonhuman Primates. National Academy Press, Washintong, D.C.

NSF International. 2002. Class II (Laminar Flow) Biosafety cabinetry. NSF/ANSI standard 49-2002. NSF International, Ann Arbor, Mich.

Occupational Safe and Health Administration (OSHA). 2003. Occupational exposure to tuberculosis. Notice. Fed. Regist. 68:75767-75775.

Occupational Safe and Health Administration (OSHA). 2003. Personal Protective Equipment. Publication 3151-12R. OSHA Publications Office, Washington, D.C.

Occupational Safety and Health Administration. 1996. CPL 2.106 Enforcement Procedures and Scheduling for Occupational Exposure to tuberculosis. Occupational Safety and Health Administration, Washington, D.C.

Occupational Safety and Health Administration. 1997. Occupational Exposure to tuberculosis; proposed rule. Fed. Regist. 62:54159-54309

Occupational Safety and health Administration. 30 July 2004. Standard Interpretations-Tuberculosis and Respiratory Protection. R. Davis Layne, Deputy Assistant secretary.

Pike R.M.1978. Past and present hazards of working with infectious agent. Arch. Pathol. Lab. Med. 102:333-36.

Pike, R.M. 1976. Laboratory-associated infections: summary and analysis of 3921 cases. Health Lab. Sci.13:105-114.

Pike.R.M. 1979. Laboratory-associated infections: incidence, fatalities, causes, and prevention. Annu. Rev. microbial. 33:41- 66.

Reid DD. Incidence of tuberculosis among workers in medical laboratories. Br Med J 1957;2:10-4.

Riley, R. 1961. Airborne pulmonary tuberculosis. Bacteriol. Rev. 25:243-248.

Riley, R.L. 1957. Aerial dissemination of pulmonary tuberculosis. Am. Rev. Tuberc. 76:931-941.

Rozo J., and Ribón W.2010. Molecular tools for *Mycobacterium tuberculosis* genotyping. Rev. salud pública. 12 (3): 510-521.

Rubin J. Mycobacterial disinfection and control. In: Seymour S. Block Lea and Febiger editors. Disinfection, sterilization and preservation, 4th edition, Year book, 1991.377-83.

Rutala W. A., Cole E.C., Wannamaker N.S. Weber D.J. 1991. Inactivation of *Mycobacterium tuberculosis* and *Mycobacterium bovis* by 14 hospitals disinfectans. Am J Med 91:267-271S.

Sattar S.A., Best M., Springthorpe V.S., Sanani G.1995. Mycobacterial testing of disinfectants: an update. Hosp Inf, 30 suppl. 372-382.

Schwebach J.R., Jacobs W.R. Jr, Casadevall A. 2001. Sterilization of *Mycobacterium tuberculosis* Erdman samples by antimicrobial fixation in biosafety level 3 laboratory. J Clin Microbiol, 39, 769-771.

Sessler, S.M., and R.M. Hoover. 1983. Laboratory Fume Hood Noise, Heating Piping and Air Conditioning. Penton/PC Reinhold, Cleveland, Ohio.

Standars Australia/Standars New Zealand. 2002. Safety in Laboratories. Part 3: Microbiological Aspects and Containment Facilities. Australia/New Zealand Standard AS/NZS2243.3:2002. Standards Australia International Ltd., Sydney, Australia.

Traag B., Driks A., Stragier P., Bitter W., Broussard G., Hatfull G., Chu F., Adams K., Ramakrishnan L., and Losick R.2010. Do mycobacteria produce endospores? PNAS 12:878–881

U.S. Department of transportation, Pipeline and Hazardous Materials Safety Administration. 2006. Hazardous materials: infectious substances; harmonization with the United Nations recommendations; proposed rule. Fed. Regist. 71:32244-32263.

U.S. Department of transportation, Research and Special Programs Administration. 2004. Harmonization with the United Nations recommendations. International Maritime Dangerous Goods Code, and International Civil Aviation Organizations Technical Instructions; final rule. Fed Regist. 69:76043-76187.

Verhagen, L. Van den Hof, S. Mycobacterial Factors Relevant for Transmission of Tuberculosis. Journal of Infectious Diseases Advance Access published March 4, 2011.

Warren R. Koch M., Engelke E., Myburgh R., van pittus N., Victor T., and van Helden P. 2006. Safe *Mycobacterium tuberculosis* DNA extraction method that does not compromise integrity. *Journal of Clinical Microbiology,* 44: 254-256.

Wayne L.G. Mycobacterial speciation. In Kubica G.P. Wayne LG. editors. The Mycobacteria. A sourcebook. New York: Marcel-Dekker: Year book, 1984. 26-65.

Welch, D. F., A. P. Guruswamy, S. J. Sides, C. J. Shaw, and M. J. R. Gilchrist. 1993. Timely culture for mycobacteria which utilizes a microcolony method. J. Clin. Microbiol. 31:2178-2184.

Wells, W. 1934. On air-borne infection. II. Droplets and droplet nuclei. Am. J. Hyg. 20:611-18.

Wells, W. F. 1955. Airborne contagion and Air Hygiene. Harvard University Press, Cambridge, Mass.

Wheelis, M.2002. Biological warfare at the 1346 Siegui of Caffa. Emerg. Infect. Dis. 8:971-975.

World Health Organization. 1992. Expert Committee on Specifications for Pharmaceutical Preparations, Thirty-Second Report. World Health Organization, New York, N.Y.

World Health Organization. 2004. Laboratory Biosafety Manual.3rd ed. World Health Organization, Geneva, Switzerland.

World Health Organization. 2004. Transport of infectious substances. Background to the amendments adopted in the 13th revision of the United Nations Model Regulations guiding the transport of infectious substances.

World Health Organizations. 2005. Guidance on Regulations for the Transport of Infectious Substances. World Health Organization, Geneva, Switzerland.

Young, S., L. Balluz, and J. Malilay. 2004. Natural and technologic hazardous material releases during and after natural disasters: a review: Sci. Total Environ.322:3-20.

Part 2

New Approaches to the TB Diagnosis

11

New Diagnostics for *Mycobacterium tuberculosis*

Michaela Lucas[1,2], Andrew Lucas[1] and Silvana Gaudieri[1,3]
[1]*Institute for Immunology and Infectious Diseases, Murdoch University, Perth, Western Australia,*
[2]*Department of Health, Perth, Western Australia,*
[3]*School of Anatomy and Human Biology and Centre for Forensic Science, University of Western Australia, Perth, Western Australia, Australia*

1. Introduction

1.1 Tuberculosis as a global health issue and the need for reliable diagnostics in primary care settings

Mycobacterium tuberculosis (Mtb) infection is one of the leading causes of morbidity and mortality worldwide with an estimated one third of the world's population infected by Mtb resulting in about two million deaths per year (Lonnroth and Raviglione, 2008; Wallis et al., 2010). Developing countries are burdened with the highest levels of Mtb infections and conversely have the lowest financial resources available to improve this situation (Figures 1 and 2). High rates of infection are associated with poverty, low levels of public hygiene and often with a high prevalence of HIV+ individuals who are at particular risk of infection, all factors that contribute to an uncontrolled spread of Mtb infection (Corbett et al., 2006; Wright et al., 2009).

Mtb can be spread from person to person via droplet nuclei that contain Mtb organisms. Droplet nuclei are primarily produced when people with pulmonary Mtb cough or sneeze and these particles can remain in the air for long periods of time. If inhaled, these droplet nuclei can reach the alveoli within the lungs where Mtb replicates. Individuals with Mtb infection can exhibit a wide range of clinical features that challenge current diagnostic approaches including acute active pulmonary infection with infective sputum, latent disease with risk of reactivation (especially in the immune-compromised host), sputum-negative and extrapulmonary Mtb infection and childhood tuberculosis (Wallis et al., 2010). In the majority of cases an infection with Mtb cannot be cleared and is contained by an effective immune response and the infection becomes latent and asymptomatic. About 10% of latently infected individuals progress to active reactivated disease during their lifetime. Thus individuals with latent Mtb infection act as infective foci of recurrent active disease and newly infect people in close contact. This large pool of undetected and untreated disease hampers eradication programs.

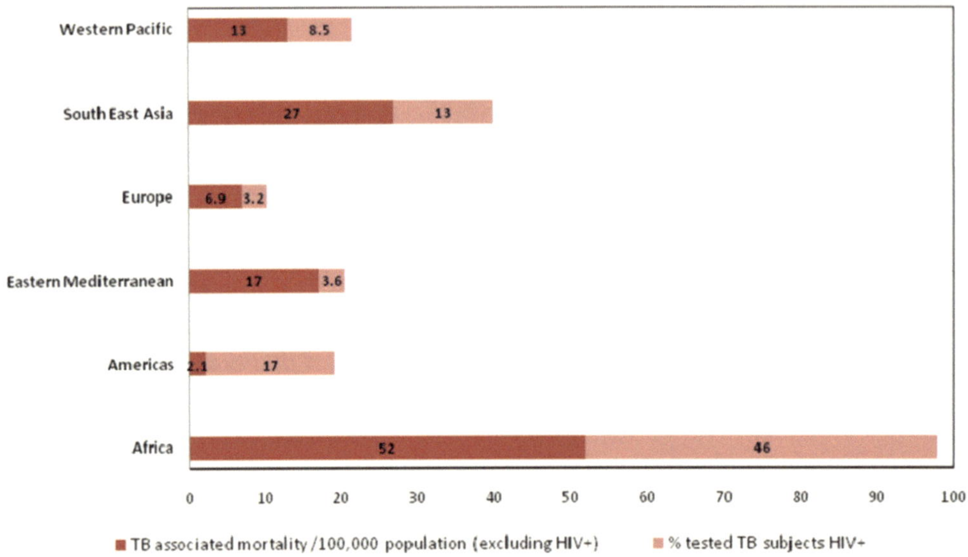

Fig. 1. Global Mtb burden of disease (2009). Data extracted from Global TB report 2010.

Global efforts to control Mtb center around improving both the rate of detection of cases and the treatment of infective subjects as reflected in the "The Stop TB strategy" published by the World Health Organisation (WHO) (WHO, 2006). The strategy aims to reverse the trend of rising incidence, halve the 1990 prevalence and mortality due to Mtb infection by 2015 and eliminate Mtb as a public health problem by 2050 (Maher et al., 2007). Successful implementation of the Stop TB strategy relies on accurate diagnostics for Mtb infection. Such an accurate diagnostic for Mtb infection should include the ability to identify adults and children with active infection, predict durable treatment success, and indicate and forecast reactivation of latent disease (Wallis et al., 2010). The ideal diagnostic tool would also need to remain trustworthy even in the setting of malnutrition and immunodeficiency and be performed within the primary care setting (Lucas et al., 2010). Given the enormity of the problem and the high prevalence in developing countries, the test(s) should also be simple and cheap. Despite major research efforts, a diagnostic assay or set of assays for Mtb infection that exhibit these properties is currently not available.

2. Current diagnostic tools for active infection: Focus on pathogen detection and early immune activation

Sputum-smear microscopy and chest radiography are still the primary tools to identify active Mtb infection in the typically resource-poor countries with a high-burden of Mtb disease (Figure 2). These tools can sometimes perform poorly and sputum is difficult to obtain from children. However, there are efforts to improve diagnostic assays available to developing countries including the development of assays that directly assay the pathogen. A summary of the main features of current diagnostics for active Mtb infection is given in Table 1.

Diagnosis of active tuberculosis

Platform/ Target	Assays	Description	Disease/ site	Disadvantages	Advantages
Sputum-Smear Microscopy	Conventional, FM, LED	Microscopic observation of stained acid-fast bacilli	Pulmonary	Sputum difficult to obtain from children, proportion of individuals smear negative, reduced sensitivity in HIV+ individuals	FM 10% more sensitive than conventional microscopy, LED FM associated with low cost, durability and no need for darkroom
Culture	Solid, Liquid	Monitor changes in media resources to detect bacterial growth	Pulmonary	Long turnaround time due to slow growth of bacteria, requires biosafety level 3 facilities	Liquid culture more sensitive than solid cultures and higher turnover rate
Biochemical	Adenosine deaminase	Detection of host enzyme released in response to intracellular pathogen	Pleuritis, pericarditis, peritonitis		ADA levels in pleural, pericardial and ascitic fluid has high specificity and sensitivity for extrapulmonary Mtb infection
Pathogen	Nucleic acid amplification tests	Detection of Mtb genetic material	Pulmonary and extra-pulmonary	Variable sensitivity especially in smear -ve and extrapulmonary disease	High specificity and positive predictive value
	Mtb antigens	Detection of circulating Mtb antigens	Pulmonary and extra-pulmonary	Variable sensitivity	Quick and relatively easy assay to perform
Serological		Detection of host humoral response to pathogen	Active and latent Mtb disease	Inconsistent estimates of sensitivity and specificity	Fast turnaround and can be used for children

Diagnosis of active tuberculosis

Platform/ Target	Assays	Description	Disease/ site	Disadvantages	Advantages
Immuno-logical markers	TST	Measurement of induration as a result of exposure to intradermal tuberculin		BCG vaccinated subjects more likely to be positive	Quick and relatively easy assay to perform
	IGRAs	Measurement of interferon gamma released from lymphocytes when stimulated with Mtb antigens		Cannot distinguish between latent and active Mtb infection, sensitivity may be lower in HIV+ subjects	High specificity and unaffected by previous BCG vaccination

References include (Wallis et al., 2010), (Daley et al., 2007; Greco et al., 2003; Mase et al., 2007), (Dinnes et al., 2007), (Jiang et al., 2007), (Flores et al., 2005; Greco et al., 2006; Ling et al., 2008), (Pai et al., 2003; Pai et al., 2004), (Sarmiento et al., 2003; Steingart et al., 2007a; Steingart et al., 2007b; Steingart et al., 2006a; Steingart et al., 2006b), (Pai et al., 2010), (Pai et al., 2008), (Goto et al., 2003; Kalantri et al., 2005), (Liang et al., 2008; Riquelme et al., 2006; Tuon et al., 2006).

Table 1. Review of current diagnostics for Mtb infection.

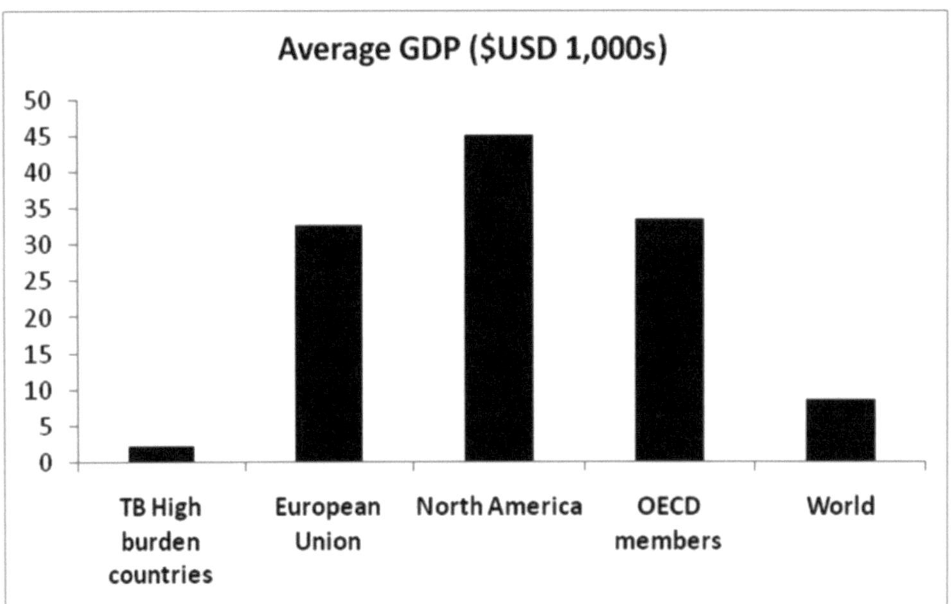

Fig. 2. Average gross national product ($USD) for 2009 for selected nations. Data extracted from Global TB report 2010 and The World Bank.

2.1 Pathogen detection

2.1.1 Microscopy

Ziehl-Neelsen sputum-smear microscopy with a conventional light microscope is commonly used to identify acid-fast bacilli in sputum to diagnose active Mtb infection in low and middle-income countries with a high prevalence of Mtb disease. This assay identifies the most infectious patients and is a quick and relatively easy procedure that is widely applicable but also requires multiple sample collections over several days (usually 3 days) and is dependent on the quality and bacterial load of the sputum specimen. The use of acid-fast fluorochrome dyes with fluorescence-based microscopy (FM) is a standard assay performed in high-income countries to detect Mtb. FM has greater sensitivity than conventional microscopy and can be performed in less time but the need for a dark room and considerable outlay costs make it less amenable for resource poor countries. The recent development of light-emitting diode (LED) fluorescence microscopy may overcome some of the difficulties associated with the widespread implementation of FM (Cuevas et al., 2011). In the setting of laboratories, which contribute to a well-functioning external quality assurance system, revised WHO guidelines for the diagnosis of pulmonary Mtb infection include the reduction in the minimum number of samples that need to be tested (from three to two), given that the inclusion of a third sample only increases sensitivity by 2-5% (Pai et al., 2008). This move could significantly reduce the local collection and testing costs and increase the successful collection rate of samples. Furthermore, the addition of simple sputum processing methods (including the use of household bleach and centrifugation) can improve sensitivity of sputum-smear microscopy. However, it is important to remember that a positive acid-fast staining result may represent the presence of non-tuberculosis mycobacteria.

2.1.2 Microbiological culture

Clinical specimens suspected of containing Mtb can be inoculated onto a culture media. Culture of Mtb on solid media (typically egg or agar-based) is more sensitive than sputum-smear microscopy for the diagnosis of active Mtb infection and can differentiate between species of mycobacteria but can take weeks to perform due to the slow growth of Mtb and related organisms. The sensitivity of cultures is generally between 80-85% with a specificity of about 98% (Prevention, 2000). The use of liquid cultures can reduce bacterial growth times (1-3 weeks compared to 3-8 weeks), can be automated and have sensitivity and specificity levels close to 100%. However, the use of such cultures requires a biosafety level 3 environment and equipment and consumables which are relatively expensive, although cheaper products may become available for developing countries (WHO, 2006).

2.1.3 Direct detection of pathogen nucleic acid

The genus Mycobacterium consists of over 80 species and many appear similar on acid-fast staining; a limitation of sputum-smear microscopy. Although cultures offer some differentiation between species, these assays have a slow turnaround time that results in a delay in diagnosing Mtb infection. Amplification and detection of Mtb DNA directly from specimens can be an efficient and sensitive method to detect Mtb infection and may also allow for the detection of mutations in the Mtb genome associated with drug resistance.

In theory, nucleic acid amplification tests (NAATs) could identify a single mycobacterium at the species level but first generation NAATs were not sufficiently reliable to replace conventional diagnostic methods for Mtb infection (Greco et al., 2006). False negative results using these assays may have been due to sampling issues (given small volumes needed for test) and possible presence in specimens of inhibitors of the amplification process. False positive results may have been due to contaminations given the inherent increased risk in these assays due to the common amplification step. Subsequent improvements using internal controls (to identify assay inhibitors) and automated systems using a single sealed tube (reduce contamination) have improved the sensitivity and specificity of these assays.

A review of several commercial NAATs showed a mean sensitivity of 96% and specificity of 85% for smear-positive cases and 66% sensitivity and 98% specificity for smear negative cases (Greco et al., 2006). Importantly, these NAATs could exclude Mtb in patients with smear positive microscopy in which environmental mycobacteria is suspected.

The fully automated Xpert Mtb device, which was developed by a consortium that included both commercial and publicly funded organisations (Cepheid Inc.; Foundation for Innovative New Diagnostics) has been endorsed by WHO for use in Mtb endemic countries (http://www.who.int/mediacentre/news/releases/2010/tb_test_20101208/en/index.html). The device does not require extensive staff training and produces results from the assay on the same day (WHO, 2006). The first assessment of the new system suggests it is highly sensitive for both smear positive and smear negative samples (Wallis et al., 2010) and the negotiation that the price per test would be reduced by 75% in countries most effected by TB should make this broadly accessible as an effective point-of-care diagnostic tool.

2.1.4 Mtb antigen detection

Assays that directly assess the presence of circulating Mtb antigens in serum, sputum, urine, cerebrospinal and pleural fluid to diagnose active Mtb disease are widely used. However, a recent review of Mtb antigen assays showed that of 47 studies examining pulmonary Mtb, the sensitivity of the assays varied from 2-100% and specificity varied from 33-100% (Flores et al., 2011). Furthermore, 21 studies examining extrapulmonary Mtb using Mtb antigen assays showed sensitivity levels varying from 0-100% and specificity from 62-100%. Most assays utilised the Mtb cell wall protein lipoarabinomannan (LAM) but some assays used multiple Mtb antigens. Interestingly, the detection of LAM in urine samples tended to have higher sensitivity in HIV+ patients than in HIV negative patients for Mtb diagnosis. However, much research is needed to improve the performance of these assays given the relative ease of translation into the primary care setting and is likely to be centred on identifying Mtb antigens that are abundantly expressed, specific to Mtb and resistant to the host's immune response.

2.2 Early immune activation markers

2.2.1 Biochemical

The diagnosis of Mtb meningitis is difficult due to the low sensitivity of identifying acid-fast bacilli in cerebrospinal fluid with microscopy and the length of time required for the culture growth of Mtb. As an alternative, the enzyme adenosine deaminase (ADA), which is widely distributed in pleural, meningeal and pericardial fluids, is used in the diagnosis of Mtb pleuritis, pericarditis and peritonitis. The host enzyme is released from lymphocytes in response to infection with intracellular pathogens (Pai et al., 2010). The biochemical assay used to quantity ADA is quick and non-invasive. A recent systematic review of 10 studies involving 1364 participants showed the ADA assay exhibited a mean sensitivity of 79% and mean specificity of 91% for Mtb meningitis (Xu et al., 2010). However, the study stresses that a negative ADA assay does not rule out Mtb meningitis and should not be used alone to make clinical decisions regarding treatment of a patient.

2.2.2 The potential role of early immune markers in the diagnosis of acute Mtb infection

Initial pathogen recognition of Mtb by macrophages occurs via toll-like receptors (TLRs), resulting in the induction of transcription of pro-inflammatory cytokine genes essential to direct the subsequent immune response (Berrington and Hawn, 2007). Mtb ligands for TLRs include CpG DNA, triggering the intracellular TLR-9, and LAM and mannosylated phosphotidylinositol acting mainly via TLR-2 (in association with TLR-1, -4 and -6) (Constantoulakis et al., 2010). Once uptake into macrophages has occurred, Mtb has unique mechanisms to survive within the phagocytes, for example by blocking biogenesis of the phagolysosome. A recent study assessed mRNA expression of a combination of these innate markers, namely TLR-2, Coronin 1, a protein which arrests the maturation of the phagolysosome within macrophages, and Sp110, a protein complex important for monocyte differentiation and apoptosis in Mtb infection. This study revealed significantly elevated levels of mRNA of all three proteins in subjects with active and latent Mtb disease as compared to healthy uninfected subjects (Chen et al., 2010). However, larger case-controlled studies are needed to confirm these findings and evaluate these factors as future diagnostic biomarkers for Mtb infection.

Another potential immune marker of Mtb infection is Neopterin. Neopterin is secreted when macrophages are activated through exposure to interferon gamma (IFN-γ) and its concentration in serum is increased in the early stages of infection whilst its levels decrease following successful treatment and increasing again upon relapse. As such it can be used as a non-specific pro-inflammatory marker for Mtb as its detection is also associated with other chronic infections that commonly coexist with Mtb, such as HIV, malaria, Hepatitis B and C (Fuchs et al., 1984; Immanuel et al., 2001; Turgut et al., 2006; Wallis et al., 1996).

Other examples of innate markers that have been shown to be increased in Mtb infection are the soluble intercellular adhesion molecules (Walzl et al., 2008), the acute phase reactant proteins (Djoba Siawaya et al., 2008), soluble urokinase plasminogen activator receptor (Eugen-Olsen et al., 2002), CXCL10/IP10 and Pentraxin 3 (Azzurri et al., 2005), and procalcitonin (Baylan et al., 2006; Kandemir et al., 2003; Nyamande and Lalloo, 2006; Prat et al., 2006; Schleicher et al., 2005).

Recently, an elegant study by Anne O'Garra and colleagues identified a 393-whole blood transcript signature for active Mtb, which correlated with clinical and radiological disease as well as treatment response. One of the surprising findings of this study was the dominant induction of genes of the IFN-γ and type I interferon pathways in neutrophils

(Berry et al., 2010). This indicates the potential power of using innate responses as surrogate markers of Mtb infection and the strength of using a combination of markers for multiplex analyses.

Despite the lack of specificity to Mtb disease associated with these innate immune markers, the measurement of these surrogate markers is technically straightforward and the assays are often readily available. It may be that by combining multiple markers distinct pathogen associated patterns will be described. Certainly the development of multiplexed assays for soluble proteins and the definition of gene expression profiles for Mtb disease by gene expression analysis (Jacobsen et al., 2007; Maertzdorf et al., 2010), such as those offered for the Luminex platform (Luminex Corp.), will continue to make this process more feasible.

3. Current diagnostic tools for latent infection: Focus on immune memory and cytokine based diagnostics

Overall, human T cell responses to Mtb involve CD4+, CD8+ and gamma-delta T cells. Akin to chronic viral infections, a broad T cell repertoire able to recognise many different types of bacterial epitopes (proteins as well as lipids) enhances the efficiency of the immune response against Mtb (Boom et al., 2003). The balance between different T helper subsets, especially Th1, T (Fox P3+) regulatory cells and Th17 helper cells may also be a key factor (Korn et al., 2007; Liang et al., 2006; Marin et al., 2010; Torrado and Cooper, 2010) and could potentially be explored for diagnostic purposes.

For some time, assays assessing the presence of Mtb specific memory CD8 and CD4 T cells have been used to identify those who previously have been infected with Mtb. Mtb-specific T cells are detectable within 2 - 3 weeks of acute infection in the peripheral blood and mark the end of the phase of rapid bacterial replication and bacterial containment. Interestingly, studies in mice suggest a late adaptive T cell response, which is linked to a delay in activation of T helper cells (Wolf et al., 2008). The measurement of Mtb specific T cells is therefore diagnostically insensitive in acute infection. This apparent problem may be overcome by the detection of Mtb-specific T cells directly at the site of infection, such as in fluid from broncho-alveolar lavage and cerebrospinal fluid, during early stages of disease in selected cohorts (Jafari et al., 2009; Thomas et al., 2008). On the other hand, the long-term maintenance of memory T cell responses to pathogens in peripheral blood (Semmo et al., 2006) make the measurements of Mtb specific T cells useful as a diagnostic cross-sectional assay to test for prior exposure to Mtb.

3.1 Tuberculin skin test and Interferon-γ release asssays (IGRA)

One of the current well established diagnostic approaches, which is based on a T cell mediated delayed hypersensitivity reaction, is the tuberculin skin test (TST). The TST is generally performed by an intradermal injection of 5 tuberculin units using purified protein derivative (PPD) following the Mantoux method. The transverse diameter of the skin induration occuring after 48-72 hours is typically measured. Therefore at least two clinic visits are required for a valid test which may prove a problem. In our recent study of Western Australian refugee children, the TST was initiated in 341 children; however reading was not possible in 37 (11%) children due to non-attendance at clinic appointments or absence of the child at scheduled home visits (Lucas et al., 2010). The interpretation of results and determination of cut-offs also varies and is infuenced by age, previous BCG vaccination and Mtb infection risk. In addition, this method is now recognised to have other limitations, such as poor specificity due to cross reactivity with both non-tuberculous mycobacteria and BCG (National Health Service, 2005) (Table 1).

More recently, measurement of IFN-γ -producing memory T cells specific for Mtb has been introduced into the clinical practice of many countries. Two blood-based IFN-γ release assays (IGRAs) are available for diagnostic use, the Quantiferon-TB gold in-tube (QFT-GIT; Cellestis, Carnegie, Australia) and the T-SPOT.TB (Oxford Immunotech,Oxford, UK). Both assays have high specificity for adult Mtb infection including in BCG-vaccinated populations (Lucas et al., 2010). Both assays measure T cell IFN-γ production in response to antigens encoded by the RD1 gene which is present in all strains of Mtb but is not present in the Mycobacterium bovis genome from which BCG is derived. This eliminates BCG cross-reactivity, however cross-reactivity to a limited number of non-Mtb mycobacteria (M. kansasii, M. szulgai, M. marinum) remains. T-SPOT.TB is an enzyme-linked immunospot (ELISpot) assay that measures the response to two antigens, early-secreted antigenic target 6 (ESAT-6) and culture filtrate protein 10 (CFP-10). The QFT-GIT assay is a whole blood IGRA assay that includes an additional Mtb-specific antigen (TB7.7). In the few head-to head comparisons of the latest generation tests, T-SPOT.TB and QFT-GIT both perform satisfactorily. Some studies however suggest that the use of the T-SPOT.TB assay may be the preferred option in subjects with primary and secondary (HIV, iatrogenic) immunodeficiencies (Lalvani, 2007; Pai et al., 2008b).

To date, there has been limited focus on high incidence paediatric populations, which are at greater risk of reactivation and extrapulmonary manifestations of Mtb, including TB meningitis. We recently published a prospective comparative study of IGRAs and TST for the diagnosis of LTBI in 524 refugee children from countries with a high prevalence of MTb that resettled to Australia (Lucas et al., 2010). This study included 182 children <5 years of age. In our study, the T-SPOT.TB and QFT-GIT had similar rates of positivity (8% and 10%, respectively) and showed good concordance when both tests gave definitive results (kappa= 0.78; $p<0.0001$). Surprisingly, both IGRAs had significant failure rates: 15% of QFT-GIT gave indeterminate results due to failed mitogen response and 14% of T-SPOT.TB results were inconclusive because of insufficient mononuclear leukocyte yields. Failure of the QFT-GIT mitogen response was associated with African ethnicity and co-morbid infections, particularly with helminths. Overall, the TST results showed low concordance (about 50%) with both IGRAs. This study highlights the influence of age, ethnicity and clinical status on IGRA results and the limitations of using these T cell based tests in refugee children.

In general, IGRAs are likely to be too complex and expensive for point-of-care testing in the Developing World, but their use in developed countries where the Mtb burden is much smaller, is currently justified. In addition, they have a role in the identification of subjects with latent Mtb prior to immunosuppressive therapy, including treatment with novel biologic drugs such as TNF-α antagonists (Bellofiore et al., 2009).

3.2 Assessment of the role of other cytokines in Mtb infection

As the cooperation between macrophages and T lymphocytes is critical for acute and long-term control of Mtb, cytokines produced during their interaction, such as IL-1, IL-2, IFN-γ, TNF-α, IL-12 and IL-23 are thought to play a critical role, all of which have potential to be used as surrogate markers of anti-Mtb immunity (Doherty et al., 2009). In addition, there is increasing evidence that during acute Mtb infection many of these pro-inflammatory cytokines are counteracted by induction of immune suppressive regulators (such as IL-10, TGF-β RII, IL1-R and IDO) in addition to upregulation of intracellular molecules, e.g. IRAK-M and suppressor of cytokine signalling (SOCS) (Almeida et al., 2009). Mtb-activated CD4+ T cells also release TNF-α which can trigger cell lysis in infected macrophages and may kill intracellular Mtb (Canaday et al., 2001) and Mtb specific TNF-α secreting CD4+ T cells have been shown to be more frequent during active than latent disease (Harari et al., 2011). In addition, IL- 18 from macrophages and DCs has recently been explored for its protective immunity against tuberculosis (Schneider et al., 2010). Newer diagnostic approaches that allow the measurement of mulitple cytokine simultaneously may aid in the diagnosis of latent infection, but also are promising tools for the identification of acute infection/re-activation/infection of Mtb.

3.3 Antibody responses to Mtb

Serological blood tests detect the host's humoral response (antibodies) to a pathogen that can remain circulating in the blood for several years. However, as with any pathogen specific immune response (antibody or T cell) this response develops after initial infection, and therefore its use at early infection timepoints is limited. Overall, these tests can be quick and inexpensive to perform using either ELISA or immunochromatographic formats. In the case of Mtb infection, serological assays would also be more practical for children, for whom sputum samples are difficult to obtain.

It is estimated that more than a million Mtb serological tests are performed each year, predominantly in high disease burden countries (Steingart et al., 2011). However, many of these assays vary in the antigens used, source and type of antigen and the class of immunoglobulin investigated. First generation antibody assays used crude mixtures of Mtb that tended to give low specificity results; most likely due to shared antigens between mycobacteria species. A review to assess the efficacy of "in-house" serological assays showed that assays with a combination of antigens gave higher sensitivity and specificity than earlier assays (Steingart et al., 2009). Furthermore, assays detecting IgG and IgA anti-Mtb antibodies gave higher sensitivity values for the detection of pulmonary Mtb than IgM-based assays. IgM-based assays may be better suited to the detection of acute Mtb infection as IgM is typically expressed early in the infection but then dissipates over time.

A recent systematic review commissioned by the WHO clearly showed that commercial serological assays for active Mtb infection exhibited substantial variation in sensitivity and specificity for pulmonary Mtb infection ((Steingart et al., 2011); Table 1). The review was based on 67 studies with 5,147 participants including 48% from low-middle income countries. Accordingly, on the 20th July 2011, WHO released a press statement warning against the use of serological tests for the diagnosis of active Mtb infection, stating that the currently available commercial serological tests exhibit low specificity and sensitivity leading to misdiagnosis, mistreatment and potential harm to public health (http://www.who.int/mediacentre/news/releases/2011/tb_20110720n/index.html).

The role of a protective antibody response in Mtb has been less investigated. Approximately 90% of patients produce antibodies to Mtb proteins with antibody profiles showing great inter-individual variation. So far, a clear correlation between antibody profiles and disease status has not been clearly established, making its use for routine diagnostics problematic (Lyashchenko et al., 1998; Wu et al., 2010). Recently, a major contribution to the field has been published by Kunnath-Velayudhan and colleagues (Kunnath-Velayudhan et al., 2010). They screened 500 sera from suspected Mtb infected subjects against the entire Mtb proteome using high-throughput microarray technology and identified signatures of antibody responses in subjects with active Mtb, with some variation across subjects, thus providing novel insights into the biology of the humoral response against Mtb and providing further steps to develop effective humoral immunodiagnostics.

4. Diagnosis of reactivation disease or low level pathogen detection

Upon inhalation of Mtb, mycobacteria are phagocytosed by alveolar macrophages that recruit mononuclear cells to the site of infection. This leads to the characteristic granuloma formation consisting of macrophages, monocytes and neutrophils. At later stages, the granuloma becomes more organised and infiltrated by lymphocytes (Russell et al., 2010). For the majority of cases Mtb is contained by the immune system. How the transition between the detection and control of acute infection to the establishment of latent Mtb infection is mediated, remains unknown. A critical factor, however, is the pathogen's ability to evade its complete elimination by the immune system. Studies have shown that even asymptomatic infected hosts harbour virulent bacteria in their tuberculous granulomas (Bouley et al., 2001; Tufariello et al., 2003). It is even possible that the granulomas paradoxically offer a niche for long-term survival of the bacteria. The barrier of activated macrophages and giant multinucleated cells that surround Mtb infected cells within granulomas are relatively impermeable to T cell infiltration although T cells remain closely associated at the site of infection (Tufariello et al., 2003). Thus paradoxically the combined efforts of the innate and adaptive immune response often contain and control the infection but fail to eliminate it. In fact the presence of Mtb antigens released into the host are thought to maintain the presence of an Mtb specific effector-memory population, which is absent in cases who have successfully eliminated the pathogen and only show evidence of a Mtb-specific central memory T cells (Millington et al., 2010). Ongoing adaptive immunity is essential in preventing reactivation of infection at a later stage (Boom et al., 2003). Reactivation disease occurs when latent bacteria from old, scarred granulomatous lesions are reactivated into an active, virulent state. A increased risk of reactivation arises when the host's immune system is compromised, which may be secondarily due to immune suppressive drugs, especially those that modify Mtb-specific immunity such as TNF-α antagonists, due to cancer, malnutrition or chronic viral infections, such as HIV. HIV+ individuals with advanced disease and low CD4+ T cell count face an approximate 10% risk per year of Mtb reactivation and co-infection of Mtb with HIV is now well documented (Shen et al., 2004). In the developing world therefore, Mtb has become one of the leading causes of death (Tufariello et al., 2003). This also highlights the problem that those with the greatest risk of reactivation are often cared for by those that are most vulnerable for Mtb infection and reinfection. Not surprisingly, this vicious cycle of reactivation/infection in developing countries has led to a flourishing Mtb spread and extensive resistance to most anti-Mtb drugs.

To-date no reliable routine diagnostics that allow pathogen recognition at low levels or immune markers that predict reactivation are available. In general, the principles underlying the diagnosis of reactivation disease will be similar to those used for the detection of early acute infection; namely pathogen based assays and assays which rely on immune markers associated with the innate immune system (see above). In addition, there are reports which suggest that a change in T cell based immunity against Mtb exists in acute and latent infection.

Casey et al., for example, expands the current technology of the T-SPOT.TB assay by measuring IFN-γ and IL-2 responses by Mtb specific T cells after stimulation with ESAT 6 and CFP 10 antigens, thus aiming to test T cells for polyfunctionality in active, treated and latent Mtb (Casey et al., 2010). The authors use a dual fluorescent ELISpot to measure two cytokines simultaneously, which could be adapted to routine –albeit expensive- clinical practice. They demonstrated that active untreated Mtb, compared to latent Mtb infection, was dominated by IFN-γ-only producing effector T cells. In addition, sequential testing of successfully treated patients revealed a shift from IFN-γ only producing T cells to a higher number of effector-memory cells secreting IL-2 and IFN-γ which confirms previous data, using a flowcytometric approach, by Caccamo et al (Caccamo et al., 2010).

5. Use of genetic studies to identify novel genes involved in Mtb pathogenesis

Recent technological advances has allowed the large-scale sampling of the human genome in a cost-effective manner and now allows researchers to examine, without a priori knowledge, genetic variations that may influence Mtb infection outcome. Furthermore, the deposit of whole genome sequences from individuals from different ethnic backgrounds into public databases allows a more comprehensive view of human genetic variation that better reflects the individuals at most risk of Mtb infection.

Genome-wide linkage studies to identify the transfer of chromosomal regions containing susceptibility genes, typically using families of affected individuals, have been performed on Mtb (reviewed in (Moller et al., 2009)). However, of the studies to date, none of the linkage peaks reach genome-wide significance. The majority of these studies targeted different populations and not surprisingly there is no obvious overlap between highlighted chromosome regions for each study.

The only reported genome-wide association study to date for Mtb involves the African TB Genetics consortium and the Wellcome Trust Case Control Consortium (Thye et al., 2010). In this study, individuals with tuberculosis and unaffected controls from the West African nations Ghana and The Gambia were genotyped for single nucleotide polymorphisms (SNPs) covering the entire genome. The initial study identified 17 loci associated with disease with a $p<10^{-5}$. However, subsequent replication studies found that the SNP rs4331426 had the highest association signal (OR 1.19; total number of individuals 11,425). Interestingly, this SNP is located within a gene-poor region of chromosome 18 (18q11.2) but does contain the gene GATA6, which encodes a transcription factor known to regulate arachidonate 15-lipoxygenase (ALOX15); a molecule involved in regulating the release of cytokines in lung epithelia cells ((Liu et al., 2009); reviewed in (Vannberg et al., 2011)). Although the role of this gene in Mtb susceptibility has not been clarified, it certainly remains a gene of interest.

But it is important to remember that Mtb is also a variable pathogen and it is likely that variation in the genetics of the host and pathogen are likely to be relevant in determining infection outcome.

6. Conclusion

Microbiological detections systems are likely to remain the gold standard for detection and identification of extracellular pathogens aided by the increasing complementary usage of PCR to shorten the time and improve the accuracy of identification. Future developments may also include screening of other less invasive sample types including volatile samples from the breath, for the presence of characteristic pathogen associated molecules or metabolic bi-products (Phillips et al., 2007). Sensitive physical detection technologies like those based on mass spectrophotometry (Metzger et al., 2010) may also make their way into larger clinical laboratories to assist in sample analysis.

Newly described cytokine networks such as those associated with inflammasome complexes (IL-1β, IL-18, IL-33) (Church et al., 2008), the IL-23/IL-17 inflammatory pathway (Kikly et al., 2006) are being studied at a basic research level and are likely to contribute additional insights into anti-pathogen immunity. The continued development of better assays for established biomarkers (e.g. monokine assay; Chakera et al., 2011) to improve sensitivity and specificity and the speed in which results are obtained or give additional insights into the immune responses to the pathogen will be central to these advances.

The complexities that underlie effective pathogen specific immunity is still incompletely understood and will continue to be informed by data generated using molecular approaches that measure changes in pathways that influence the response to infection. Advances in the CHIP technology (Weinmann et al., 2002), which involves the selection of specific DNA binding proteins by antibodies, will add additional dimension to the data being obtained and show which genetic levers are being pulled during a response to a given pathogen. Furthermore, this technology is complemented by Next-generation sequencing that will allow the detection of low frequency viral and host variants as well as transcripts. It is hoped that insights generated by such approaches, along with further iterations of these technologies will result in more sophisticated approaches and tools to be developed, affordable to the countries burdened with the highest levels of Mtb.

7. References

Almeida, A. S., P. M. Lago, et al. (2009). "Tuberculosis is associated with a down-modulatory lung immune response that impairs Th1-type immunity." J Immunol 183(1): 718-31.

Azzurri, A., O. Y. Sow, et al. (2005). "IFN-gamma-inducible protein 10 and pentraxin 3 plasma levels are tools for monitoring inflammation and disease activity in Mycobacterium tuberculosis infection." Microbes Infect 7(1): 1-8.

Baylan, O., A. Balkan, et al. (2006). "The predictive value of serum procalcitonin levels in adult patients with active pulmonary tuberculosis." Jpn J Infect Dis 59(3): 164-7.

Bellofiore, B., A. Matarese, et al. (2009). "Prevention of tuberculosis in patients taking tumor necrosis factor-alpha blockers." J Rheumatol Suppl 83: 76-7.

Berrington, W. R. and T. R. Hawn (2007). "Mycobacterium tuberculosis, macrophages, and the innate immune response: does common variation matter?" Immunol Rev 219: 167-86.

Berry, M. P., C. M. Graham, et al. (2010). "An interferon-inducible neutrophil-driven blood transcriptional signature in human tuberculosis." Nature 466(7309): 973-7.

Boom, W. H., D. H. Canaday, et al. (2003). "Human immunity to M. tuberculosis: T cell subsets and antigen processing." Tuberculosis (Edinb) 83(1-3): 98-106.

Bouley, D. M., N. Ghori, et al. (2001). "Dynamic nature of host-pathogen interactions in Mycobacterium marinum granulomas." Infect Immun 69(12): 7820-31.

Caccamo, N., G. Guggino, et al. (2010). "Multifunctional CD4(+) T cells correlate with active Mycobacterium tuberculosis infection." Eur J Immunol 40(8): 2211-20.

Canaday, D. H., R. J. Wilkinson, et al. (2001). "CD4(+) and CD8(+) T cells kill intracellular Mycobacterium tuberculosis by a perforin and Fas/Fas ligand-independent mechanism." J Immunol 167(5): 2734-42.

Casey, R., D. Blumenkrantz, et al. (2010). "Enumeration of functional T-cell subsets by fluorescence-immunospot defines signatures of pathogen burden in tuberculosis." PLoS One 5(12): e15619.

Chakera A, Bennett SC, et al. (2011). "A whole blood monokine-based reporter assay provides a sensitive and robust measurement of the antigen-specific T cell response." J Transl Med. 9(1):143.

Chen, Y. C., C. C. Hsiao, et al. (2010). "Toll-like receptor 2 gene polymorphisms, pulmonary tuberculosis, and natural killer cell counts." BMC Med Genet 11: 17.

Church, L. D., G. P. Cook, et al. (2008). "Primer: inflammasomes and interleukin 1beta in inflammatory disorders." Nat Clin Pract Rheumatol 4(1): 34-42.

Constantoulakis, P., E. Filiou, et al. (2010). "In vivo expression of innate immunity markers in patients with Mycobacterium tuberculosis infection." BMC Infect Dis 10: 243.

Corbett, E. L., B. Marston, et al. (2006). "Tuberculosis in sub-Saharan Africa: opportunities, challenges, and change in the era of antiretroviral treatment." Lancet 367(9514): 926-37.

Cuevas, L. E., N. Al-Sonboli, et al. (2011). "LED fluorescence microscopy for the diagnosis of pulmonary tuberculosis: a multi-country cross-sectional evaluation." PLoS Med 8(7): e1001057.

Daley, P., S. Thomas, et al. (2007). "Nucleic acid amplification tests for the diagnosis of tuberculous lymphadenitis: a systematic review." Int J Tuberc Lung Dis 11(11): 1166-76.

Dinnes, J., J. Deeks, et al. (2007). "A systematic review of rapid diagnostic tests for the detection of tuberculosis infection." Health Technol Assess 11(3): 1-196.

Djoba Siawaya, J. F., N. B. Bapela, et al. (2008). "Immune parameters as markers of tuberculosis extent of disease and early prediction of anti-tuberculosis chemotherapy response." J Infect 56(5): 340-7.

Doherty, M., R. S. Wallis, et al. (2009). "Biomarkers for tuberculosis disease status and diagnosis." Curr Opin Pulm Med 15(3): 181-7.

Eugen-Olsen, J., P. Gustafson, et al. (2002). "The serum level of soluble urokinase receptor is elevated in tuberculosis patients and predicts mortality during treatment: a community study from Guinea-Bissau." Int J Tuberc Lung Dis 6(8): 686-92.

Flores, L., K. Steingart, et al. (2011). "Antigen detection tests for the diagnosis of tuberculosis: A systematic review and meta-analysis." Clin Vaccine Immunol.

Flores, L. L., M. Pai, et al. (2005). "In-house nucleic acid amplification tests for the detection of Mycobacterium tuberculosis in sputum specimens: meta-analysis and meta-regression." BMC Microbiol 5: 55.

Fuchs, D., A. Hausen, et al. (1984). "Neopterin as an index of immune response in patients with tuberculosis." Lung 162(6): 337-46.

Goto, M., Y. Noguchi, et al. (2003). "Diagnostic value of adenosine deaminase in tuberculous pleural effusion: a meta-analysis." Ann Clin Biochem 40(Pt 4): 374-81.

Greco, S., E. Girardi, et al. (2003). "Adenosine deaminase and interferon gamma measurements for the diagnosis of tuberculous pleurisy: a meta-analysis." Int J Tuberc Lung Dis 7(8): 777-86.

Greco, S., E. Girardi, et al. (2006). "Current evidence on diagnostic accuracy of commercially based nucleic acid amplification tests for the diagnosis of pulmonary tuberculosis." Thorax 61(9): 783-90.

Harari, A., V. Rozot, et al. (2011). "Dominant TNF-alpha+ Mycobacterium tuberculosis-specific CD4+ T cell responses discriminate between latent infection and active disease." Nat Med 17(3): 372-6.

Immanuel, C., R. Rajeswari, et al. (2001). "Serial evaluation of serum neopterin in HIV seronegative patients treated for tuberculosis." Int J Tuberc Lung Dis 5(2): 185-90.

Jacobsen, M., D. Repsilber, et al. (2007). "Candidate biomarkers for discrimination between infection and disease caused by Mycobacterium tuberculosis." J Mol Med 85(6): 613-21.

Jafari, C., S. Thijsen, et al. (2009). "Bronchoalveolar lavage enzyme-linked immunospot for a rapid diagnosis of tuberculosis: a Tuberculosis Network European Trialsgroup study." Am J Respir Crit Care Med 180(7): 666-73.

Jiang, J., H. Z. Shi, et al. (2007). "Diagnostic value of interferon-gamma in tuberculous pleurisy: a metaanalysis." Chest 131(4): 1133-41.

Kalantri, S., M. Pai, et al. (2005). "Bacteriophage- based tests for the detection of Mycobacterium tuberculosis in clinical specimens: a systematic review and meta-analysis." BMC Infect Dis 5: 59.

Kandemir, O., B. Uluba, et al. (2003). "Elevation of procalcitonin level in patients with pulmonary tuberculosis and in medical staff with close patient contact." Arch Med Res 34(4): 311-4.

Kikly, K., L. Liu, et al. (2006). "The IL-23/Th(17) axis: therapeutic targets for autoimmune inflammation." Curr Opin Immunol 18(6): 670-5.

Korn, T., E. Bettelli, et al. (2007). "IL-21 initiates an alternative pathway to induce proinflammatory T(H)17 cells." Nature 448(7152): 484-7.

Kunnath-Velayudhan, S., H. Salamon, et al. (2010). "Dynamic antibody responses to the Mycobacterium tuberculosis proteome." Proc Natl Acad Sci U S A 107(33): 14703-8.

Lalvani, A. (2007). "Diagnosing tuberculosis infection in the 21st century: new tools to tackle an old enemy." Chest 131(6): 1898-906.

Liang, Q. L., H. Z. Shi, et al. (2008). "Diagnostic accuracy of adenosine deaminase in tuberculous pleurisy: a meta-analysis." Respir Med 102(5): 744-54.

Liang, S. C., X. Y. Tan, et al. (2006). "Interleukin (IL)-22 and IL-17 are coexpressed by Th17 cells and cooperatively enhance expression of antimicrobial peptides." J Exp Med 203(10): 2271-9.

Ling, D. I., L. L. Flores, et al. (2008). "Commercial nucleic-acid amplification tests for diagnosis of pulmonary tuberculosis in respiratory specimens: meta-analysis and meta-regression." PLoS One 3(2): e1536.

Liu, C., D. Xu, et al. (2009). "15-Lipoxygenase-1 induces expression and release of chemokines in cultured human lung epithelial cells." Am J Physiol Lung Cell Mol Physiol 297(1): L196-203.

Lonnroth, K. and M. Raviglione (2008). "Global epidemiology of tuberculosis: prospects for control." Semin Respir Crit Care Med 29(5): 481-91.

Lucas, M., P. Nicol, et al. (2010). "A prospective large-scale study of methods for the detection of latent Mycobacterium tuberculosis infection in refugee children." Thorax 65(5): 442-8.

Lyashchenko, K., R. Colangeli, et al. (1998). "Heterogeneous antibody responses in tuberculosis." Infect Immun 66(8): 3936-40.

Maertzdorf, J., D. Repsilber, et al. (2010). "Human gene expression profiles of susceptibility and resistance in tuberculosis." Genes Immun.

Maher, D., C. Dye, et al. (2007). "Planning to improve global health: the next decade of tuberculosis control." Bull World Health Organ 85(5): 341-7.

Marin, N. D., S. C. Paris, et al. (2010). "Regulatory T cell frequency and modulation of IFN-gamma and IL-17 in active and latent tuberculosis." Tuberculosis (Edinb) 90(4): 252-61.

Mase, S. R., A. Ramsay, et al. (2007). "Yield of serial sputum specimen examinations in the diagnosis of pulmonary tuberculosis: a systematic review." Int J Tuberc Lung Dis 11(5): 485-95.

Metzger, J., T. Kirsch, et al. (2010). "Urinary excretion of twenty peptides forms an early and accurate diagnostic pattern of acute kidney injury." Kidney Int 78(12): 1252-62.

Millington, K. A., S. Gooding, et al. (2010). "Mycobacterium tuberculosis-specific cellular immune profiles suggest bacillary persistence decades after spontaneous cure in untreated tuberculosis." J Infect Dis 202(11): 1685-9.

Moller, M., E. de Wit, et al. (2009). "Past, present and future directions in human genetic susceptibility to tuberculosis." FEMS Immunol Med Microbiol 58(1): 3-26.

National Health Service, U. (2005). The Mantoux test: Administration, reading and interpretation. London, Department of Health Publications: 1-6.

Nyamande, K. and U. G. Lalloo (2006). "Serum procalcitonin distinguishes CAP due to bacteria, Mycobacterium tuberculosis and PJP." Int J Tuberc Lung Dis 10(5): 510-5.

Pai, M., L. L. Flores, et al. (2003). "Diagnostic accuracy of nucleic acid amplification tests for tuberculous meningitis: a systematic review and meta-analysis." Lancet Infect Dis 3(10): 633-43.

Pai, M., J. Minion, et al. (2010). "New and improved tuberculosis diagnostics: evidence, policy, practice, and impact." Curr Opin Pulm Med 16(3): 271-84.

Pai, M., A. Ramsay, et al. (2008). "Evidence-based tuberculosis diagnosis." PLoS Med 5(7): e156.

Pai, M., L. W. Riley, et al. (2004). "Interferon-gamma assays in the immunodiagnosis of tuberculosis: a systematic review." Lancet Infect Dis 4(12): 761-76.

Pai, M., A. Zwerling, et al. (2008). "Systematic review: T-cell-based assays for the diagnosis of latent tuberculosis infection: an update." Ann Intern Med 149(3): 177-84.

Phillips, M., R. N. Cataneo, et al. (2007). "Volatile biomarkers of pulmonary tuberculosis in the breath." Tuberculosis (Edinburgh, Scotland) 87: 44-52.

Prat, C., J. Dominguez, et al. (2006). "Procalcitonin and neopterin correlation with aetiology and severity of pneumonia." J Infect 52(3): 169-77.

Prevention. (2000). "Diagnostic Standards and Classification of Tuberculosis in Adults and Children. This official statement of the American Thoracic Society and the Centers for Disease Control and Prevention was adopted by the ATS Board of Directors, July 1999. This statement was endorsed by the Council of the Infectious Disease Society of America, September 1999." Am J Respir Crit Care Med 161(4 Pt 1): 1376-95.

Riquelme, A., M. Calvo, et al. (2006). "Value of adenosine deaminase (ADA) in ascitic fluid for the diagnosis of tuberculous peritonitis: a meta-analysis." J Clin Gastroenterol 40(8): 705-10.

Russell, D. G., C. E. Barry, 3rd, et al. (2010). "Tuberculosis: what we don't know can, and does, hurt us." Science 328(5980): 852-6.

Sarmiento, O. L., K. A. Weigle, et al. (2003). "Assessment by meta-analysis of PCR for diagnosis of smear-negative pulmonary tuberculosis." J Clin Microbiol 41(7): 3233-40.

Schleicher, G. K., V. Herbert, et al. (2005). "Procalcitonin and C-reactive protein levels in HIV-positive subjects with tuberculosis and pneumonia." Eur Respir J 25(4): 688-92.

Schneider, B. E., D. Korbel, et al. (2010). "A role for IL-18 in protective immunity against Mycobacterium tuberculosis." Eur J Immunol 40(2): 396-405.

Semmo, N., M. Lucas, et al. (2006). "Maintenance of HCV-specific T-cell responses in antibody-deficient patients a decade after early therapy." Blood 107(11): 4570-1.

Shen, Y., L. Shen, et al. (2004). "Clinical latency and reactivation of AIDS-related mycobacterial infections." J Virol 78(24): 14023-32.

Steingart, K. R., N. Dendukuri, et al. (2009). "Performance of purified antigens for serodiagnosis of pulmonary tuberculosis: a meta-analysis." Clin Vaccine Immunol 16(2): 260-76.

Steingart, K. R., L. L. Flores, et al. (2011). "Commercial serological tests for the diagnosis of active pulmonary and extrapulmonary tuberculosis: an updated systematic review and meta-analysis." PLoS Med 8(8): e1001062.

Steingart, K. R., M. Henry, et al. (2007). "Commercial serological antibody detection tests for the diagnosis of pulmonary tuberculosis: a systematic review." PLoS Med 4(6): e202.

Steingart, K. R., M. Henry, et al. (2007). "A systematic review of commercial serological antibody detection tests for the diagnosis of extrapulmonary tuberculosis." Thorax 62(10): 911-8.

Steingart, K. R., M. Henry, et al. (2006). "Fluorescence versus conventional sputum smear microscopy for tuberculosis: a systematic review." Lancet Infect Dis 6(9): 570-81.

Steingart, K. R., V. Ng, et al. (2006). "Sputum processing methods to improve the sensitivity of smear microscopy for tuberculosis: a systematic review." Lancet Infect Dis 6(10): 664-74.
Thomas, M. M., T. S. Hinks, et al. (2008). "Rapid diagnosis of Mycobacterium tuberculosis meningitis by enumeration of cerebrospinal fluid antigen-specific T-cells." Int J Tuberc Lung Dis 12(6): 651-7.
Thye, T., F. O. Vannberg, et al. (2010). "Genome-wide association analyses identifies a susceptibility locus for tuberculosis on chromosome 18q11.2." Nat Genet 42(9): 739-41.
Torrado, E. and A. M. Cooper (2010). "IL-17 and Th17 cells in tuberculosis." Cytokine Growth Factor Rev 21(6): 455-62.
Tufariello, J. M., J. Chan, et al. (2003). "Latent tuberculosis: mechanisms of host and bacillus that contribute to persistent infection." Lancet Infect Dis 3(9): 578-90.
Tuon, F. F., M. N. Litvoc, et al. (2006). "Adenosine deaminase and tuberculous pericarditis--a systematic review with meta-analysis." Acta Trop 99(1): 67-74.
Turgut, T., H. Akbulut, et al. (2006). "Serum interleukin-2 and neopterin levels as useful markers for treatment of active pulmonary tuberculosis." Tohoku J Exp Med 209(4): 321-8.
Vannberg, F. O., S. J. Chapman, et al. (2011). "Human genetic susceptibility to intracellular pathogens." Immunol Rev 240(1): 105-16.
Wallis, R. S., M. S. Helfand, et al. (1996). "Immune activation, allergic drug toxicity and mortality in HIV-positive tuberculosis." Tuber Lung Dis 77(6): 516-23.
Wallis, R. S., M. Pai, et al. (2010). "Biomarkers and diagnostics for tuberculosis: progress, needs, and translation into practice." Lancet 375(9729): 1920-37.
Walzl, G., K. Ronacher, et al. (2008). "Biomarkers for TB treatment response: challenges and future strategies." J Infect 57(2): 103-9.
Weinmann, A. S., P. S. Yan, et al. (2002). "Isolating human transcription factor targets by coupling chromatin immunoprecipitation and CpG island microarray analysis." Genes Dev 16(2): 235-44.
WHO (2006) "The stop TB strategy."
Wolf, A. J., L. Desvignes, et al. (2008). "Initiation of the adaptive immune response to Mycobacterium tuberculosis depends on antigen production in the local lymph node, not the lungs." J Exp Med 205(1): 105-15.
Wright, A., M. Zignol, et al. (2009). "Epidemiology of antituberculosis drug resistance 2002-07: an updated analysis of the Global Project on Anti-Tuberculosis Drug Resistance Surveillance." Lancet 373(9678): 1861-73.
Wu, X., Y. Yang, et al. (2010). "Humoral immune responses against the Mycobacterium tuberculosis 38-kilodalton, MTB48, and CFP-10/ESAT-6 antigens in tuberculosis." Clin Vaccine Immunol 17(3): 372-5.
Xu, H. B., R. H. Jiang, et al. (2010). "Diagnostic value of adenosine deaminase in cerebrospinal fluid for tuberculous meningitis: a meta-analysis." Int J Tuberc Lung Dis 14(11): 1382-7.

12

Nanodiagnostics for Tuberculosis

Bruno Veigas, Gonçalo Doria and Pedro V. Baptista*
CIGMH, Departamento de Ciências da Vida, Faculdade de Ciências e Tecnologia,
Universidade Nova de Lisboa
Portugal

1. Introduction

Tuberculosis (TB) remains one of the most serious infectious diseases in the world requiring new and more effective diagnostics and treatments (World Health Organization [WHO], 2010). Several approaches have been developed to improve TB diagnostics, reducing the time from weeks to a few days that still require demanding expertise technical personal for labor intensive and expensive methods, which hamper application in resource-poor countries where the main TB epidemic is observed. Nanotechnology has triggered the development of new and cheaper approaches for biomolecular recognition that may circumvent the current limitations of conventional molecular diagnostic methods used in the global fight against TB. This new era of molecular nanodiagnostics may provide a rapid and sensitive detection of the main TB etiologic agent in humans, i.e. *Mycobacterium tuberculosis*.

Nanodiagnostics can be defined as the use of nano-sized materials, devices or systems for diagnostics purposes. Biological tests measuring the presence or activity of selected analytes become quicker, more sensitive and more flexible when nanoscale particles are put to work as tags or labels, with numerous advantages over more traditional procedures, for example fluorescence and chemiluminescence technology. Here we will provide a closer look into nanodiagnostics systems developed for TB diagnostics and/or *M. tuberculosis* detection and characterization, such as nanoparticle-based systems (e.g. gold, silver, silica and quantum dots) and nanocantilevers. These techniques are already showing to be more sensitive and specific than conventional commercial molecular diagnostics methodologies although many aspects of nanodiagnostics for TB still need further evaluation and validation. Current advances in nanofabrication may enable the construction of cheap and full-automated devices, extending the limits of current molecular diagnostics and enable point- of-care diagnostics.

2. Tuberculosis

Tuberculosis is caused by *M. tuberculosis*, a member of the *Mycobacterium tuberculosis* complex (MTBC) and, according to the most current statistics of the World Health

---

* Corresponding Author

Organization, remains one of the most serious infectious diseases in the world, being responsible for 1.7 million deaths and 9.4 million new cases in 2009 alone (WHO, 2010). The emergence of multidrug-resistant TB also represents a serious threat to the TB control and an increasing public health problem (Deun et al., 2010), leading to a global need for rapid drug susceptibility testing. Single nucleotide sequence variations (mutations and/or polymorphisms) within *M. tuberculosis* genome have been associated with antibiotic resistance for all first-line drugs (isoniazid, rifampin, pyrazinamide, ethambutol, and streptomycin), and for several second-line and newer drugs (ethionamide, fluoroquinolones, macrolides, and nitroimidazopyrans), making these sequences ideal targets for the development of molecular drug susceptibility testing (Abebe et al., 2011; Miller et al., 1994; Musser, 1995; Soini & Musser, 2001; Telenti et al., 1993).

The mainstay for TB diagnostics in endemic developing countries is sputum smear microscopy (Perkins, 2009). However, the sensitivity of this technology is low as it can only detect roughly half of all active cases of tuberculosis when properly used - in people with co-infections and in children the sensitivity is even lower. Moreover, though routinely described as a simple technology, microscopy is actually complex, and highly dependent on the training and diligence of the technician, requiring multiple examinations which may take weeks to complete, with the consequence that many patients drop out during the diagnostic process. Several diagnostic approaches have brought incremental improvements for the direct detection, species identification and drug susceptibility testing of mycobacteria that are capable of reducing the laboratorial time from weeks to a few days (Barnard et al., 2008; D'Amato et al., 1995; De Beenhouwer et al., 1995; Griffith et al., 2007; Hillemann et al., 2005; Hirano et al., 1999; Moore et al., 2006; Park et al., 2002; Rossau et al., 1997; Sharma et al., 2003; Traore et al., 2000). Most of these approaches for direct detection of TB and drug susceptibility from clinical specimens, including several commercial tests, rely on complex and expensive DNA amplification based procedures (e.g. PCR), whereas the need is for affordable, simple and high-throughput systems with the possibility to use small amounts of sample (Cheng et al., 2005; Das et al., 2010; Shamputa et al., 2004; Watterson et al., 1998). These molecular recognition assays still need to make the way to widespread utilization in some technological advanced countries, which will definitely delay the required validation and setup for simplified platforms for general use at more remote and less equipped areas.

Some of the diagnostic tools expected to be introduced into control programs will be incremental improvements on existing technologies while others will be radically new. The speed and extent of adoption of new technologies will depend on the balance between the benefits they bring and the degree of disruption their implementation causes. For instance, a simplified microscopy method may see greater adoption than a novel alternative that necessitates changes in the way testing or case notification are carried out. On the other hand, a new method that rapidly identifies all smear-positive and many smear-negative cases might, if suitably robust and specific, see widespread use and could substantially replace microscopy. Point-of-care diagnosis is instrumental to TB control because, despite having the necessary treatment, strategies in some regions are rather ineffective (see South Africa as an example). Identifying new cases very quickly and getting patients immediately on to treatment are crucial in addressing this pandemic. New diagnostic tools for drug resistant TB (TB that is resistant to drugs - multi-drug resistant TB, MDR-TB) are urgently needed for reducing diagnostic time from months to days.

Several new technologies are under development, which will enable the presumptive diagnosis of MDR-TB in just one to two days, compared with two or more months when using conventional culture and drug susceptibility tests. Rapid diagnosis of MDR-TB will have several benefits: earlier treatment of patients, reduction of time spent on inappropriate and ineffective treatment (thereby promoting the development of further drug resistance), and reduction of MDR-TB spreading in congregate settings.

3. Nanodiagnostics for TB

Nanotechnology introduced new paradigms for molecular diagnostics - nanodiagnostics, where the increased sensitivity, specificity, speed and reduced cost constitutes an appealing alternative to conventional techniques (Azzazy et al., 2006). Because we are dealing with nanometer sized objects and/or nanometer scale, bulk matter physics does not apply and amazing and extraordinary new properties arise. This interesting field relies on the knowledge and technological developments emerging from transdisciplinary research efforts that bring together a plethora of expertise from areas as diverse as Materials Science, Physics, Biology and Biotechnology, Chemistry and Medicine. From the intersection of these complementarities new and radical approaches can be explored towards application in platforms for biomolecular recognition (e.g. nucleic acids, antibodies, proteins, etc.) that can be miniaturized for point of care utilization and/or for enhanced portability for small laboratory settings in remote areas without the standard access to conventional laboratory equipment and apparatus. Nanodiagnostics have redefined the standards for molecular diagnostics, triggering the development of new approaches in biomolecular recognition and analytical systems, where the most promising approaches include nanoparticles (NPs), nanotubes, nanopores and nanocantilever technologies (Baptista et al., 2008; Branton et al., 2008; Jain, 2007; Rosi & Mirkin, 2005; Wang et al., 2009). Their potential arises from recognition events occurring at one-to-one interactions between analytes and signal-generating nanostructures, allowing for an increased sensitivity and specificity at lower costs.

Different nanodiagnostics systems have been developed for the molecular diagnostics of TB. Despite the wide range of nanoscale systems being used for biomolecular assays in general (e.g. electromechanical, electrochemical) (Azzazy et al., 2006; Das et al., 2010; Jain, 2007), nanoparticle based systems, such as gold, silver, silica and quantum dots (QDs), have been the most widely used for TB diagnostics due to their unique physicochemical properties, that offer greater sensitivity than conventional reporter molecules and can be easily tuned and functionalized by simple chemistry modulation and derivatization (Azzazy, 2009). Table 1 summarizes existing nanotechnology based systems applied to TB diagnostics.

3.1 Nanoparticles

Nanoparticles are typically in the size range of 1–100 nm and can have different shapes and compositions (Liu, 2006). They are structurally robust and have very specific size dependent properties that differ considerably from those observed on microparticles or bulk materials. Depending on their size and composition they exhibit peculiar properties, such as quantum confinement in semiconductor nanocrystals, surface plasmon resonance (SPR) in some metal NPs and superparamagnetism in magnetic materials (Vollath, 2008). They also provide large

Technology	Description	Application(s)	Reference(s)
Noble metal NPs	Detection relies on the evaluation of SPR change upon aggregation and the concomitant colorimetric changes that can be assessed by the naked eye.	> Specific detection of *M tuberculosis* complex, *M. avium* complex, *M. avium subsp. paratuberculosis*, *M. bovis* and *M. tuberculosis*. > Detection of *rpo*B mutations associated with drug resistance.	Baptista et al., 2006; Costa et al., 2010; Liandris et al., 2009; Silva et al., 2008, 2010; Soo et al., 2009; Veigas et al., 2010
Magnetic NPs	Detection by measurement of the spin-spin relaxation time. Minimal sample preparation needed, without the need for sample amplification.	> High sensitive detection of *bacillus Calmette-Guérin*.	Kaittanis et al., 2007; Lee et al., 2009
Quantum Dots	Fluorescence detection of inorganic fluorophores with size-dependent optical properties, bright and narrow fluorescence. Highly sensitive. Optimal for multiplex assays.	> Conjugation of streptavidin-coated QDs with specific bacteriophage. > Integration with magnetic NPs for the detection of *M. tuberculosis* and *M. avium subsp. paratuberculosis*.	Rotem et al., 2006; Gazouli et al., 2010
Silica NPs	Fluorescence detection of NPs with large quantities of fluorophore molecules inside a polymer or silica matrix. Easy conjugation with several biomolecules and fluorophore making. Ideal for multiplex assays.	> Detection of *M. tuberculosis* by combining luminescent NPs and indirect immunofluorescence microscopy. > Improved two-color flow-cytometry assay by a combination of thc bioconjugated fluorescent silica NPs and SYBR Green I to avoid false positives.	Qin et al., 2007, 2008

Technology	Description	Application(s)	Reference(s)
Electro-chemical devices	Electrochemical nanofabricated sensors. Portable microfluidic nuclear magnetic resonance biosensor for rapid, quantitative, and multiplexed detection of biological targets. Reduced cost of the automated sensitive detection. Ideal for point-of-care applications.	> Specific detection of *M. tuberculosis* by nanostructured zinc oxide (nsZnO) films. > Amorphous/ nanocrystalline biosensor integrated into an optoelectronic platform for the specific identification of *M. tuberculosis* complex members.	Das et al., 2010; Lee et al., 2010; Wang et al., 1997; Prabhakar et al., 2008;

Table 1. Nanotechnology systems for TB diagnostics

surface to volume ratio with the same size range of biomolecules and cellular organelles, allowing a nearly one-on-one interaction between the NP and the biomolecule of interest (Azzazy et al., 2006, 2007; Jain, 2005) and making them of high potential for use in *in vitro* diagnostics. The most promising NPs already applied to TB diagnostics are gold, magnetic and silica NPs, and QDs. Size-dependent properties of the NPs also enable modification of the surface for conjugation with various biomolecules allowing for a wide range of bioassay applications (Salata, 2004).

3.1.1 Noble metal nanoparticles

Nobel metal NPs have attracted considerable attention in molecular diagnostic applications due to their simplicity and versatility, becoming a critical component in the development of nanotechnology-based detection of pathogens (Liu, 2006). Gold NPs (AuNPs), in particular, have been extensively used due to their unique optical properties with their typical bright red color in colloidal solutions associated with a well-defined SPR band in the visible region of the spectrum (Halfpenny & Wright, 2010). This SPR is originated from the collective oscillation of conduction band electrons at the NPs' surface induced by the interacting electromagnetic radiation of light. The SPR band is weakly dependent on size of the NP and refractive index of the surrounding media, but changes considerably with the composition, shape and inter-particle distance (Johnson et al., 2007). In the latter case, the aggregation of AuNPs leads to a pronounced color transition from red to blue due to plasmon coupling between NPs (Jain, 2007). Another remarkable property of AuNPs is the easiness of chemical functionalization via the use of thiol-ligands (e.g. thiol-modified oligonucleotides, antibodies or other biomolecules) that form quasi-covalent bonds with the NP's gold surface, rendering gold nanoprobes for specific target recognition (Daniel & Astruc, 2004).

Most AuNPs based methods rely on the colorimetric changes of the colloidal solution upon aggregation either mediated by a change to the dielectric medium or by recognition of a specific target. The design of these systems is centered in the ability of complementary targets to balance and control inter-particle attractive and repulsive forces, which determine whether AuNPs are stabilized or aggregated and, consequently, the SPR band and color of the solution remains unaltered or changes, respectively. For example, a specific complementary target can hybridize to the gold nanoprobes and promote an inter-particle cross-linking aggregation (e.g. when using two nanoprobes with contiguous target recognition) or stabilize the nanoprobes against the changes of the dielectric medium, which otherwise would induce a non-cross-linking aggregation of the nanoprobes in the absence of a complementary target (e.g. exploring the differential salt induced non-cross-linking aggregation of the nanoprobes) (Baptista et al., 2005).

The first application of AuNPs for the molecular diagnostics of *M. tuberculosis* was introduced by Baptista et al. (Baptista et al., 2006). The method consists in differential stabilization of gold nanoprobes in the presence of different DNA targets. The presence of a complementary target prevents nanoprobe aggregation and the solution remains red, while non-complementary/mismatched targets or their absence do not prevent gold nanoprobe aggregation, resulting in a visible change of color from red to blue. The gold nanoprobes were functionalized with thiol-modified oligonucleotides harboring a sequence derived from the *M. tuberculosis* RNA polymerase β-subunit gene sequence suitable for mycobacteria identification. The methodology was tested in clinical samples demonstrating high efficiency when combined with an initial round of PCR for target amplification (Baptista et al., 2006) - see Figure 1.

The attained results have shown a 100% concordance with the available commercial molecular TB diagnostics test INNO-LiPA Rif.TB. Following optimization towards detection of single base mismatches (Doria et al., 2010), this strategy was applied to the rapid detection of MTBC strains and simultaneous characterization of the presence of mutations associated with rifampicin resistance (Veigas et al., 2010). This low-complexity assay enabled the detection of mutations D516V and S531L from MTBC clinical specimens with remarkable sensitivity in just a few hours. Based on the molecular signatures of MTBC members and the most common mutations associated with RIF resistance in *M. tuberculosis*, a two-step approach based on the PCR amplification of a fragment of *rpo*B gene and subsequent hybridization with specific nanoprobes, namely a probe for the rpoB locus shared by all the members of the MTBC and a probe specific to MTBC members, was developed. Three additional sets of probes specific for the most common point mutations associated with RIF resistance (D516V; H526D; S531L) were also designed and synthesized. Each set composed of two probes: one complementary to the wild-type sequence and the other complementary to the mutation. A limit of detection could be set at 75 nM, however, for robust single base mismatch determination, 117 nM of DNA target were used per assay. This non-cross-linking approach correctly detected the presence of DNA from members of the MTBC in 83.3% of all samples, when compared to the INNO-LiPA Rif.TB assay. By means of a set of two probes for each mutation associated to RIF resistance to be screened (mutations in codons 516, 526 and 531 of the rpoB gene), it was possible to correctly score the presence of at least one of the mutations in 81% of all samples also screened via the INNO-LiPA Rif.TB assay. Following PCR amplification, the method takes only 90 min to yield a colorimetric result which, through the use of a suitable photodetector (e.g. UV/visible spectrophotometer, microplate reader, etc.), may be used in medium throughput analysis at a peripheral laboratory or point-of-care. Fast and reliable identification of MTBC members and mutations within the *rpo*B gene is of great advantage as it is a secondary marker for isoniazid resistance allowing to predict, with a high degree of confidence, whether the strain is indeed a multidrug-resistant TB (Hillemann et al., 2005).

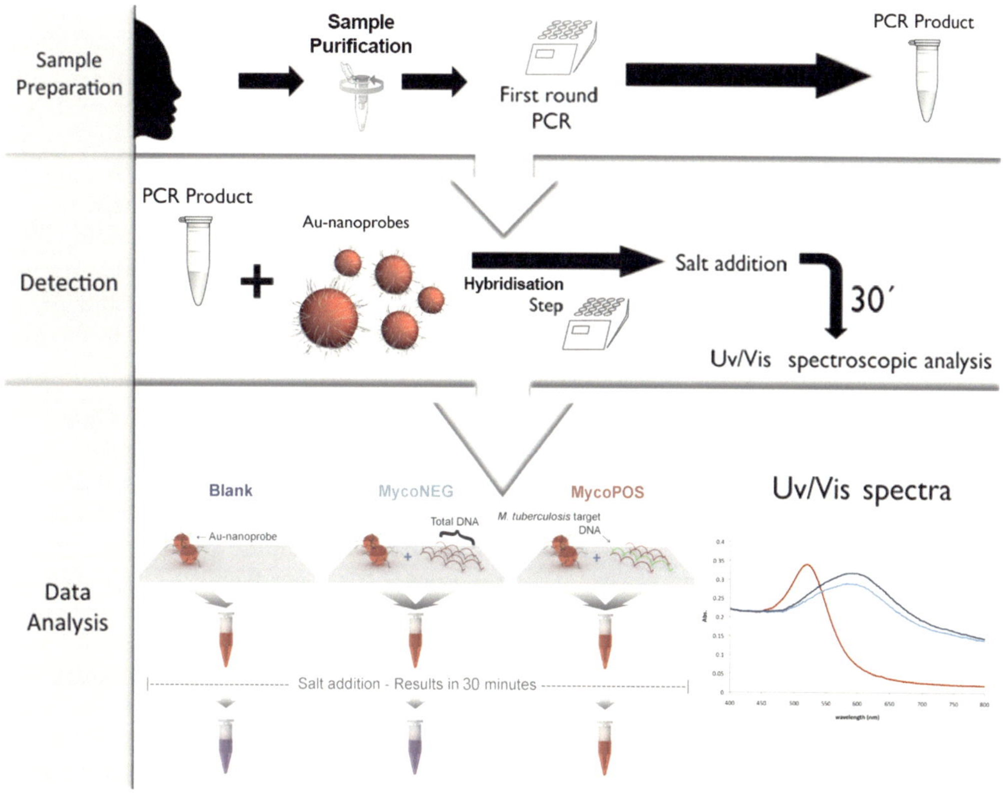

Fig. 1. Non-cross-linking detection of MTBC members. A DNA sample is extracted from a patient and amplified by a first round PCR. The resulting PCR product is characterized using gold nanoprobes and following a non-cross-linking approach that consists of a visual comparison between solutions before and after salt induced nanoprobe aggregation: 'Blank', nanoprobe alone; 'MycoNEG', nanoprobe in the presence of a non-complementary DNA sequence; and 'MycoPOS', nanoprobe in the presence of a complementary DNA sequence.

Optimization of the above strategy allowed detection and identification of members of the MTBC at the species level. Three different nanoprobes based on the *gyr*B *locus*, allowed the specific identification of MTBC, *M. bovis* and *M. tuberculosis* (Costa et al., 2010). Based on the conserved *gyr*B gene sequence between species from the MTBC, a set of primers was used to PCR amplify a specific 1020 bp fragment of the gene from MTBC species only. *In silico* alignment of the *gyr*B gene sequences showed three regions that allowed discrimination between MTBC members. As proof-of-concept, one probe was designed to identify this genomic region shared by all the members of the MTBC, and two probes were designed to specifically identify *M. tuberculosis* and *M. bovis*, respectively. The MTBC probe positively identified the members of the MTBC used in the assay, while clearly discriminating the non-members. The *M. tuberculosis* and *M. bovis* probes unequivocally identified the respective species. Also, a blind assay using mycobacteria strains isolated from fifteen different clinical samples showed 100% concordance with the results attained by the *gyr*B-PCR-RFLP method.

Towards a point-of-care application, Baptista and co-workers further integrated the non-cross-linking nanoprobe-based method in an innovative optoelectronic platform that allows an analytical measurement of the colorimetric changes, hence to detect a target without the need of experienced personnel. The device integrates an amorphous/nanocrystalline biosensor and a light emission source with the non-cross-linking method for specific DNA detection. This low cost, fast and simple optoelectronic platform was optimized for the specific identification of MTBC members and the consequent improvement of the laboratorial diagnostics algorithms of TB (Bernacka-Wojcik, et al., 2010; Silva et al., 2008, 2010). The integration of these technologies together with the possibility of miniaturization are of utmost importance for the development of an integrated biosensor suitable for peripheral laboratories and/or point-of-care diagnostics, providing a new tool in the fight against TB.

Recently, Liandris et al. have developed a non-cross-linking approach to the detection of TB without the need of target amplification (Liandris et al., 2009). The method relied on the same non-cross-linking hybridization approach of Baptista and co-workers, whereas the aggregation of the gold nanoprobes was induced by an increasing acid concentration instead of salt. The detection is based on the fact that double and single-stranded oligonucleotides have different electrostatic properties. After hybridization, single-stranded DNA becomes double-stranded DNA. As a result, the double-stranded DNA cannot uncoil sufficiently like the single-stranded DNA to expose its bases toward the gold nanoprobe. Therefore, the nanoprobe undergoes aggregation in an acidic environment. Liandris and coworkers designed an array of gold nanoprobes to collectively detect the main mycobacterial pathogens in clinical samples, namely MTBC, *M. avium* complex and *M. avium* subsp. *paratuberculosis*. A nanoprobe harboring 20 nucleotides was designed to harbor a conserved genus region sequence of 16s–23s ITS DNA of the most common mycobacterial pathogens. In order to obtain an indication of the method's performance on clinical samples, the assay was tested for the detection of *M. avium* subsp. *paratuberculosis* DNA in feces. For this purpose, 12 fecal samples were collected from an equal number of goats from a herd with a well-established record of *M. avium* subsp. *paratuberculosis* and the results were compared to those obtained by a real-time PCR assay. The quantification was performed using *M. avium* subsp. *paratuberculosis* DNA of known concentration, and the standard curve as obtained by real-time PCR. The evaluation of the specificity and repeatability of this non-cross-linking approach indicated a reliable and highly specific detection of a broad spectrum of mycobacteria without cross reactions with related bacteria (the concordance of the two methods with connection to real-time PCR positive and negative sample was defined respectively as 87.5% and 100%). Moreover, the methodology demonstrated to be highly sensitive, where even the lowest concentration of the targeted sequence was easily detected by simple visual observation of the test and the control tubes (Liandris et al., 2009).

Following a cross-linking approach, Soo et al. designed a set of gold nanoprobes to specifically hybridize with target DNAs of MTBC and *M. tuberculosis* strains (Soo et al., 2009). The nanoprobes were oriented in a tail-to-tail arrangement, one probe functionalized via a thiol moiety located at the 5′end of the sequence and other at 3′ end, with both sequences being contiguous to each other. This way the hybridization of the nanoprobes with the complementary target resulted in the formation of a polymeric cross-linked network, bringing the AuNPs close enough to induce a color change from red to blue (Beermann et al., 2007; Li et al., 2006; Liandris et al., 2009; Storhoff et al., 2005). The efficacy of such cross-linking assay was evaluated by analyzing sputum specimens. Results were compared with traditional culture and biochemical identification methods together with patients clinical assessments. The detection limit of this assay was measured using IS6110 DNA amplified from *M. tuberculosis* H37Rv chromosome. This methodology was able to detect as low as 0.5 pmol of DNA target within two hours. The assay comprises two main steps, namely, the target DNA amplification by single or nested PCR, followed by nanoprobe detection. The gold nanoprobes are added to the heat denatured PCR products, and incubated at 55ºC for DNA hybridization with increased stringency. In the presence of complementary DNA the nanoprobes aggregated upon hybridization to the target, resulting in decrease in absorbance of the solution at 525 nm. On the other hand, the color and absorbance pattern did not change when specific complementary target DNAs were absent in the solution. The methodology was evaluated by directly and simultaneously detecting MTBC and *M. tuberculosis* from 600 clinical strains and comparing the results with those from conventional culture methods and biochemical identification in combination with clinical assessment. The assay presented 96.6% sensitivity and 98.9% specificity towards detection of MTBC, and 94.7% sensitivity and 99.6% specificity for detection of *M. tuberculosis*.

3.1.2 Magnetic nanoparticles

Magnetic properties are largely dependent on the composition and molecular structure of the NPs (Lu et al., 2007). Different materials can exhibit diamagnetic, paramagnetic or ferromagnetic behavior (Sato et al., 2003). In most cases, the particles range from 1 to 100 nm in size and may display supermagnetism when the thermal energy is enough to change the direction of magnetization of the NPs (Neubergera et al., 2005). Superparamagnetic NPs made of magnetic materials (e.g. iron, nickel, cobalt, or alloys of magnetic metals) are preferred for biomedical applications, due to the fact that they behave non-magnetically when they are not under the influence of an external magnetic field, thus preventing undesired self-magnetic agglomeration. In the presence of an external magnetic field gradient, the large magnetic moments of all the atoms align with the field and the superparamagnetic NPs can be manipulated to interact with different biomolecules (Jain, 2007). Removing the external magnetic field causes the NPs to lose their alignment with the field and relax into random directions of magnetization. To make the superparamagnetic NPs biocompatible, they are coated with a material such as silica or polyethylene glycol, and then functionalized with the relevant targeting biomolecule for the desired application, such as antibodies, proteins or oligonucleotides (Jain, 2005). As an example, superparamagnetic NPs have been used in the development of a magnetic immunoassay. The presence of a target analyte allows the superparamagnetic NPs to bind to a magnetic sensor in a sandwich conformation, which creates a local magnetic field that is detected by the sensor once an applied external field is used to induce a magnetic moment in the superparamagnetic NPs, (Sato et al., 2003).

Kaitanis and coworkers designed superparamagnetic iron oxide nanoprobes coupled with a magnetic relaxation methodology to detect *Mycobacterium avium* spp. *paratuberculosis*, in milk and blood (Kaittanis et al., 2007). The methodology could quickly quantify the bacterial target with high sensitivity, and was not susceptible to interferences caused by other bacteria. The principle underlying the detection by these nanosensors is their ability to change between disperse and clustered (or assembled) state upon target interaction, with a concomitant change in the spin-spin relaxation time of the solution's water protons. This approach, apart from sensitive and fast, is independent of the sample's optical properties and requires minimum sample preparation. More recently, Lee et al. developed a very similar methodology where bacteria were targeted by highly magnetic NPs with a large Fe core and a thin ferrite shell NPs, concentrated into a microfluidic chamber, and detected by nuclear magnetic resonance (Lee et al., 2009). The clinical utility of this diagnostic platform was evaluated by detecting TB using the *bacillus* Calmette-Guérin (BCG) as a surrogate for *M. tuberculosis*. Following liquefaction, the samples were subjected to standard TB diagnostic tests, namely culture and acid-fast bacilli smear microscopy, to be compared with the magnetic NPs-based nuclear magnetic resonance measurements. This methodology shown similar results to those attained with the standard culture-based methods (detection limit of ~20 colony forming units) with the advantage to be less prone to human error and less labor-intensive. The nuclear magnetic resonance-based detection was much faster (< 30 min) and performed on a single microfluidic chip, markedly contrasting with the culture-based test that was time-consuming (> 2 weeks) and facility-dependent (e.g. incubators).

Both these methodologies are in their first stages of development and present great advantages over current techniques such as speed, easiness of procedure and minimum sample preparation.

3.1.3 Quantum dots

Quantum dots are inorganic fluorophores with size-dependent optical properties, exhibiting strong light absorbance, bright and narrow symmetric emission bands and high photo stability, due to three-dimensional quantum confinement effects (Chan et al., 2002; Yezhelyev et al., 2006). The size and composition of QDs determine their emission wavelength and color (Coto-García et al., 2011; Michalet et al., 2005; Sukhanova & Nabiev, 2008). Moreover, the QDs can maintain these properties upon conjugation to biomolecules (Alivisatos et al., 2005; Fortina et al., 2005; Salata, 2004) making them preferred fluorescent probes for imaging applications (Halfpenny & Wright, 2010). The fact that QDs do not depend on the presence of a variety of different fluorescence dyes also allows their application for multiplexing analysis (Azzazy & Mansour, 2009). Although QDs are typically insoluble in water, they can be made biocompatible by several strategies including silanization and coating with a polymer shell, thus enabling their utilization in biological systems. Target specificity is achieved by conjugating them to a variety of biomolecules, such as antibodies, streptavidin and oligonucleotides, enabling their application in conventional molecular biological methodologies, such as fluorescent *in situ* hybridization (FISH), immunological assays or northern/southern/western blots (Michalet et al., 2005). In fact, QDs have already been used in a number of biological applications including studies of protein trafficking, DNA detection and dynamic studies of cell mobility (Zrazhevskiy et al., 2010). Rotem and coworkers reported the use of QDs for the detection of pathogenic bacteria combining *in vivo* biotinylation of engineered host-specific bacteriophage with the conjugation of the phage to streptavidin-coated fluorescent QDs (Rotem et al., 2006).

Although the proof of concept only used a single phage–host system, the method may be expanded for the detection of multiple bacterial strains by their specific phages. This concept could be applied to any slow growing pathogen, such as *M. tuberculosis* for TB diagnostics.

Only recently QDs have been used for the detection and imaging of respiratory pathogens and, in particular, for TB diagnostics. Gazouli and coworkers developed and evaluated a detection assay for specific DNA sequences combining fluorescent semiconductor QDs with magnetic beads allowing for a fast identification of two members of the *Mycobacterium* genus (*M. tuberculosis* and *M. avium* subsp. *paratuberculosis*) without the need for DNA amplification (Gazouli et al., 2010). The assay involves two biotinylated oligonucleotide probes to recognize and detect specific complementary mycobacterial target DNA through a sandwich like hybridization. Five 30-bp-long genus-specific probes were designed for the detection of *Mycobacterium* based on the 23S rRNA gene, which is highly conserved among the mycobacterial species. For the detection of *M. tuberculosis* and *M. avium* subsp. *paratuberculosis*, 2 sets of five 30-bp-long probes were designed based on IS6110 and IS900, respectively. Cadmium selenite QDs conjugated with streptavidin and species-specific probes were used to produce a fluorescent signal, while the magnetic beads conjugated with streptavidin and genus-specific probes were used to isolate and concentrate the DNA targets. The minimum detection limit of the assay was defined to be 12.5 ng of DNA diluted in a sample volume of 20 µl. In order to obtain an indication of the method's performance with clinical samples, the system was compared with conventional diagnostics methodologies, namely Ziehl-Neelsen staining and real-time PCR. Additionally, to assess the performance of the assay with clinical material, DNA isolated from bronchoalveolar lavage samples, formalin-fixed paraffin-embedded tissues or feces was used for the detection of *M. tuberculosis* and *M. avium* subsp. *paratuberculosis*. With regard to *M. tuberculosis*, the assessment relied on DNA isolated from bronchoalveolar lavage samples from 48 patients with clinical tuberculosis and 12 bronchoalveolar lavage samples from healthy individuals, both confirmed by culture and real-time PCR, with the exception of a bronchoalveolar lavage sample that reacted negatively by the latter method. The overall concordance of this assay was 84.61% and 100% with regard to positive and negative results, respectively. This approach of capturing and detection in two steps by different building blocks minimizes false-positives associated with low specificity. Given that the capture and detection probes of the QD assay are complementary to different genes of the mycobacterial genome, the chances of false-negative results due to DNA fragmentation are inevitably increased. Nonetheless, this weakness can be circumvented by the use of a different set of DNA probes that anneal closer to each other, allowing an assessment that minimizes false-positive results associated with low specificity (Gazouli et al., 2010). Additionally, the method avoids the drawback of PCR-based diagnostic assays that are prone to false-negative results generated by inhibitors commonly found in clinical samples such as feces.

3.1.4 Silica nanoparticles

Fluorescence-based detection techniques have been extensively used in both biological research and clinical diagnostics, due to the extremely high sensitivity. Dye-doped silica NPs contain large quantities of dye (fluorophore) molecules inside a polymer or silica matrix, amplifying the fluorescence of each interaction event. This signal enhancement facilitates ultrasensitive analyte determination otherwise undetectable with conventional fluorescence labeling techniques. Furthermore, the polymer and silica matrix serves as a protective shell, reducing photo-bleaching (Zhao et al., 2007) and allows a high versatility towards different surface modification protocols (Tan et al., 2004). These silica NPs are also more hydrophilic, biocompatible and not subject to microbial degradation, swelling or porosity changes with varying pH (Jain et al., 1998). Several systems based in silica NPs have been widely applied in biological imaging and ultrasensitive bioassays, including cell staining (Santra et al., 2001a), DNA detection (He et al., 2006; Zhao et al., 2003), cell surface receptor targeting (Her et al., 2006; Santra et al., 2001a, 2001b, 2004), and ultrasensitive detection of pathogens (Zhao et al., 2004). Moreover, these NPs can also be conjugated with QDs in a core shell like structure, taking advantage of the capabilities of QDs and taking advantage of silica chemistries versatility, while reducing toxicity (Qin et al., 2007).

The first application of dye-doped silica NPs for TB molecular diagnostics was published by Qin and co-workers, where a rapid immunological method combining highly luminescent RuBpy-doped silica NPs with indirect immunofluorescence microscopy allowed for detection of *M. tuberculosis* in both mixed bacterial and sputum samples (Qin et al., 2007). Later on, this approach was improved by using two-color flow-cytometry and adding SYBR Green I to avoid false positives (Qin et al., 2008). Briefly, *M. tuberculosis* is first recognized by the antibody-conjugated RuBpy-doped silica NPs, and then stained with a nucleic acid dye SYBR Green I to discriminate bacterial cells from background particles, followed by multiparameter determination with flow-cytometry. This way, the population of *M. tuberculosis* dual stained with antibody-conjugated RuBpy-doped silica NPs and SYBR-I could be discerned as a distinct population and the false positives caused by aggregates of NP-bioconjugates and nonspecific binding of NP-bioconjugates to background debris could be decreased dramatically, when compared with the initial one-color approach. Moreover, the decrease of false positives also allowed achieving a higher sensitivity for detection of *M. tuberculosis*. This later dual-color approach allowed for detection of TB in buffer and spiked urine, with higher sensitivities than the conventional flow cytometry techniques, maintaining the same simplicity, speed and usability.

3.2 Nano-fabricated devices

Several biosensors for the determination of short sequences from the *M. tuberculosis* DNA have been described (Buijtels et al., 2008; Csako, 2006; McGlennen, 2001). Wang and co-workers developed a sensor that relies on the modification of the carbon-paste transducer oligonucleotide probe and their hybridization to complementary strands from the *M. tuberculosis* DNA (Wang et al., 1997). Chronopotentiometry was employed as transducer and the sensor allowed detection down to nanograms per milliliter of *M. tuberculosis* DNA. Prabhakar et al. used cysteine modified NH_2-end peptide nucleic acid probes and 5'-thiol end labeled DNA probes immobilized onto BK-7 gold coated glass plates for specific detection of *M. tuberculosis* using SPR (Prabhakar et al., 2008). More recently, Das and co-workers developed nanostructured zinc oxide films on conducting indium–tin–oxide coated glass plate to immobilize a DNA probe and specifically detect *M. tuberculosis* based on the strong electrostatic interactions between ZnO and the complementary target (Das et al., 2010). The presence of nanostructured ZnO films allowed to increase the electro-active surface area for DNA molecules loading and detect genomic target DNA up to 100 pM, which enables the direct detection of pathogens in clinical samples at point of care.

These nanofabricated sensors have the capability of reducing the costs of the automated sensitive detection, making them ideal for point-of-care applications. Moreover, these platforms demonstrate the most promising trends in bioanalytical and biochemical methods, the fusion of different approaches, methods and technologies into a single platform.

3.3 Nano-electromechanical devices – nanocantilevers

Nanocantilevers are one of the most promising nanotechnologies for identification of biomolecules capable of providing label-free detection with high sensitivity and specificity (Craighead, 2007). These systems can operate either statically, by measuring absolute cantilever deflection, or dynamically, by measuring resonance frequency shifts. In the *static mode*, the main parameter measured is the differential surface stress produced when molecular adsorption is produced on one side of the cantilever (Fritz et al., 2000). In *dynamic mode*, sensing relies on the observation of the dynamical properties of a resonant cantilever (e.g. vibration amplitude, resonance frequency), which has been increasingly applied for mass sensing (Craighead, 2007; Waggoner & Craighead, 2007). Sensors based on static operation have demonstrated their potential for selective detection of DNA and proteins in liquid. Mass sensors based on dynamic mode can potentially achieve sub-femtomolar sensitivity (Llic et al., 2005). The ultrahigh mass sensitivity is counterbalanced with a very low selectivity due to the device contamination with non-sought molecules and salt debris (Varshney et al., 2008). Thus, in practice small bio-molecules, such as proteins or oligonucleotides, can be detected at low concentrations. Recent developments merged this nanotechnology with AuNPs as sensitizing agents (Wittenberg & Haynes, 2009). These NPs act as mass enhancers, allowing detection of biomolecules at the femtomolar level and beyond, while maintaining the possibility of performing parallel analyses and working with minute sample volumes. Despite these advantages, to our knowledge, nano-electromechanical systems have not yet been applied to the diagnostics of TB.

4. Conclusions

In the last decades we witnessed the development of nanotechnology in isolated fields of research, introducing new and revolutionary approaches for molecular detection. Today the most promising advances are made at the interface, merging two or more technological architectures for new hybrid approaches, circumventing current limitations of each existing techniques for biomolecule analysis protocols. Tremendous advancements in the development and performance of new technological approaches for the rapid diagnostics of TB and prediction of drug resistance have been made in the last few years. The obvious advantages of nanodiagnostics based schemes are their ability to provide results within hours, with increased sensitivities and specificities at a fraction of a cost when compared to conventional microbiological and molecular biology methodologies, such as sputum smear microscopy and nucleic acid amplification based techniques. Nevertheless, thus far, only a very small number of these new nanodiagnostics platforms have been translated to the clinical setting for TB molecular diagnostics. The great efforts put into the development of proof-of-concept approaches most of the time lack the connection and the robustness to make an impact in the analytical laboratory and very few techniques are available for direct application in respiratory specimens (Lee et al., 2009, 2010). It is expected that in the next few years, some of the strategies depicted throughout this short chapter can take their rightful place at the front line of fighting TB.

Future trends in nanodiagnostics will continue through miniaturization of biochip technology to the nanoscale range for point-of-care diagnostics with a sample-in answer-out approach that hampers user-error, thus enabling their use by non-specialized personnel.

5. Acknowledgment

The authors thank CIGMH - FCT/MCTES for financial support.

6. References

Abebe, G., Paasch, F., Apers, L., Rigouts, L., & Colebunders, R., (2011). Tuberculosis drug resistance testing by molecular methods: Opportunities and challenges in resource limited settings, *Journal of Microbiological Methods,* vol. 84, no. 2, pp. 155-160

Alivisatos, A.P., Gu, W., & Larabell, C., (2005). Quantum dots as cellular probes, *Annual Review of Biomedical Engineering,* vol. 7, pp. 55–76

Azzazy, H.M.E., & Mansour, M.M.H., (2009). In vitro diagnostic prospects of nanoparticles, *Clinica Chimica Acta,* vol. 403, pp. 1-8

Azzazy, H.M.E., Mansour, M.M.H., & Kazmierczak, S.C., (2006). Nanodiagnostics: A new frontier for clinical laboratory medicine, *Clinical Chemistry,* vol. 52, no. 7, pp. 1238-1246

Azzazy, H.M.E., Mansour, M.M.H., & Kazmierczak, S.C., (2007). From diagnostics to therapy: Prospects of quantum dots, *Clinical Biochemistry,* vol. 40, pp. 917–927

Baptista, P.V., Doria, G., Henriques, D., Pereira, E., & Franco, R., (2005). Colorimetric detection of eukaryotic gene expression with DNA-derivatized gold nanoparticles, *Journal of* Biotechnology, vol. 119, pp. 111-117

Baptista, P.V., Koziol-Montewka, M., Paluch-Oles, J., Doria, G., & Franco, R., (2006). Gold-nanoparticle-probe-based assay for rapid and direct detection of *Mycobacterium tuberculosis* DNA in clinical samples, *Clinical Chemistry,* vol. 52, pp. 1433-1434

Baptista, P.V., Pereira, E., Eaton, P., Doria, G., Miranda, A., Gomes, I., Quaresma, P., & Franco, R., (2008). Gold nanoparticles for the development of clinical diagnosis methods, *Analytical and Bioanalytical Chemistry,* vol. 391, no. 3, pp. 943-950

Barnard, M., Albert, H., Coetzee, G., O'Brien, R., & Bosman, M.E., (2008). Rapid molecular screening for multidrug-resistant tuberculosis in a high-volume public health laboratory in South Africa, *American Journal of Respiratory and Critical Care Medicine,* vol. 177, pp. 787-792

Beermann, B., Carrillo-Nava, E., Scheffer, A., Buscher, W., Jawalekar, A.M., Seela, F., & Hinz, H.J., (2007). Association temperature governs structure and apparent thermodynamics of DNA-gold nanoparticles, *Biophysical Chemistry,* vol. 126, no. 1-3, pp. 124-131

Bernacka-Wojcik, I., Senadeera, R., Wojcik, P.J., Silva, L.B., Doria, G., Baptista, P.V., Aguas, H., Fortunato, E., Martins, R., (2010). Inkjet printed and "doctor blade" TiO2 photodetectors for DNA biosensors, *Biosensors & Bioelectronics*, vol. 25, no. 5, pp. 1229-1234

Branton, D., Deamer, D.W., Marziali, A., Bayley, H., Benner, S.A., Butler, T., Di Ventra, M., Garaj, S., Hibbs, A., Huang, X., Jovanovich, S.B., Krstic, P.S., Lindsay, S., Ling, X.S., Mastrangelo, C.H., Meller, A., Oliver, J.S., Pershin, Y.V., Ramsey, J.M., Riehn, R., Soni, G.V., Tabard-Cossa, V., Wanunu, M., Wiggin, M., & Schloss, J.A., (2008). The potential and challenges of nanopore sequencing, *Nature Biotecnhology*, vol. 26, pp. 1146-1153

Buijtels, P.C., Willemse-Erix, H.F., Petit, P.L., Endtz, H.P., Puppels, G.J., Verbrugh, H.A., van Belkum, A., van Soolingen, D., & Maquelin, K., (2008). Rapid identification of mycobacteria by Raman spectroscopy, *Journal of Clinical Microbiology*, vol. 46, no. 3, pp. 961-965

Chan, W.C.W., Maxwell, D.J., Gao, X., Bailey, R.E., Han, M., & Ni, S., (2002). Luminescent quantum dots for multiplexed biological detection and imaging, *Current Opinion in Biotechnology*, vol. 13, no. 1, pp. 40-46

Cheng, V.C.C., Yew, W.W., & Yuen, K.Y., (2005). Molecular diagnostics in tuberculosis, *European Journal of Clinical Microbiology & Infectious Diseases*, vol. 24, pp. 711-720

Costa, P., Amaro, A., Botelho, A., Inácio, J., & Baptista, P.V., (2010). Gold nanoprobes assay for identification of mycobacteria from the *Mycobacterium tuberculosis* complex, *Clinical Microbiology and Infection*, vol. 16, no. 9, pp. 1464-1469

Coto-García, A.M., Sotelo-González, E., Fernández-Argüelles, M.T., Pereiro, R., Costa-Fernández, J.M., & Sanz-Medel, A., (2011). Nanoparticles as fluorescent labels for optical imaging and sensing in genomics and proteomics, *Analitical and Bioanalitical Chemistry*, vol. 399, no. 1, pp. 29-42

Craighead, H.C., (2007). Nanomechanical systems: measuring more than mass, *Nature Nanotechnology*, vol. 2, no. 1, pp. 18-19

Csako, G., (2006). Present and future of rapid and/or high-throughput methods for nucleic acid testing, *Clinica Chimica Acta*, vol. 363, no. 1-3, pp. 6-31

D'Amato, R.F., Wallman, A.A., Hochstein, L.H., Colaninno, P.M., Scardamaglia, M., Ardila, E., Ghouri, M., Kim, K., Patel, R.C., & Miller, A., (1995). Rapid diagnosis of pulmonary tuberculosis by using Roche AMPLICOR Mycobacterium tuberculosis PCR test, *Journal of Clinical Microbiology*, vol. 33, no. 7, pp. 1832–1834

Daniel, M.C., & Astruc, D., (2004). Gold nanoparticles: Assembly, supramolecular chemistry, quantum-size-related properties, and applications toward biology, catalysis, and nanotechnology, *Chemical Reviews*, vol. 104, no. 1, pp. 293-346

Das, M., Sumana, G., Nagarajan, R., & Malhotra, B.D., (2010). Application of nanostructured ZnO films for electrochemical DNA biosensor, *Thin Solid Films*, vol. 519, pp. 1196-1201

Deun, A.V., Martin, A., & Palomino, J.C., (2010). Diagnosis of drug-resistant tuberculosis: reliability and rapidity of detection, *International Journal of Tuberculosis and Lung Disease*, vol. 14, no. 2, pp. 131-140

De Beenhouwer, H., Lhiang, Z., Jannes, G., Mijs, W., Machtelinckx, L., Rossau, R., Traore, H., & Portaels, F., (1995). Rapid detection of rifampicin resistance in sputum and biopsy specimens from tuberculosis patients by PCR and line probe assay, *Tubercle and Lung Disease*, vol. 76, no. 5, pp. 425-430

Doria, G., Baumgartner, B.G:, Franco, R., & Baptista, P.V., (2010). Optimizing Au-nanoprobes for specific sequence discrimination, *Coloids and Surfaces B, Biointerfaces*, vol. 77, no. 1, pp. 122-124

Elghanian, R., Storhoff, J.J., Mucic, R.C., Letsinger, R.L., & Mirkin, C.A., (1997). Selective colorimetric detection of polynucleotides based on the distance-dependent optical properties of gold nanoparticles, *Science*, vol. 277, no. 5329, pp. 1078-1081

Fortina, P., Kricka, L.J., Surrey, S., & Grodzinski, P., (2005). Nanobiotechnology: the promise and reality of new approaches to molecular recognition, *Trends Biotechnology*, vol. 23, pp. 168-173

Fritz, J., Baller, M.K., Lang, H.P., Rothuizen, H., Vettiger, P., Meyer, E., Guntherodt, H.J., Gerber, C., & Gimzewski, J.K., (2000). Translating biomolecular recognition into nanomechanics, *Science,* vol. 288, no. 5464, pp. 316-318

Gazouli, M., Liandris, E., Andreadou, M., Sechi, L.A., Masala, S., Paccagnini, D., & Ikonomopoulos, J., (2010). Specific detection of unamplified Mycobacterial DNA by use of fluorescent semiconductor quantum dots and magnetic beads, *Journal of Clinical Microbiology*, vol.48, no. 8, pp. 2830–2835

Griffith, D.E., Aksamit, T., Brown-Elliott, B.A., Catanzaro, A., Daley, C., Gordin, F., Holland, S.M., Horsburgh, R., Huitt, G., Iademarco, M.F., Iseman, M., Olivier, K., Ruoss, S., von Reyn, C.F., Wallace, R.J., & Winthrop, K., (2007). An official ATS/IDSA statement: Diagnosis, treatment, and prevention of nontuberculous Mycobacterial diseases, *American Journal of Respiratory and Critical Care Medicine*, vol. 175, pp. 367-416

Halfpenny, K.C., & Wright, D.W., (2010). Nanoparticle detection of respiratory infection, *Wiley Interdisciplinary Reviews. Nanomedicine and Nanobiotecnhology*, vol. 2, no. 3, pp. 277-290

He, X.X., Chen, J.Y., Wang, K.M., Tan, W.H., & Qin, D.L., (2006). Preparation and properties of Cy3 doped core-shell silica fluorescent nanoparticles, *Chemical Journal of Chinese Universities*, vol. 27, no. 10, pp. 1835–1839

Hillemann, D., Weizenegger, M., Kubica, T., Richter, E., & Niemann, S., (2005). Use of the genotype MTBDR assay for rapid detection of rifampin and isoniazid resistance in Mycobacterium tuberculosis complex isolates, *Journal of Clinical Microbiology*, vol. 43, no. 8, pp.3699-3703

Hirano, K., Abe, C., & Takahashi, M., (1999). Mutations in the *rpo*B gene of rifampin-resistant *Mycobacterium tuberculosis* strains isolated mostly in Asian countries and their rapid detection by line probe assay, *Journal of Clinical Microbiology*, vol. 37, no. 8, pp. 2663-2666

Jain, K.K., (2005). Nanotechnology in clinical laboratory diagnostics, *Clinica Chimica Acta*, vol. 328, no. 2 pp. 37–54

Jain, K.K., (2007). Applications of nanobiotechnology in clinical diagnostics, *Clinical Chemistry*, vol. 53, no. 11, pp. 2002–2009

Jain, T.K., Roy, I., De, T.K., & Maitra, A., (1998). Nanometer silica particles encapsulating active compounds: A novel ceramic drug carrier, *Journal of the American Chemical Society*, vol. 120, no. 43, pp. 11092–11095

Johnson, C.J., Zhukovsky, N., Cass, A.E.G., & Nagy, J.M., (2007). Proteomics, nanotechnology and molecular diagnostics, *Proteomics,* vol. 8, pp. 715-730

Kaittanis, C., Naser, S.A., & Perez, J.M., (2007). One-step, nanoparticle-mediated bacterial detection with magnetic relaxation, *Nano Letters*, vol. 7, no. 2, pp. 380-383

Lee, H., Yoon, T.J., & Weissleder, R., (2009). Ultrasensitive detection of bacteria using core-shell nanoparticles and a NMR-filter system, *Angewandte Chemie International Edition*, vol. 48, no. 31, pp. 5657-5660

Lee, W.G., Kim, Y.G., Chung, B.G., Demirci, U., & Khademhosseini, A., (2010). Nano/Microfluidics for diagnosis of infectious diseases in developing countries, *Advanced Drug Delivery Reviews*, vol. 62, pp. 449–457

Li, Y., Wark, A.W., Lee, H.J., & Corn, R.M., (2006). Single-nucleotide polymorphism genotyping by nanoparticle-enhanced surface plasmon resonance imaging measurements of surface ligation reactions, *Analalitical Chemistry*, vol. 78, pp. 3158–3164

Liandris, E., Gazouli, M., Andreadou, M., Comor, M., Abazovic, N., Sechi, L.A., & Ikonomopoulos, J., (2009). Direct detection of unamplified DNA from pathogenic mycobacteria using DNA-derivatized gold nanoparticles, *Journal of Microbiological Methods*, vol. 78, no. 3, pp. 260–264

Liu, W.T., (2006). Nanoparticles and their biological and environmental applications, *Journal of Bioscience and Bioengineering*, vol. 102, no. 1, pp. 1-7

Llic, B., Yang, Y., Aubin, K., Reichenbach, R., Krylov, S., & Craighead, H.G., (2005). Enumeration of DNA molecules bound to a nanomechanical oscillator, *Nanoletters*, vol. 5, no. 5, pp. 925-929

Lu, A.H., Salabas, E.L., & Schüth, F., (2007). Magnetic nanoparticles: synthesis, protection, functionalization, and application, *Angewandte Chemie International Edition*, vol. 46, no. 8, pp. 1222-1244

McGlennen, R.C., (2001). Miniaturization technologies for molecular diagnostics", *Clinical Chemistry*, vol. 47, pp. 393-402

Michalet, X., Pinaud, F.F., Bentolila, L.A., Tsay, J.M., Doose, S., Li, J.J., Sundaresan, G., Wu, A.M., Gambhir, S.S., & Weiss, S., (2005). Quantum dots for live cells, in vivo imaging, and diagnostics, *Science*, vol. 307, no. 5709, pp. 538–544

Miller, L.P., Crawford, J.T., & Shinnick, T.M., (1994). The *rpoB* gene of *Mycobacterium tuberculosis, Antimicrobial Agents and Chemotherapy*, vol. 38, no. 4, pp. 805–811

Moore, D.A., Evans, C.A., Gilman, R.H., Caviedes, L., Coronel, J., Vivar, A., Sanchez, E., Piñedo, Y., Saravia, J.C., Salazar, C., Oberhelman, R., Hollm-Delgado, M.G., LaChira, D., Escombe, A.R., & Friedland, J.S., (2006). Microscopic-observation drug-susceptibility assay for the diagnosis of TB, *The New England Journal of Medicine*, vol. 355, no. 15, pp. 1539-1550

Musser, J.M., (1995). Antimicrobial agent resistance in Mycobacteria: molecular genetic insights, *Clinical Microbiology Reviews*, vol. 8, no. 4, pp. 496-514

Neubergera, T., Schöpf, B., Hofmannb, H., Hofmannc, M., & von Rechenberga, B., (2005). Superparamagnetic nanoparticles for biomedical applications: Possibilities and limitations of a new drug delivery system, *Journal of Magnetism and Magnetic Materials*, vol. 293, no. 1, pp. 483–496

Park, W.G., Bishai, W.R., Chaisson, R.E., & Dorman, S.E., (2002). Performance of the microscopic observation drug susceptibility assay in drug susceptibility testing for *Mycobacterium tuberculosis, Journal of Clinical Microbiology*, vol. 40, no. 12, pp. 4750-4752

Perkins, M.D. (2009). New diagnostics for tuberculosis, In: *Tuberculosis: A comprehensive clinical reference*, Schaaf, H.S., Zumla, A.I., Grange, J.M., Raviglione, M.C., Yew, W.W., Starke, J.R., Pai, M. & Donald, P.R., pp. 227-236, W.B. Saunders, ISBN:978-1-4160-3988-4 , Edinburgh

Prabhakar, N., Singh, H., & Malhotra, B.D., (2008). Nucleic acid immobilized polypyrrole-polyvinylsulphonate film for *Mycobacterium tuberculosis* detection, *Electrochemistry Communications*, vol. 10, no. 6, pp. 821-826

Qin, D., He, X., Wang, K., & Tan, W.H., (2008). Using fluorescent nanoparticles and SYBR Green I based two-color flow cytometry to determine *Mycobacterium tuberculosis* avoiding false positives", *Biosensors and Bioelectronics*, vol. 24, no. 4, pp. 626-631

Qin, D., He, X., Wang, K., Zhao, X.J., Tan, W.H., & Chen, J., (2007). Fluorescent nanoparticle-based indirect immunofluorescence microscopy for detection of *Mycobacterium tuberculosis*, *Journal of Biomedicine and Biotechnology*, vol. 2007, no. 89364

Rosi, N.L., & Mirkin, C.A., (2005). Nanostructures in biodiagnostics, *Chemical Reviews*, vol. 105, no. 4, pp. 1547-1562

Rossau, R., Traore, H., De Beenhouwer, H., Mijs, W., Jannes, G., De Rijk, P., & Portaels, F., (1997). Evaluation of the INNO-LiPA Rif. TB assay, a reverse hybridization assay for the simultaneous detection of *Mycobacterium tuberculosis* complex and its resistance to rifampin, *Antimicrobial Agents and Chemotherapy*, vol. 41, no. 10, pp. 2093-2098

Rotem, E., McKinstry, M., Hwang, J., Oppenheim, A.B., Fekete, R.A., Giulian, G., Merril, C., Nagashima, K., & Adhya, S., (2006). High-sensitivity bacterial detection using biotin-tagged phage and quantum-dot nanocomplexes, *Proceedings of the National Academy of Sciences of the United States of America*. Vol. 103, no. 13, pp. 4841-4845

Salata, O.V., (2004). Applications of nanoparticles in biology and medicine, *Journal of Nanobiotechnology*, vol. 2, no. 3, doi:10.1186/1477-3155-2-3

Santra, S., Liesenfeld, B., Dutta, D., Chatel, D., Batich, C.D., Tan, W.H., Moudgil, B.M., & Mericle, R.A., (2005). Folate conjugated fluorescent silica nanoparticles for labeling neoplastic cells, *Journal of Nanoscience and Nanotechnology*, vol. 5, no. 6, pp. 899– 904

Santra, S., Wang, K.M., Tapec, R., & Tan, W.H., (2001a). Development of novel dye-doped silica nanoparticles for biomarker application, *Journal of Biomedical Optics*, vol. 6, no. 2, pp. 160–166

Santra, S., Yang, H., Dutta, D., Stanley, J.T., Holloway, P.H., Tan, W.H., Moudgil, B.M., & Mericle, R.A., (2004). TAT conjugated, FITC doped silica nanoparticles for bioimaging applications, *Chemical Communications*, no. 24, pp. 2810–2811

Santra, S., Zhang, P., Wang, K.M., Tapec, R., & Tan, W.H., (2001b). Conjugation of biomolecules with luminophore-doped silica nanoparticles for photostable biomarkers, *Analytical Chemistry*, vol. 73, no. 20, pp. 4988–4993

Sato, K., Hosokawa, K., & Maeda, M., (2003). Rapid aggregation of gold nanoparticles induced by non-cross-linking DNA hybridization, *Journal of the American Chemical Society*, vol. 125, no.1, pp. 8102-8103

Shamputa, I.C:, Rigouts, L., & Portaels, F., (2004). Molecular genetic methods for diagnosis and antibiotic resistance detection of mycobacteria from clinical specimens, *Acta Pathologica, Microbiologica et Immunologica Scandinavica*, vol. 112, pp. 728-752

Sharma, M., Sethi, S., Mishra, B., Sengupta, C., & Sharma, S.K., (2003). Rapid detection of mutations in rpoB gene of rifampicin resistant *Mycobacterium tuberculosis* strains by line probe assay, *Indian Journal of Medical Research,* vol. 117, pp. 76-80

Silva, L.B., Baptista, P.V., Raniero, L., Doria, G., Martins, R., & Fortunato, E., (2008). Characterization of optoelectronic platform using an amorphous/nanocrystalline silicon biosensor for the specific identification of nucleic acid sequences based on gold nanoparticle probes, *Sensors and Actuators B,* vol. 132, pp. 508–511

Silva, L.B., Veigas, B., Doria, G., Costa, P., Inácio, J., Martins, R., Fortunato, E., & Baptista, P.V., (2010). Portable optoelectronic biosensing platform for identification of mycobacteria from the *Mycobacterium tuberculosis* complex, *Biosensors & Bioelectronics,* vol. 26, no. 5, pp. 2012-2017

Soini, H., & Musser, J.M., (2001). Molecular diagnosis of Mycobacteria, *Clinical Chemistry,* vol.47, no. 5, pp. 809–814

Soo, P.C., Horng, Y.T:, Chang, K.C., Wang, J.Y., Hsueh, P.R., Chuang, C.Y., Lu, C.C., & Lai, H.C., (2009). A simple gold nanoparticle probes assay for identification of *Mycobacterium tuberculosis* and *Mycobacterium tuberculosis* complex from clinical specimens, *Molecular Cell Probes,* vol. 23, no. 5, pp. 240-246

Storhoff, J.J., Lucas, A.D., Garimella, V., Bao, Y.P., & Müller, U.R., (2005). Homogeneous detection of unamplified genomic DNA sequences based on colorimetric scatter of gold nanoparticle probes", *Nature Biotechnology,* vol 22, no. 7, pp, 883-887

Sukhanova, A., & Nabiev, I., (2008). Fluorescent nanocrystal-encoded microbeads for multiplexed cancer imaging and diagnosis, *Critical Reviews in Oncology/Hematology,* vol. 68, no. 1, pp. 39–59

Tan, W., Wang, K., He, X., Zhao, X.J., Drake, T., Wang, L., & Bagwe, R.P., (2004). Bionanotechnology based on silica nanoparticles, *Medicinal Research Reviews,* vol. 24, no. 5, pp. 621-63

Telenti, A., Imboden, P., Marchesi, F., Matter, L., Schopfer, K., Bodmer, T., Lowrie, D., Colston, M.J., & Cole, S., (1993). Detection of rifampicin-resistance mutations in *Mycobacterium tuberculosis, The Lancet,* vol. 341, no. 8846, pp. 647-651

Traore, H., Fissette, K., Bastian, I., Devleeschouwer, M., & Portaels, F., (2000). Detection of rifampicin resistance in *Mycobacterium tuberculosis* isolates from diverse countries by a commercial line probe assay as an initial indicator of multidrug resistance", *International Journal of Tuberculosis and Lung Disease,* vol. 4, no. 5, pp. 481-484

Varshney, M., Waggoner, P.S., Tan, C.P., Aubin, K., Montagna, R.A., & Craighead, H.G., (2008). Prion protein detection using nanomechanical resonator arrays and secondary mass labeling, *Analytical chemistry,* vol. 80, no. 6, pp. 2141-2148

Veigas, B., Machado, D., Perdigão, J., Portugal, I., Couto, I., Viveiros, M., & Baptista, P.V., (2010). Au-nanoprobes for detection of SNPs associated with antibiotic resistance in *Mycobacterium tuberculosis, Nanotechnology,* vol. 21, no. 41, pp. 5101-5108

Vollath, D., (2008) *Nanomaterials: an introduction to synthesis, properties and applications* (1st edition), Wiley-VCH, ISBN:978-3-527-31531-4, Weinheim

Waggoner, P.S., & Craighead, H.G., (2007). Micro and nanomechanical sensors for environmental, chemical, and biological detection, *Lab on a Chip,* vol. 7, no. 10, pp.1238-1255

Wang, H., Yang, R., Yang, L., Tan, W., (2009). Nucleic acid conjugated nanomaterials for enhanced molecular recognition, *ACS Nano,* vol. 3, no. 9, pp. 2451-2460

Wang, J., Rivas, G., Cai, X., Dontha, N., Shiraishi, H., Luo, D., & Valera, F.S., (1997). Sequence-specific electrochemical biosensing of M. tuberculosis DNA, *Analytica Chimica Acta*, vol. 337, no. 1, pp. 41-48

Watterson, S.A., Wilson, S.M., Yates, M.D., & Drobniewski, F.A:, (1998). Comparison of three molecular assays for rapid detection of rifampin resistance in *Mycobacterium tuberculosis*, *Journal of Clinical Microbiology*, vol. 36, no. 7, pp. 1969-1973

WHO (2010) *Global tuberculosis control: WHO Report 2010*, WHO Press, ISBN 978-92-4-156406-9, Geneva

Wittenberg, N.J., Haynes, C.L., (2009). Using nanoparticles to push the limits of detection, *Wiley Interdisciplinary Reviews, Nanomedicine and Biotecnhology*, vol. 1 , no. 2, pp. 237-254

Yezhelyev, M.V., Gao, X., Xing, Y., Al-Hajj, A., Nie, S., & O'Regan, R.M., (2006). Emerging use of nanoparticles in diagnosis and treatment of breast cancer, *The Lancet Oncology*, vol. 7, no. 8, pp. 657-667

Zhao, W., Wang, L., & Tan, W., (2007). Fluorescent nanoparticle for bacteria and DNA detection, *Advances in Experimental Medicine and Biology*, vol 620, pp. 129-135

Zhao, X.J., Hilliard, L.R., Mechery, S.J., Wang, Y., Bagwe, R.P., Jin, S., Tan, W.H., (2004). A rapid bioassay for single bacterial cell quantitation using bioconjugated nanoparticles, *Proceedings of the National Academy of Sciences of the United States of America*, vol. 101, no. 42, pp. 15027– 15032

Zhao, X.J., Tapec-Dytioco, R., & Tan, W.H., (2003) Ultrasensitive DNA detection using highly fluorescent bioconjugated nanoparticles, *Journal of the American Chemical Society*, vol. 125, no. 38, pp. 11474–11475

Zrazhevskiy, P., Sena, M., Gao, X., (2010). Designing multifunctional quantum dots for bioimaging, detection, and drug delivery. *Chemical Society Reviews*, vol. 39, no. 11, pp. 4326-4354

13

Sputum Smear Microscopy for Tuberculosis: Evaluation of Autofocus Functions and Automatic Identification of Tuberculosis Mycobacterium

Cicero F. F. Costa Filho and Marly G. F. Costa
Centre for Electronic and Information Technology/Federal University of Amazonas
Brazil

1. Introduction

Since 1997 the World Health Organization has published an annual report on global control of tuberculosis (TB) with the purpose of providing a comprehensive and up-to-date assessment of the TB epidemic. According to the Global TB control report of 2010 (World Health Organization [WHO], 2010), the global burden of disease caused by TB in 2009 is as follows: 9.4 million incident cases, 14 million prevalent cases, 1.3 million deaths among non HIV-positive people and 0.38 million deaths among HIV positive people.

The absolute number of cases continues to increase from year to year. The slow reduction in incident rates per capita is outweighed by increases in population. The greatest number of cases are in Asia (55%) and Africa (30%). Other regions have lower numbers of cases: Eastern Mediterranean Region (7%), European Region (4%) and American Region (3%). The main effort of WHO today concerning TB is to attain the targets included in the Millennium Development Goals (MDGs).

Adopted by world leaders in 2000, the MDGs are a blueprint that guides the efforts of the United Nations Development Program and various and various aid agencies, providing concrete, numerical benchmarks for tackling extreme poverty in its many dimensions to be achieved by 2015. The MDGs define 8 goals (United Nations [UN], 2010) with 21 targets that are measured by 60 indicators. TB falls under the 6th goal related to fighting disease epidemics, aiming to: "Combat HIV/AIDS, Malaria and other diseases". Within this goal the following target refers to TB: "Halt and begin to reverse the incidence of malaria and other major diseases". Related to this target, the following indicator refers to TB: Halt and begin to reverse TB incidence by 2015; Reduce prevalence and deaths due to TB by 50% compared with a baseline of 1990.

To achieve these indicators the WHO adopted a Partnership Global Plan to Stop TB (WHO, 2011). Launched in January 2006, it includes sputum smear microscopy as the main diagnostic tool. Indeed, one of the targets of this plan is stated as follows: "A treatment success rate among sputum smear positive case of 90%". The main reason for sputum smear microscopy to be included is that it is the main non-invasive technique employed for TB diagnosis. Other non-invasive techniques include culture and chest radiography.

Sputum smear microscopy has several operational advantages over culture as a diagnostic tool (Luelmo, 2004): "The results are available soon, correlate with infectiousness, and identify both patients at high risk of death from tuberculosis if untreated and patients who require more drugs in the initial treatment regimen because of greater bacterial load". In addition sputum smear microscopy has an important role in follow up of TB treatment. Only when the smears are negative can the intensive phase of the treatment be suspended.

Despite the historical importance of chest radiography in TB diagnosis, it is not used today as a diagnostic tool alone. The following reasons justify this practice: 1) Some other diseases of the lung show a similar appearance in radiographic picture. Consequently radiographic exam is not specific to TB; 2) Lesions of pulmonary tuberculosis can take almost any form in a radiographic image (American Thoracic Society [ATS], 2000) .

Two main facts enable the use of sputum smear microscopy for TB diagnosis. The first one is that special dyes allow to differentiating the bacillus from the background. The second one is that there is a positive correlation between the number of bacillus in the smear and the probability of their being identified by microscopy.

To support the last statement, Table 1 (David, 1976, as cited in Toman, 2004a) shows the positive correlation that exists between the number of bacillus present in a sputum specimen, the number of bacillus in a smear and the probability of finding theses bacillus by microscopy. For this study 0.01 ml of sputum was placed on a slide and spread over an area of 200mm^2. The magnification of the microscope used allowed for observing 10.000 fields on this slide.

No. of bacilli observed	Estimated concentration of bacilli per ml of especimen	Probability of a positive result
0 in 100 or more field	<1000	<10%
1-2 in 300 fields	5000-10000	50%
1-9 in 100 fields	about 30 000	80%
1-9 in 10 fields	about 50 000	90%
1-9 per field	about 100 000	96.2%
10 or more per field	about 500 000	99.95%

Table 1. Number of observed bacilli, concentration of bacilli in sputum specimen (culture results) and probability of a positive result

Two techniques are used for TB diagnostic with sputum smear microscopy: Fluorescence microscopy and conventional microscopy. Fluorescence microscopy uses an acid-fast fluorochrome dye (eg, auramine O or auramine-rhodamine), while conventional microscopy uses the carbolfuchsin Ziehl-Neelsen - ZN or Kinyoun acid-fast stains. While the first one uses an intense light source, such as a halogen or high-pressure mercury vapor lamp, the second one uses a conventional artificial light source.

1. Fluorescence microscopy has the following main advantages over conventional microscopy: 1) Fluorescence microscopy uses a lower power objective lens (typically 25x), while conventional microscopy uses a higher power objective lens (typically 100x). As a consequence fluorescence microscopy allows the same area of a smear to be scanned in a much shorter time than with conventional microscopy (Bennedesen & Larsen, 1966);
2. Fluorescence microscopy is on average 10% more sensitive than conventional microscopy (Steingart et. al., 2006).

The main shortcomings of fluorescence microscopy are: 1) The relatively high costs of the microscopy unit and its maintenance when compared with the conventional microscopy unit; 2) The handling and maintenance of the optical equipment require advanced technical skill (Toman, 2004b).

The sensitivity of tuberculosis diagnostic through sputum smear analysis reported in the literature varies greatly. While reported sensitivities of conventional microscopy range from 0.32 to 0.94, reported sensitivities of fluorescence microscopy range from 0.52 to 0.97. On average the specificity of fluorescence microscopy is similar to conventional microscopy and range from 0.94 to 1 (Steingart et. al., 2006).

In addition to the huge variability in sensitivity, the manual screening for bacillus identification is a labor-intensive task that consumes between 40 minutes and 3 hours, depending on patient's level of infection and it is needed to analyse 40-100 images (Sotaquirá, 2009).

Automatic methods for bacilli screening were first developed for fluorescence microscopy images (Veropoulos et. al., 1998; Forero et. al., 2003). The first methods for automatic bacilli screening in conventional microscopy were published only in 2008 (Costa et. al., 2008; Sadaphal et. al., 2008; Raof et. al., 2008). Some other methods for automatic bacilli screening were published in recent years (Forero, 2004, 2006; Lenseigne et. al., 2007; Sotaquira et. al., 2009; Makkapati, et. al., 2009; Khutlang et. al., 2010).

Some authors (Forero et. al., 2006; Sotaquira, 2009; Khutlang, 2010) claimed that the main advantages of an automatic bacilli screening over a manual one are better reproducible values for sensitivity and specificity and a faster screening process. Table 2 shows reported values for sensitivity, specificity and time waste for one image analysis using automatic methods.

The sensitivity and specificity values previously cited for manual screening methods refer to tuberculosis diagnosis. The sensitivity and specificity values for automatic methods shown in Table 2 refer to object classification as bacillus or not bacillus. Therefore, a rigorous comparison of sensitivities and specificities between manual and automatic screening methods could not be done.

Only one paper of Table 2 cited time wasted for one image analysis, 1.87s. To compute the time consumed with a TB automatic diagnosis it is necessary to take into account the number of images needed to achieve a correct diagnosis. As previously cited, in order to achieve a correct diagnosis, it is necessary to analyze between 20 and 100 fields of one slide. With an automatic procedure, it is also necessary to take into account the time spent with focusing computations, image acquisition and microscopy displacement. According to

Santos (Santos et. al., 1997) focusing computations takes 1.8s per field, while acquisition takes 0.7s, including 0.5s for slide movement. Assuming that no parallel process occurs and considering the worst case scenario of 100 images we have the time spent with an automatic diagnosis (T_{ad}) given by:

$$T_{ad} = 100x(1.87 + 1.8 + 0.7) = 437s \cong 7\ minutes \quad (1)$$

This value is a few times smaller than the value of 40 minutes previously cited for a TB manual diagnostic with sputum smear microscopy.

Author	Microscopy	Sensitivity (%)	Specificity (%)	Time for one image analysis (seconds)	Computer
Veropoulos, 1998	Fluorescence	93.53	98.79	not cited	--
Forero, 2006	Fluorescence	97.89	94.67	not cited	--
Sotaquira, 2009	Conventional	90.90	100	1.87	Intel processor of 2 GHz and 512 MB of RAM
Khutlang, 2010	Conventional	97.77	99.13	not cited	--

Table 2. Sensitivity, Specificity and time for one image analysis

Steps involved in automated microscopy include those shown if Figure 2. In the following sections, we analyze some of these steps. In section 2 we address the problem of auto focusing, discussing the main functions used in auto focusing methods. In the third section we discuss the main differences between the methods used for bacilli segmentation and classification in fluorescence microscopy and conventional microscopy.

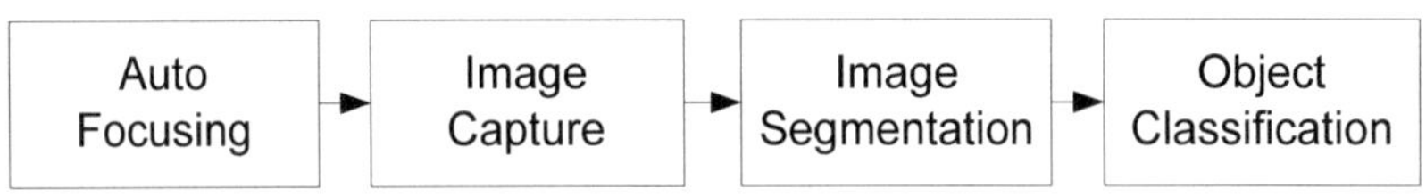

Fig. 2. Steps involved in automated bacilli recognition

2. Autofocus evaluation functions

Automatic microscopy is accomplished through coupling an electronic camera to a microscope. Auto focusing of electronic cameras is accomplished by searching for the lens position that gives the best focused image (Subbaro &. Tyan, 1995). A focused image can be thought of as one that, for a set of images captured with different microscope stages, presents the best average focus over an entire field of view. In a frequency viewpoint, a focused image can be thought of as one that has more high frequency components. It is important that samples be well prepared, resulting in thin structures, because thick samples present structures with different foci. An auto focusing process employs a focus measure and a procedure to determine the best focused image. A focus measure can be defined as follow: "First, the image for which the focus measure needs to be computed is normalized for brightness by dividing the image by its mean brightness. Then, it is convolved with a focus measure filter (FMF). Then, the energy (sum of squared values) of the filtered image is computed. This energy is the focus measure" (Subbaro &. Tyan, 1998). An important conclusion concerning focus measures, established by the same authors, is that the best focus measure could be different for different objects depending on both image content and noise characteristic. In other words, there is no best focus measure that can be used for auto focusing of different image types. Because of this, it is important to find the best focus measure that can be used in TB auto focusing. In this section we will revise the main focus measure functions used in automatic microscopy.

The main focus measures functions used in auto focusing can be divided into four groups:

Functions Based on Image Differentiation

Different FMF have been used for image differentiation:

Threshold Absolute Gradient: This function computes and accumulates the first difference between a pixel and its neighbor with a distance of one, when the difference is larger than a threshold.

$$F_{th\_grad} = \sum_M \sum_N |g(i,j+1) - g(i,j)| \quad (2)$$

$$while\ |g(i,j+1) - g(i,j)| \geq \theta$$

Squared Gradient: Similar to the previous function but with squared difference. The larger differences influence the results more.

$$F_{sq\_grad} = \sum_M \sum_N |g(i,j+1) - g(i,j)|^2 \quad (3)$$

$$while\ |g(i,j+1) - g(i,j)| \geq \theta$$

Tenenbaum Gradient (Krotkov, 1987): This function uses the Sobel operator.

$$F_{tenen} = \sum_M \sum_N T[g(i,j)] \quad (4)$$

$$T[g(i,j)] = G_x^2(i,j) + G_y^2(i,j)$$

$$G_x(i,j), G_y(i,j) = Image\ convolution\ with\ Sobel\ operators$$

Brenner Gradient (Brenner et. al., 1971): This function computes the first difference between a pixel and its neighbor with a distance of two.

$$F_{brenner} = \sum_M \sum_N |g(i,j+2) - g(i,j)|^2 \quad (5)$$

$$while\ |g(i,j+1) - g(i,j)| \geq \theta$$

Energy of Image Laplacian: This function implements the image convolution with a Laplace mask.

$$F_{Laplace} = \sum_M \sum_N \left(g(i,j+1) + g(i,j-1) + g(i+1,j) + g(i-1,j) - 4g(i,j)\right)^2 \quad (6)$$

First order Gaussian Derivative (Geusebroeck et. al., 2000): This function involves image convolution with the derivative of a Gaussian smooth filter.

$$F_{Gaussian} = \frac{1}{NM} \sum_N \sum_M \left(g(i,j) * G_x(x,y,\sigma)\right)^2 + \left(g(i,j) * G_y(x,y,\sigma)\right)^2$$

$$G_x(x,y,\sigma)\ and\ G_y(x,y,\sigma)\ are\ the\ first\ order\ Gassuain\ derivatives\ in\ the\ x\ and\ y\ directions$$

σ *is the standard deviation* $\cong (d/2)/\sqrt{3}$, d= bacillus width

Statistics-Based Functions

These functions evaluate the contrast of an image:

Variance: This function measures the variation in image gray level of pixels.

$$F_{var} = \frac{1}{MN}\sum_M \sum_N |g(i,j) - \bar{g}| \tag{7}$$

Normalized Variance: This function compensates for the differences in bright levels among different images

$$F_{var} = \frac{1}{MN\bar{g}}\sum_M \sum_N |g(i,j) - \bar{g}| \tag{8}$$

Functions Based on Histogram

Entropy: The entropy function is a measure of information content

$$F_{entr} = -\sum_l p_l log p_l \tag{9}$$

$$p_l \textit{ is the relative frequency of gray level } l$$

Variance of Log Histogram: This function emphasizes the bright pixels in the image by multiplying the variance by the logarithm

$$F_{var\_log} = \sum_l \left(l - E_{log}\{l\}\right) log p_l \tag{10}$$

$$E_{log}\{l\} = \sum_l l log p_l \textit{ is the expected value of } \log \textit{histogram}$$

Functions Based on Correlation Measurement

These functions were proposed by Vollath (Vollath, 1998) and, according to the author, had good performance in noise presence.

Autocorrelation (Vollath's F_4):

$$F_{autocorr} = \sum_M \sum_N g(i+1,j)g(i,j) - \sum_M \sum_N g(i+2,j)g(i,j) \tag{11}$$

Standard Deviation-Based Correlation (Vollath's F_5):

$$F_{autocorr} = \sum_M \sum_N g(i+1,j)g(i,j) - MN\bar{g}^2 \tag{12}$$

Some measures based on frequency content have been proposed, such as the wavelet transform (Kautsky et. al., 2002). Nevertheless it did not present good results in TB auto focusing.

It should be observed that some of these functions depend on threshold, while some others do not depend on any parameter. Some of these functions were used for TB auto focusing. Table 3 shows published papers involving TB auto focusing, detailing the focus measure employed in each one.

The papers of Russel (Russel & Douglas, 2007) and Kimura (Kimura Junior et. al., 2010) were careful to consider slides with different background contents. For example, Kimura divided the TB conventional microscopy images into two groups: Images with high density background content and images with low density background content. Figure 3(a) shows an image with high density background content and Figure 3(b) an image with low density background content. In both groups the variance and normalized variance functions showed the best performance. Osibote (Osibote et. al., 2010) also obtained a better performance with the normalized variance function.

Authors	Microscopy Type	Evaluation Functions	Results
Forero et. al. (2004)	Fluorescence	Variance, Energy of Image Laplacian, Wavelet Transform, Autocorrelation, Variance of Log Histogram	The best results were obtained with Variance of Log Histogram Function. Other measure produced meaningful results
Russel & Douglas (2007)	Conventional	Energy of Image Laplacian, First Order Gaussian Derivative, Variance of Log Histogram	The best results were obtained with Energy Laplacian Function. Compared with manual focus: average difference = 1.45μm. Standard deviation = 1.88μm.
Kimura Junior et. al. (2010)	Conventional	Brenner Gradient, Energy of Image Laplacian, Wavelet Transform, Variance, Normalized Variance, Autocorrelation, Standard Deviation-Based Correlation, Entropy, Variance of Log Histogram	The best results were obtained with Variance and Normalized Variance. Entropy was the quickest function. Wavelet function was the slower function.
Osibote et. al. (2010)	Conventional	Normalized Variance, Brenner Gradient, Energy of Image Laplacian, Autocorrelation, Tenembaum Gradient	The best results were obtained with Normalized Variance Function

Table 3. Published papers involving TB auto focusing

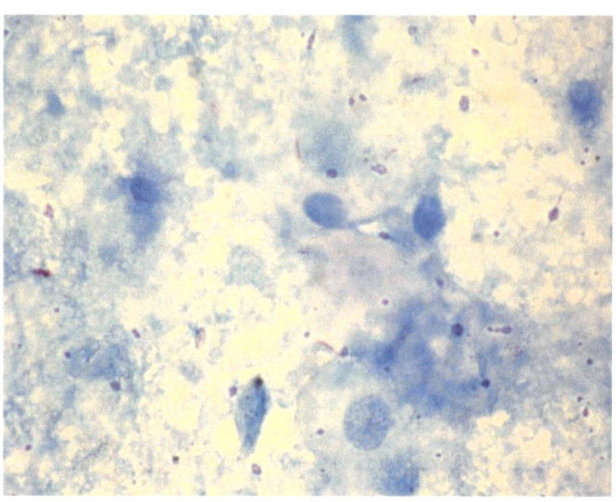
(a)

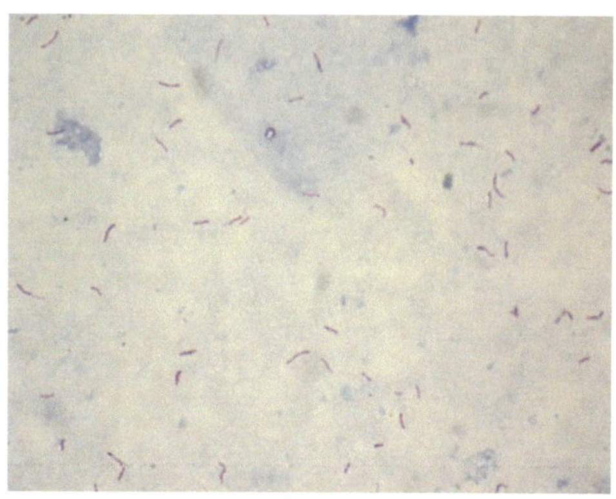
(b)

Fig. 3. Images with different density background content. (a) high density background content; (b) low density background content

The shape of a focus function typically resembles a Gaussian curve as shown if Figure 4.

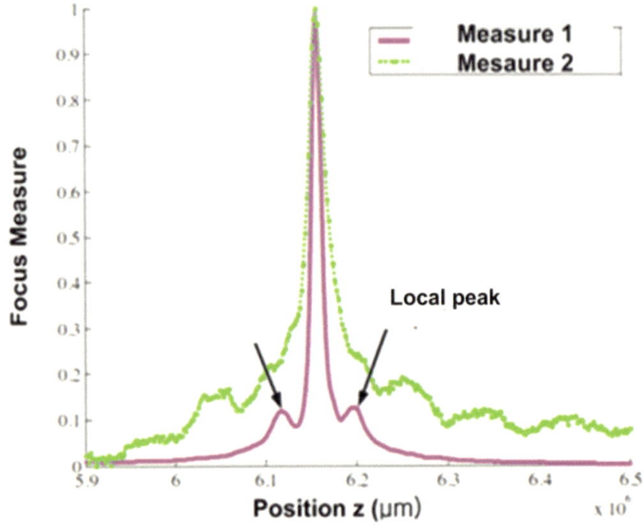

Fig. 4. Typical shape of a focus function

The horizontal coordinate of the graph of Figure 4 corresponds to the z position of the microscope vertical axis. To plot the focus function it is necessary to vary this z position and obtain a stack of points described in equation (13). The z position movement for obtaining the image stack is illustrated in Figure 5.

$$\text{Stack} = \{(FM_1, z_1), (FM_2,z_2),........(FM_{n/2}z_{n/2})....(FM_{n-1}z_{n-1})\ (FM_n,z_n)\} \quad (13)$$

Where: FM_i = Focus measure at position z_i

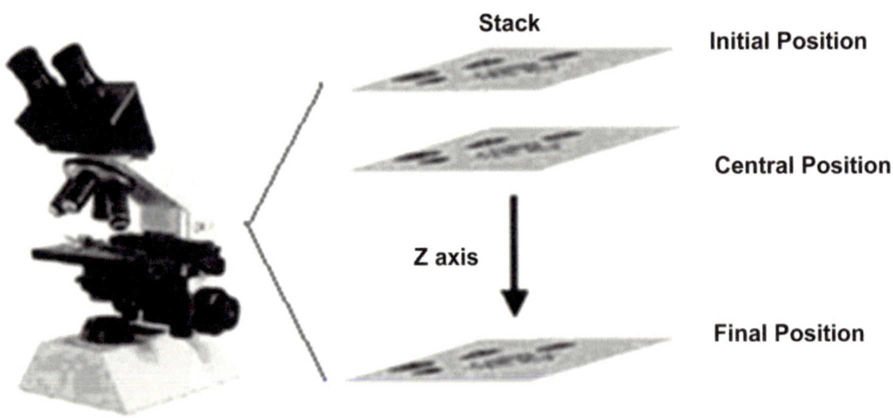

Fig. 5. Z position movement for obtaining the image stack

The in-focus image normally is the central image of the stack. Varying the z position changes the image sharpness and hence the degree of focus. Each image in a stack, therefore, is at a different focus level. For focus measure computation, images are converted from RGB to gray scale. The performance of a focus measure is frequently evaluated using the focus curve and according to four features (Firestone at. al., 1991), defined as:

1. Accuracy: expressed here as the number of steps by which the maximum of a particular focus function departs from the correct focal position;

Range: the number of steps between the two neighboring local minima around the global maximum;

Number of false maxima: number of spurious focus function maxima;

Width: computed at 50% of the height focus curve. This criterion describes the sharpness or narrowness of the peak.

Santos et al. (1997) introduced a 5th feature, Execution Time, as follows:

Execution Time: the time taken for an algorithm to compute the focus plot and locate the position of maximum focus.

According to Santos (Santos et. al., 1997) a quantitative evaluation may compare a focus curve to an ideal function with respect to each of these features. The authors define an ideal focus function as having a value of 0 for execution time, accuracy, width and number of false maxima and a range determined by multiplying the number of images in the stack used to plot the focus function and the step size between each position in the stack (adjustment step of the microscopy). To obtain a measure of how a focus measure departs from an ideal behavior the following algorithm is used:

1. A series of focus measure curves is obtained (these series should contain images with different background content). The mean and the standard deviation of each feature in the series are obtained.
2. The five feature values of each image series are normalized by subtracting the corresponding mean and dividing by the standard deviation. This produces values for the different features that can be compared as they all now have mean zero and standard deviation equal to unity.
3. For each feature the distance from the ideal function is computed. First the differences between the feature value in the function and in the ideal function are obtained. Then the square root of the addition of the squares of these results is computed.
4. Finally, to produce a final figure of this function, the mean value of the five distances is obtained.

When doing a TB diagnosis with sputum smear microscopy, a bacilli count on a number of fields of one slide is necessary. A time-consuming autofocus procedure determines the optimal focus through the acquisition of the focus function for each field. To reduce lens motion and achieve faster autofocus times the following procedure proposed by Osibote (Osibote et. al., 2010) can be used:

1. Obtaining the focus position for the first field of the slide through the acquisition of a full image stack of the focus measure, ensuring a perfect evaluation of this field to avoid locating the optimal focus in a false minimum position;
2. Adopt a simplified procedure to determine the optimal focus position in subsequent fields, using the optimal focus position of the previous field as a reference. For this purpose the procedure proposed by Yanzdafar (Yanzdafar et. al., 2008) can be used.

3. Automated sputum smear microscopy

According to Forero (Forero et. al., 2006) bacilli are structures that have a length between 1 and 10 μm and a width between 0.2 and 0.6 μm presenting a straight, curve or bent shape, as shown if Figure 6.

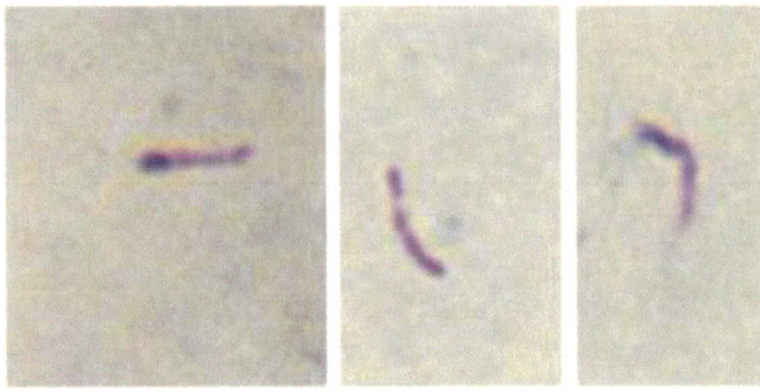

Fig. 6. Different shapes of bacilli

Depending on the staining procedures used, the bacilli assume different appearances. When the sputum smear is stained with an acid-fast fluorochrome dye, as is the case when fluorescence microscopy is used, the bacilli fluoresce in the range between green and yellow up to white, while the background is dark. Otherwise, when the sputum smear is stained with carbolfuchsin Ziehl-Neelsen - ZN or Kinyoun acid-fast stains, as is the case when conventional microscopy is used, the bacilli may have different colours, varying from light fuchsia to dark purple. In Figure 7 we show images of both microscopy types.

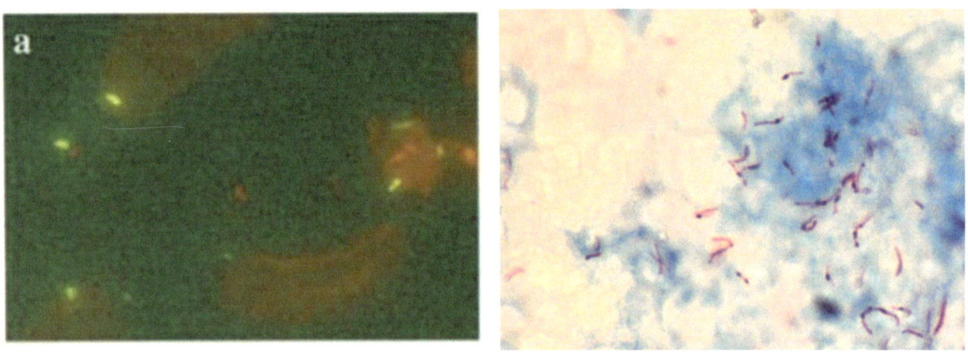

Fig. 7. Fluorescence microscopy (after Forero et al., 2004) and conventional microscopy sputum smear image

The block diagram of Figure 2 shows the main steps involved in automated bacilli recognition. Table 4 shows the main methods used in the literature for each step of this block diagram.

As shown in Figure 2, after image capture, bacilli segmentation is performed. The segmentation procedures adopted in both types of images shown in Figure 7 are completely different from each other.

In fluorescence microscopy images, the bacilli are easily separated from the background with a threshold operation. Afterwards, the segmentation is performed using edge detection operators, such as canny operators (Veropoulos et. al., 1998; Forero et. al., 2004). Intermediate steps for edge linking and boundary tracing are also employed. Figure 8 shows the results of the segmentation procedure used by Forero (Forero et. al., 2004) when applied to the image on the left side of Figure 7.

In conventional microscopy images, the bacilli are not easily separated from the background with a threshold operation. In this case, for bacilli segmentation, colour space techniques are used. As shown in Table 4, the techniques found in the literature vary: histogram based techniques, Bayesian pixel classifiers, KNN pixel classifiers, etc. The colour spaces used also vary: RGB, YCbCr and Lab

Author	Microscopy	Bacilli segmentation	Bacilli Classification	Results
Veropoulos et. al, 1998	Fluorescence	Edge detection techniques: Canny operator	**Shape Descriptors:** 15 Fourier descriptors; **Classifier:** Back-propagation (BP), RBF networks, KNN, Kernel Regression (KR)	**Accuracy:** BP - 97.57% RBF - 88.06% KNN - 91.80 KR - 95.24%
Forero et. al, 2004	Fluorescence	Edge detection techniques (Canny operator) + Adaptive color thresholding (RGB color space)	**Shape Descriptors:** compactness, eccentricity and Hu's moments descriptors; **Classifier:** Classification tree	**Specificity, Sensitivity:** 99.74%, 73.33% 94.96%, 86.66%
Forero et. al, 2006	Fluorescence	Edge detection techniques (Canny operator) + Adaptive color thresholding	**Shape Descriptors:** Hu's moments descriptors; **Classifier:** Gaussian mixture models	**Specificity, Sensitivity:** 97.89%, 94.67% 98.10%, 92.9%
Costa et. al., 2008	Conventional	**Color space techniques:** Adaptive global threshold; **Color space:** RGB	Size filters	**Sensitivity:** 76.65% **False Positive Rate:** 12%
Sadaphal et. al., 2008	Conventional	**Color space techniques:** Bayesian segmentation; **Color space:** RGB	**Shape Descriptors:** Axis ratio, eccentricity; **Classifier:** Classification tree	No information
Raof et. al., 2008	Conventional	**Color space techniques:** Thresholding; **Color space:** RGB		No information
Sotaquirá et. al. , 2009	Conventional	**Color space techniques:** First derivative of histogram; **Color space:** YCbCr, Lab		**Accuracy:** 96.3% **False detection:** 9.78%
Khutlang et. al. (2010)	Coventional	**Color space techniques:** Pixel classifiers (Baye's, Linear regression, quadratic discriminant); **Color space:** RGB	**Shape Descriptors:** Fourier features, color moments, eccentricity, compactness; **Classifier:** Probabilistic neural network, kNN, SVM	**Accuracy:** 98.55% **Sensitivity:** 97.77% **Specificity:** 99.13%

Table 4. Published papers involving Automated Sputum Smear Microscopy

After the segmentation step is finished, not only bacilli are segmented. Some structures fluoresce the same way as bacilli in fluorescence microscopy images. Similarly some structures have the same colour properties as bacilli in conventional microscopy images. confused with bacilli. These structures, also called noise, could be debris or cells present in the background. To illustrate this point, near the lower left corner of Figure 7, a circular structure can be seen that fluoresces the same way as a bacillus, but because of its circular shape could not be classified as one. Nevertheless, this structure is segmented the same way as a bacillus, as shown in Figure 8.

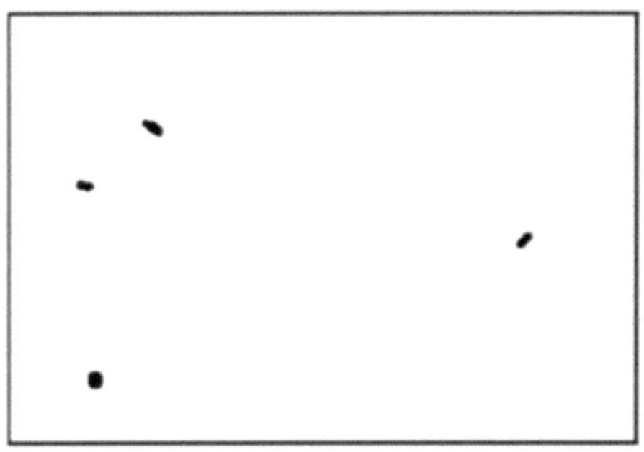

Fig. 8. Objects resulting from segmentation procedures applied in the left image of Figure 7.

To separate noise from bacilli in the segmented images an additional step, called object classification in the block diagram of Figure 2 is normally employed. For this purpose classifiers using shape descriptors are used. As the bacilli may have different sizes, positions and orientations, the shape descriptors used must be rotation, translation and scale invariant. As shown in Table 4, the most used descriptors used are: compactness, eccentricity, Hu's moments and Fourier Descriptors. Varied classifiers such as classification trees, Support Vector Machines and Neural Networks were employed by some authors in order to recognize the bacilli.

The results presented in Table 4 show that, in bacilli detection, results for sensitivity and specificity as good as 97.77% and 99.13% are cited. It is noteworthy, however that the authors who cited these values, do not consider touching bacilli. In some cases, as the one shown in Figure 9, these bacilli are present in large quantities. Disregarding these bacilli implies a different count of what is done by manual means. Because of this, we believe that other ways of removing noise than those that use shape descriptors must be investigated.

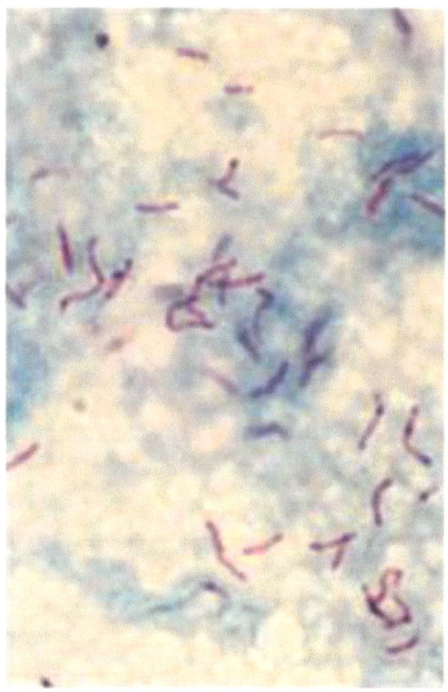

Fig. 9. Conventional microscopy image showing some examples of touching bacilli

4. References

ATS (2000). Diagnostic standards and classification of tuberculosis in adults and children. *American Journal of Respiratory and Critical Care Medicine*, Vol. 161, pp. 1376-1395, ISSN 1073-449X

Brenner, J.F., Dew, B.S., Horton, J.B., King, J.B., Netrath, P.W. & Sellers, W.B. (1971), An automated microscope for cytologic research, *Journal of Histochemistry and Cytochemistry*, Vol. 24, pp 100-111, ISSN 0022-1554

Bennedsen, J. & Larsen, S. O. (1966), Examination for tubercle bacilli by fluorescence, *Scandinavian Journal of Respiratory Disease*, Vol. 47, pp.114–20, ISSN 0036-5572

Costa, M. G. F., Costa Filho, C. F. F., Sena, J. F., Salen, J. & Lima, M. O. (2008), Automatic identification of mycobacterium tuberculosis with conventional light microscopy, *Proceedings of the 30th Annual International Conference of the IEEE EMBS*, pp. 382-385,Vancouver, British Columbia, Canada

Firestone, L., Cook, K., Culp, K., Talsania, N. & Preston Jr, K. (1991), Comparison of autofocus methods for automated microscopy, *Cytometry*, Vol. 12, pp.195-206

Forero, M. G. & Cristóbal, G. (2003), Automatic identification techniques of tuberculosis bacteria, *Proc. SPIE*, Vol. 5203, pp. 71–81, ISSN 0277-786X

Forero, M.G., Sroubek, F. & Cristóbal, G. (2004). Identification of tuberculosis bacteria based on shape and color, *Real Time Imaging*, Vol. 10, pp. 251–262, ISSN 1077-2014

Forero, M.G., Cristóbal, G. & Desco, M. (2006), Automatic identification of Mycobacterium tuberculosis by Gaussian mixture models, *Journal of Microscopy*, Vol. 223, pp. 120–132, ISSN 0022-2720

Geusebrock, J., Cornelissen, F., Smeulders, A.W.M. & Geerts, G. (2000), Robust auto focusing in microscopy, *Cytometry*, Vol. 39, pp.1-9, ISSN 0196-4763

Kautsky, J., Flusser, .J, Zitova, B. S. & Imberova, S., (2002), A new waveletbased measure of image focus. *Pattern Recognition Letters*, Vol. 23, pp. 1785–1794.

Khutlang, R., Krishnan, S., Dendere, R., Whitelaw, A., Veropoulos, K., Learmonth, G. & Douglas, T. S. (2010), Classification of Mycobacterium tuberculosis in Images of ZN-Stained Sputum Smears, *IEEE Transactions on Information Technology in Biomedicine*, Vol. 14, No. 4, pp. 949-957, ISSN 1089-7771

Kimura Junior, A., Costa, M., Costa Filho, C. F. F., Fujimoto, L. B.M. & Salem, J. (2010), Evaluation of autofocus functions of conventional sputum smear microscopy for tuberculosis, *32th Annual International IEEE EMBS Conference*, pp. 3041-3044

Krotkov, E. (1987), Focusing, *International Journal of Computer Vision*, Vol. 1, pp. 223-227, ISSN 0920-5691

Lenseigne, B., Brodin, P., Christophe, T. & Genovesio, A. (2007), Support vector machines for automatic detection of tuberculosis bacteria in confocal microscopy images, *Proceedings of 4th IEEE International Symposium on Biomedical Imaging*, pp. 85-88, ISBN 0-7803-7585-8, Arlington, VA, USA

Luelmo, F. (2004), What is the role of sputum microscopy in patients attending health facilities?, In: *Toman's Tuberculosis Case detection, treatment, and monitoring –questions and answers*, T. Frieden, pp. 7-10, World Health Organization, ISBN 9241546034, Hong Kong, China

Makkapati, V., Agrawal, R. & Acharya, R. (2009), Segmentation and Classification of Tuberculosis Bacilli from ZN-stained Sputum Smear Images, *Proceddings of 5th Annual IEEE Conference on Automation Science and Engineering*, pp. 217-220, ISBN 978-1-60566-750-8 , Bangalore, India

Osibote, O.A., Dendere, R., Krishnan, S. & Douglas, T.S. (2010), Automated focusing in bright-field microscopy for tuberculosis detection, *Journal of Microscopy*, Vol. 240, 2, pp.155-163, ISSN 0022-2720

Raof, R. A. A., Salleh, Z., Sahidan, S. I., Mashor, M. Y., Md Noor, S. S., Idris, F. M. & Hasan, H. (2008), Color Thresholding Method For Image Segmentation Algorithm of Ziehl-Neelsen Sputum Slide Images, *Proceedings of 5th International Conference on Electrical Engineering, Computing Science and Automatic Control*, pp. 212-217, ISBN 978-1-4244-2499-3, Mexico City, Mexico

Russel, M.J & Douglas, T. S. (2007), Evaluation of autofocus algorithms for tuberculosis microscopy, *29th Annual International IEEE EMBS Conference*, pp. 3489-3492

Sadaphal, P, Rao, J., Comstock, G.W. & Beg, M.F. (2008), Image processing techniques for identifying Mycobacterium tuberculosis in Ziehl-Neelsen stains. *International Journal of Tuberculosis Lung Disease*, Vol. 12, n. 5, pp. 579-582, ISSN 1027-3719.

Santos, A., Ortiz-Solorzano, C.; Vaquero, J.; Malpica, N.; Pozo, F. Del (1997), Evaluation of autofocus functions in molecular cytogenetic analysis. *Journal of Microscopy*, Vol. 188, pp. 264–272, ISSN 0022-2720

Sotaquirá, M., Rueda, L. & Narvaez, R. (2009), Detection and quantification of bacilli and clusters present in sputum smear samples: a novel algorithm for pulmonary tuberculosis diagnosis, *Proceedings of International Conference on Digital Image Processing*, pp. 117-121, ISBN 978-0-7695-3565-4 , Bankoc, Thailand

Steingart, K. R., Henry, M., Ng, V., Hopewell, P. C., Ramsay, A., Cunningham, J., Urbanczik, R., Perkins, M., Aziz, M. A. & Pai, M. (2006), Fluorescence versus conventional sputum smear microscopy for tuberculosis: a systematic review, *Lancet Infectious Deseases*, Vol. 6, pp. 570-581, ISSN 1473-3099

Subbarao, M. & Tyan, J. K. (1995), The Optimal Focus Measure for Passive Autofocusing and Depth-from-Focus, *Proc. SPIE Conf. Viedometrics IV*, Vol. 2, 598, pp. 89-99, Philadelphia, ISBN 0-8194-1321-6

Subbarao, M. & Tyan, J. K. (1998), Selecting the Optimal Focus Measure for Autofocusing and Depth-From-Focus, *IEEE Transactions on Pattern Analysis and Machine Intelligence*, Vol. 20, 8, pp. 864-870, ISSN 0162-8828

UN, The Millennium Development Goals Report 2010 (2010), 18/05/2011, Available from: <http://www.un.org/millenniumgoals/reports.shtml >

Toman, K. (2004a), How reliable is smear microscopy?, In: *Toman's Tuberculosis Case detection, treatment, and monitoring –questions and answers*, T. Frieden, pp. 7-10, World Health Organization, ISBN 9241546034, Hong Kong, China

Toman, K. (2004b), What are the advantages and disadvantages of fluorescence microscopy?, In: *Toman's Tuberculosis Case detection, treatment, and monitoring – questions and answers*, T. Frieden, pp. 7-10, World Health Organization, ISBN 9241546034, Hong Kong, China

Veropoulos, K., Campbell, C., Learmonth, G., Knight, B., & Simpson, J (1998), The Automated Identification of Tubercle Bacilli using Image Processing and Neural Computing Techniques, *Proceedings of 8th International Conference on Artificial Neural Networks*, Vol. 2, pp. 797-802, ISBN 3540762639 ,Skövde, Sweden,.

Vollath, D. (1988), The influence of the scene parameters and of noise on the behaviour of automatic focusing algorithms, *Journal of Microscopy*, Vol. 151, pp.133-146

WHO, Global TB Control report (2010). 18/05/2011, Available from: <http://www.who.int/tb/publications/global_report/2010/en/index.html >

Yazdanfar, S., Kenny, K.B., Tasimi, K., Corwin, A.D., Dixon, E.L. & Filkins R.J. (2008), Simple and robust image-based auto focusing for digital microscopy. *Optics Express*. Vol. 16, pp. 8670–8677.

14

The Use of Phage for Detection, Antibiotic Sensitivity Testing and Enumeration

Catherine Rees[1] and George Botsaris[2]
[1]*University of Nottingham and*
[2]*Cyprus University of Technology*
[1]*United Kingdom*
[2]*Cyprus*

1. Introduction

Bacteriophage are bacterial viruses which may attack and destroy bacterial cells. While many have a narrow host range and are used in sub-typing techniques, some infect many members of a genus or species and these have been used to develop rapid detection methods for a variety of bacterial pathogens (Rees and Loessner, 2008). The use of bacteriophage (or phage) in assays for detecting bacteria was first reported over half a century ago when an assay to detect *Salmonella* using phage Felix 01 was described by Cherry et al. (1954). Since then other bacteriophage-based detection methods have been developed that take advantage of the specificity of the host-phage interaction and its ability, once inside the host, to replicate rapidly. This is particularly useful when studying slow-growing organisms such as *Mycobacterium tuberculosis* and other slow growing mycobacteria such as *Mycobacterium avium* subsp. *paratuberculosis* (see Stanley et al., 2007; Grant & Rees, 2009, Botsaris et al., 2010). This chapter will provide an introduction to phage biology and will then describe the different phage-based detection methods that have been described for *M. tuberculosis* - including one that has been developed into a commercial product. In addition adaptations of the phage test are described that allow the antibiotic sensitivity of isolates to be rapidly determined, and also how a further modification can be used to allow rapid estimation of viable cell number. However, all these indirect methods have their limitations and these too will be discussed in each case.

2. Mycobacteriophage

Mycobacteriophage, which are phage that infect any members of the *Mycobacterium* genus, were first isolated and characterized by Gardner and Weiser in 1947 and further investigation was prompted in the 1950s by their utility in typing of clinical isolates. Phage typing is a method used to sub-type members of a bacterial species based the sensitivity of a particular host strain to a panel of bacteriophage that have been shown to have a limited host range within the group (see Rees and Loessner, 2008, for a description of this method). So far over 200 different mycobacteriophage have been described, infecting a broad variety of mycobacterial hosts and these have been isolated from a variety of environmental sources, such as soil or surface water (Froman et al., 1954; Caroli & Avio, 1975), and stool and resection specimens of patients with tuberculosis or sarcoidosis (Mankiewicz, 1961; Mankiewicz & Liivak, 1967). The collection of Mycobacteriophage is continually being expanded due to an education programme developed by researchers at the University of Pittsburgh, supported by the Howard Hughes Medical Institute Science Education Alliance. This has recently resulted in the publication of a multi-author paper describing the isolation, sequencing and comparative genomic analysis of 18 new mycobacteriophages isolated from geographically distinct locations by freshmen attending Universities across within the United States (Pope et al., 2011).

Like all viruses, phage consist of a nucleic acid core and a protein coat, and considerable variation in structure has been reported. However all mycobacteriophage that have been described to date are double-stranded DNA viruses consisting of icosahedral heads with a tail which may be either short or long and either flexible (Siphoviridae) or contractile (Myoviridae) (Hatfull et al., 2008; see Figure 1). These tail structures play an essential role in host cell recognition and penetration of the bacterial cell wall structure. The comparative genomic analysis of mycobacteriophage reveals that they have relatively large genomes (average length approx. 70 kbp), contain large numbers of previously unidentified genes, and are highly diverse at both the nucleotide and amino acid sequence levels (Pedulla et al., 2003; Hatfull et al., 2010; Pope et al., 2011). Once inside the host cell the phage take over the host cell biosynthetic machinery and use this to replicate themselves, usually producing hundreds of progeny phage per infected cell (Figure 2). At the end of the replication cycle many phage produce enzymes (lysins) which degrade the cell wall and result in the lysis of the host cell and release of the progeny phage. However some phage do not always enter this lytic cycle. Instead, after entering the cell, they can enter a dormant state resulting in a latent infection. This state is known as lysogeny, but these lysogenic (or temperate) phage can be induced back into the lytic cycle, often in response to environmental conditions that either damage cellular structures or induce a stress response in the host cell (Figure 2). Both lytic and lysogenic Mycobacteriophage have been identified.

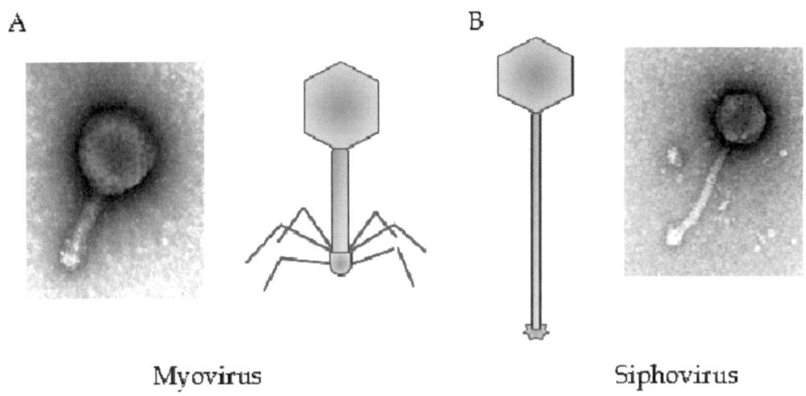

Fig. 1. Common Morphotypes of Mycobacteriophage
Myoviridae (panel A) typically have short, rigid contractile tails which often have associated tail fibres. Siphoviridae (panle B) have longer, flexible, non-contractile tails which termimates in a base-plate structure and tail fibres are absent. Both types of phage have double stranded DNA genomes. The majority of Mycobacteriophage are Siphoviridae.

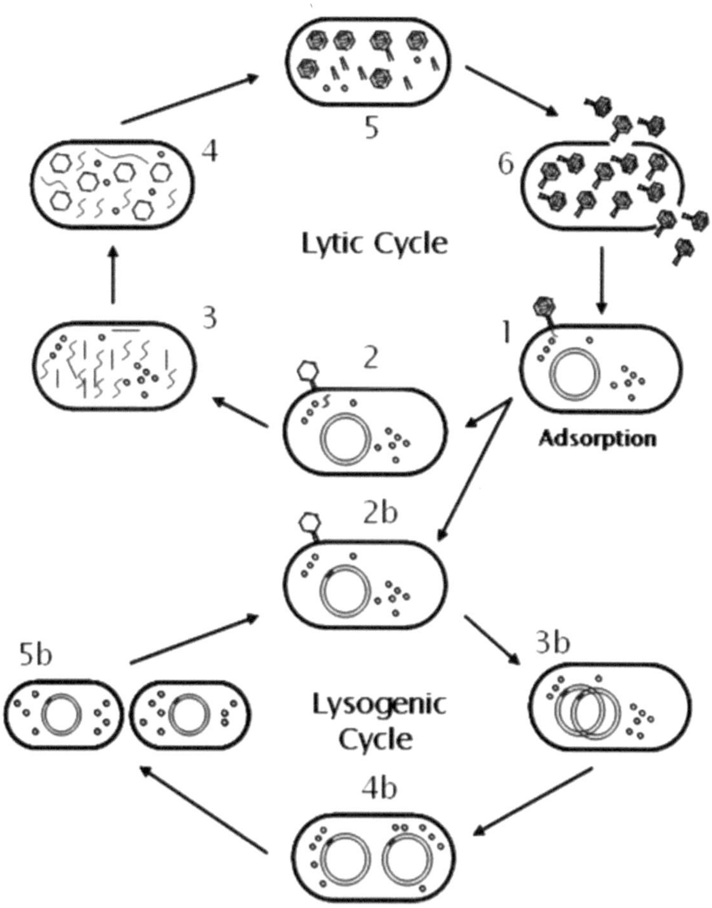

Fig. 2. The Bacteriophage Replication Cycle
Schematic representation of the Lytic and the Lysogenic Cycles. Lytic Cycle: Infection is mediated via receptors found in the phage tail structures. During infection the bacteriophage inserts the genomic DNA located inside the virus capsid into the cell (1 & 2) and then it takes over the cell replication machinery and directs the synthesis of bacteriophage nucleic acids and proteins (3 & 4 and 5). Finally the phage produces enzymes (lysins) that breaks open the cell and the mature bacteriophage particles are released (6). Lysogenic Cycle: adsorption occurs in the same way (1) but the bacteriophage DNA is not replicated and instead integrates into the host cell's genome (2b). It is then replicated along with the host cell DNA at cell division and the lytic genes are not expressed (3b and 4b). When the cell divides a copy of the bacteriophage DNA is transferred along with the host chromosome (5b). Following induction into the lytic phase, the integrated phage DNA is excised from the host cell genome and the lytic genes are then expressed leading to phage replication.

3. Use of phage in detection assays

Mycobacteriophage have been used to detect slow fastidious mycobacteria, such as members of the TB complex. The main two techniques developed for detection of mycobacteria using phage are recombinant Reporter Phage and the Phage Amplification Assay (PAA), also known as Phage Amplified Biologically (PhaB) assay. These two methods differ in how the host cell is detected at the end of the assay and both are described in more detail in the following sections.

3.1 Reporter Phage assays for mycobacteria

The Reporter Phage detection method uses genetic engineering to introduce a reporter gene into a phage genome. Since genes are not expressed inside the virion particle, no signal is produced from the reporter gene until it enters a host cell during infection. At this point the reporter gene is expressed along with the phage replication genes and this can be detected to indicate that an infection event has occurred (see Figure 3). The limitation here is the packaging constraint of the phage being used; this is the natural limit on the size of phage genome that can be packaged into a phage head. If the size of the gene being introduced into the phage exceeds the packaging constraint, the recombinant phage particles are defective. However the firefly luciferase reporter gene (*Fflux* or *luc*) has been successfully introduced into a number of mycobacteria phage (Jacobs et al., 1993; Sarkis et a., 1995; Pearson et al., 1996; Riska et al., 1997). This enzyme requires a source of ATP to produce light (bioluminescence), and this is provided by the infected cell. When the luciferin substrate for the enzyme is added (exogenously) the light can be sensitively detected by a luminometer.

The first Mycobacterial Reporter Phage described were based on the lytic phage TM4 since it was argued that a lytic phage would not be able to enter the dormant lysogenic state and therefore would produce high levels of reporter signal. However but it was found that these lysed the *Mycobacterium* cells too rapidly so that only low levels of luciferase were produced. This reduced the limit of detection when using this phage to approximately 10^4 mycobacterial cells (Jacobs et al., 1993). The same group also constructed a reporter phage using the temperate phage L5 and found that when the phage integrated into the chromosome there was prolonged expression of the reporter gene and this then reduced the limit of detection to approximately 10^2 cells after a 40 h incubation period, or 10^3 cells after 20 h (Sarkis et al., 1995). Although this demonstrated for the first time that reporter phage could be used to rapidly and sensitively detect Mycobacteria, this phage had a limited host range and therefore could not be developed as a practical test for *M. tuberculosis*. Instead the TM4-based reporter phage was improved by changing the site of insertion of the *Fflux* gene in the phage genome and isolating mutants of the phage to improve host range. This lead to the isolation of a TM4-based reporter phage that could detect as few as 120 *Mycobacterium bovis* BCG after 12 h of incubation (Carriere et al., 1997) which is significantly faster than any culture-based method can achieve and when tested on clinical samples it was shown that smear-positive sputum samples could be detected within 24-48 h (Riska et al., 1997). One limitation of the Reporter Phage assay for direct identification of *M. tuberculosis* in clinical samples is that these phage are able to infect a number of species of *Mycobacterium*, for instance TM4 also infects *M. bovis* and members of the *M. avium* complex (Timme and Brennan, 1984). This results in reduced specificity of the assay and hence produces false-positive test results. To overcome this, the reporter phage have been used in combination with p-nitro-a-acetylamino-b-hydroxy propiophenone (NAP) which specifically inhibits the growth of *M. tuberculosis* complex bacteria (Eidus et al. 1960). Parallel samples, with and without the addition of NAP, are used and the results of the Reporter Phage assay compared. If light is produced from both samples then the organism detected is not M. tuberculosis. However if light is suppressed in the sample containing NAP, this indicates that *M. tuberculosis* cells have been detected (Riska et al. 1997). Using this combination of tests, Banaiee et al. (2001) reported that 94% of strains tested could be correctly identified.

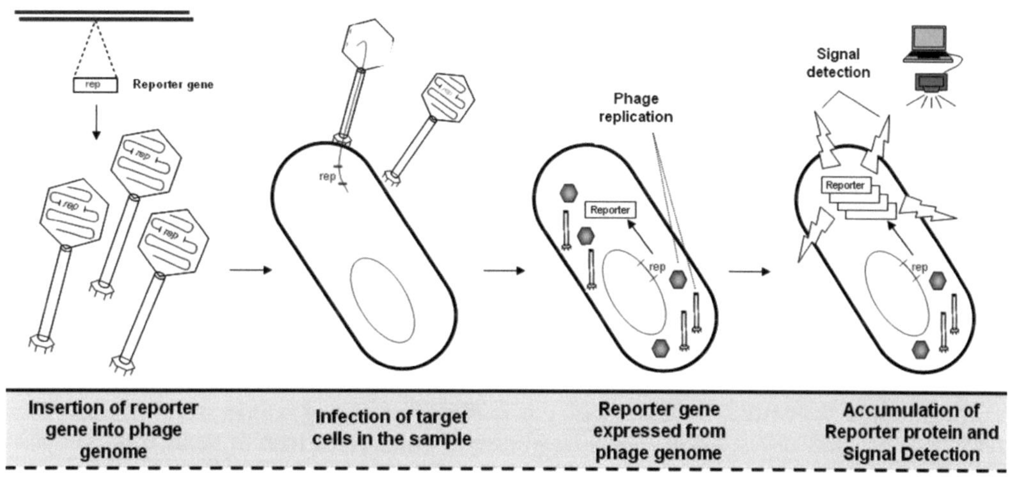

Fig. 3. General Schematic for Reporter Phage Assays
Schematic representation for Reporter Phage Assays. Following the insertion of the reporter gene into the phage genome the phage infects the targeted host cell. The reporter gene is then expressed from the phage genome and as the reporter protein accumulates the signal is detected.

Although these initial reports were promising there have been very few recent reports of the use of reporter phage as a diagnostic tool for TB. Recently, Dusthackeer et al. (2008) reported the construction of a new *Fflux* Reporter Phage using the temperate phage, Che12 - again arguing that integration of these phage would produce more sustained light levels - and also using promoters to direct the expression of the *Fflux* that were predicted to be more highly expressed in dormant bacilli (isocitrate lyase (*icl*) and alpha crystallin protein (*acr*)). They also re-engineered the promoter sequences gene in the defective TM4-based phage phAE129 (Carriere et al., 1997) to determine if light output could be improved. Interestingly, by comparing the results obtained for the two phage they showed that while these promoters did increase light output when the phage infected dormant cells, the Che12 Reporter Phage only poorly infected dormant bacilli. This is probably because it lacks a peptidoglycan hydrolase TM3 motif found in the TM4 tape- measure protein and this is required to allow phage to efficiently infect *M. smegmatis* in stationary phase when it has a thicker or more highly cross-linked peptidoglycan layer.

Two new Reporter Phage constructs have also been described which have been engineered to contain genes encoding the fluorescent proteins GFP or ZsYellow (Piuri et al., 2009). These were introduced into the conditionally-replicating TM4 derivative phAE87 under the control of the constitutive *M. bovis* BCG Hsp60 promoter to create the fluorophage phAE87::*hsp60-EGFP* and phAE87::*hsp60-ZsYellow*. However these were evaluated for use as a rapid, semi-automoated method for determining antibiotic sensitivity of *M. tuberculosis* isolates rather than as a detection method (see section 4) and this seems to be now accepted as the most useful application of the Reporter Phage in TB diagnostics.

However there may still be examples where the Reporter Phage may provide a useful tool for the detection of other types of pathogenic Mycobacteria. For instance Sasahara et al. (2004) described the use of Reporter Phage for the detection of the cattle pathogen *Mycobacterium avium* subspecies *paratuberculosis* (MAP). Using phage phAE85 >1000 cells /mL were detectable within 24-48 h. When applied to milk, the authors reported that MAP was detectable at 100 cells/ml in skim milk and 1,000 cells/ml in whole milk. While this is a useful demonstration of the rapid detection of pathogenic Mycobacteria in a food matrix, it is unlikely that this will be adopted as a rapid testing method by the food industry since these Reporter Phage are considered to be GMOs and any laboratory using them is required to work according to the local GM regulations, and the cost of implementing these is not generally compatible with food microbiology testing.

3.2 Phage amplification assays

Unlike the Reporter Phage assays, the PAA or PhaB assays do not use recombinant phage. In these assays a positive indication of the presence of mycobacteria is the formation of plaques at the end of the assay. There have been several variations of these types of assay published but the general principle is a phage protection assay (see Rees and Loessner, 2008). To initiate the assays the sample containing the target cell is first mixed with a high titre of the bacteriophage. The samples are then incubated to allow time for cell infection to occur and for the phage to enter the eclipse phase. At this point any exogenous phage that have not entered an appropriate host cell are destroyed by the addition of a virucide. Various chemicals have been described that can be used as the virucide, but the essential feature of the chemical chosen is fast inactivation of phage particles while having no effect on the viability of the host cells (Stewart et al., 1998). These internalized phage now must be detected, and in its simplest form the phage released at the end of the lytic cycle are detected by the formation of plaques (areas of no growth) in a bacterial lawn. Many of the Mycobacteria phage, such as TM4 and D29, have a broad host range and can also infect the fast growing, non-pathogen *M. smegmatis*. Hence this is often used as a rapidly growing host to produce lawns of bacterial to detect the newly released phage (see Figure 4).

This assay has been produced as commercial kits (the *FAST*plaqueTB™ or Phage Tek MB assays; www.biotec.com) and also "in house" versions have been described (McNerney et al., 2004) and its performance has been extensively reviewed (see Kalantri et al., 2005; Palomino, 2005; Dinnes et al., 2007). The assessment of the performance of these tests have been variable, with some groups reporting that that they perform very well (Albert et al., 2002; Muzaffar et al., 2002; Shenai et al., 2002; Kiraz et al., 2007) while others have reported problems with sample contamination leading to loss of results (Mbulo et al. 2004; Bonnet et al., 2009), and hence decreased sensitivity of the test. This problem has been addressed by the manufacturers by the introduction of an antibiotic supplement containing nystatin, oxacillin and aztreonam (NOA) which suppresses the growth of a wide range of Gram-positive and Gram-negative bacteria and yet does not lead to significant reduction in assay sensitivity while increasing the proportion of interpretable results obtained (Albert et al., 2007; Mole et al., 2007). Although the phage assay is simple to perform, inexpensive and does not require any sophisticated or dedicated equipment, it does require the samples to be

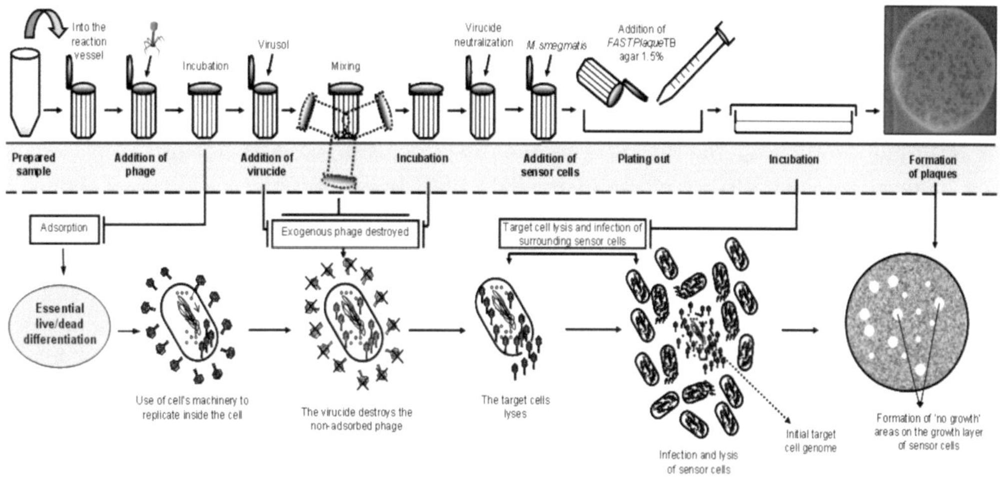

Fig. 4. Diagram of Phage Amplification Assay
Grapic representation of the phage amplification assay. On the top the processing steps of the assay are presented and on the bottom the scientific details of the assay are shown. Following the appropriate sampling preparation the assay is carried out following the procedure described and presented in this figure.

transferred to a dedicated microbiology laboratory. This was perceived to be a disadvantage over conventional sputum smear testing when diagnosis was being performed in clinics in remote areas where reliable, temperature controlled transportation of samples is difficult (Mbulo et al., 2004; Prakash et al., 2009).

The issue of specificity of the phage test arises from the fact that the test utilizes the broad host range of phage D29 to allow both slow growing and fast growing Mycobacteria to be infected. As discussed in relation to the Reporter Phage assays, additional tests are therefore required to determine if the cell detected is TB or a non-tuberculosis *Mycobacterium* spp. For the commercial phage assays a cut-off of 20 plaques is applied, which is the expected number of plaques that will result from the presence of non-pathogenic Mycobacteria that have been fortuitously introduced into sputum, so that samples with fewer than 20 plaques are scored as negative. Patients with active disease generally produced samples with much higher plaque numbers due to growth of the bacteria. However Stanley et al. (2007) have demonstrated that PCR can also be used to increase the specificity of the D29 phage amplification assay.

In this report the assay was being used for the detection of MAP in raw milk samples, but the presence of other pathogenic or non-pathogenic Mycobacteria in these samples could not be ruled out. To overcome this problem, DNA was extracted from the center of the plaques formed at the end of the assay and used for PCR amplification of signature sequences so that the identity of the cell detected by the phage could be determined (see Figure 4). Since *M. tuberculosis* and *M. bovis* were both likely to be present in raw milk samples a multiplex plaque PCR assay was developed to allow simultaneous discrimination between these three organisms. The signature sequences chosen were all multicopy *IS* elements (MAP, IS*900*; TB complex IS*6110* and IS*1081*) with the size of the PCR product indicating which element had been amplified. Combining the phage assay with PCR provides a significant advantage over direct PCR detection methods since the phage test provides live/dead discrimination while the PCR assay achieves definitive molecular molecular identification of the cell detected.

By reducing sample loss due to contamination by the introduction of antibiotic supplements and increasing the specificity of the phage-based test by combining with PCR, it should be possible that a rapid and robust assay format can be achieved. However the need to perform PCR increases the complexity, cost and time required to complete the assay and the usefulness of this combination assay has yet to be evaluated for clinical cases of TB.

4. Antibiotic sensitivity testing

While the usefulness of phage detection tests for direct identification of *M. tuberculosis* in clinical samples remains questionable, the use of both Reporter Phage and PAA/PhaB assays for determining antibiotic susceptibility of clinical isolates has proven to be more a valuable tool. The principle of these tests was first outlined by Jacobs et al. (1993) using Reporter Phage when they demonstrated that phage growth and gene expression was inhibited if rifampicin was added to antibiotic-sensitive cells whereas if the cells were resistant to the antibiotic, signal generation was unaffected. They showed that the reporter gene signal could be detected within minutes of infection of *M. tuberculosis* with a Fflux Reporter Phage, and by comparing the results of Reporter Phage infection in the presence and absence of the antibiotic, the sensitivity of *M. tuberculosis* isolates could be determined within days. As before, this type of assay is not specific to *M. tuberculosis* and Williams et al. (1999) described the use of *Fflux* Reporter phage to rapidly determination of drug susceptibilities of MAP giving faster results and, in this case, also being used to determine the minimum inhibitory concentration (MIC) of the antibiotics tested more rapidly and accurately.

Similar assays have been developed for the non-recombinant phage assays by showing that phage growth is inhibited, but in this case it is the formation of plaques that is inhibited rather than the signal from a reporter gene (Wilson et al., 1997 and reviewed in Minion and Pai, 2010), and again these have been produced as a commercial test (*FAST*plaque-Response™; www.biotec.com) which can be used on direct patient specimens as well as indirect isolates. Other assay formats using microtitre plates and alternative methods of detecting phage growth have also been described (Gali et al., 2003; McNerney et al., 2007;, which have been designed to shorten the time required for testing. Most recently Bainee et al., (2008) have described a microtitre format Reporter Phage assay that can be semi-automated. Isolates were inoculated in to the wells of the microtitre dish, treated with either rifampicin (RIF), isoniazid (INH) or no antibiotic and then incubated for 40 h before samples were infected with the TM4-based Reporter Phage phAE142. After 3 h of infection the light levels in each well are determined using a microplate luminometer and the sensitivity of the strains determined by comparing the light levels of the treated and control samples. This method was shown to be able to determine both the RIF and INH resistance of clinical isolates of M. tuberculosis with a median test result time of 2 days.

Minion and Pai (2010) carried out a meta-analysis of 31 studies describing the use of the different phage assays used to determine rifampicin resistance and concluded that the

Reporter Phage assays had the highest accuracy (sensitivity = 99.3%, specificity = 98.6%), with in-house phage amplification assays also performing well (sensitivity = 98.5%, specificity = 97.9%). Estimates from studies evaluating the commercial *FAST*plaque kits were slightly lower (sensitivity = 95.5%, specificity = 95.0%); however, this difference was not statistically significant (based on overlapping confidence intervals) from the LRP and in-house assays (Minion and Pai, 2010). However this report did highlight the fact that the phage-based methods currently provide the fastest phenotypic assay for antibiotic susceptibility testing and if levels of technical failure can be reduced these assays could be a useful clinical tool to improve patient outcomes.

5. Enumeration assays

Perhaps the most overlooked potential of these phage based assays is as a research tool for the rapid evaluation of viable count of laboratory cultures. Simple modifications of the Phage Amplification assay allow cell number to be rapidly determined, with results being available within 24 h. This method was first reported by Stanley et al. (2007) in a paper describing the development of a phage amplification assay for MAP. In this case 10-fold serial dilutions of MAP cultures were prepared and a sample of each dilution tested using the Phage Amplification assay and it was found that the number of plaques detected correlated well with the number of MAP cells in the test sample (Stanley, 2005). Rather than diluting the sample and testing each one, a modification of the *FAST*plaque assay method was devised that allowed the viable count of a sample containing an unknown number of cells. In this case the sample is simply diluted immediately prior to plating so that the plaque number can be accurately counted and then the number of cells present in the original sample determined according to the dilution factor (Botsaris et al., 2009; Figure 5).

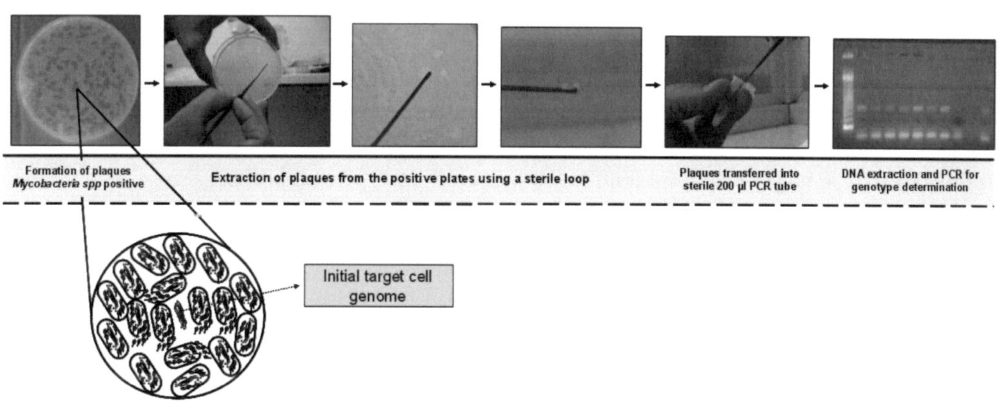

Fig. 5. Extraction of Plaques and Molecular Identification
Schematic representation of the plaque extraction method. The plaques containing the genome of the initial targeted cell are extracted using a sterile loop. The loop is used to cut gently all 4 sides of the plaque area and then the plaque is gently lifted and placed into a PCR tube for DNA extraction.

It is clear that there is not always a 1:1 relationship between the cfu and pfu counts obtained, however results for a given isolate grown under the same conditions seem to be relatively constant (Stanley, 2005). Foddai et al. (2009) described the optimisation of the MAP Phage Amplification assay to accurately detect and enumerate MAP cells. They investigated the optimal buffer conditions for D29 phage infection of MAP cells, determined the minimal time for D29 incubation with MAP to produce extracellular phage (burst time) and the incubation time required before virucide treatment and assessed the impact of changing these parameters on the correlation between plaque count and corresponding colony count. To achieve a correlation closer to 1:1 between pfu/ml and cfu/ml value when detecting MAP, the authors suggested modifications to the standard protocol including supplementing the medium with 2 mM calcium chloride to enhance phage infection, incubating cells at 37 °C overnight before infection with D29 and extending the time allowed for phage infection to 2 h so that phage successfully infect a higher percentage of cells.

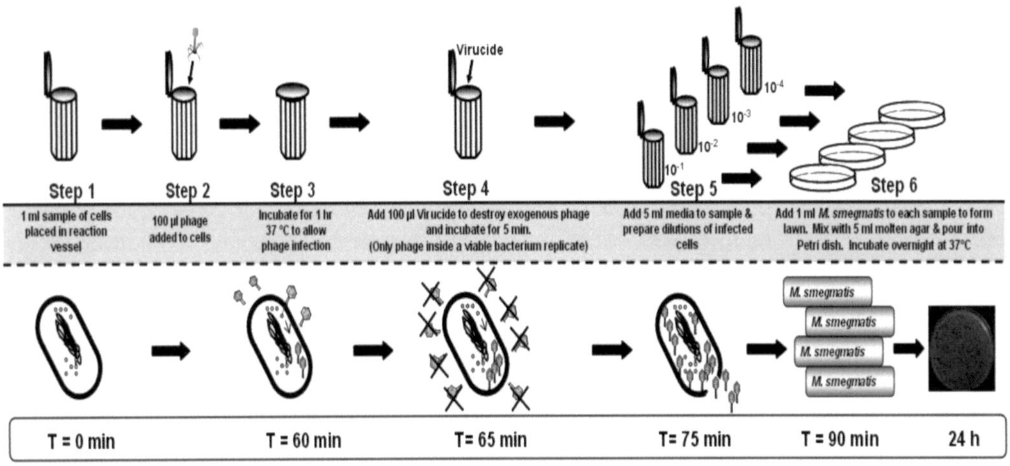

Fig. 6. Modification of the PAA for Enumeration of cells
Enumeration of cells using the PAA. 1 ml of the sample is infected with phage. Following adsorption exogenous phage are destroyed by the addition of a virucide which is then neutralised. Serial dilutions are made and plated on a lawn of M. smegmatis cells. Plaques (representing the target cells) are enumerated after overnight incubation.

A limited number of reports of the use of phage for enumeration have appeared in the literature - all for MAP rather than for *M. tuberculosis* - but these do demonstrate the usefulness of the method, especially when following inactivation kinetics. Altic et al. (2007) used the FPTB assay in UV inactivation studies and the authors observed that the colony counts were consistently 1 to 2 log_{10} higher than the plaque counts. However the rate of inactivation measured by both culture and Phage Amplification Assay were identical, so that even though a proportion of the population was detected, these cells were inactivated in the same rate as the rest of the culture. Similarly Donaghy et al. (2009) used the Phage Amplification assay to monitor UV inactivation of MAP using a novel pilot-scale UV treatment for milk. Again there was a discrepancy between the cfu and pfu values obtained, and some evidence of large differences in the infectivity of different strains of MAP, but despite this the inactivation curves obtained were identical and the pfu data was available within 24 h whereas the culture results required up to 18 weeks for growth of the colonies. This demonstrates the power of the phage-based assays to provide rapid data to allow development of experimental design to initiate new areas of research. Once the normal pfu:cfu ratio has been established for a particular strain grown under a particular condition, the phage assay can be used to rapidly determine the number of viable cells present in a sample without the need for extended periods of incubation.

6. Conclusion

The use of bacteriophage to type bacterial cells has been accepted as a standard microbiological method for many decades. First reports of the use of this technique for Mycobacteria appear in the 1960's and it continued to be used as a standard method for investigations of epidemiological investigations until the 1980's (see Snider et al., 1984). However the advent of molecular methods of identification and subtyping has made such phage-based methods obsolete. The difficulty of culturing with these slow growing and fastidious bacteria may have driven the development of alternative methods for detection and identification. To this end the rapid growth of phage within these cells has been exploited to produce a range of different assay methods and assay formats, all with the aim of producing rapid, simple, economic tests that can be adopted in areas where more expensive molecular diagnostic tests cannot be supported. However to date none of these has gained widespread acceptance in the clinical setting. Perhaps this is because all of these methods still require a degree of staff expertise to be able to perform the tests and therefore they do not yet fulfil the criteria required to be of use in less developed countries. However there is potential for these assays to be used effectively as an adjunct to standard culture methods to further our understanding of Mycobacteria, and perhaps as our understanding of the phage-host interaction increases we may be able to solve some of the limitations of the current phage based assays and allow them to eventually realise their potential in combating human disease.

7. References

Albert, H., Heydenrych, A., Brookes, R., Mole, R.J., Harley, B., et al. (2002) Performance of a rapid phage-based test, *FASTPlaque*TB, to diagnose pulmonary tuberculosis from sputum specimens in South Africa. *Int J Tuberc Lung Dis.* 6: 529–537.

Albert, H., A.P. Trollip, K. Linley, C. Abrahams, T. Seaman and R.J. Mole. (2007) Development of an antimicrobial formulation for control of specimen-related contamination in phage-based diagnostic testing for tuberculosis. *Journal of Applied Microbiology*. 103: 892–899

Altic L.C., Rowe M.T., and Grant I.R. (2007) UV Light inactivation of *Mycobacterium avium* subsp. *paratuberculosis* in milk as assessed by *FASTPlaque*TB phage assay and culture. *Applied and Environmental Microbiology*. 73: 3728–3733

Banaiee, N., Bobadilla-del-Valle, M., Bardarov, S.Jr, Riska, P.F., Small, P.M., et al. (2001) Luciferase reporter mycobacteriophages for detection, identification, and antibiotic susceptibility testing of *Mycobacterium tuberculosis* in Mexico. *Journal of Clinical Microbiology*. 39: 3883–3888

Banaiee, N., V. January, C. Barthus, M. Lambrick, D. RoDiti, M.A. Behr, W.R. Jacobs Jr., & L.M. Steyn (2008) Evaluation of a semi-automated reporter phage assay for susceptibility testing of *Mycobacterium tuberculosis* isolates in South Africa. *Tuberculosis*. 88: 64–68

Bonnet, M.,Gagnidze, L., Varaine, F.,Ramsay, A., Githui, W, & Guerin, P. J. (2009) Evaluation of *FASTPlaque*TB (TM) to diagnose smear-negative tuberculosis in a peripheral clinic in Kenya. *International Journal of Tuberculosis and Lung Disease*. 13 (9): 1112-1118

Botsaris, G., Stanley, E. and Rees, C. (2009) Use of Phage Amplification Assay to rapidly enumerate viable MAP and other Mycobacteria. *Proceedings of 10th ICP* - 2009: 94

Botsaris, G., Slana, I., Liapi, M., Dodd, C., Economides, C., Rees, C. and Pavlik, I. (2010) Rapid detection methods for viable *Mycobacterium avium* subspecies *paratuberculosis* in milk and cheese. *International Journal of Food Microbiology*. 141: S87-S90.

Caroli, G., and Avio, C.M. (1975) Isolation of mycobacteriophages from surface water. *Annali Sclavo*. 17: 568

Carriere, C., Riska, P.F., Zimhony, O., Kriakov, J., Bardarov, S., Burns, J., Chan, J., and Jacobs, W.R. (1997) Conditionally replicating luciferase reporter phages: Improved sensitivity for rapid detection and assessment of drug susceptibility of *Mycobacterium tuberculosis*. *J. Clin. Microbiol.* 35:3232-3239

Cherry, W.B., Davis, B.R., Edwards, P.R., and Hogan, R.B. (1954) A simple procedure for the identification of the genus *Salmonella* by means of a specific bacteriophage. *Journal of Laboratory and Clinical Medicine*. 44: 51–55

Dinnes, J., Deeks, J., Kunst, H., Gibson, A., Cummins, E., Waugh, N., Drobniewski, F., Lalvani, A. (2007) A systematic review of rapid diagnostic tests for the detection of tuberculosis infection. *Health Technol Assess* 11(3): 1-196

Donaghy, J., M. Keyser, J. Johnston, F.P. Cilliers, P.A. Gouws and M.T. Rowe (2009) Inactivation of *Mycobacterium avium* ssp. *paratuberculosis* in milk by UV treatment. *Letters in Applied Microbiology*. 49: 217–221

Dusthackeer A., Kumar V., Subbian S., Sivaramakrishnan G., Zhu G., Subramanyam B., Hassan S., Nagamaiaha, S., Chan, J., Paranji Rama N. (2008) Construction and evaluation of luciferase reporter phages for the detection of active and non-replicating tubercle bacilli. *Journal of Microbiological Methods*. 73 (1): 18-25.

Eidus, L., Diena, B.B. and Greenberg, L. (1960) The use of p-nitro-aacetlyamino-beta-hydroxy-propiophenone (NAP) in the differentiation of mycobacteria. *Am Rev Respir Dis*. 81: 759–760.

Foddai, A., Elliott, C.T., and Grant, I.R. (2009) Optimization of a phage amplification assay to permit accurate enumeration of viable *Mycobacterium avium* subsp. *paratuberculosis* cells. *Applied and Environmental Microbiology*. 75: 3896-3902

Froman, S., Will, D.W. and Bogen, E. (1954) Bacteriophage active against virulent *Mycobacterium tuberculosis*. Isolation and activity. *American Journal of Public Health*. 44: 1326–1333

Galí, N., Domínguez, J., Blanco, S., Prat, C., Quesada, M. D., Matas, L., & Ausina, V. (2003) Utility of an in-house mycobacteriophage-based assay for rapid detection of rifampin resistance in *Mycobacterium tuberculosis* clinical isolates. *J Clin Microbiol*. 41(6):2647-9.

Gardner, G., M. and Weiser, R., S. (1947) A bacteriophage for *Mycobacterium smegmatis*. Proceedings of the Society for Experimental Biology and Medicine. 66: 205–206

Grant, I.R. and Rees, C.E.D. (2009) *Mycobacterium avium* subspecies *paratuberculosis*. In: *Molecular detection of food borne pathogens*. Ed. Dongyou Liu. pp 225-239

Hatfull, G. F., Cresawn, S. G., Hendrix R. W. (2008) Comparative genomics of the mycobacteriophages: insights into bacteriophage evolution. *Research in Microbiology*, 159(5):332-339

Hatfull, G. F., Jacobs-Sera, D., Lawrence, J. G., Pope, W. H., Russell, D. A., et al. (2010) Comparative Genomic Analysis of 60 Mycobacteriophage Genomes: Genome Clustering, Gene Acquisition, and Gene Size. *Journal of Molecular Biology*. 397: 119-143

Jacobs, W.R.Jr., Barletta, R.G., Udani, R., Chan, J., Kalkut, G., Sosne, G., Kieser, T., Sarkis, G.J., Hatfull, G.F. and Bloom, B.R. (1993) Rapid assessment of drug susceptibilities of *Mycobacterium tuberculosis* by means of luciferase reporter phages. *Science*. 260: 819–822

Kiraz, N.; Et, L. Akgun, Y., Kasifoglu, N., & Kiremitci, A. (2007) Rapid detection of Mycobacterium tuberculosis from sputum specimens using the FASTPlaqueTB test. *International Journal of Tuberculosis and Lung Disease*. 11(8): 904-908

McNerney, R., Kambashi, B. S., Kinkese, J., Tembwe, R. and Godfrey-Faussett P. (2004) Development of a Bacteriophage Phage Replication Assay for Diagnosis of Pulmonary Tuberculosis. *Journal of Clinical Microbiology*, 42 (5):2115-2120

McNerney R, Mallard K, Urassa H M, Lemma E, & Donoghue H.D. (2007) Colorimetric phage-based assay for detection of rifampin-resistant *Mycobacterium tuberculosis*. *J Clin Microbiol*. 45: 1330–1332.

Mankiewicz, E., and Liivak, M. (1967) Mycobacteriophages isolated from human sources. *Nature*. 216: 485-486

Mankiewicz, E. (1961) Mycobacteriophages isolated from persons with tuberculous and non-tuberculous conditions. *Nature*. 191: 1416

Mbulo, G.M., Kambashi, B.S., Kinkese, J., Tembwe, R., Shumba, B., Godfrey-Faussett, P., McNerney, R. (2004) Comparison of two bacteriophage tests and nucleic acid amplification for the diagnosis of pulmonary tuberculosis in sub-Saharan Africa. *International Journal of Tuberculosis and Lung Disease*. 8: 1342–1347.

Minion, J., Pai, M. (2010) Bacteriophage assays for rifampicin resistance detection in *Mycobacterium tuberculosis*: updated meta-analysis. *International Journal of Tuberculosis and Lung Disease*. 14:941–951

Mole, R. J. and Maskell, T. W. O'C. (2001). Phage as a diagnostic—the use of phage in TB diagnosis. *Journal of Chemical Technology and Biotechnology*. 76: 683–688

Mole, R. A. Trollip, C. Abrahams, M. Bosman & H. Albert. (2007) Improved contamination control for a rapid phage-based rifampicin resistance test for *Mycobacterium tuberculosis*. *Journal of Medical Microbiology*. 56, 1334–1339

Muzaffar R, Batool S, Aziz F, Naqvi A, Rizvi A. (2002) Evaluation of the FASTPlaqueTB assay for direct detection of *Mycobacterium tuberculosis* in sputum specimens. *International Journal of Tuberculosis and Lung Disease* 6: 635–640.

Palomino J.C. (2005) Nonconventional and new methods in the diagnosis of tuberculosis: feasibility and applicability in the field. *Eur Respir J*. 26: 339–350

Pearson, R.E., Jurgensen, S., Sarkis, G.J., Hatfull, G.F. and Jacobs, W.R.Jr. (1996) Construction of D29 shuttle phasmids and luciferase reporter phages for detection of mycobacteria. *Gene* 183: 129–136

Pedulla, M.L., Ford, M.E., Houtz, J.M., Karthikeyan, T., Wadsworth, C., Lewis, J.A., et al. (2005) Bacteriophage-based tests for the detection of *Mycobacterium tuberculosis* in clinical specimens: a systematic review and metaanalysis. *BMC Infectious Diseases*. 5:59

Keenan, L., Bardarov, S., Kriakov, J., Lawrence, J.G., Jacobs, W.R. Jr., Hendrix, R.W. and Hatfull, G.F. (2003) Origins of highly mosaic mycobacteriophage genomes. *Cell.* 113: 171-182

Piuri, M., Jacobs, W. R., Jr & Hatfull, G. F. (2009). Fluoromycobacteriophages for rapid, specific, and sensitive antibiotic susceptibility testing of *Mycobacterium tuberculosis. PLoS One.* 4, e4870

Pope, W.,H., Jacobs-Sera, D., Russell, D. A., Peebles, C. L., Al-Atrache, Z., et al. (2011) Expanding the Diversity of Mycobacteriophages: Insights into Genome Architecture and Evolution. *PLoS ONE* 6(1): e16329.

Prakash, S., Katiyar, S. K., Purwar, S., Singh, J. P. (2009) Clinical evaluation of the mycobacteriophage-based assay in rapid detection of *Mycobacterium tuberculosis* in respiratory specimens. *Indian Journal of Medical Microbiology.* 27 (2): 134-8

Rees C.E.D and M.J. Loessner. (2008) Phage Identification of Bacteria, In: *Practical Handbook of Microbiology*".2nd edition E. Goldman & L. Green CRC Press, pp85-99.

Riska, P.F., Jacobs, W.R.,Jr, Bloom, B.R., McKitrick, J. and Chan, J. (1997) Specific identification of *Mycobacterium tuberculosis* with the luciferase reporter mycobacteriophage: use of p-nitro--acetylamino-ß-hydroxy propiophenone. *Journal of Clinical Microbiology.* 35: 3225-3231

Sarkis, G.J., Jacobs, W.R., and Hatfull, G.F. (1995) L5 Luciferase reporter mycobacteriophages - A sensitive tool for the detection and assay of live Mycobacteria. *Molec. Microbiol.*, 15:1055-1067

Sasahara, K.C., Gray, M.J., Shin, S.J. and Boor, K.J. (2004) Detection of viable *Mycobacterium avium* subsp. *paratuberculosis* using luciferase reporter systems. *Foodborne Pathogens and Disease.* 1: 258-266

Shenai, S., Rodrigues, C., and Mehta, A.P. (2002) Evaluation of a new phage amplification technology for rapid diagnosis of tuberculosis. *Indian Journal of Medical Microbiology.* 20: 194-199

Snider, D. E. Jr., Jones, W. D., Good, R. C. (1984) The usefulness of phage typing *Mycobacterium tuberculosis* isolates. *Am Rev Respir Dis.* 130(6):1095-9.

Stanley E. (2005) The development of a rapid detection method for *Mycobacterium avium* subspecies *paratuberculosis* in milk PhD Thesis, University of Nottingham.

Stanley, E.C., Mole, R.J., Smith, R.J., Glenn, S.M., Barer, M.R., McGowan, M. and Rees, C.E.D. (2007) Development of a new, combined rapid method using phage and PCR for detection and identification of viable *Mycobacterium paratuberculosis* bacteria within 48 hours, *Applied and Environmental Microbiology.* 73: 1851-1857

Stewart, G.S., Jassim, S.A., Denyer, S.P., Newby, P., Linley, K., Dhir, V.K. (1998) The specific and sensitive detection of bacterial pathogens within 4 h using bacteriophage amplification. *J Appl Microbiol.* 84(5):777-83.

Timme, T.L. and Brennan, P.J. (1984) Induction of bacteriophages from members of the *Mycobacterium avium, Mycobacterium intracellulare, Mycobacterium scrofulaceum* serocomplex. *J Gen Microbiol.* 130, 2059-2066.

Williams, S.L., Harris, N.B. and Barletta, R.G. (1999) Development of a firefly luciferase-based assay for determining antimicrobial susceptibility of *Mycobacterium avium* subsp. *paratuberculosis. Journal of Clinical Microbiology.* 37: 304-309

Wilson, S. M., Al-Suwaidi, Z., McNerney, R., Porter, J., and Drobniewski, F. (1997) Evaluation of a new rapid bacteriophage-based method for the drug susceptibility testing of *Mycobacterium tuberculosis. Nat Med.* 3: 465- 468.

15

Molecular Imaging in TB: From the Bench to the Clinic

Nuria Andreu[1], Paul T. Elkington[1] and Siouxsie Wiles[1,2]
[1]*Imperial College London,*
[2]*University of Auckland,*
[1]*United Kingdom*
[2]*New Zealand*

1. Introduction

Despite all efforts, tuberculosis (TB) still constitutes a serious global health threat with 9.4 million new cases and 1.7 million deaths worldwide in 2009 (World Health Organisation, 2010). Furthermore, an estimated one third of the worlds' population is infected with the bacterium responsible, *Mycobacterium tuberculosis*. The main handicaps in fighting TB include a vaccine which works poorly in the most affected populations, and an arduous treatment regimen, involving a combination of several drugs taken over many months. This is further complicated by the emergence of multi-drug resistant (MDR) and extensively drug-resistant (XDR) *M. tuberculosis* strains, which require even longer treatment times with less well-tolerated drugs. Eradication of TB will require the development of new drugs and vaccines, alongside improved methods for diagnosis and monitoring treatment efficacy. With the vast burden of disease falling in resource poor settings, the challenge will also be to develop methodologies that can be deployed with minimal investment in infrastructure, maintenance and staff expertise.

Recent decades have seen the emergence of the new discipline of molecular imaging. In essence, molecular imaging enables the non-invasive visualisation, characterisation, and quantification of biological processes taking place within intact living subjects, be it a mouse or man (Filippi & Rocca, 2011; Horky & Treves, 2011; Pysz et al., 2010; Sandhu et al., 2010). Imaging has long been applied to managing TB; simple chest x-rays have allowed clinicians to visualise TB in people for over a century (Singh & Nath, 1994). However, the new molecular imaging techniques are revolutionising medical research, with the potential to translate into significant changes in clinical practice. In this chapter we describe the new generation of imaging modalities and how these are being applied to eradicating TB, from the laboratory bench and in to the clinic.

2. Molecular imaging modalities

Molecular imaging is broadly defined as the visualisation, characterisation and quantification of biological processes, at the cellular and subcellular level, within living subjects. Importantly, the non-invasive nature of the techniques enables the study of disease processes longitudinally within the same subjects, a powerful tool indeed for elucidating host-pathogen interactions and treatment efficacy. A number of imaging modalities have emerged, which vary in their methods of image generation, spatial resolution, depth penetration and detection thresholds (Table 1). As a result each modality has different advantages and disadvantages (Table 2), suggesting the techniques should be used to complement each other to answer specific research questions.

Modality	Image generation	Spatial resolution	Depth penetration
Computed tomography (CT)	x-rays	50-200 μm	No limit
Magnetic resonance imaging (MRI)	Radiowaves	25-100 μm	No limit
Positron emission tomography (PET)	High energy γ-rays	1-2 mm	No limit
Single photon emission (SPE) CT	Lower energy γ-rays	1-2 mm	No limit
Optical	Visible light	2-5 mm	1-2 cm

Table 1. Features of currently employed imaging modalities (Adapted from Massoud & Gambhir, 2003)

2.1 Computed Tomography (CT)

CT imaging combines low-dose x-rays and computing to produce reconstructions of the internal organs and tissues. This is possible because diverse tissue types differentially absorb x-rays as they pass through the body. CT is not a molecular imaging tool per se, but can provide important information on anatomical changes which arise as a result of disease processes. Widely used in clinical settings, there are now a number of miniaturised machines suitable for scanning of small animals (often referred to as micro-CT). To collect data, the subject is placed on a motorised table, which then moves into the lead-encased CT machine. Inside, an x-ray source and a set of x-ray detectors rotate 360 degrees around the subject in synchrony. At every angle, the detectors record the x-rays passing through the subject to provide a digital projection which is collected and sent to a computer. The x-ray source produces a narrow, fan-shaped beam, with widths ranging from 1 to 20 mm. In axial CT, which is commonly used for head scans, the table is stationary during a rotation, after which it is moved along for the next slice. In helical CT, which is commonly used for body scans, the table moves continuously as the x-ray source and detectors rotate, producing a spiral or helical scan. Clinical machines typically have multiple rows of detectors operating side by side, so that many slices (currently up to 64) can be imaged simultaneously, reducing the overall scanning time. As an alternative to the fan-shaped x-ray beam, small animal scanners may instead use a cone-shaped beam, where the scanned subject is captured completely in one rotation, speeding up the imaging process. The data are processed by computer to produce a series of image slices representing two-dimensional (2D) or three-dimensional (3D) views of the target organ or body region.

Modality	Advantages	Disadvantages
CT	Unlimited depth penetration High spatial resolution Whole body imaging of animals and humans Short aquisition times (minutes) Anatomical imaging	Radiation exposure Poor soft tissue contrast Moderately expensive
MRI	Unlimited depth penetration High spatial resolution Whole body imaging of animals and humans Good soft tissue contrast Non-ionising radiation Anatomical imaging	Expensive Long acquisition times (minutes to hours) Limited sensitivity
PET	Unlimited depth penetration Whole body imaging of animals and humans Can be combined with CT for anatomical imaging	Radiation exposure Expensive Long acquisition times (minutes to hours) Low spatial resolution PET cyclotron or generator needed
SPECT	Unlimited depth penetration Whole body imaging of animals and humans Can be combined with CT for anatomical imaging Can distinguish between radionuclides, so multiple processes can be imaged simultaneously	Radiation exposure Long acquisition times (minutes to hours) Low spatial resolution
Optical	Short aquisition times Highly sensitive and quantitative Whole body imaging of animals Can be combined with CT for anatomical imaging of animals Inexpensive	Limited depth penetration Whole body imaging of humans not possible

Table 2. Advantages and disadvantages of imaging modalities (Adapted from Massoud & Gambhir, 2003)

The spatial resolution of CT is primarily limited by scanning times, the size of the x-ray source, and the sensitivity of the detection system. In addition, CT has relatively poor soft tissue contrast; generally, iodinated molecules are applied as contrast agents, owing to the high x-ray absorption coefficient of iodine (McClennan, 1994). Current iodine-based contrast agents have several limitations, including adverse reactions, renal toxicity, vascular permeation and rapid renal clearance resulting in limited imaging times. As a result, alternative contrast agents have been suggested, such as polymer-coated Bi_2S_3 (Rabin et al., 2006) or gold nanoparticles (Hainfield et al., 2006). Indeed, gadolinium chelate-coated gold nanoparticles have been reported as dual imaging probes for CT and magnetic resonance imaging (MRI) (Alric et al, 2008). Tissue contrast can also be improved by using a dual-energy x-ray method in which the projection data are acquired using two different x-ray spectra (Taschereau et al., 2010). However, one of the major limitations of CT is radiation exposure, and while the doses are low, they are not negligible and this can limit repeated imaging of the subject.

2.2 Magnetic Resonance Imaging (MRI)

MRI is based on the interactions of atoms and molecules in a tissue of interest, upon exposure to a magnetic field. In addition to providing detailed structural images, MRI can obtain physiological information through the use of specific contrast agents. While the proton ^{1}H is most widely used in MRI, due to the abundance of water within soft tissues, other paramagnetic atoms such as ^{13}C, ^{17}O, ^{19}F, ^{23}Na and ^{31}P are also useful. Within an MRI scanner, a strong 'coiled' magnet produces a magnetic field with a gradient in the X, Y and Z directions, which causes nuclei to align themselves. The device also contains a radiofrequency (RF) coil which is used to produce a temporary RF pulse, resulting in a change in nuclei alignment. Following the pulse, the protons return to their baseline orientation (known as relaxation) which is detected as a change in electromagnetic flux.

The behaviour of the energy inserted into the system is described by two relaxation constants: the longitudinal relaxation time (T1) or the transverse relaxation time (T2). Different tissues have different relaxation times and this can be used to produce endogenous contrast between different tissues. Addition of exogenous contrast agents can further enhance tissue contrast by selectively shortening either T1 or T2 in a tissue of interest. According to their magnetic properties, contrast agents can be classified as paramagnetic (for example, gadolinium based agents) or superparamagnetic (for example, iron oxide nanoparticles) (reviewed in Geraldes & Laurent, 2009). Depending on their biodistribution patterns, different contrast agents can also be utilised to image specific anatomical regions. MRI is becoming widely used in both clinical and preclinical settings, with dedicated MRI machines available for humans and rodents. An advantage of MRI is that it does not involve ionising radiation, has unlimited depth penetration and good soft tissue contrast. However, it is expensive and scanning times are typically long, from minutes to hours.

2.3 Positron Emission Tomography (PET)

PET imaging involves the visualisation of a radiotracer, a biomarker labelled with a positron emitter. The positron emitters typically used are isotopes with short half-lives (several hours to a few minutes), such as ^{11}C, ^{13}N, ^{15}On and ^{18}F. Radiotracers are typically made to reflect compounds normally used by the body, such as glucose or ammonia, or molecules that bind to specific receptors. Once the radiotracer is injected into a subject, it therefore distributes based on its similarity to the original biomarker compound. The most commonly used radiotracer is an analogue of glucose labelled with ^{18}F, [^{18}F]-2-fluoro-deoxy-D-glucose, ([^{18}F]-FDG). A major advantage of PET imaging is that it can be used to trace the fate of any compound, provided it can be radiolabeled with a PET isotope. As a result, the processes that can be probed using PET imaging are virtually limitless, and radiotracers for new target molecules and processes continue to be developed. For a summary of available PET radiotracers see Pysz et al., 2010. Dedicated clinical and small animal PET scanners are now available.

PET imaging is based on the fact that the incorporated radionucleotide undergoes positive β decay and emits a positron. The positron travels a few mm before it annihilates with an electron to emit a pair of photons moving in approximately opposite directions. These photons are then detected by the scanning device. As the photons are travelling at approximately 180° to each other, it is possible to localise their source along a straight line of coincidence known as a line of response (LOR). The distribution pattern of the LORs is then used to reconstruct an image of the radioactivity distribution within the subject. One minor limitation of utilising photons is that they are differentially attenuated as they traverse different thicknesses of tissue. This attenuation results in the reconstruction of structures deep within the body as having falsely low uptake of the radiotracer. However this attenuation can be corrected for by combining PET with CT imaging.

Despite the great promise of PET imaging, there are a number of significant disadvantages. One is the use of ionising radiation, although this is minimised by the use of radioisotopes with short half-lives. However, these short half-lives require both costly cyclotron generators and chemical synthesis apparatus within close proximity to the scanning facility for the production of the radiotracers. This certainly limits the use of the technology within resource poor settings. Furthermore, scanning times are typically long, from minutes to hours, and the technique provides low spatial resolution.

2.4 Single Photon Emission Computed Tomography (SPECT)

Like PET, SPECT imaging is based on the distribution and uptake of a radiolabelled tracer after injection into a subject. Unlike PET tracers, SPECT radionucleotides undergo radioactive decay and emit γ-rays of a particular energy, which are then captured by an external detector. A number of 2D projections are captured from multiple angles which, when combined, form a 3D image. Radiotracers based upon radioactive metals, such as ^{111}In, ^{188}Re, ^{131}I, and ^{133}Xe, are often used. For a summary of available SPECT radiotracers see Pysz et al., 2010. PET and SPECT imaging share many of the same advantages and disadvantages. However, while PET is more sensitive, SPECT imaging is much cheaper largely thanks to the availability of different radiotracers which are longer lived and easier to obtain. Moreover, different SPECT radiotracers have different energies enabling multiple tracers to be used to image different processes.

2.5 Optical Imaging

The electromagnetic radiation we refer to as light undergoes a range of interactions when propagating through tissue. Importantly, these interactions depend on the structural arrangement and physical properties of the micro-environment. Such interactions have led to the development of the field of optical imaging which encompasses a wide variety of methods and approaches (Table 3), from visualising tissue anatomy on the microscopic scale (Zonios et al., 2001) to the 3D localisation of a photonic signal in whole animals using fluorescence molecular tomography (Ntziachristos, 2006).

In this chapter we will focus on biophotonic imaging (BPI), a preclinical imaging technique based on the ability of light to travel through flesh. This principle is easily demonstrated by placing a torch underneath ones hand and observing the light emerging through the fingers. BPI involves the detection of visible light which arises from either the excitation of a fluorescent protein (FP), or molecule, or from an enzyme-catalysed oxidation reaction (a phenomenon known as bioluminescence).

Resolution	Technique	Contrast	Depth
	Epi microscopy	A, Fl	20 μm
Microscopic	Confocal microscopy	Fl	500 μm
	Multi-photon microscopy	Fl	800 μm
	Optical projection tomography	A, Fl	15 mm
Mesoscopic	Optical coherence tomography	S	2 mm
	Laser speckle imaging	S	1 mm
	Hyperspectral imaging	A, S, Fl	<5 mm
	Endoscopy	A, S, Fl	<5 mm
	Fluorescence reflectance imaging (FRI)	A, Fl	<7 mm
Macroscopic	Diffuse optical tomography (DOT)	A, Fl	<20 cm
	Fluorescence resonance imaging (FRI)	A, Fl	<7 mm
	Fluorescence molecular tomography (FMT)	Fl	<20 cm
	Biophotonic Imaging (BPI)	Fl, E	< 3cm

Key: A, Absorption; Fl, fluorescence; S, Scattering; E, Emission.

Table 3. Optical imaging techniques (taken from N. Andreu et al., 2011).

Bioluminescence arises from the oxidation of a substrate (a luciferin) by an enzyme (a luciferase), which usually requires energy (in the form of $FMNH_2$ and ATP) and oxygen. Luciferin and luciferase are generic terms as none of the major classes share sequence homology. Most widely studied are the systems belonging to luminous beetles in the family Lampyridae (such as the firefly *Photinus pyralis*), the sea pansy *Renilla reniformans*, the marine copepod *Gaussia princeps* and numerous luminous bacteria (such as *Vibrio* sp. and *Photorhabdus luminescens*). In contrast, fluorescence arises when a fluorescent compound is irradiated with light of a suitable wavelength. This leads to the transition of an electron in the molecule to a higher energy state, a process known as excitation. This process is almost instantaneous, taking around 10^{-15} seconds. Upon return of the electron to a lower energy level (around 10 ns), light of lower energy is emitted, giving the fluorescent signal.

Although the emitted light may be dim, it can be detected externally using sensitive photon detectors such as those based on cooled, or intensified, charge coupled device (CCD) cameras, mounted within light-tight specimen chambers. As light passes through a range of tissue types (including skin, muscle and bone) it is possible to observe and quantify the spatial and temporal distribution of light production from within living subjects (N. Andreu et al, 2011). In general, imaging of luminescence is much more sensitive than imaging fluorescence as a result of better signal-to-noise ratios. This is mainly due to the high levels of background fluorescence *in vivo* compared to luminescence, due to endogenously produced fluorophores such as keratin, porphyrins, NAD(P)H, collagen and elastin (Troy et al., 2004). A major limitation of BPI is the limited depth penetration through tissue. Hence BPI is currently only applied to imaging small animals, although visualisation of bioluminescence from within infant monkeys (the long-tailed macaque, *Macaca fascicularis*) has been reported (Tarantal et al., 2006). Alternatively, the light could potentially be detected internally using an endoscopic device, such as reported by Hsiung and colleagues to image colonic pathology (Hsiung et al., 2008). The advantages of BPI are that it is inexpensive, sensitive and requires short imaging times.

3. Use of molecular imaging in animal models of TB

M. tuberculosis, the infectious agent of TB, can infect many animals in addition to its natural human host. Although the study of TB in patients is extremely useful, a detailed analysis of the pathogenesis and the interactions of *M. tuberculosis* with the host requires the use of well-defined models that can be infected in a controlled manner. Furthermore, animal models can be easily manipulated, can be used in statistically significant numbers, and the results are obtained in a relatively short time frame. In addition, they are particularly useful in drug and vaccine efficacy testing before moving the most promising candidates to clinical studies.

For both practical and economical reasons, laboratory mice remain the most extensively used animal model of TB: they are easy to manipulate and house, there is a wide range of mutant and genetically modified strains, and there are many immunological reagents available. However, latent infection is difficult to achieve in the mouse model, and the pathology, with poorly organised granulomas, differs considerably to that observed in humans. By contrast, guinea pigs and particularly rabbits display a spectrum of pathology that better represents the human disease. Moreover, guinea pigs are extremely susceptible to *M. tuberculosis* infection and relatively inexpensive compared to other larger animal models, which makes this model very useful for vaccine efficacy studies. Even so, studies with guinea pigs and rabbits are limited by the narrow range of immunological reagents available. This is not the case in non-human primates, which are the closest model to humans in terms of pathology and disease development and therefore constitute the most relevant model to predict treatment and vaccine efficacy. Nevertheless, work with non-human primates presents many limitations regarding space requirements, animal availability, and costs. In summary, each animal model presents both advantages and disadvantages which must be carefully considered when designing a new study. A more detailed description of these animal models of TB can be found elsewhere (Dharmadhikari & Nardell, 2008; Flynn, 2006; Gupta & Katoch, 2005).

The use of animals in research is accompanied by ethical responsibilities and most countries promote the three Rs: replacement, reduction and refinement. Replacement refers to methods that avoid the use of animals, for example, *in silico* computer modelling, or using established human and animal cell lines and non-mammalian models such as the nematode *Caenorhabditis elegans* or the embryo of the zebrafish, *Danio rerio*. Reduction refers to methods which minimise the use of animals and enable researchers to obtain comparable levels of information from fewer animals or to obtain more information from the same number of animals, thereby reducing the future use of animals. Refinement refers to improvements to scientific procedures and husbandry which minimise actual or potential pain, suffering, distress or lasting harm and/or improve animal welfare. Molecular imaging is a very powerful tool for implementation of two of the 3Rs, refinement and reduction. Using traditional disease models, infected animals are sacrificed at defined time points and tissues excised for determination of pathogen numbers and localisation. In contrast, the non-destructive nature of molecular imaging allows the course of an infection to be monitored simply by repeated imaging of the same group of animals. Importantly, this allows disease progression to be followed with extreme accuracy, while allowing each animal to act as its own control. Furthermore, we have demonstrated that BPI can provide real time information on the effectiveness of the inoculation method (Wiles et al., 2007). As a result, errors in administration can be detected immediately (N. Andreu et al., 2011) and animals eliminated from further study - thus minimising any potential pain, suffering and distress for the animal and reducing variation by removing flawed scientific data.

One major drawback to working with *M. tuberculosis* is the slow growth of the organism. This lengthens the time required to carry out *in vivo* experiments extraordinarily, and delays the quantification of bacterial burdens by about four weeks, which is the time required for *M. tuberculosis* to form visible colonies on agar. Therefore, the use of molecular imaging to track infection dynamics in real time would be a major advantage as it would enable researchers to make on-the-spot decisions, shortening the length of the experiment if clear differences (for example, between control and vaccinated groups) were observed. There is, therefore, an increasing interest in the development of molecular imaging techniques in animal models of TB. Moreover, the developments and knowledge acquired through the use of these techniques in animal models may eventually translate into the clinic.

3.1 Computed Tomography (CT)

CT imaging has mostly been used as a complementary technique to PET and SPECT imaging (see sections 3.3 and 3.4), as it gives high-resolution anatomical information for a better localisation of the radionuclide signal. However, CT has also been evaluated as an imaging method on its own to assess disease burden in macaques (Lewinsohn et al., 2006). To this end, four animals were infected by bronchoscopy instillation of *M. tuberculosis*, and disease progression was monitored every four weeks clinically (weight, body temperature, complete blood count and erythrocyte sedimentation rate), immunologically (ELISPOT), bacteriologically (quantitative *M. tuberculosis* culture from bronchoalveolar lavage), and by CT imaging. In addition, a necropsy was performed at the end of the experiment (12 weeks post-infection) which included histopathology and bacterial burden quantification from selected organs. Clinical indicators failed to provide information about disease progression, as most of them were fairly constant through the whole experiment. Most bacterial cultures from bronchoalveolar lavage were positive, although some cultures were negative even though CT imaging and post-mortem analysis showed infection. Even bacterial cultures from post-mortem lung samples were not consistently positive, which was attributed to a non-uniform infection of the lungs and therefore biased tissue sampling. In contrast, CT imaging provided a reliable readout of disease progression in the whole lung and also allowed monitoring of other organs, such as the liver and spleen. Moreover, different types of lesions were observed, and progression of the lesions from small nodules to cavitation and necrosis was evident. CT findings were corroborated by post-mortem histopathology and, together with immunological monitoring, provided a non-invasive, accurate, and rapid assessment of TB in this animal model. It is important to note that even though a CT scanner was not available in the animal biosafety level 3 (BSL3) containment facility, the authors were able to image infected animals in a scanner localised within a non-containment facility, by transporting and imaging the anesthetised macaques in a box fitted with HEPA filters. This is a solution that has also been adopted for other imaging techniques like PET/CT, SPECT/CT and BPI (see below).

3.2 Magnetic Resonance Imaging (MRI)

To our knowledge, MRI was the first molecular imaging method reported for an animal model of TB, when Kraft and colleagues used the technique to assess lesion distribution and lesion numbers as an indication of disease burden in BCG-vaccinated and unvaccinated guinea pigs infected with *M. tuberculosis* by the aerosol route (Kraft et al., 2004). 3D lung images were reconstructed from images taken of 2 mm slices of formalin-fixed and agarose-embedded lungs, and lung volumes, lymph node volumes and total nodular burden were quantified. Small nodules were observed 15 days post-infection, which developed into granulomatous lesions 20 days later. Lesions were uniformly distributed in the lungs, which suggested that aerosol delivery of *M. tuberculosis* results in a homogenous infection. Additionally, lesions numbers supported the hypothesis that a single bacillus establishes a single lesion. In terms of vaccine efficacy, the authors found the same number of lesions in vaccinated and unvaccinated animals but the lesions were smaller in the vaccinated group, thus suggesting that BCG has an effect on disease development rather than on the initial establishment of the infection. All in all, they found that MRI was a useful method to assess disease burden in terms of lesion distribution, size and number. The main limitation was a low sensitivity when dealing with very small (< 1 mm) lesions.

More recently, the same laboratory used MRI to assess treatment efficacy in guinea pigs infected with *M. tuberculosis* (Ordway et al., 2010). The treatment had a dramatic effect on bacterial load with a 4-6 log decrease in viable counts (as determined by colony forming units [CFUs]) both in the lungs and lymph nodes in just 25 days. However, the effect on lesion burden, as quantified by MRI, was slower and could only be detected in the lungs after 50 days of therapy (Figure 1). In addition, the lesions in the lymph nodes of the treated group were smaller, although the differences with the untreated group were only obvious at later time points. These results were corroborated by histological analysis, although the number of lesions in the lungs of the treated animals was already lower than in the control group by day 25.

MRI has also been applied to studies in non-human primates (Sharpe et al., 2009, 2010). Disease burden in this animal model has been traditionally assessed by a range of ante- and post-mortem methods such as clinical signs (behaviour, weight, and body temperature), laboratory markers (haemoglobin levels, erythrocyte sedimentation rate, and immunology),

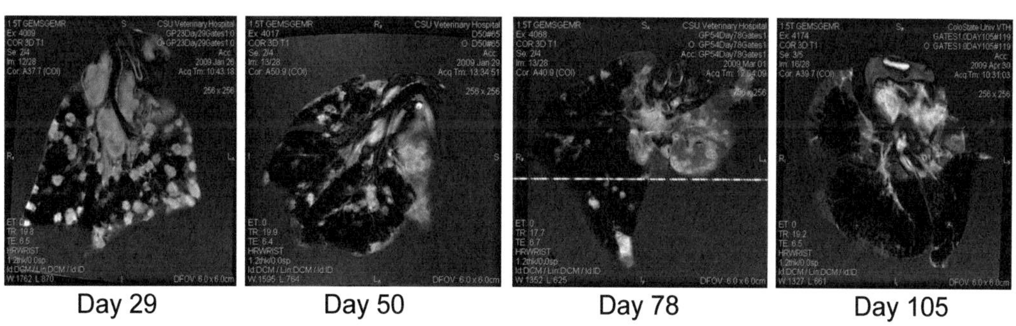

Fig. 1. MRI showing lesions resolving/disappearing during treatment of *M. tuberculosis*-infected guinea pigs with a cocktail of anti-TB drugs (given as days post-treatment).

chest x-ray, gross pathology, and histology. However, most of these methods are qualitative and subjective. Moreover, the most common alternative method, the quantitative estimation of total lesion numbers in the lung by manual counting, is laborious and particularly difficult in animals with more severe disease, as individual lesions become difficult to distinguish. Sharpe and colleagues used MRI and stereology (a statistical method that extracts quantitative information of a 3D structure from measurements made on planar sections of the material) to quantify lesion volume relative to lung volume in macaques infected with a range of doses of *M. tuberculosis* by the aerosol route (Sharpe et al., 2009). Similarly to what was previously seen in guinea pigs, the authors observed a uniform distribution of lesions in the lungs. In addition, the lesion-to-lung volume ratio increased with the infectious dose, and this ratio revealed subtle differences in the level of pulmonary disease and correlated well with other measures of disease burden. By contrast, methods such as gross pathology and chest x-ray were less sensitive and did not differentiate between the levels of disease in the animals exposed to the highest infectious doses. In conclusion, MRI together with stereology makes up a sensitive, quantitative, systematic and consistent method to assess disease burden in the macaque model of tuberculosis. Moreover, when MRI was compared with more traditional methods to measure vaccine efficacy, it was found that MRI combined with stereology was the only readout that distinguished between the unvaccinated and the vaccinated groups, and it was even able to show differences between survivor and non-survivor animals within the vaccinated groups, thus highlighting the sensitivity of the method (Sharpe et al., 2010).

In summary, the use of MRI appears to be a reliable method to assess disease burden in the lungs of *M. tuberculosis*-infected animals. However, it should be noted that the studies described here were performed on fixed lungs where the bacteria had been inactivated, as the use of MRI under BSL3 containment was not available. Initially, the whole lung was fixed and used for imaging to reduce sample error. As a result the tissue could not be used for other procedures, such as determination of bacterial load. However, the results discussed above illustrate that aerosol delivery of *M. tuberculosis* results in an even distribution of the lesions in the lungs and, therefore, samples can be taken and used for other techniques without compromising its reliability. Similarly to what has been done to image live animals by CT scanning, MRI of live animals could be done by using a sealed box with filters to transport the animals to the MRI facility and contain them during imaging. When available, MRI of live animals will allow longitudinal monitoring of disease progression, and real-time observation of vaccine and drug efficacy. The *ex vivo* results discussed here, together with the excellent soft tissue contrast of MRI and the development of faster MRI devices that reduce the artefacts induced by respiratory motion, suggest that *in vivo* MRI may become a very useful technique for the study of TB in animal models.

3.3 Positron Emission Tomography (PET)

Another technique which is gaining popularity in TB research is PET combined with CT imaging (PET/CT). The PET radiotracer [^{18}F]-FDG is used to image inflammation at the infection site, as it accumulates in inflammatory cells such as neutrophils and activated macrophages. This technology has been used to image TB infection (Figure 2) and to assess drug treatment efficacy in mice (Davis et al., 2009b). The authors infected two strains of mice, BALB/c (which develop diffused granulomas) and C3HeB/FeJ (which develop well-defined necrotic granulomas), and evaluated three different treatments: (i) first line tuberculosis regimen (rifampin + pyrazinamide + isoniazid), (ii) a more bactericidal regimen (rifampin + pyrazinamide + moxifloxacin), and (iii) a bacteriostatic regimen (ethambutol). The animals were imaged and CFUs obtained at different time points during the 12 weeks of treatment. Furthermore, one group of BALB/c mice was followed for 22 weeks after completion of the bactericidal treatments to assess relapse of the infection. For the imaging, anesthetised mice were contained in a sealed device with holes for passage of gases fitted with 0.22 μm filters. In both mouse models, CFU counts perfectly reflected the efficiency of the three treatments being evaluated, with a faster decrease in bacterial numbers when moxifloxacin was used instead of isoniazid, and stabilization of bacterial burden when mice were treated with ethambutol only.

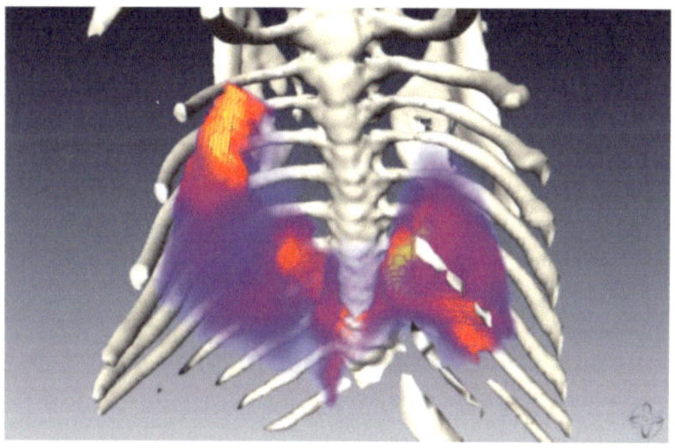

Fig. 2. 3D co-registered PET and CT images from a live C3HeB/FeJ mouse infected with a low-dose aerosol of *M. tuberculosis*. The brightness of the lesions represents FDG activity, with brighter lesions being more active. The heart also takes up FDG and can therefore be seen on the left. The bony structure (rib cage and scapula), shown in grey, were extracted from the CT (Davis, S.L. & Jain, S.K.; unpublished data).

The use of PET/CT imaging allowed differentiation between the bacteriostatic and bactericidal treatments, as the [^{18}F]-FDG activity was higher in the mice treated with ethambutol. However, unexpectedly, [^{18}F]-FDG activity was higher in mice treated with moxifloxacin than in those treated with isoniazid during the first four weeks of treatment. The authors suggested that this could be due to the limited statistical power of the study since only three mice per group were used, or that it could be an inherent limitation of using [^{18}F]-FDG, whereby an increased killing of *M. tuberculosis* would cause an increased Tumour Necrosis Factor (TNF)-mediated inflammation and therefore increased [^{18}F]-FDG activity even though bacterial numbers were decreasing. Relapse was detected in both groups of mice by PET imaging and by CFU counts. In summary, PET/CT allowed the non-invasive monitoring of disease progression in real-time. Moreover, individual lesions could be observed in the C3HeB/FeJ mouse model; as treatment response has been suggested to be lesion-dependent, the possibility of monitoring individual lesions would be very useful. However, it is important to take into account that this method does not specifically image infection but only measures inflammation which, as illustrated by the treatment results of this work, does not always correlate with bacterial burden. Nevertheless, this method has some advantages over using, for example, CFU counts: it uses a reduced number of animals, and the same animals can be repeatedly imaged which allows a more easy detection of untimed events such as relapse.

PET/CT imaging is also being used in non-human primates, although the results have only been presented in meetings and no peer-reviewed article has been published to date. For example, PET/CT has been used to monitor disease progression and drug efficacy in macaques (Lin et al., 2009). Using CT imaging, lesions as small as 1 mm were detected in the lungs and lymph nodes of infected animals. Moreover, lesion progression could be followed over time. Interestingly, co-registered [^{18}F]-FDG–PET images revealed that individual granulomas differed in their [^{18}F]-FDG affinity: whereas some granulomas exhibited high uptake values, others seemed devoid of [^{18}F]-FDG. The imaging results were complemented with post-mortem histology and bacterial burden analysis of individual lesions. The authors found a complex, lesion-specific response to drug treatment that included changes in [^{18}F]-FDG avidity. These remarkable results show that even though PET and CT are two complementary techniques, images should be first analysed separately, and that caution should be taken when interpreting the results of PET activity in terms of [^{18}F]-FDG accumulation.

3.4 Single Photon Emission Computed Tomography (SPECT)

SPECT/CT has also been used for imaging of TB infection in mice (Davis et al., 2009a). The authors used the radiotracer 1-(2'deoxy-2'-fluoro-β-D-arabinofuranosyl)-5-[^{125}I]-iodouracil ([^{125}I]-FIAU), a nucleoside analogue, together with an engineered *M. tuberculosis* strain that stably expressed the enzyme thymidine kinase (TK) which phosphorylates [^{125}I]-FIAU leading to its accumulation within the bacteria. In contrast to [^{18}F]-FDG–PET imaging, this technique specifically images the bacteria instead of the inflammatory response, as [^{125}I]-FIAU is a poor substrate for mammalian TK. Using this technique, the authors were able to image individual necrotic granulomas in the lungs of C3HeB/FeJ infected mice (Figure 3). The presence of the lesions was subsequently corroborated by histopathology. However, the limit of detection was found to be $5x10^6$ to $1x10^7$ CFUs, a rather high bacterial burden for mice infected with *M. tuberculosis*. The authors suggested that the sensitivity of the method could be improved by increasing the expression of TK in the bacilli or by using more

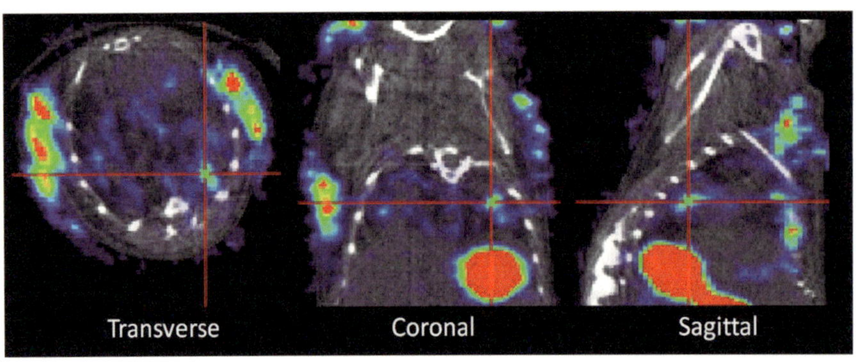

Fig. 3. Co-registered SPECT and CT images from a live C3HeB/FeJ mouse infected with a low-dose aerosol of an *M. tuberculosis* strain expressing bacterial thymidine kinase (TK) under the control of a strong mycobacterial promoter. TB lesions were imaged 8-weeks after this infection, using [^{125}I]-FIAU, a nucleoside analog substrate for bacterial TK. The FIAU-SPECT signal localizes to the TB lesion (crosshairs) in the lungs, indicating uptake of FIAU by the bacteria (Davis, S.L. & Jain, S.K.; unpublished data).

sensitive (and expensive) radionuclides such as ^{123}I or ^{124}I. Other limitations of the technique include: the limited blood supply at the centre of the granulomas could limit accessibility to imaging substrates; TK requires ATP, which could be restricted in latent bacteria; and the presence of non-specific signal in tissues such as liver, gall bladder, or stomach, that either metabolize or excrete FIAU or its iodinated derivatives.

3.5 Biophotonic Imaging (BPI)

Bioluminescence imaging is one of the most widely used imaging techniques in the study of infectious diseases (N. Andreu et al., 2011). Luciferases have been used in mycobacterial research for more than 20 years; the two most widely used are the firefly luciferase (FFluc) and the luciferase of the bacterium *Vibrio harveyi* (LuxAB). Both luciferases produce light in the presence of a combination of a substrate and a cofactor, namely D-luciferin and ATP (for FFluc) and n-decanal and $FMNH_2$ (for LuxAB). As the co-factors are only found in live cells, the production of light by the luciferases provides a sensitive indicator of cell viability. The bacterial luciferase system has a major advantage when compared with the FFluc: the genes for the synthesis of the substrate are known and can be co-expressed with the *luxAB* genes as a convenient gene set (*luxCABDE*) that renders the bacteria autoluminescent, that is, no external addition of substrate is needed for light production. Light-emitting mycobacteria have been used as an easier and faster approach than commonly used methods to assess bacterial numbers *in vitro* and in macrophages, for example, in drug screening assays (Arain et al., 1996). The first approach to use luminescent mycobacteria in animal models consisted of measuring luminescence *ex vivo* in organ homogenates (Hickey et al., 1996). This method generated results in a much quicker time frame than using CFU counts and has been applied to drug and vaccine efficacy testing (Hickey et al., 1996; Snewin et al., 1999).

More recently, a recombinant *M. bovis* BCG strain expressing the bacterial luciferase enzyme LuxAB has been used to monitor mycobacterial infection *in vivo* (Heuts et al., 2009). In this work, only the luciferase genes were expressed and, therefore, the n-decanal substrate had to be injected before imaging. Although n-decanal is very toxic, the authors were able to deliver it dissolved in a mixture of olive oil and ethanol by injection into the mouse peritoneum. To assess the usefulness of the system, immunodeficient $RAG2^{-/-}/\gamma cR^{-/-}$ mice were intravenously infected with the luminescent BCG strain, and bioluminescence imaging was performed at different time points for 11 weeks. A signal coming from the spleen was detected four weeks post-infection, when the bacterial load was around $5x10^7$ CFUs. The signal increased over time and extended to the abdomen of the animal but no signal was observed in the lungs, even though CFU counting showed a bacterial burden in this organ of 10^7 CFUs at eight weeks post-infection. However, luminescence was detected in the excised lungs, suggesting that tissue attenuation was responsible for the failure to detect the signal in the whole animal. The same luminescent BCG strain was also used to assess drug efficacy and the host immune response. A reduction in light emission, which paralleled the reduction in bacterial numbers, was observed in treated mice compared to the untreated mice, as well as in inmunocompetent BALB/c and T-cell reconstituted $RAG2^{-/-}/\gamma cR^{-/-}$ mice compared to immunosupressed $RAG2^{-/-}/\gamma cR^{-/-}$ mice. Therefore, bioluminescence imaging allows monitoring of mycobacterial infection in mice. However, the system was not useful for imaging infection in the lungs, and a toxic substrate had to be administered to the mice before imaging.

To overcome these difficulties, our group has recently optimised the expression of FFluc and the complete bacterial luciferase system in *M. tuberculosis* (N. Andreu et al., 2010). The resulting mycobacterial strains express either the optimised gene encoding FFluc (which is the brightest luciferase and uses a non-toxic substrate) or the optimised *luxCABDE* gene set from *Photorhabdus luminescens* (which results in autoluminescent strains that do not need the exogenous addition of substrate to produce light). Both *M. tuberculosis* strains were imaged *in vivo* in the lungs and spleens of infected mice (Figure 4), with limits of detection of around 10^5-10^6 CFU per lung and 10^5 CFU per spleen, whereas as few as 10^4 CFU can be imaged in the dissected organs (our unpublished results). Further work will assess the usefulness of these luminescent mycobacteria in drug efficacy testing and in other small animal models such as guinea pigs.

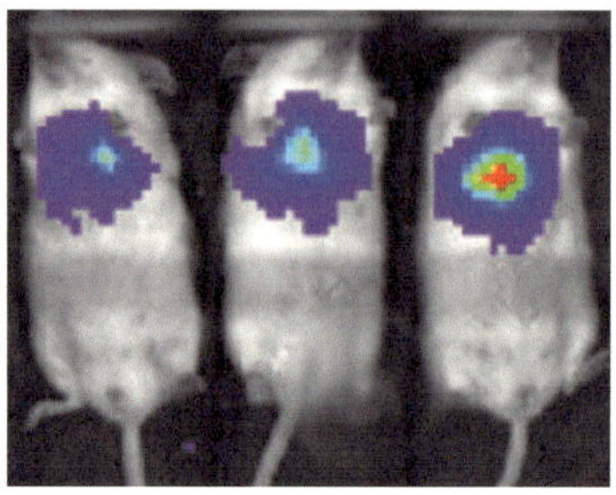

Fig. 4. Visualisation of bioluminescent bacteria within living mice infected with *FFluc*-expressing *M. tuberculosis* after administration of luciferin. The image was obtained using an IVIS Spectrum and is displayed as a pseudocolour image, where red represents the most intense light emission while blue correspond to the weakest signal (Andreu, N. & Wiles, S; unpublished data).

Fluorescence imaging has had a more limited use in the study of infectious diseases, although it has been widely applied to other research fields such as cancer research (N. Andreu et al., 2011). In a first attempt to develop fluorescence imaging of *M. tuberculosis* infection, a GFP-expressing *M. tuberculosis* strain was used to infect mice and guinea pigs, and five weeks post-infection the lungs were imaged using a photon imager (Sugawara et al., 2006). Granulomas as small as 1 mm of diameter were detected, and the results were corroborated by histopathology examination. The same fluorescence technique was used to visualize granulomas in a latent model of TB in guinea pigs (Sugawara et al., 2009). In this case, the animals were subcutaneously infected with *M. tuberculosis* and the infection was followed for 10 months. No clinical signs of infection were evident in any of the animals for the length of the experiment, although the bacteriological analysis of lungs and spleens 180 and 300 days post-infection showed the presence of a few bacteria. Similarly, even though no granulomas were detected by gross pathology examination, microgranulomas were observed in the histological analysis. According to the authors, these small lesions corresponded to the fluorescent spots detected by photon imaging of sliced lungs and spleens. More work is still needed to validate these results and to be able to use this technology *in vivo*.

FPs that emit light in the far-red region of the spectrum are more appropriate for *in vivo* imaging than for example GFP, as red light is less affected by absorption and scattering when travelling through tissues. This is exemplified by the finding that as few as 10^5 CFUs of a BCG strain that expressed tdTomato (excitation 554 nm, emission 581 nm) can be detected after being subcutaneously injected into mice, in comparison to 10^7 CFUs of BCG expressing enhanced GFP (EGFP) (excitation 484 nm, emission 510 nm) (Kong et al., 2009). Therefore, far-red reporters show a lot of promise for fluorescence *in vivo* imaging of *M. tuberculosis* infection in animal models, and the expression of several red FPs in mycobacteria has recently been optimised (Carroll et al., 2010).

The strategies presented above use recombinant bacteria that express an exogenous FP. A much more versatile strategy consists of using an activatable fluorescent agent that is non-fluorescent in its native (quenched) state but produces fluorescence through enzyme-mediated release of its fluorochrome. This strategy has been widely used in cancer and inflammation research but, until recently, not in infectious diseases. Using a near-infrared fluorogenic substrate for β-lactamase, an enzyme that is endogenously expressed by *M. tuberculosis* but not by eukaryotic cells, it is possible to detect 10^6 CFUs of *M. tuberculosis* subcutaneously injected in mice (Kong et al., 2010). The maximal signal was produced 48 h after substrate injection, and no signal was detected 48 h later, which suggests that repetitive imaging of the same animals can be done every 96 h. Surprisingly, the limit of the detection in the lungs of live animals was 10^4 CFUs, which is far lower than the limit of detection subcutaneously, even though the lungs are localised much deeper in the body. The signal was localised laterally, close to the armpit of the animal, and 3D fluorescence molecular tomography (FMT) and imaging of the excised lungs proved that the lungs were the source of the signal. The amount of fluorescence correlated with bacterial numbers when the imaging was performed 24 h post-substrate administration, but at later time-points substrate accumulation lead to a similar level of fluorescence independently of bacterial numbers. In addition, the technique was used to assess drug efficacy by imaging treated and untreated mice, showing that the signal increased in the untreated group while it decreased in the treated group. Although much work needs to be done to assess the usefulness of the technique, one can imagine many potential applications not only in *in vivo* imaging but also *in vitro* using fluorescence microscropy or FACS, as well as for TB diagnosis (e.g. detection of bacilli in sputum or imaging tuberculosis in patients). However, a limitation that needs to be considered is the fact that other bacteria, such as *Pseudomonas aeruginosa* or *Staphylococcus aureus*, also express β-lactamase and therefore may give a false signal. Thus, alternative fluorogenic substrates that are activated by other endogenous enzymes are currently under study; for example, certain trehalose analogues that are substrates for the *M. tuberculosis* mycolyltransesterases Ag85A, Ag85B and Ag85C (Backus et al., 2011).

4. Imaging TB in human disease

4.1 Radiography

The plain radiograph was first described in 1895 by Röntgen, at the same time that the TB pandemic was peaking in wealthy Western countries such as Victorian England. Consequently, there is a long experience and literature of plain radiographic imaging of TB, which has been reviewed previously (McAdams et al., 1995; J. Andreu et al., 2004; Curvo-Semedo et al., 2005). In summary, TB can cause a wide array of chest x-ray appearances, but classically causes consolidation and cavitation in the apices of the upper lobes. TB can also cause disease at the apices of the lower lobes, which appears in the mid-zone on chest radiograph (Figure 5). However, TB can result in a wide range of other features, such as miliary disease with small millet seed-sized nodules throughout the lungs, pleural effusions, mediastinal lymphadenopathy and extrapulmonary disease. In the era of HIV infection, where the host immune system is compromised, the appearances of pulmonary TB are often atypical (Kwan & Ernst, 2011), ranging from classical cavitation to areas of pneumonia to a normal chest x-ray even in the presence of a high mycobacterial load. This illustrates the importance of the adaptive immune response in driving lung inflammation, resulting in consolidation and tissue destruction.

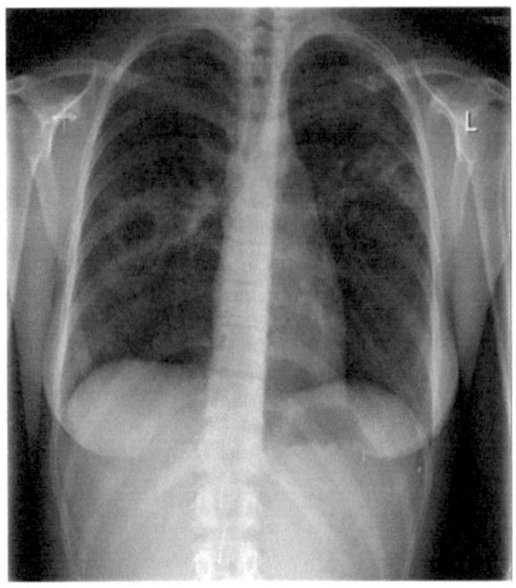

Fig. 5. Radiograph illustrating right mid zone cavitation on a 17 year old patient with pulmonary TB.

As TB is treated, areas of consolidation tend to gradually resolve, leaving an area of fibrosis or scar tissue which persists for life. Cavities remain even after cure, because the lung cannot reconstruct the intricate extracellular matrix after it has been destroyed. However, it is well recognised that radiographic appearances may often worsen before they improve (Leung, 1999), and similarly some lesions may increase in size and density while others appear to resolve. Even in HIV negative patients with drug-sensitive disease, such "paradoxical" reactions may occur (Cheng, 2002). This demonstrates the different behaviour of inflammatory lesions even in the same patient, and one challenge for modern imaging techniques is to define the molecular mechanisms underlying this immune response to improve our understanding of what constitutes an effective as opposed to deleterious immune response to TB.

4.2 Computed Tomography (CT)

CT involves cross-sectional imaging of patients and so permits a much greater degree of resolution of anatomical structures, although it results in a higher radiation dose and higher cost than plain radiography. CT can demonstrate cavity formation with much greater sensitivity and will demonstrate subtle changes which may be missed on plain chest x-rays (Figure 6 [left panel]). For example, filling of small airways with inflammatory debris may result in a "tree-in-bud" pattern (Figure 6 [right panel], arrow), which should immediately alert the physician to the possibility of mycobacterial infection. Therefore, CT scanning provides information of changes at a much more precise anatomical level than plain radiography, but does not give information about the molecular events occurring at the site of infection.

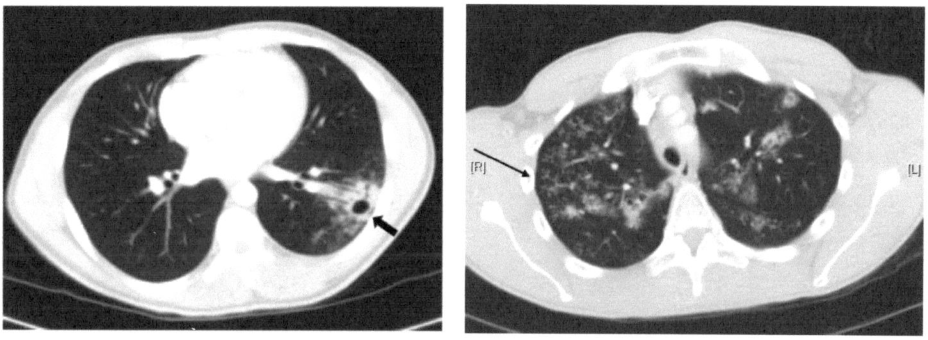

Fig. 6. CT imaging reveals a small left mid zone cavity (indicated by arrow) that was not visible on plain chest x-ray (left panel) and a tree-in-bud bronchial filling in a 33 year old man with pulmonary TB (right panel), which appears as branched opacities in the lung field adjacent to arrowhead.

4.3 Magnetic Resonance Imaging (MRI)

MRI provides the best imaging of the meninges and spinal cord, and so is useful in the diagnosis of cerebral TB, TB meningitis and paraspinal TB abscesses. MRI is a rapidly developing area, and so may emerge as a modality which can provide insight into molecular events in TB. The advantage of MRI is that it involves no ionizing radiation and provides excellent anatomical resolution. New MRI modalities to investigate inflammatory diseases are under development (Pirko et al., 2004), but these have not yet entered the clinical arena for investigation in TB.

4.4 Positron Emission Tomography (PET)

PET imaging is a widely used nuclear medicine technique which has the potential to study pathological events at a molecular level before extensive anatomical changes are observed on plain radiography. PET imaging is commonly combined with CT scanning in patients to provide both functional and anatomical information. [^{18}F]-FDG accumulates in metabolically active cells after phosphorylation, and so is taken up by metabolically active macrophages within the TB granuloma and other inflammatory foci. A primary limitation of PET imaging for TB is the high cost and low availability in developing world. Increased PET uptake is well described in both pulmonary and extrapulmonary TB lesions (Matsuura et al., 2000; Bakheet et al., 1998; C.M. Yang et al., 2003), and can cause diagnostic uncertainty with malignancy and other infections (Chen et al., 2004; Li et al., 2008).

PET scanning is clinically useful in certain patients with TB. For example, when patients have normal radiology but symptoms highly suggestive of active TB, PET scans may identify occult foci of infection which can then be sampled to confirm the diagnosis and for culture (Figure 7, arrow). Furthermore, PET imaging has been proposed for monitoring the resolution of TB disease (Hofmeyr et al., 2007), although the benefit must be weighed against the increased radiation exposure. Current research questions which need to be addressed are whether PET imaging can be useful to define cure, especially in the context of drug-resistant TB where treatment regimes may exceed 18 months, and also investigate whether active foci can be identified in patients with clinically "latent" disease.

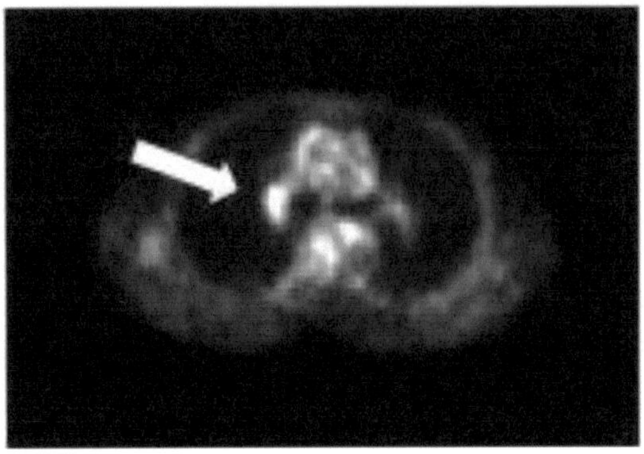

Fig. 7. PET imaging reveals increased uptake of [^{18}F]-FDG in a right hilar lymph node, appearing as bright white (as indicated by arrow).

In addition to [^{18}F]-FDG, a wide array of radiopharmaceuticals have been developed at the preclinical level which might be applied to TB (Signore & Glaudemans, 2011). However, the potential of these in man have not yet been confirmed. For example, radiolabelling the antibiotic ciprofloxacin looked promising initially to investigate cryptic foci of infection (Britton et al., 2002), but has not entered clinical practice widely. The ability to detect a wide range of pathophysiological markers suggests that PET imaging may emerge as a powerful modality to investigate the biology of TB in man, but currently most prospective candidates require further study in model systems before clinical studies in man can be considered.

4.5 Single Photon Emission Computed Tomography (SPECT)

A number of SPECT radiotracers have been applied to the management of TB including ^{99m}Tc-methoxyisobutylisonitrile (^{99m}Tc-MIBI) (Ahmadihosseini, 2008), ^{67}Ga (Liu et al., 2007) and ^{111}In-octreotide (Vanhagen et al., 1994). ^{99m}Tc-MIBI is a widely used myocardial perfusion agent, which can accumulate in tumours and inflammatory lesions (Aktolun et al., 1991; Caner et al., 1992; Kao et al., 1994; A. Yang et al, 2007). Ahmadihosseini and colleagues studied 36 patients with either proven active or inactive treated pulmonary TB and found that ^{99m}Tc-MIBI uptake was increased in 23 out of 24 patients (95.8%) with active pulmonary TB but none of those with inactive TB (Ahmadihosseini et al., 2008). *M. tuberculosis* has been demonstrated to have significantly higher ^{99m}Tc-MIBI uptake compared with fibroblasts and myocytes cultures (Stefanescu et al., 2007), suggesting the bacilli themselves contribute to the signal detected on ^{99m}Tc-MIBI SPECT images.

A number of studies have found positive SPECT images in sputum smear negative patients subsequently found to have a positive sputum culture for *M. tuberculosis* (Ahmadihosseini et al., 2008; Önsel et al., 1996; Stefanescu et al., 2006), suggesting that SPECT imaging may be very useful while awaiting culture results. However, as previously stated, many benign and malignant etiologies can also demonstrate ^{99m}Tc-MIBI uptake (Aktolun et al., 1991; Caner et al., 1992; Kao et al., 1994; A. Yang et al, 2007), which significantly decreases the value of this radiotracer in the differential diagnosis of pulmonary TB from other lung pathologies.

5. Future prospects

A fundamental challenge of TB research is to develop applications which are useful in resource poor settings and can be deployed with minimal investment in infrastructure, maintenance and staff expertise. Furthermore, any application needs to be equally applicable in urban and rural settings. Most modern imaging techniques are useful in the developed world, but are not available to the vast majority of patients with TB who live in resource-poor settings.

However, the detailed study of a small number of patients may identify pathophysiological markers of TB which can then be simplified to develop new diagnostic and therapeutic approaches applicable in resource poor settings. Ironically, when one considers molecular imaging of TB in this light, developing an imaging technique based on plain chest radiography is currently the only widely deliverable approach in the near future. For example, if a highly radio-dense specific TB ligand was developed, a diagnostic test might involve taking an initial chest x-ray, injecting the labelled ligand, and then taking a second x-ray to identify high uptake in the region of TB. This might be useful in the common clinical scenario when a patient presents with upper zone fibrosis, which may be caused by either old self-healed TB or new active TB. If the patient is sputum smear negative, an expensive and invasive bronchoalveolar lavage is required, so a non-invasive test to determine disease activity would be useful.

Another frequent clinical scenario is a patient with immunological evidence of infection, but with a normal chest x-ray and a cryptic location of disease. An investigation whereby one could locate the site of disease for aspiration and culture analysis would be clinically useful. This assay might either rely on antimycobacterial ligands, potentially using the "dock and lock" strategy (Goldenberg et al., 2007), whereby a primary antibody is first injected which docks on the mycobacterial target, and then 24 hours later a second radiolabelled antibody is injected which locks onto the primary antibody, or alternatively might focus on the host immune response, such as looking for increased metalloproteinase activity at the site of disease (Elkington et al., 2011).

In additional to diagnosis, a secondary role of imaging is to determine the prognostic and therapeutic correlates of host immunity. Currently, standard treatment lasts for six months. A recent trial comparing short-course therapy for four months in patients with low risk features was stopped because of increased recurrence in the short course treatment group (Daley, 2010). We need better markers to identify patients who will respond rapidly to treatment and imaging modalities to define mycobacterial load, the effectiveness of the host immune response and TB cure.

6. Conclusions

It is clear that molecular imaging technologies will play an important role in improving our understanding of the host-pathogen interactions that occur in animal models of TB, and should speed up preclinical testing of novel vaccine candidates and therapeutic regimes. In the clinical setting, standard radiographic imaging is likely to remain the mainstay of TB management in humans, with PET imaging emerging as a useful adjunct in specific cases. Indeed, molecular imaging in human TB also has the potential to provide valuable insights into disease pathogenesis, and to aid in the development of new diagnostic approaches and treatment options. However, it remains to be discovered whether approaches currently at preclinical development can be rolled out to the regions of the world where TB is pandemic. We hope that the detailed investigation of small number of patients using cutting-edge technologies may identify pathological markers which can then be developed into simpler, plain radiograph based assays which fulfil the requirements of a truly valuable TB diagnostic.

7. Acknowledgements

This work has been supported in part by a grant to the Imaging TB consortium from the Bill and Melinda Gates Foundation TB Drug Accelerator Program. PE is funded by the UK National Institute for Health Research (NIHR) and is grateful for support from the NIHR Biomedical Research Centre (BRC) scheme at Imperial College London. SW is funded by a Sir Charles Hercus Fellowship from the Health Research Council of New Zealand. The authors would like to thank Prof. Ian Orme (Colorado State University) and Dr. Sanjay Jain MD (Johns Hopkins) for the provision of figures.

8. References

Ahmadihosseini, H., Sadeghi, R., Zakavi, R., Kakhki, V.R. & Kakhki, A.H. (2008). Application of technetium-99m-sestamibi in differentiation of active from inactive pulmonary tuberculosis using a single photon emission computed tomography method. *Nuclear Medicine Communications*, Vol. 29, No. 8, August 2008, pp. 690-694, ISSN 0143-3636

Aktolun, C., Demirel, D., Kir, M., Bayhan, H. & Maden, H.A. (1991). Technetium-99m-MIBI and thallium-201 uptake in pulmonary actinomycosis. *Journal of Nuclear Medicine*, Vol. 32, No. 7, July 1991, pp. 1429–1431, ISSN 0161-5505

Alric, C., Taleb, J., Le Duc, G., Mandon, C., Billotey, C., Le Meur-Herland, A., Brochard, T., Vocanson, F., Janier, M., Perriat, P., Roux, S. & Tillement, O. (2008). Gadolinium chelate coated gold nanoparticles as contrast agents for both X-ray computed tomography and magnetic resonance imaging. *Journal of the American Chemical Society*, Vol. 130, No. 18, May 2008, pp. 5908-5915, ISSN 0002-7863

Andreu, J., Caceres, J., Pallisa, E., and Martinez-Rodriguez, M. (2004). Radiological manifestations of pulmonary tuberculosis. *European Journal of Radiology*, Vol. 51, No. 2, August 2004, pp. 139-149, doi:10.1016/j.ejrad.2004.03.009, ISSN 0720-048X

Andreu, N., Zelmer, A., Fletcher, T., Elkington, P.T., Ward, T.H., Ripoll, J., Parish, T., Bancroft, G.J., Schaible, U., Robertson, B.D. & Wiles, S. (2010). Optimisation of bioluminescent reporters for use with mycobacteria. *PLoS One,* Vol. 5, No. 5, May 2010, e10777, ISSN 1932-6203

Andreu, N., Zelmer, A. & Wiles, S. (2011). Non-invasive biophotonic imaging for studies of infectious disease. *FEMS Microbiology Reviews*, Vol. 35, No. 2, March 2011, pp. 360-394, ISSN 0168-6445

Arain, T. M., Resconi, A.E., Singh, D.C. & Stover, C.K. (1996). Reporter gene technology to assess activity of antimycobacterial agents in macrophages. *Antimicrobial Agents and Chemotherapy*, Vol. 40, No. 6, June 1996, pp. 1542-1544, ISSN 1098-6596

Backus, K.M., Boshoff, H.I., Barry, C.S., Boutureira, O., Patel, M.K., D'Hooge, F., Lee, S.S., Via, L.E., Tahlan, K., Barry, C.E. III & Davis, B.G. (2011). Uptake of unnatural trehalose analogs as a reporter for *Mycobacterium tuberculosis*. *Nature Chemical Biology*, Vol. 7, No. 4, April 2011, pp. 228-235, ISSN 1552-4450

Bakheet, S.M., Powe, J., Ezzat, A., & Rostom, A. (1998). F-18-FDG uptake in tuberculosis. *Clinical Nuclear Medicine*, Vol. 23, No. 11, November 1998, pp. 739-742, ISSN 0143-3636

Britton, K.E., Wareham, D.W., Das, S.S., Solanki, K.K., Amaral, H., Bhatnagar, A., Katamihardja, A.H., Malamitsi, J., Moustafa, H.M., Soroa, V.E., Sundram, F.X. & Padhy, A.K. (2002). Imaging bacterial infection with (99m)Tc-ciprofloxacin (Infecton). *Journal of Clinical Pathology*, Vol. 55, No. 11, November 2001, pp. 817-823, ISSN 0021-9746

Caner, B., Kitapcl, M., Unlu, M., Erbengi, G., Calikoğlu, T., Göğüş, T. & Bekdik, C. (1992). Technetium-99m-MIBI uptake in benign and malignant bone lesions' a comparative study with technetium-99m-MDP. *Journal of Nuclear Medicine*, Vol. 33, No. 3, March 1992; pp. 319–324, ISSN 0161-5505

Carroll, P., Schreuder, L.J., Muwanguzi-Karugaba, J., Wiles, S., Robertson, B.D., Ripoll, J., Ward, T.H., Bancroft, G.J., Schaible, U.E. & Parish, T. (2010). Sensitive detection of gene expression in mycobacteria under replicating and non-replicating conditions using optimized far-red reporters. *PLoS One*, Vol. 5, No. 3, March 2010, e9823, ISSN 1932-6203

Chen, Y.K., Shen, Y.Y. & Kao, C.H. (2004). Abnormal FDG PET imaging in tuberculosis appearing like lymphoma. *Clinical Nuclear Medicine*, Vol. 29, No. 2, February 2004, pp. 124, ISSN 0363-9762

Cheng, V.C., Ho, P.L., Lee, R.A., Chan, K.S., Chan, K.K., Woo, P.C., Lau, S.K., & Yuen, K.Y. (2002). Clinical spectrum of paradoxical deterioration during antituberculosis therapy in non-HIV-infected patients. *European Journal of Clinical Microbiology & Infectious Diseases*, Vol. 21, No. 11, November 2002, pp. 803-809, ISSN 0934-9723

Curvo-Semedo, L., Teixeira, L. & Caseiro-Alves, F. (2005). Tuberculosis of the chest. *European Journal of Radiology*, Vol. 55, No. 2, August 2005, pp. 158-172, doi:10.1016/j.ejrad.2005.04.014, ISSN 0720-048X

Daley, C.L. (2010). Update in tuberculosis 2009. *American Journal of Respiratory and Critical Care Medicine*, Vol. 181, No. 6, March 2010, pp. 550-555, ISSN 1073-449X

Davis, S.L., Be, N.A., Lamichhane, G., Nimmagadda, S., Pomper, M.G., Bishai, W.R. & Jain, S.K. (2009a). Bacterial thymidine kinase as a non-invasive imaging reporter for *Mycobacterium tuberculosis* in live animals. *PLoS One*, Vol.4, No.7, July 2009, e6297, ISSN 1932-6203

Davis, S.L., Nuermberger, E.L., Um, P.K., Vidal, C., Jedynak, B., Pomper, M.G., Bishai, W.R. & Jain, S.K. (2009b). Noninvasive pulmonary [18F]-2-fluoro-deoxy-D-glucose positron emission tomography correlates with bactericidal activity of tuberculosis drug treatment. *Antimicrobial Agents and Chemotherapy*, Vol.53, No.11, November 2009, pp. 4879-4884, ISSN 1098-6596

Dharmadhikari, A.S. & Nardell, E.A. (2008). What animal models teach humans about tuberculosis. *American Journal of Respiratory Cell and Molecular Biology*, Vol.39, No. 5, November 2008, pp. 503-508, ISSN 1535-4989

Elkington, P., Shiomi, T., Breen, R., Nuttall, R.K., Ugarte-Gil, C.A., Walker, N.F., Saraiva, L., Pedersen, B., Mauri, F., Lipman, M., Edwards, D.R., Robertson, B.D., D'Armiento, J. & Friedland, J.S. (2011). MMP-1 drives immunopathology in human tuberculosis and transgenic mice. *Journal of Clinical Investigation*, Vol. 121, No. 5, May 2011, pp. 1827-1833, ISSN 00219738

Filippi, M. & Rocca, M.A. (2011). MR imaging of multiple sclerosis. *Radiology*, Vol. 259, No. 3, June 2011, pp. 659-681, ISSN 0033-8419

Flynn, J.L. (2006). Lessons from experimental *Mycobacterium tuberculosis* infections. *Microbes and Infection*, Vol. 8, No. 4, April 2006, pp. 1179-1188, ISSN 1286-4579

Goldenberg, D.M., Chatal, J.F., Barbet, J., Boerman, O. & Sharkey, R.M. (2007). Cancer imaging and therapy with bispecific antibody pretargeting. *Update on Cancer Therapeutics*, Vol. 2, No. 1, March 2007, pp. 19-31, ISSN 1872-115X

Geraldes, C.F. & Laurent, S. (2009). Classification and basic properties of contrast agents for magnetic resonance imaging. *Contrast Media & Molecular Imaging*, Vol. 4, No. 1, January-February 2009, pp. 1-23, DOI: 10.1002/cmmi.265, ISSN 1555-4317

Gupta, U.D. & Katoch, V.M. (2005) Animal models of tuberculosis. *Tuberculosis (Edinburgh)*, Vol. 85, No. 5-6, September-November 2005, pp. 277-293, ISSN 1472-9792

Hainfeld, J.F., Slatkin, D.N., Focella, T.M. & Smilowitz, H.M. (2006). Gold nanoparticles: a new X-ray contrast agent. *British Journal of Radiology*, Vol. 79, No. 939, March 2006, pp. 248-253, ISSN 0007-1285

Heuts, F., Carow, B., Wigzell, H. & Rottenberg, M.E. (2009). Use of non-invasive bioluminescent imaging to assess mycobacterial dissemination in mice, treatment with bactericidal drugs and protective immunity. *Microbes and Infection*, Vol. 11, No. 14-15, December 2009, pp. 1114-1121, ISSN 1286-4579

Hickey, M.J., Arain, T.M., Shawar, R.M., Humble, D.J., Langhorne, M.H., Morgenroth, J.N. & Stover, C.K. (1996). Luciferase in vivo expression technology: use of recombinant mycobacterial reporter strains to evaluate antimycobacterial activity in mice. *Antimicrobial Agents and Chemotherapy*, Vol. 40, No. 2, February 1996, pp. 400-407, ISSN 1098-6596

Hofmeyr, A., Lau, W.F. & Slavin, M.A. 2007. *Mycobacterium tuberculosis* infection in patients with cancer, the role of 18-fluorodeoxyglucose positron emission tomography for diagnosis and monitoring treatment response. *Tuberculosis (Edinburgh)*, Vol. 87, No. 5, September 2007, pp. 459-463, ISSN 1472-9792

Horky, L.L. & Treves, S.T. (2011). PET and SPECT in brain tumors and epilepsy. *Neurosurgery Clinics of North America*, Vol. 22, No. 2, April 2011, pp. 169-184, ISSN 1042-3680

Hsiung, P.L., Hardy, J., Friedland, S., Soetikno, R., Du, C.B., Wu, A.P., Sahbaie, P., Crawford, J.M., Lowe, A.W., Contag, C.H. & Wang, T.D. (2008). Detection of colonic dysplasia in vivo using a targeted heptapeptide and confocal microendoscopy. *Nature Medicine*, Vol. 14, No. 4, April 2008, pp. 454-458, 1078-8956

Kao, C.H., Wang, S.J. & Liu, T.J. (1994). The use of technetium-99m-rnethoxyisobutylisonitrile breast scintigraphy to evaluate palpable breast masses.

European Journal of Nuclear Medicine, Vol. 2, No. 5, May 1994, pp. 432–436, ISSN 1619-7089

Kong, Y., Subbian, S., Cirillo, S.L. & Cirillo, J.D. (2009). Application of optical imaging to study of extrapulmonary spread by tuberculosis. *Tuberculosis (Edinburgh)*, Vol. 89, Suppl. 1, December 2009, pp. S15-S17, ISSN 1472-9792

Kong, Y., Yao, H., Ren, H., Subbian, S., Cirillo, S.L., Sacchettini, J.C., Rao, J. & Cirillo, J.D. (2010). Imaging tuberculosis with endogenous beta-lactamase reporter enzyme fluorescence in live mice. *Proceedings of the National Academy of Sciences of the United States of America*, Vol. 107, No. 27, July 2010, pp. 12239-12244, ISSN 1091-6490

Kraft, S. L.; Dailey, D.; Kovach, M.; Stasiak, K. L.; Bennett, J.; McFarland, C. T.; McMurray, D. N., Izzo, A. A.; Orme, I. M. & Basaraba, R. J. (2004) Magnetic resonance imaging of pulmonary lesions in guinea pigs infected with *Mycobacterium tuberculosis*. *Infection and Immunity*, Vol.72, No.10, pp. 5963–5971, ISSN 1098-5522

Kwan, C.K. & Ernst, J.D. (2011). HIV and tuberculosis: a deadly human syndemic. *Clinical Microbiology Reviews*, Vol. 24, No. 2, April 2011, pp. 351-376. ISSN 0893-8512

Leung, A.N. (1999). Pulmonary tuberculosis: the essentials. *Radiology*, Vol. 210, No. 2, February 1999, pp. 307-322, ISSN 0033-8419

Lewinsohn, D.M., Tydeman, I.S., Frieder, M., Grotzke, J.E., Lines, R.A., Ahmed, S., Prongay, K.D., Primack, S.L., Colgin, L.M., Lewis, A.D. & Lewinsohn, D.A. (2006) High resolution radiographic and fine immunologic definition of TB disease progression in the rhesus macaque. *Microbes and Infection*, Vol.8, No.11, pp. 2587-2598, ISSN 1286-4579

Li, Y.J., Zhang, Y., Gao, S. & Bai, R.J. (2008). Systemic disseminated tuberculosis mimicking malignancy on F-18 FDG PET-CT. *Clinical Nuclear Medicine*, Vol. 33, No. 1, January 2008, pp. 49-51, ISSN 0363-9762

Lin, P.L., Carney, J., Tomko, J.A., Frye, L.J., Coleman, T., Scanga, C.A., Lopresti, B.J., Mountz, J.M., Klein, E., Barry, C.E. & Flynn, J.L. (2009). Using PET/CT imaging to monitor tuberculosis progression and its response to chemotherapy in experimentally infected non-human primates. *World Molecular Imaging Congress*, Presentation number 0158, Montreal, Canada, September 2009

Liu, S.F., Liu, J.W., Lin, M.C., Lee, C.H., Huang, H.H. & Lai, Y.F. (2007). Monitoring treatment responses in patients with pulmonary TB using serial lung gallium-67 scintigraphy. *American Journal of Roentgenology*, Vol. 188, No. 5, May 2007, pp. 403–408, ISSN 0361-803X

Massoud, T.F. & Gambhir, S.S. (2003). Molecular imaging in living subjects: seeing fundamental biological processes in a new light. *Genes and Development*, Vol. 17, No. 5, March 2003, pp. 545-580, ISSN 0890-9369

Matsuura, E., Umehara, F., Hashiguchi, T., Fujimoto, N., Okada, Y. & Osame, M. (2000). Marked increase of matrix metalloproteinase 9 in cerebrospinal fluid of patients with fungal or tuberculous meningoencephalitis. *Journal of the Neurological Sciences*, Vol. 173, No. 1, February 2000, pp. 45-52, ISSN 0022-510X

McAdams, H.P., Erasmus, J. & Winter, J.A. (1995). Radiologic manifestations of pulmonary tuberculosis. *Radiologic Clinics of North America*, Vol. 33, No. 4, July 1995, pp. 655-678, ISSN 0033-8389

McClennan, B.L. (1994). Adverse reactions to iodinated contrast media. Recognition and response. *Investigative Radiology*, Vol. 29, Suppl. 1, May 1994, pp.S46-50, ISSN 0020-9996

Ntziachristos, V. (2006). Fluorescence molecular imaging. *Annual Review of Biomedical Engineering*, Vol. 8, August 2006, pp. 1-33, ISSN 1523-9829

Önsel, C., Sönmezoglu, K., Camsari, G., Atay, S., Cetin, S., Erdil, Y.T., Uslu, I., Uzun, A., Kanmaz, B. & Sayman, H.B. (1996). Technetium-99m-MIBI scintigraphy in pulmonary tuberculosis. *Journal of Nuclear Medicine*, Vol. 37, No. 2, February 1996, pp. 233–238, ISSN 0161-5505

Ordway, D.J., Shanley, C.A., Caraway, M.L., Orme, E.A., Bucy, D.S., Hascall-Dove, L., Henao-Tamayo, M., Harton, M.R., Shang, S., Ackart, D. Kraft, S.L., Lenaerts, A.J., Basaraba, R.J. & Orme, I.M. (2010). Evaluation of standard chemotherapy in the guinea pig model of tuberculosis. *Antimicrobial Agents and Chemotherapy*, Vol. 54, No. 5, May 2010, pp. 1820-1833, ISSN 1098-6596

Pirko, I., Johnson, A., Ciric, B., Gamez, J., Macura, S.I., Pease, L.R. & Rodriguez, M. (2004). In vivo magnetic resonance imaging of immune cells in the central nervous system with superparamagnetic antibodies. *FASEB Journal* (the official publication of the Federation of American Societies for Experimental Biology), Vol. 18, No. 1, January 2004, pp. 179-182, ISSN 0892-6638

Pysz, M.A., Gambhir, S.S. & Willmann, J.K. (2010). Molecular imaging: current status and emerging strategies. *Clinical Radiology*, Vol. 65, No. 7, July 2010, pp. 500-516, ISSN 0009-9260

Rabin, O., Manuel Perez, J., Grimm, J., Wojtkiewicz, G. & Weissleder, R. (2006). An X-ray computed tomography imaging agent based on long-circulating bismuth sulphide nanoparticles. *Nature Materials*, Vol. 5, No. 2, February 2006, pp. 118-122, ISSN 1476-1122

Sandhu, G.S., Solorio, L., Broome, A.M., Salem, N., Kolthammer, J., Shah, T., Flask, C. & Duerk, J.L. (2010). Whole animal imaging. *Wiley Interdisciplinary Reviews. Systems Biology and Medicine*, Vol. 2, No. 4, July-August 2010, pp. 398-421, ISSN 1939-005X

Sharpe, S.A., Eschelbach, E., Basaraba, R.J., Gleeson, F., Hall, G.A., McIntyre, A., Williams, A., Kraft, S.L., Clark, S., Gooch, K., Hatch, G., Orme, I.M., Marsh, P.D. & Dennis, M.J. (2009). Determination of lesion volume by MRI and stereology in a macaque model of tuberculosis. *Tuberculosis (Edinburgh)*, Vol. 89, No. 6, November 2009, pp. 405-416, ISSN 1472-9792

Sharpe, S.A., McShane, H., Dennis, M.J., Basaraba, R.J., Gleeson, F., Hall, G., McIntyre, A., Gooch, K., Clark, S., Beveridge, N.E., Nuth, E., White, A., Marriott, A., Dowall, S., Hill, A.V., Williams, A. & Marsh, P.D. (2010). Establishment of an aerosol challenge model of tuberculosis in rhesus macaques and an evaluation of endpoints for vaccine testing. *Clinical and Vaccine Immunology*, Vol.17, No.8, August 2010, pp. 1170-1182, ISSN 1556-679X

Signore, A. & Glaudemans, A.W. (2011). The molecular imaging approach to image infections and inflammation by nuclear medicine techniques. *Annals of Nuclear Medicine*, DOI: 10.1007/s12149-011-0521-z, Epub ahead of print: Aug 12, ISSN 0914-7187

Singh, S.P. & Nath, H. (1994). Early radiology of pulmonary tuberculosis. *American Journal of Roentgenology*, Vol. 162, No. 4, April 1994, pp. 846, ISSN 0361-803X

Snewin, V.A., Gares, M.P., Gaora, P.O., Hasan, Z., Brown, I.N. & Young, D.B. (1999). Assessment of immunity to mycobacterial infection with luciferase reporter constructs. *Infection and Immunity*, Vol. 67, No. 9, September 1999, pp. 4586-4593, ISSN 1098-5522

Stefanescu, C., Rusu, V., Boisteanu, D., Azoicai, D., Costin, M., Oleniuc, D., Hurjui, M. & Sattish, P. (2006). 99mTc isonitrils biophysical aspects in pulmonary tuberculosis. Part I. In vivo evaluation of 99mTc MIBI and 99mTc tetrofosmin biophysical localization mechanisms. *Revista Medico Chirurgicala a Societatii de Medici si Naturalisti din Iasi*, Vol. 110, No. 4, October-December 2006, pp. 944–949, ISSN 0300-8738

Stefanescu, C., Rusu, V., Azoici, D. & Hurjui, I. (2007). 99mTc isonitrils biophysical aspects in pulmonary tuberculosis. Part II. In vitro evaluation of 99mTc MIBI cellular uptake mechanism. *Revista Medico Chirurgicala a Societatii de Medici si Naturalisti din Iasi*, Vol. 111, No. 1, January-March 2007, pp. 210–215, ISSN 0300-8738

Sugawara, I., Mizuno, S., Tatsumi, T. & Taniyama, T. (2006) Imaging of pulmonary granulomas using a photon imager. *Japanese Journal of Infectious Diseases*, Vol. 59, No. 5, October 2006, pp. 332-333, ISSN 1344-6304

Tarantal, A.F., Lee, C.C., Jimenez, D.F. & Cherry, S.R. (2006). Fetal gene transfer using lentiviral vectors: in vivo detection of gene expression by microPET and optical imaging in fetal and infant monkeys. *Human Gene Therapy*, Vol. 17, No. 12, December 2006, pp. 1254-1261, ISSN 1043-0342

Taschereau, R., Silverman, R.W. & Chatzijoannou, A.F. (2010). Dual-energy attenuation coefficient decomposition with differential filtration and application to a micro-CT scanner. *Physics in Medicine and Biology*, Vol. 55, No. 4, February 2010, pp. 1141-1155, ISSN 0031-9155

Troy, T., Jekic-McMullen, D., Sambucetti, L. & Rice, B. (2004). Quantitative comparison of the sensitivity of detection of fluorescent and bioluminescent reporters in animal models. *Molecular Imaging*, Vol. 3, No. 1, January 2004, pp. 9-23, ISSN 1535-3508

Wiles, S., Crepin, V.F., Childs, G., Frankel, G. & Kerton, A. (2007). Use of biophotonic imaging as a training aid for administration of substances in laboratory rodents. *Laboratory Animals*, Vol. 41, No. 3, July 2007, pp. 321-328, ISSN 0023-6772

Vanhagen, P.M., Krenning, E.P., Reubi, J.C., Kwekkeboom, D.J., Bakker, W.H., Mulder, A.H., Laissue, I., Hoogstede, H.C. & Lamberts, S.W. (1994). Somatostatin analogue scintigraphy in granulomatous diseases. *European Journal of Nuclear Medicine*, Vol. 21, No. 6, June 1994, pp. 497–502, ISSN 1619-7089

World Health Organisation. (2010). Global tuberculosis control 2010: WHO Press, 2010

Yang, A., Xue, J., Li, X., Yu, Y., Deng, H., Hu, G., Meng, X. & Li, J. (2007). Experimental and clinical observations of 99mTc-MIBI uptake correlate with P-glycoprotein expression in lung cancer. *Nuclear Medicine Communications*, Vol. 28, No. 9, September 2007, pp. 696–703, ISSN 0143-3636

Yang, C.M., Hsu, C.H., Lee, C.M. & Wang, F.C. (2003). Intense uptake of [F-18]-fluoro-2 deoxy-D-glucose in active pulmonary tuberculosis. *Annals of Nuclear Medicine*, Vol. 17, No. 5, July 2003, pp. 407-410, ISSN 0914-7187

Zonios, G., Bykowski, J. & Kollias, N. (2001). Skin melanin, hemoglobin, and light scattering properties can be quantitatively assessed in vivo using diffuse reflectance spectroscopy. *Journal of Investigative Dermatology*, Vol. 117, No. 6, December 2001, pp. 1452-1457, ISSN 0022-202X

16

Data Mining Techniques in the Diagnosis of Tuberculosis

T. Asha[1], S. Natarajan[2] and K. N. B. Murthy[3]
[1]*Department of Information Science & Engineering,*
Bangalore Institute of Technology,
[2,3]*Department of Information Science and Engineering,*
PES Institute of Technology,
India

1. Introduction

Data mining is the knowledge discovery process which helps in extracting interesting patterns from large amount of data. With the amount of data doubling every three years, data mining is becoming an increasingly important tool to transform these data into information. It is commonly used in a wide range of profiling practices, such as marketing, surveillance, fraud detection, medical and scientific discovery (J.Han & M.Kamber,2006).

Humans have been manually extracting patterns from data for centuries, but the increasing volume of data in modern times has called for more automated approaches. As data sets have grown in size and complexity, direct hands-on data analysis has increasingly been augmented with indirect, automatic data processing. This has been aided by other discoveries in computer science, such as neural networks, clustering, genetic algorithms (1950s), decision trees (1960s) and support vector machines (1980s). Data mining (DM) is the process of applying these methods to data with the intention of uncovering hidden patterns.

1.1 Data mining process

Generally KDD is an iterative and interactive process involving several steps. This KDD process was chosen (Figure 1) according to UNESCO definition because of its simplicity and comprehensiveness.

1.1.1 Problem identification and definition

The first step is to understand the application domain and to formulate the problem. This step is clearly a prerequisite for extracting useful knowledge and for choosing appropriate data mining methods in the third step according to the application target and the nature of data.

1.1.2 Obtaining and preprocessing data

The second step is to collect and pre-process the data. Today's real-world databases are susceptible to noisy, missing, and inconsistent data due to their typically huge size (often several gigabytes or more), and their likely origin from multiple, heterogeneous sources. Low quality data will lead to low quality mining results. Data pre-processing is an essential step for knowledge and data mining. Data pre-processing include the data integration, removal of noise or outliers, the treatment of missing data, data transformation and reduction of data etc. This step usually takes the most time needed for the whole KDD process.

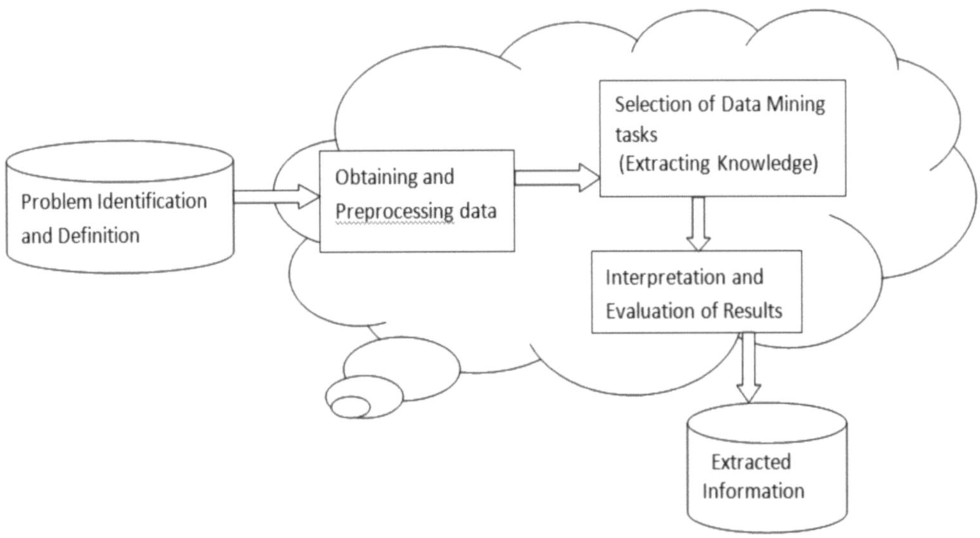

Fig. 1. Structure of Data Mining (KDD) Process

1.1.3 Selection of data mining / knowledge discovery in database

The third step is data mining that extracts patterns and models hidden in data. This is an essential process where intelligent methods are applied in order to extract data patterns. In this step we have to first select data mining tasks and then data mining method. The major classes of data mining methods are predictive modeling such as classification and regression; segmentation (clustering) and association rules which are explained in detail in the next section.

1.1.4 Interpretation and evaluation of results

The fourth step is to interpret (post-process) discovered knowledge, especially the interpretation in terms of description and prediction which is the two primary goals of discovery system in practice. Experiments show that discovered patterns or models from data are not always of interest or direct use, and the KDD process is necessarily iterative with judgement of discovered knowledge. One standard way to evaluate induced rules is to divide the data into two sets, training on the first set and testing on the second. One can repeat this process a number of times with different splits, and then average the results to estimate the rules performance.

1.1.5 Using discovered knowledge

The final step is to put the discovered knowledge in practical use. Putting the results in practical use is certainly the ultimate goal of the knowledge discovery. The information achieved can be used later to explain current or historical phenomenon, predict the future, and help decision-makers make policy from the existed facts (ho, nd).

1.2 Data mining tasks and functionalities

Data Mining functionalities are specifically of two categories: descriptive data mining and predictive data mining. Descriptive methods find human-interpretable patterns that describe the data. Predictive methods perform inference on the current data in order to make predictions (J.Han & M.Kamber, 2006).

The predictive tasks of data mining are:

- Classification - Arranges the data into predefined groups. For example an email program might attempt to classify an email as legitimate or spam. Common algorithms include Decision Tree Learning, Nearest neighbor, Naive Bayesian classification and Neural Network.
- Regression -Attempts to find a function which models the data with the least error.

The descriptive tasks of data mining are:

- Association rule learning - Searches for relationships between variables. For example a supermarket might gather data on customer purchasing habits. Using association rule learning, the supermarket can determine which products are frequently bought together and use this information for marketing purposes. This is sometimes referred to as "market basket analysis".
- Clustering - Is like classification but the groups are not predefined, so the algorithm will try to group similar items together.

Data mining finds its applications in various fields. **Web mining -** is the application of data mining techniques to discover patterns from the Web. According to analysis targets, web mining can be divided into three different types, which are Web Usage Mining (WUM), Web Content Mining (WCM) and Web Structure Mining (WSM). It is called **Spatial Data mining** if we apply data mining techniques to spatial data. **Multimedia Data mining**- is the application of data mining techniques to multimedia data such as audio, video, image, graphics etc. **Text mining**- applying data mining techniques on unstructured or semi-structured text data such as news group, email, documents. Bioinformatics and Bio-data analysis on biological data.

Data mining draws ideas from many fields such as Machine learning/Artificial Intelligence, Pattern Recognition, Statistics, and Database Systems. In recent years, data mining has been widely used in the area of genetics, medicine, bioinformatics with its applications applied to biomedical data as facilitated by domain ontologies and mining clinical trial data which is also called medical data mining.

Different types of medical data are now available on the web, where DM algorithms and applications can be applied, helping in easy diagnosis. Efficient and scalable algorithms can be implemented both in sequential and parallel mode thus improving the performance. Such type of mining is called medical data mining.

1.3 Medical data mining

In recent years, data mining has been widely used in the area of genetics and medicine, called medical data mining. In the past two decades we have witnessed revolutionary changes in biomedical research and bio-technology. There is an explosive growth of bio-medical data, ranging from those collected in pharmaceutical studies and cancer therapy investigations to those identified in genomics and proteomics research. The rapid progress of biotechnology and bio-data analysis methods has led to the emergence and fast growth of a promising new field: Bioinformatics. On the other hand, recent progress in data mining research has led to the developments of numerous efficient and scalable methods for mining interesting patterns and knowledge in large databases, ranging from efficient classification methods to clustering, outlier analysis, frequent, sequential and structured pattern analysis methods, and visualization and spatial/temporal data analysis tools. The question becomes how to bridge the two fields, Data Mining and Bioinformatics, for successful data mining in biomedical data. Especially, we should analyze how data mining may help efficient and effective bio-medical data analysis and outline some research problems that may motivate the further developments of powerful data mining tools for bio data or medical data analysis.

Data mining is a process that involves aggregating raw data stored in a database and analyzing them to identify trends, patterns and anomalies. Medical data mining is an active research area under data mining since medical databases have accumulated large quantities of information about patients and their clinical conditions. Relationships and patterns hidden in this data can provide new medical knowledge as has been proved in a number of medical data mining applications. A Doctor quickly swung into action after a renowned pharmaceutical company in the USA announced in 2001 that it was withdrawing a cholesterol-lowering drug following the deaths of more than 30 people. Using his medical records database, his staff was able to identify all patients taking the cholesterol-lowering drug and notify them within 24 hours of the announcement. What the doctor did is technically known as Data Mining. Very few doctors, however, were able to act on the situation, because they did not have accessible raw data in the electronic format.

Not only does disciplined storage of medical data helps the physicians and healthcare institutions, but it also helps pharmaceutical companies to mine the data to see the trends in diseases. It also helps prioritize product development and clinical trials based on the accurate demands visible from the data that is mined.

Various data mining tasks can be applied on different diseases data set. This helps even the doctor to identify hidden associations between various symptoms. Research has been carried out on gene data, proteonomic data and attributes related to diseases covering even risk factors. Prediction of diseases has also been done on scanned images leading to medical imaging, which is the fastest growing area. Lot of Research has been carried out leading to breast cancer, liver diseases and other types of cancer and also diseases related to heart. There are very few articles related to Tuberculosis.

2. Tuberculosis

Tuberculosis (TB) is a common and often deadly infectious disease caused by mycobacterium; in humans it is mainly *Mycobacterium tuberculosis*. It usually spreads through the air and attacks low immune bodies such as patients with Human Immunodeficiency Virus (HIV). It is a disease which can affect virtually all organs, not sparing even the relatively inaccessible sites. The microorganisms usually enter the body by inhalation through the lungs. They spread from the initial location in the lungs to other parts of the body via the blood stream. They present a diagnostic dilemma even for physicians with a great deal of experience in this disease. Hence Tuberculosis (TB) is a contagious bacterial disease caused by mycobacterium which affects usually lungs and is often co-infected with HIV/AIDS.

It is a great problem for most developing countries because of the low diagnosis and treatment opportunities. Tuberculosis has the highest mortality level among the diseases caused by a single type of microorganism. Thus, tuberculosis is a great health concern all over the world, and in India as well (wikipedia.org).

Symptoms of TB depend on where in the body the TB bacteria are growing. TB bacteria usually grow in the lungs. TB in the lungs may cause symptoms such as a bad cough that lasts 3 weeks or longer pain in the chest coughing up blood or sputum. Other symptoms of active TB disease are: weakness or fatigue, weight loss, no appetite, chills, fever and sweating at night.

Although common and deadly in the third world, Tuberculosis was almost non-existent in the developed world, but has been making a recent resurgence. Certain drug-resistant strains are emerging and people with immune suppression such as AIDS or poor health are becoming carriers.

2.1 Data set description

The medical dataset we are using includes 700 real records of patients suffering from TB obtained from a city hospital. The entire dataset is put in one file having many records. Each record corresponds to most relevant information of one patient. Initial queries by doctor as symptoms and some required test details of patients have been considered as main attributes. Totally there are 12 attributes (symptoms) and last attribute is considered as class in case of Associative Classification. The symptoms of each patient such as age, chronic cough(weeks), loss of weight, intermittent fever(days), night sweats, Sputum, Bloodcough, chestpain, HIV, radiographic findings, wheezing and TBtype are considered as attributes.

Table 1 shows names of 12 attributes considered along with their Data Types (DT). Type N- indicates numerical and C is categorical.

3. Association Rule Mining

Association Rule Mining (ARM) is an important problem in the rapidly growing field called data mining and knowledge discovery in databases (KDD). The task of association rule mining is to mine a set of highly correlated attributes/features shared among a large number of records in a given database. For example, consider the sales database of a bookstore, where the records represent customers and the attributes represent books. The mined patterns are the set of books most frequently bought together by the customer. An example could be that, 60% of the people who buy Design and Analysis of Algorithms also buy Data Structure. The store can use this knowledge for promotions, self-placement etc. There are many application areas for association rule mining techniques, which include catalog design, store layout, customer segmentation, telecommunication alarm diagnosis and so on.

No	**Name**	**DT**
1	Age	N
2	chroniccough(weeks)	N
3	weightloss	C
4	intermittentfever(days)	N
5	nightsweats	C
6	Bloodcough	C
7	chestpain	C
8	HIV	C
9	Radiographicfindings	C
10	Sputum	C
11	wheezing	C
12	TBType	C

Table 1. List of Attributes and their Datatypes

3.1 Definition of association rule

Here we give the classical definition of association rules. Let $\{ t_1, t_2,\ldots..t_n\}$ be a set of transactions and let I be a set of items, $I=\{ I_1,I_2,\ldots.I_m \}$. An association rule is an implication of the form $X \rightarrow Y$, where X, Y are disjoint subsets of item I and $X \cap Y = \phi$. X is called the *antecedent* and Y is called the *consequent* of the rule. In general, a set of items such as the antecedent or consequent of a rule is called an *Itemset*. Each *itemset* has an associated measure of statistical significance called *support*. *support(x)=s* is the fraction of the transactions in the database containing X. The rule has a measure of strength called *confidence* defined as the ratio *support(X* $\cup$ *Y) / support(X)* (J.Han & M.Kamber, 2006).

Given a set of transactions T, the goal of association rule mining is to find all rules having support ≥ *minsup* threshold and confidence ≥ *minconf* threshold.

Mining Association rule is a Two-step approach:

- Frequent Itemset Generation
  - Generate all itemsets whose support ≥ minsup.
- Rule Generation
  - Generate high confidence rules from each frequent itemset, where each rule is a binary partitioning of a frequent itemset.

Frequent Itemset Generation

The two important algorithms for frequent itemset generation are Apriori algorithm (first proposed by Agrawal, Imielinski and swami VLDB 1994) and Frequent pattern tree growth (FP-Tree) (FPgrowth—Han, Pei & Yin @SIGMOD'00).

Apriori algorithm employs two actions join step and prune step as explained in the following algorithm to find frequent itemsets.

- Apriori principle: It states that if an itemset is frequent, then all of its subsets must also be frequent
- Apriori principle holds due to the following property of the support measure:
  - Support of an itemset never exceeds the support of its subsets
  - $\forall X, Y : (X \subseteq Y) \Rightarrow s(X) \geq s(Y)$
- This is known as the anti-monotone property of support

Apriori algorithm

- Let k=1
- Generate frequent itemsets of length 1
- Repeat until no new frequent itemsets are identified
  - Generate length (k+1) candidate itemsets from length k frequent itemsets [join step]
  - Prune candidate itemsets containing subsets of length k that are infrequent [prune step]
  - Count the support of each candidate by scanning the DB
  - Eliminate candidates that are infrequent, leaving only those that are frequent

Rule Generation

Once the frequent itemsets from transactions in a database D have been found, it is straightforward to generate strong association rules from them where strong association rules satisfy both minimum support and minimum confidence. This is calculated from the following equation

$$\text{Confidence(A->B)} = \text{support\_count}(A \cup B) / \text{support\_count}(A)$$

Based on the above equation association rules can be generated as follows:

- For each frequent itemset l, generate all non empty subsets of l.
- For every nonempty subset s of l, output the rule " s -> (l-s)" if support_count(l) / support_count(s) is greater than or equal to min_conf, where min_conf is the minimum confidence threshold.

Challenges of Apriori

- Multiple scans of transaction database
- Huge number of candidates
- Tedious workload of support counting for candidates

Improving Apriori: general ideas

- Reduce passes of transaction database scans
- Shrink number of candidates
- Facilitate support counting of candidates

Since the processing of the Apriori algorithm requires plenty of time, its computational efficiency is a very important issue. In order to improve the efficiency of Apriori, many researchers have proposed modified association rule-related algorithms.

Advantages of frequent itemset generation and rule generation

- Finding inherent regularities in data
  - What products were often purchased together?— Beer and diapers?!
  - What are the subsequent purchases after buying a PC?
  - What kinds of DNA are sensitive to this new drug?
  - Can we automatically classify web documents?
- Applications
  - Basket data analysis, cross-marketing, catalog design, sale campaign analysis, Web log (click stream) analysis, and DNA sequence analysis.

3.2 Tuberculosis association rules

Tuberculosis association rules can be generated by applying data mining ARM technique with the following steps:

- Pre-processing the dataset by discretizing and normalizing
- Generating rules by applying apriori on preprocessed range data

3.2.1 Pre-processing

Incomplete, noisy, and inconsistent data are common among real world databases. Hence it is necessary to preprocess such data before using it. The most common topics under data preprocessing are Data cleaning, Data integration, Data Transformation, Data reduction, Data discretization and automatic generation of concept hierarchies.

Discretization and Normalization are the two data transformation procedures that help in representing the data and their relationships precisely in a tabular format that makes the database easy to understand and operationally efficient. This also reduces data redundancy and enhances performance.

The above TB attributes are normalized and discretized to a suitable binary format. A categorical data field has a value selected from an available list of values. Such data items can be normalized by allocating a unique column number to each possible value. Numerical data fields are discretized by taking values that are within some range defined by minimum and maximum limits. In such cases we can divide the given range into a number of sub-ranges and allocate a unique column number to each sub-range respectively.

Here we give a small example of five patients medical records with five attributes. Table 2 shows original data. Table 3 contains schema of how the attributes are mapped to individual column numbers. Table 4 is the final translated or normalized data.

Age	Chronic cough(weeks)	Weight loss	HIV	Sputum
17	3	Yes	Negative	Yes
13	6	Yes	Negative	Yes
45	6	Null	Negative	Yes
32	Null	Yes	Positive	Null
22	Null	Yes	Positive	Yes

Table 2. Original (raw) Data

Age < 25	Age >= 25	Chronic cough (weeks)< 4	4 <= Chronic cough (weeks) < 8	Chronic cough (weeks) = Null	Weight loss = Yes
1	2	3	4	5	6

Weight loss = Null	HIV = Positive	HIV = Negative	Sputum = Yes	Sputum = Null
7	8	9	10	11

Table 3. Schema Table

In the above tables, note that Age is a numerical attribute and its cut off point is <25 & >=25. Similarly HIV is a categorical attribute where positive value is assigned one number and negative another. The value Null for categorical attribute weightloss is equivalent to No and is assigned a unique number. By using the schema table above we map each tuple in the original data of table 2 to a resulting normalized table shown in table 4. Resulting table has the same number of columns as the original table but filled with unique integer values.

Age	Chronic cough(weeks)	Weight loss	HIV	Sputum
1	3	6	9	10
1	4	6	9	10
2	4	7	9	10
2	5	6	8	11
1	5	6	8	10

Table 4. Normalized Table

3.2.2 TB rules generation

a. **Frequent Itemsets from TB data:** The following figure 2 and 3 shows some of the frequent itemsets generated with 70% support, 90% confidence and 60% support,

[1] {chroniccough(weeks)<39.0} = 692
[2] {weightloss=null} = 550
[3] {chroniccough(weeks)<39.0 weightloss=null} = 544
[4] {intermittentfever(days)<91.25} = 669
[5] {chroniccough(weeks)<39.0 intermittentfever(days)<91.25} = 664
[6] {weightloss=null intermittentfever(days)<91.25} = 530
[7] {chroniccough(weeks)<39.0 weightloss=null intermittentfever(days)<91.25} = 526
[8] {nightsweats=null} = 496
[9] {Bloodcough=null} = 671
[10] {chroniccough(weeks)<39.0 Bloodcough=null} = 663
[11] {weightloss=null Bloodcough=null} = 534
[12] {chroniccough(weeks)<39.0 weightloss=null Bloodcough=null} = 528
[13] {intermittentfever(days)<91.25 Bloodcough=null} = 645
[14] {chestpain=null} = 570
[15 {chroniccough(weeks)<39.0 chestpain=null} = 564
[16] {intermittentfever(days)<91.25 chestpain=null} = 542
[17] {chroniccough(weeks)<39.0 intermittentfever(days)<91.25 chestpain=null} = 539
[18] {Bloodcough=null chestpain=null} = 546

Fig. 2. Frequent Itemsets with 70%support and 90% confidence

80%confidence. The Format of the rule is: [N] {I} = S, where N is a sequential number, I is the item set converted from normalized numerical value to schema text (symptoms) and S the support.

[1] {chroniccough(weeks)<39.0} = 692
[2] {weightloss=null} = 550
[3] {chroniccough(weeks)<39.0 weightloss=null} = 544
[4] {intermittentfever(days)<91.25} = 669
[5] {Bloodcough=null} = 671
[6] {chroniccough(weeks)<39.0 Bloodcough=null} = 663
[7] {weightloss=null Bloodcough=null} = 534
[8] {chestpain=null} = 570
[9] {chroniccough(weeks)<39.0 chestpain=null} = 564
[10] {weightloss=null chestpain=null} = 454
[11] {HIV=Negative} = 465
[12] {chroniccough(weeks)<39.0 HIV=Negative} = 459
[13] {intermittentfever(days)<91.25 HIV=Negative} = 455
[14] {chroniccough(weeks)<39.0 intermittentfever(days)<91.25 HIV=Negative} = 450
[15] {Bloodcough=null HIV=Negative} = 452
[16] {Sputum=yes} = 422
[17] {TBtype=PTB} = 472
[18] {chroniccough(weeks)<39.0 TBtype=PTB} = 466
[19] {intermittentfever(days)<91.25 TBtype=PTB} = 462
[20] {HIV=Negative TBtype=PTB} = 465
[21] {chroniccough(weeks)<39.0 HIV=Negative TBtype=PTB} = 459
[22] {intermittentfever(days)<91.25 HIV=Negative TBtype=PTB} = 455
[23] {intermittentfever(days)<91.25 Bloodcough=null HIV=Negative TBtype=PTB} = 442
[24] {chroniccough(weeks)<39.0 intermittentfever(days)<91.25 Bloodcough=null HIV=Negative TBtype=PTB} = 437

Fig. 3. Frequent Itemsets with 60%support and 80% confidence

b. Discovered TB Association rules

Several medically important association rules are obtained after applying apriori algorithm to the normalized table. It takes the frequent itemsets in figure 2 and 3 and generates rules as shown in figure 4 and 5 respectively. Each association rule shows the relation between one symptom with the other. Data set was first tested by fixing support=70% and confidence=90%.We could get very few association rules, some are listed in figure 4. Rule 7 in figure 4 describes that if weightloss equals null and intermittent fever is less than 91 days implies Bloodcough is null with 97.5% confidence. Most of the rules show the relationship between only few attributes like weightloss, intermittent fever, Bloodcough and chest pain. All the attributes were not shown here. Next with 60% support and 80% confidence we could get large number of association rules, few listed in figure 5 that provides more relationship with many frequent attributes. Rule 1 in figure 5 says if HIV status is negative their TBtype is Pulmonary Tuberculosis (PTB) with 100% confidence. Rule 5 shows the relationship between intermittent fever, Bloodcough, HIV and PTB. Though all the rules

(1) {intermittentfever(days)<91.25 chestpain=null} -> {chroniccough(weeks)<39.0} 99.44

(2) {intermittentfever(days)<91.25 Bloodcough=null chestpain=null} -> {chroniccough(weeks)<39.0} 99.42

(3) {nightsweats=null} -> {chroniccough(weeks)<39.0} 98.99

(4) {chestpain=null} -> {chroniccough(weeks)<39.0} 98.94

(5) {weightloss=null} -> {chroniccough(weeks)<39.0} 98.9

(6) {Bloodcough=null} -> {chroniccough(weeks)<39.0} 98.8

(7) {weightloss=null intermittentfever(days)<91.25} -> {Bloodcough=null} 97.54

(8) {chroniccough(weeks)<39.0 weightloss=null intermittentfever(days)<91.25} -> {Bloodcough=null} 97.52

(9) {chroniccough(weeks)<39.0 weightloss=null Bloodcough=null} -> {intermittentfever(days)<91.25} 97.15

(10) {weightloss=null} -> {Bloodcough=null} 97.09

(11) {Bloodcough=null chestpain=null} -> {chroniccough(weeks)<39.0 intermittentfever(days)<91.25} 95.05

(12) {chestpain=null} -> {chroniccough(weeks)<39.0 Bloodcough=null} 94.73

(13) {chroniccough(weeks)<39.0 chestpain=null} -> {intermittentfever(days)<91.25 Bloodcough=null} 92.02

(14) {chestpain=null} -> {intermittentfever(days)<91.25 Bloodcough=null} 91.57

(15) {chestpain=null} -> {chroniccough(weeks)<39.0 intermittentfever(days)<91.25 Bloodcough=null} 91.05

Fig. 4. Rule generation with 70%support and 90% confidence

(1) {HIV=Negative} -> {TBtype=PTB} 100.0

(2) {chroniccough(weeks)<39.0 HIV=Negative} -> {TBtype=PTB} 100.0

(3) {chroniccough(weeks)<39.0 intermittentfever(days)<91.25 HIV=Negative} -> {TBtype=PTB} 100.0

(4) {Bloodcough=null HIV=Negative} -> {TBtype=PTB} 100.0

(5) {intermittentfever(days)<91.25 Bloodcough=null HIV=Negative} -> {TBtype=PTB} 100.0

(6) {HIV=Negative TBtype=PTB} -> {chroniccough(weeks)<39.0} 98.7

(7) {Bloodcough=null TBtype=PTB} -> {chroniccough(weeks)<39.0} 98.69

(8) {chroniccough(weeks)<39.0 nightsweats=null Bloodcough=null} -> {intermittentfever(days)<91.25} 98.1

(9) {chroniccough(weeks)<39.0 TBtype=PTB} -> {intermittentfever(days)<91.25} 98.06

(10) {TBtype=PTB} -> {chroniccough(weeks)<39.0 intermittentfever(days)<91.25} 96.82

(11) {weightloss=null Bloodcough=null} -> {intermittentfever(days)<91.25} 96.81

(12) {Bloodcough=null TBtype=PTB} -> {chroniccough(weeks)<39.0 intermittentfever(days)<91.25 HIV=Negative} 95.2

(13) {chroniccough(weeks)<39.0 weightloss=null} -> {chestpain=null} 82.53

Fig. 5. Rule generation with 60% support and 80% confidence

may not be interesting to users, only few rules like explained above gives very good description and some hidden relationship may also be found.

We could see from the following output that left side (Antecedent) and right side (consequent) of the rule keep on interchanging repeatedly, which can be pruned by applying some conditions on both antecedent and consequent of a rule.

The format is: (N) ANTECEDENT -> CONSEQUENT CONFIDENCE (%)

4. Associative classification

Association Rule Mining (ARM) as explained in section 3 is one of the most popular approaches in data mining and if used in the medical domain has a great potential to improve disease prediction. This results in large number of descriptive rules. Therefore ARM can be integrated within classification task to generate a single system called as Associative classification (AC) which is a better alternative for predictive analytics.

Classification based on association rules has been proved as very competitive (Liu.B et al., 1998). The general idea is to generate a set of association rules with a fixed consequent (involving the class attribute) and then use subsets of these rules to classify new examples. This approach has the advantage of searching a larger portion of the rule version space, since no search heuristics are employed, in contrast to Decision Tree and traditional classification rule induction. The extra search is done in a controlled manner enabled by the good computational behaviour of association rule discovery algorithms. Another advantage is that the produced rich rule set can be used in a variety of ways without relearning, which can be used to improve the classification accuracy (Jorge and Azevedo, 2005).

The procedure of associative classification rule mining as shown in figure 6 is not much different from that of general association rule mining. A typical associative classification system is constructed in two stages: 1) discovering all the event association rules (in which the frequency of occurrences is significant according to some tests); 2) generating classification rules from the association patterns to build a classifier. In the first stage, the learning target is to discover the association rules inherent in a database, but generating frequent itemsets may prove to be quite expensive. The number of rules generated from association rule discovery is quite large. Hence rule pruning is required. Moreover, to avoid the problem of overfitting, proper rule pruning method is to be employed. Ranking of the rules is also important. When a test instance has more than one potentially applicable rules, rule ranking is necessary to prefer one rule over the others. In the second stage, the task is to select a set of relevant association rules discovered to construct a classifier given the predicting attribute.

For example given a rule X -> Y, AC will only consider rules having a target class as the consequent. This means the new integration focuses on a subset of association rules, whose right hand-sides are restricted to the classification class attribute. This type of rule is called Class Association Rules (CARs). While normal association rule allows more than one condition as its consequent and any item from *X* can be the consequent, CARs generated in AC limit the consequent to one fixed target class for each rule and item from *X* are forbid to appear as the class label. In order to perform AC, a classifier will first mine CARs from a given transaction and later select the most predictive rule to perform a classifier (Chien and Chen, 2010). AC generates CARs depending on the frequent item generation technique in mining rules. Despite its benefit, AC does propose challenges in its classification performance. The most important thing is to the approach in mining appropriate CARs for the classification and its pruning technology since AC will generate large number of frequent item sets due to its pruning algorithm. Its prominent pitfalls are in its incapability of handling numerical data.

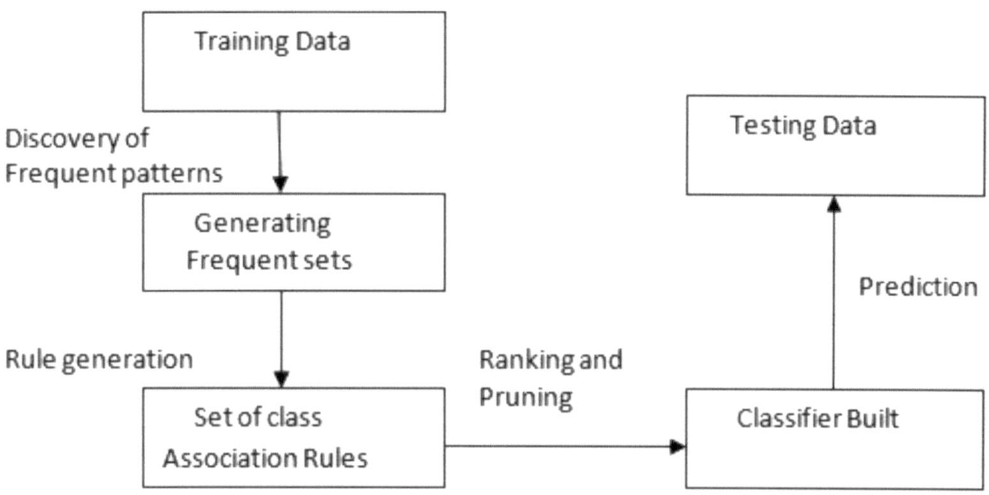

Fig. 6. Associative classification procedure

4.1 Associative Classification Algorithms

Different approaches have been proposed for associative classification that has been found to outperform traditional classification algorithms. Some of AC algorithms include Classification based on Association (CBA), Classification based on Multiple Association Rules (CMAR), and Classification based on Predictive Association Rules (CPAR-Chien and Chen, 2010). Generally, AC consists of three main phases, which are rule generation, rule pruning, and classification (Do et al., 2009; Tang and Liao, 2007).The performance, however, might differ depending on the algorithm employed in any of these three phases.

4.1.1 CBA

The first AC algorithm was introduced by (Liu. B et al., 1998), namely CBA. The algorithm is based on the Apriori association rule algorithm in generating CARs. These rules are later pruned and only one most suitable rule will be used to classify the test set. Essentially, the CBA algorithm performs three tasks. First, it mines all CARs. Second, it produces a classifier from CARs, and finally, it mines normal association rules.

1. Generation of CARs

In CBA, the classification Association rules (CARs) are found iteratively in an apriori algorithm-like fashion. At first, frequent 1-rule itemsets are generated and are pruned. Using this iteratively, other frequent rule itemsets are also found. They are then pruned to get complete set of Classification association rules.

2. Building classifier (Ranking and Pruning Rules)

To prune the rules, CBA uses pessimistic error based pruning method in C4.5. The rule ranking is defined as below:

Given two rules r_i and r_j, $r_i > r_j$ (i.e., r_i precedes r_j or r_i has higher precedence over r_j) if one of the following holds good:

1. The confidence of r_i is greater than that of r_j
2. Their confidences are the same but support of r_i is greater than that of r_j
3. Both the confidences and supports of r_i and r_j are the same, but r_i is generated before r_j

After rule ranking, each training instance is covered by the rule having highest precedence among the rules that can cover the case. Every rule correctly classifies at least one training instance. The rules that do not cover any training instance are removed. The training instances that do not fall into any of the observed classes are added to a default class.

The multiple capabilities in CBA solve a number of problems in traditional classification systems. Since traditional classifiers only generate a small subset of rules that exists in data to form a classifier, the discovered rules may not be interesting. Also, to generate more rules we would need the classification system to load the entire database into the main memory. But because CBA generate all rules, the algorithm is more successful in finding interesting rules and the system also allows the data to reside on disk. However, in CBA, the rule generation process might degrade the accuracy of the classifier due to its randomness in selecting the most suitable rule to form the classifier model. CBA inherits Apriori multiple scan features that generates large number of rules, which is costly in terms of large computational time.

4.1.2 CMAR

CMAR is later introduced as the extension to CBA (Li et al., 2001). The CMAR algorithm implements FP-Growth algorithm instead of Apriori in generating its frequent itemset.

Next, the subset of matching rules are used to classify a test instance instead of one rule, and this in turn produces better accuracy.

The CMAR algorithm generates and evaluates rules in a similar way as CBA, but uses a more efficient FPtree structure. A major difference is that it uses multiple rules in prediction with associated weights.

The CMAR algorithm (as described in Li et al., 2001) uses an FP-growth algorithm (Han & Kamber, 2000) to produce a set of CARs and uses CBA method for rule ranking. It prunes rules using high confidence, highly related rules and analyzes the correlation among them using Chi-Squared testing. To test the resulting classifier Li et al. propose the following process.

Given a record r in the test set:

1. Collect all rules that satisfy r, and if consequents of all rules are all identical, or only one rule, classify record according to the consequents.
2. Else group rules according to classifier and determine the combined effect of the rules in each group, the classifier associated with the "strongest group" is then selected. The strength of a group is calculated using a *Weighted Chi Squared* (WCS) measure. Following algorithm shows steps for rule pruning.

Selecting rules based on database:

1. Sort rules in the rank descending order;
2. For each data object in the training data set, set its cover-count to 0;
3. While both the training data set and rule set are not empty, for each rule R in rank descending order, find all data objects matching rule R. If R can correctly classify at least one object then select R and increase the cover-count of those objects matching R by 1. A data object is removed if its cover-count passes coverage threshold δ;

Nonetheless, when the datasets are large, both rule generation and rule selection in CBA and CMAR are time consuming. The CPAR and other predictive mining algorithms overcome this problem by generating a small set of predictive rules directly from the dataset based on the rule prediction and coverage analysis, as opposed to generating candidate rules.

4.1.3 CPAR

CPAR is an improvement to CBA and CMAR (Thabtah et al., 2005; Thabtah, 2007). It is proposed by Chen, Yin and Huang in 2005.The core of CPAR and other predictive mining algorithms is the predictive rule mining capability, whereby after an instance has been correctly covered by a rule, instead of removing it, its weight is decreased by multiplying a factor. This is essentially a greedy approach in rule generation, which is more efficient than generating all candidate rules.

CPAR may choose a number of attributes if those attributes have similar best gain. This is done by first calculating the gain and applying a GAIN_SIMILARITY_RATIO to this. All attributes with gain better than Local Gain Threshold (LGT) are then selected for further processing.

The Local Gain Threshold (LGT) is given by the formula:

LGT = bestGain * GAIN_SIMILARITY_RATIO

Where, GAIN_SIMILARITY_RATIO is a constant whose value is 0.99.

CPAR takes as input a (space separated) binary valued data set R and produces a set of CARs. The resulting classifier comprises a linked-list of rules ordered according to Laplace accuracy. CPAR also uses a dynamic programming approach to avoid repeated calculation in rule generation, which in turn is more economical. More importantly, CPAR selects best *k* rules in prediction.

4.2 Predictive accuracy and rules of associative classifiers

Difference between ARM and AC with reference to results is that the former generates only large number of descriptive rules whereas the latter generate fewer rules along with their performance measure thru accuracy.

CBA generates around 81 rules once it is pruned we get only two rules with an accuracy of 81.14%.

1. { chroniccough(weeks)>23} ->{ TBtype=PTB}
2. { HIV = {Negative}} -> {TBtype=PTB}

CMAR generated about 1091 rules and the pruned output is only 38 rules with an accuracy of 99.1428%. Few are listed below:

1. {HIV = {Negative} } -> { TBtype=PTB}
2. {Bloodcough = {null} HIV = {Negative} } -> {TBtype=PTB}
3. {chroniccough(weeks) <= 22 Bloodcough = {null} HIV = {Negative} } ->TBtype=PTB
4. {HIV = {positive} Sputum = {null}} -> {TBtype=retroviralPTB}
5. {Age>36 HIV = {positive} Sputum = {null}} -> {TBtype=retroviralPTB}
6. {Age>36 chroniccough(weeks)<=22 chestpain={null} HIV={positive} } -> {TBtype=retroviralPTB}

CPAR after pruning could produce only 4 rules with an accuracy of 99.14%.

1. {wheezing = {yes} HIV = {positive}} -> TBtype=retroviralPTB
2. {HIV = {Negative} } -> {TBtype=PTB}
3. {weightloss = {yes} HIV = {positive}} -> {TBtype=retroviralPTB}
4. {HIV = {positive}} -> {TBtype=retroviralPTB}

When compared to both ARM and AC rules, it can be seen that AC rules are smaller and better in description and also CPAR provides better rules compared to all algorithms.

5. Summary

In this chapter two data mining techniques which help in the diagnosis of Tuberculosis have been discussed. Medical databases have accumulated large quantities of information about patients and their clinical conditions and digital era has provided the availability of these information in abundance. Data mining is a knowledge discovery process that helps in extracting relationships and patterns hidden in this data and can provide a new medical knowledge to doctors in their treatment procedure.

Association Rule Mining (ARM) is one of the most popular approaches in data mining and if used in the medical domain has a great potential to improve disease prediction. It shows doctor the hidden disease symptoms associated with one another. There are many algorithms associated with ARM and the most popular is Apiori. It works in two phases- first is frequent itemset generation where all the items in a database above some minimum specified threshold called support will be generated. Second one is rule generation which generates from the frequent sets, an association rule of the form X->Y based on some minimum confidence. We can say that whenever X appears there is a chance that Y also appears along with it with minimum confidence threshold. These concepts are applied on TB dataset which reveals important association between the symptoms. But this method results in large number of repetitive rules.

Associative classification (AC) is another data mining approach that integrates association rule mining and classification. It uses association rule mining algorithm, such as Apriori or Frequent pattern growth , to generate the complete set of association rules. Then it selects a small set of high quality rules and uses this rule set for prediction. This method results in smaller number rules compared to ARM.

Three important algorithms of AC such as CBA, CMAR and CPAR have been discussed in the chapter. Almost every algorithm contains two major data mining steps, an association rule (AR) mining stage- rules generated here are called as classification association rules (CARs) and a classification stage which uses the mined rules from the first stage directly. The second stage chooses rules with high priority from the CARs to cover training set. The difference between them is based on the priority evaluation of rules which usually depends on the confidence, support, rule length or common quality standard of classification rules. CPAR is better in rule generation compared to others. TB rules and accuracy are compared for every associative classification algorithm

Though the entire rules may not help doctors, few rules may describe the relationship between one symptom with the other and also sometimes it can reveal hidden relationship.

6. References

Agrawal, R., Imielinski, T. and Swami, A. "Mining association rules between sets of items in large databases", In *Proceedings of the 1993 ACM SIGMOD international conference on Management of data* (SIGMOD 93). ACM, New York ,USA ,22(2), 207-216.1993.

Ali. A. El-Solh, M.D., Chiu-Bin Hsiao, M.D., Susan Goodnough RN, et al " Predicting Active pulmonary Tuberculosis using an Artificial Neural network ," CHEST journal 116(4), 968-973,1999.

Antonie, M.-L., Za¨ıane, O. R. and Holte, R.C. "Learning to use a learned model: A two-stage approach to classification", In *Proceedings of the Sixth International Conference on Data Mining (ICDM '06,* IEEE Computer Society*).* Washington, DC, USA, 33–42, 2006.

A. Jorge and P. J. Azevedo,"An Experiment with Association Rules and Classification: Post-Bagging and Conviction", In A. G. Hoffmann, H. Motoda, and T. Scheffer, editors, Discovery Science, volume 3735 of Lecture Notes in Computer Science, pages 137–149. Springer, 2005.

Bavani Arunasalam and Sanjay Chawla ,"CCCS: A Top-down Associative Classifier for Imbalanced Class Distribution", In *Proceedings of 12th ACM SIGKDD international conference on Knowledge discovery and data mining(KDD'06,* August 20–23 *).* Philadelphia, Pennsylvania, 517-522, 2006.

Carlos Ordonez, Cesar A. Santana , Levien de Braal, "Discovering interesting association rules in medical data," Proc. ACM DMKD 2000 , 78-85 ,2000.

Carlos Ordonez, Edward omiecinski, Cesar A. Santana, et al "Mining Constrained Association Rules to Predict Heart Diseases," Proc. ICDM Nov., 433-440 ,2001.

Carlos Ordonez, "Association Rule Discovery With the Train and Test Approach for Heart Disease prediction'' IEEE Transactions on Information Technology in Biomedicine ,10(2), 334-343,2006.

Chen, T. J., Chou, L. F. and. Hwang, S. J "Application of a data mining technique to analyze coprescription patterns for antacids in Taiwan," *Clin.Ther.*, 25(9), 2453–2463, 2003.

Elisabeth Georgii, Lothar Richter, Ulrich Ruckert and Stefan Kramer "Analyzing Microarray data using quantitative association rules, " Bioinformatics , 21(2) , 123-129, 2005.

Imberman, S., Domanski, B., Thompson, H. "Using dependency/association rules to find indications for computed tomography in a head trauma dataset, " *Artificial Intelligence in Medicine*, Elsevier, 26(1), 55-68,2002.

Keivan Kianmehr, Reda Alhajj, "A class association rule-based classification framework and its application to gene expression data Export," *Artificial Intelligence in Medicine*, Elsevier, 44(1), 7-25,2008.

Kesari Verma and O. P. Vyas. Classification Based On Calendar Based Temporal Association Rule. ADIT Journal Of Engineering, VOL. 2, NO.1, December 2005.

Krzysztof J. Cios, William Moore,G "Uniqueness of medical data mining" *Artificial Intelligence in Medicine,* Elsevier, 26(1), 1–24,2002.

Li, W., Han, J. and Pei, J. ,Cmar: Accurate and efficient classification based on multiple class-association rules. In *Proceedings of the 2001 IEEE International Conference on Data Mining(ICDM '01).* IEEE Computer Society, Washington, DC, USA, 369–376. 2001.

Liu, B., Hsu, W. and Ma, Y.,"Integrating Classification and Association Rule Mining", In *ACM Int. Conf. on Knowledge Discovery and Data Mining (SIGKDD '98),* New York City, NY, 80–86, 1998.

Murat Karabatak, Cevdet Ince, M. "A new feature selection method based on association rules for diagnosis of erythemato-squamous diseases," Expert Systems with Applications:, Elsevier, 36(10), 12500-12505,2009.

Naderi Dehkordi, M. H. Shenassa,"CLoPAR: Classification based on Predictive Association Rules",. In Proceedings of 3rd International IEEE Conference Intelligent Systems. September 2006.

NIU Qiang, XIA Shi-Xiong, ZHANG Lei.,"Association Classification based on Compactness of Rules. In *Proceedings of Second International Workshop on Knowledge Discovery and Data Mining(WKDD).* Moscow, 245-247, 2009.

Orhan Er., Feyzullah Temurtas, Tantrikulu, A.C., "Tuberculosis disease diagnosis using Artificial Neural networks, " Journal of Medical Systems, category: online submission, Springer, DOI 10.1007/s10916-008-9241-x ,2008.

Parameshvyas Laxminarayan, Sergio A. Alvarez, Carolina Ruiz, and Majaz Moonis, " Mining Statistically Significant Associations for Exploratory Analysis of Human Sleep Data," IEEE Transactions on Information Technology in Biomedicine, 10(3) ,440-450, 2006.

Rakesh Agrawal and Ramakrishnan Srikant, " Fast algorithms for mining association rules in large databases ," Proc. VLDB conference Sept 12-15, 487-499 ,1994.

Roddick, J. F., Fule, P. and. Graco, W. J "Exploratory medical knowledge discovery: Experiences and issues," *SIGKDD Explorations,* 5(1), 94–99 ,2003.

Sabeti, M., Sadreddini, M. H., Tahmores Nezhad, J., "EEG Signal Classification Using An Association Rule-Based Classifier", In *Proceedings of IEEE International Conference on Signal Processing and Communications (ICSPC 24-27 November2007).* Dubai, United Arab Emirates, pp. 620-623, 2007.

Sebban, M. , Mokrousov, I., Rastogi, N. and Sola, C. " A data-mining approach to spacer oligo nucleotide typing of Mycobacterium tuberculosis," Bioinformatics, 18(2), 235-243,2002.

Tamura, Makio , D'haeseleer, Patrik "Microbial genotype-phenotype mapping by class association rule mining," Bioinformatics, 24(13), 1523-1529,2008.

T. D. Do, S.C. Hui, and A. C. M. Fong,"Associative Classification with Artificial Immune System", IEEE Transactions on Evolutionary Computation 13(2):217-228, 2009.

Thabtah, F.,"A review of associative classification mining", *Journal of Knowl. Eng. Rev.,* 2(1), 37–65, 2007.

Thabtah, F., Cowling, P. and Peng, Y., "MCAR: multi-class classification based on association rule approach", In *Proceeding of the Third IEEE International Conference on Computer Systems and Applications.* Cairo, Egypt, 1–7, 2005.

Viet Phan-Luong and Rabah Messouci. "Building Classifiers with Association Rules based on Small Key Itemsets", In *Proceedings of 2nd International Conference on Digital Information Management.* Lyon, 1, 200-205, 2007.

Yanbo, J., Wang , Qin Xin and Frans Coenen. "Novel Rule Weighting Approach in Classification Association Rule Mining", In *Proceedings of the Seventh IEEE International Conference on Data Mining Workshops* (ICDMW). 271-276,2007.

Y. W. C. Chien and Y. L. Chen, "Mining Associative Classification Rules with Stock Trading Data – A GA- based Method", Knowledge-based Systems, 23(6):605-614, 2010.

Z. Tang and Q. Liao, "A New Class-based Associative Classification Algorithm", International Journal of Applied Mathematics, 2007.

Books

[1] Ian H Witten and Eibe Frank. 2001. Data mining practical machine learning tools and techniques. Morgan Kaufmann publishers.

[2] J. Han and M. Kamber 2006 Data mining: concepts and techniques. Morgan Kaufmann publishers, Sanfrancisco, 47-97.

17

Immunological Diagnosis of Active and Latent TB

Beata Shiratori, Hiroki Saitoh, Umme Ruman Siddiqi, Jingge Zhao, Haorile Chagan-Yasutan, Motoki Usuzawa, Chie Nakajima[1], Yasuhiko Suzuki[1] and Toshio Hattori
Tohoku University, Graduate School of Medicine
[1]Hokkaido University, Research Center for Zoonosis Control
Japan

1. Introduction

Immunological diagnosis of tuberculosis (TB) is based on the immune responses against Mycobacterium tuberculosis (MTB). Immunological diagnosis can detect both active and latent TB, and can detect not only pulmonary TB but also extra-pulmonary TB. Compared to conventional diagnosis, immunological diagnostic tests have eminent advantages. On the other hand, there are still some limitations. As is known, various mycobacteria share homologous proteins, that lead to immunological cross reaction. To correctly detect TB infection, we need to choose a method that initiates the anti-MTB immune response properly. Human immunodeficiency virus (HIV) infection weakens the immune response, which may lead to false-negative results. HIV infection accompanied by TB is another urgent issue in global health. In this chapter, we will explain the immunological responses to MTB and the immunological interaction between HIV and TB. We will then introduce each diagnosis from the immunological point of view, and describe novel assays which we are now developing.

2. Immunological response to MTB

In this section, we describe the immune response to MTB and MTB/HIV co-infection.

2.1 Innate immunity and adaptive immunity

When the immune system encounters foreign organisms, it works to eliminate them and both innate immunity and adaptive immunity are engaged in this process (Murphy, 2011). In this section, we will briefly describe the immune responses to give the theoretical basis for the immunological diagnosis of TB.

Innate immunity is a non-specific response to pathogen and is the first line of defence against microorganisms. When macrophages recognize foreign organisms, the cells ingest and digest them. Receptors on the cell surface, especially those of toll-like receptor family, are involved in this process. Then macrophages express digested fragments on their surface promoting the initiation of the secondary response, the adaptive immunity.

Adaptive immunity is antigen specific and creates immunological memory. Responding T cells are functionally divided into T-helper cells 1 (Th1) and T-helper cells 2 (Th2), which are activated by antigen presentation through major histocompatibility complex class II (MHC II) on macrophages. Th1 cells stimulate T cell populations that secrete interferon gamma (IFN-γ) and interleukin-2 (IL-2) to activate cytotoxic T cells and, finally, to eliminate foreign organisms. This response is known as cell mediated immunity. Th2 cells secrete interleukin-4 (IL-4) to stimulate B cells, which produce antibody against the pathogen. This response is known as humoral immunity. Immunological diagnosis is based on the adaptive immune response to a targeted pathogen. If we detect or measure the activation of the immune response induced by MTB, we can diagnose MTB infection.

Recently, Th17 cells, which are responsible for inflammation, and T regulatory (Treg) populations, which suppress a variety of immune responses, have received much attention.

2.2 Immunological responses to MTB

MTB enters our body through the airway in droplet nuclei and is phagocytosed by alveolar macrophages. Macrophages digest MTB to connect MHC II molecules in the cell and fragments of MTB, then present their complex on the cell surface. Antigen presentation generates adaptive immunity(Walzl et al., 2011).

Th1 cells are activated and produce cytokines, such as IFN-γ and IL-2. These cytokines activate cytotoxic T cells and macrophages. IFN-γ enhances the anti-microbial activity of macrophages.

Th2 cells, producing IL-4, promote TB specific antibody production by B cells. These interactions lead to the generation of memory cells. There are two main populations of memory cells, effector memory T cells (which may be transiently present in the blood if bacteria are cleared) and central memory T cells (which may remain for life but may not provide protection in all individuals). The recently developed IGRA test measures IFN-γ produced by effector memory T cells (Horsburgh & Rubin, 2011).

Despite these sophiscated immune responses, they often fail to eliminate MTB from the body and the bacteria may exist in a quiescent state for a prolonged period. Such a state is called latent tuberculosis infection (LTBI). In 10% of infected individuals, active TB develops and more than 80% of new cases of TB result from reactivation of the primary infection. The increase of HIV rates facilitates the reactivation of TB due to the imunosuppression.

2.3 TB with HIV infection

This lethal combination of TB/HIV is anything but rare; demographic analyses have estimated that over 60 % of the population in the sub-Saharan region has been infected by MTB, which has become a leading cause of mortality among HIV patients. At the end of 2009, TB infection was reported to be responsible for 13% of HIV deaths (Science Daily, 2009). Retrospective studies concluded that, among HIV/TB patients, 7% to 45% of them probably develop symptoms homogeneous with Immune Reconstitution Inflammatory Syndrome (IRIS) (Murdoch et al., 2007; Shelburne et al., 2005). Therefore, exploring the relationship between TB and HIV become necessary.

Since HIV virus can weaken the immune system, LTBI can be activated resulting in pulmonary or extrapulmonary TB. A variety of immune cells and immune cytokines are involved in the reactivation of LTBI. Some cytokines, such as interleukin-8 (IL-8) and interleukin-12β (IL-12β), may be used as biomarkers to monitor the immune reaction to LTBI (Wu et al., 2007) and possibly shed light on preventing of LTBI progression in HIV patients (Walzl et al., 2011). So far, various biomarkers to characterize LTBI and TB in HIV patients have been proposed. Without medical intervention, HIV infection will progress to acquired immune deficiency syndrome (AIDS), accompanied by multi-microbial infections, including TB infection, which often proves lethal.

2.3.1 Mechanism of immunological interaction of HIV and TB

Infection with HIV enhances the susceptibility to MTB infection. Because the occurrence of these two diseases is heavily dependent on the immune system, their interactions are more complex than previously understood. Previously, we studied the plasma levels of two matricelluar proteins such as galectin-9 (GAL-9) and osteopontin (OPN) in AIDS patients complicated with various opprotunistic infections (Chagan-Yasutan et al., 2009). The levels of both molecules were high in all the patients but only the level of GAL-9 decreased and that of OPN remained high after Highly Active Antiretroviral Therapy (HAART). Also, As Figure 1 shows, it was noted that the GAL-9 level was exceptionally high in acute HIV infected individuals (Chagan-Yasutan et al., 2009). The cellular receptor for GAL-9 is the T-cell immunoglobulin domain and mucin domain 3 (Tim-3) and Tim-3 is expressed on Th1 cells. Mycobacterium tuberculosis-infected macrophages express GAL-9 and the Tim-3 GAL-9 interaction leads to macrophage activation and stimulates the bactericidal activity by inducing caspase-1–dependent interleukin-1β (IL-1β) secretion. Therefore, Th1 cell surface molecule Tim-3 may have evolved to inhibit the growth of intracellular pathogens via its ligand GAL-9, which is also known to inhibit the expansion of effector Th1 cells (Jayaraman et al., 2010). Therefore, only one case of MTB associated with acute HIV was reported (Crowley et al., 2011).

In contrast, chronic HIV infected individuals succumb to various opportunistic infections and pulmonary TB is known to occur when CD4+ T cell numbers are still high, indicating that the immune system plays a role in the development of pulmonary TB (Holmes et al., 2005). Similarly, T cell epitopes of different strains representative of global diversity are highly conserved in MTB (Comas et al., 2010). Due to the conserved epitopes, the host can maintain MTB for a long time as latent infection and can transmit it to the next generation. It is also suspected that CD4+ T cells have an essential role in tissue damage that results in cavity formation, which enhances aerosol infection. In HIV endemic areas, the situation becomes more complex if the CD4+ T cells numbers increase after HAART and then recovery of the immune system is variable (Fig 2).

2.3.2 Network among LTBI and HIV

A. Healthy Individuals. For immunologically potent people, the reaction to invading microbes consists of innate and adaptive immune mechanisms. Genome research has

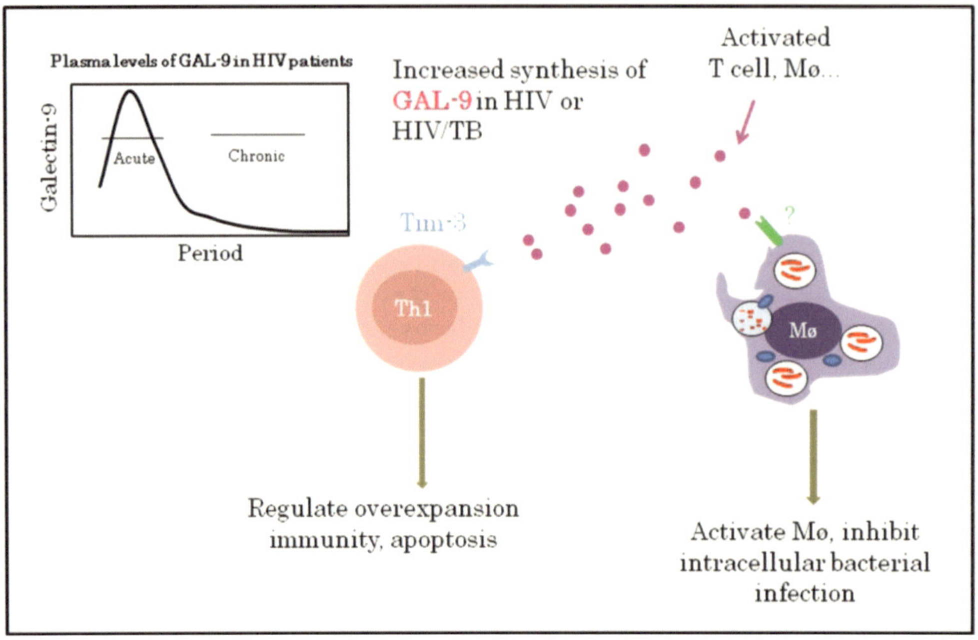

Fig. 1. Proposed biological effects of GAL-9 in HIV or HIV/TB infection.
The plasma levels of GAL-9 were elevated in chronic AIDS patients as well as in TB patients (non-published data), but were exceptionally high in acute HIV infection (Chagan-Yasutan et al., 2009). It was reported that GAL-9 interacts with its Tim-3 ligand to regulate the overexpansion of Th1 cells to induce apoptosis (Zhu et al., 2005; Kashio et al., 2003). In TB, however it was speculated that GAL-9 contributes to the activation of macrophage cells (Mø) and then inhibits intracellular bacterial infection by caspase-1 dependent IL-1β production (Jayaraman et al., 2010).

revealed that TB epitopes binding to human CD4 + T cells are conserved (Comas et al., 2010). Accordingly, during the long history of fighting against TB, human beings have evolved a spectrum of potential TB-specific naive CD4+ T cells, which can be activated as soon as TB invades and transformed to TB effective CD4+ T cells to fight against TB bacilli, some of which would transform into central memory T cells (CMT) after TB is controlled. Such CMT cells are capable of quick proliferation once they confront TB. During infection, these TB antigen specific CD4 + T cells make up a certain percentage of CD4+ T cells; the percentage could be affected by the volume of CMT and individual differences in gene expression profiles (Maertzdorf et al., 2011).

B. LTBI (Latent tuberculosis infection) Individuals. Thirty percents of the population in the world is infected by MTB. However, effector CD4+ T cells protect LTBI individuals from developing active TB. In this case CMT act as a backup to proliferate of effector CD4+ T cells. Observation of this TB-specific reaction can be simplified by monitoring the IFN-γ level in IGRA (Rueda et al., 2010). Apart from IFN-γ, other biomarkers including CD154 and CD107 also indicate a TB-specific reaction (Streitz et al., 2011). IFN-γ has multiple effects on the immune system to control TB. As IFN-γ is secreted by TB effector CD4+ Th1 cells, it could mediate cytotoxic T cells to recognize and damage TB-infected macrophage cells. IFN-γ also enhances MHC II on macrophages. Other cytokines such as IL-2 and IL-4 could act in synergy with IFN-γ to control LTBI. However, 10% of them eventually progress to active TB (Day et al., 2011).

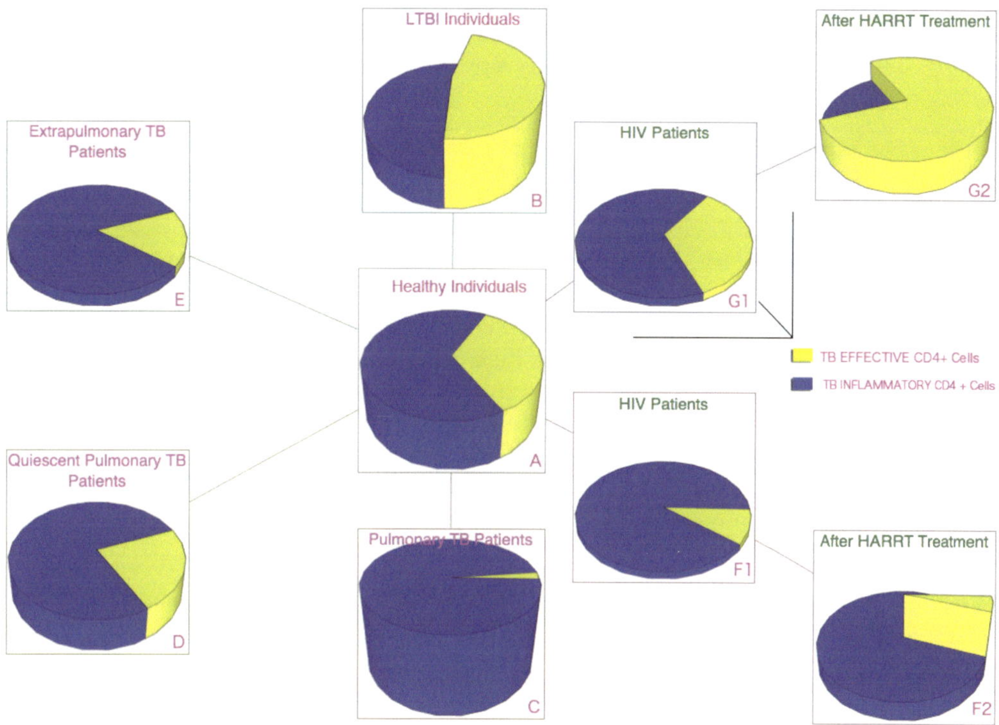

Fig. 2. Schematic network among LTBI and HIV.
The horizontal plane indicates the make up of inflammatory CD4+ cells and TB effective CD4 + T cells (Effector memory T cells), which are coloured in blue and yellow, respectively. The overall reaction of different cells to TB is described according to the volumes of the different colours, the vertical lengths of which indicate biomarkers that rise up or descend resulting from TB reaction. Such schema and many exceptional cases are present in HIV/AIDS and tuberculosis.

C. Pulmonary TB. A pulmonary cavity is a typical sign of pulmonary TB. A recent paper reported that CD4+ T cells could be an essential factor for TB cavity formation (Russell et al., 2010). Patients of pulmonary TB have been reported to have mainstream TNF-α TB specific CD4+ T cells, which can lead to an inflammatory reaction (Indicated by blue colour in vertical direction of C) in active TB patients. A recent study based on 101 TB and LTBI individuals described that TNF-α specific CD4+ T cells might be an important biomarker for diagnosing active TB. In the majority of active TB patients TNF-α can be detected in the MTB antigen stimulated cells. Flow-cytometry showed that inflammatory-related CD4+ T cells represent 37.4% of total CD4+ T cells (indicated by area between blue and yellow colour in C) is the cut-off of LTBI becoming active TB (Harari et al., 2011). And such TNF-α TB specific CD4+ T cells activate other inflammatory cells. However, IFN-inducible neutrophils may also play an essential role in eliciting inflammatory CD4+ T cells.

Neutrophils corresponding to IFN-α,β and γ modulate an inflammatory reaction in active TB patients (Berry et al., 2010).

D. Extrapulmonary TB. Due to the small number of inflammatory CD4+ T cells, TB lacks the ability to form cavities in the lungs and lead to multi-organ or systemic infection. Such patients are frequently found among those with AIDS and patients on immunosuppressive therapy. Interestingly, extrapulmonary TB is a prominent risk factor for IRIS. (Manosuthi et al., 2006)

E. The stage between LTBI and active TB infection. It features opacities in the lungs, but sputum and IGRAs test are negative.

F1, G1. HIV-infected Patients. In Sub-Saharan region, frequently seen cases are LTBI individuals infected by HIV. Asymptomatic HIV can last by 2 years to 10 years in normal individuals after infection. As a result of HIV infection, CD4+ cells drop progressively. After HIV infection, the virus targets all CD4+ T cells including effector, inflammatory and CMT CD4+ T cells and anti-HIV drugs restores their function. F1 indicates those patients who didn't carry larger number of CMT cells and could not produce enough effector CD4+ T cells after TB stimulation. G1 indicates that those patients with a large pool of TB CMTs or who has been infected by LTBI prior to HIV infection and then carried more LTBI stimulating specific effector CD4+ T cells or memory T cells (Mueller et al., 2008). F1, G1 will finally process to extrapulmonary TB (indicated by E), if no medication intervenes.

F1-F2. HIV Patients during HAART treatment. In macaque experiment, SHIV was found to preferentially infect CMT cells (He et al., 2011). When HAART treatment is applied, CD4+ T cells count will rise. Occasionally, such rise causes IRIS, because CMT cell count will bounce up and effector CD4+ T cells will show increased activity. However MTB specific inflammatory CD4+ T cells will dominate their large number. (Indicated by proportional volume between blue and yellow). As TB Inflammatory CD4+ T cells lead the reaction, patients have similar prognoses as pulmonary TB (Indicated by C) (Worodria et al., 2011).

G1-G2. HIV Patients after HAART treatment. HAART will rapidly reconstitute the immune surveillance (indicated by elevation of yellow column) (Hua et al., 2011). The occurrence of TB therefore decreases (Sant'Anna et al., 2009).

Net work

C-F1-F2. TB and HIV stimulate specific inflammatory T cells to produce TNF-α which, in turn, help them to progress at faster rate (Sorathiya et al., 2010). The patients can be treated by anti-TB therapy followed by HAART. Occasionally, paradoxical TB IRIS[1] occurs, probably caused by MTB specific inflammatory CD4+ T cells. MCP-1 (monocyte chemotactic protein 1) was found to be a reliable candidate biomarker to screen patients who may develop to paradoxical IRIS (Haddow et al., 2011). B-G1-G2. HAART strengthen immune responses against MTB and can decrease the occurrence of TB (Middelkoop et al., 2011, Hua

---

[1] Definition of TB IRIS: 'paradoxical' worsening of symptoms of known disease, either at a new body site or at the original body site, with an incidence of 8–43% of TB-co-infected individuals starting ART; or 'unmasking' of occult Mycobacterium tuberculosis infection, in which infection was not clinically apparent prior to ART but presents floridly during ART, affecting around 5% among those starting ART without known TB infection in South Africa.

et al., 2011). Notably, HAART unmasking TB manifestation can be found in some cases and C-reactive protein (CRP) was reported to be helpful to detect the development of unmasking TB-IRIS cases (Haddow et al., 2011).

3. Immunological diagnosis

Over decades, there have been attempts to find new diagnostic tools, that are sensitive and specific, simple, inexpensive and able to distinguish latent tuberculosis from active tuberculosis as well as MTB infected individuals from uninfected ones.

3.1 Tuberculin skin test

Tuberculin skin test, also called as Mantoux skin test, has been used for the diagnosis of tuberculosis for more than a century. Despite the numbers of logistic and performance problems and poor specificity, TST is still performed as a routine diagnostic method. The purified protein derivative (PPD) antigens, that are used for TST are highly homologous to antigens of Mycobacterium bovis bacillus Calmette-Guerin (BCG) vaccine and non-tuberculosis mycobacteria (NTM) antigens. These and other factors may lead to false-positive or false negative TST results.

Although other antigens have been evaluated as a skin test reagents e.g.molybdopterin-64 (MPT-64) and molybdopterin-59 (MPT-59), none of them proved superior to tuberculin skin test (Wilcke et al., 1996).

False-positive reactions	**False-negative reactions**
✓ Infection with NTM ✓ Previous BCG vaccination ✓ Incorrect method of TST administration ✓ Incorrect interpretation of reaction ✓ Incorrect bottle of antigen used	✓ Cutaneus anergy ✓ Recent TB infection ✓ Very old TB infection ✓ Very young age (less than 6 months old) ✓ Recent live-virus vaccination (e.g., measles and chicken pox) ✓ Incorrect method of TST administration ✓ Incorrect interpretation of reaction

Table 1. False-positive and false-negative TST reactions. (CDC, 2010)

3.2 Interferon Gamma Releasing Assay (IGRA)

Because IFN-γ is a cytokine that plays a critical role in resistance to Mycobacterium tuberculosis infection and MTB infected individuals respond to MTB antigen stimulation by releasing increased amounts of this cytokine from effector memory cells, methods based on measuring the IFN-γ production by antigen stimulated human T lymphocytes have been developed. There are two new blood tests on the market, the enzyme-linked immunospot assay (ELISpot) (T-SPOT®.TB, Oxford Immunotec, Oxford, UK) and the enzyme-linked immunosorbent assay (ELISA) (QuantiFERON-TB Gold In-Tube, QFT-GIT, Cellestis, Carnegie, Australia). Both IGRAs have high sensitivity and specificity, for QFT-GIT 81%-

92.6% and 98.8%-99.2% and for T-SPOT®.TB 87.5%-95.6% and 86.3%-99.9%, respectively (Diel et al., 2008; Harada et al., 2008; Oxford Immunotec, 2011). Firstly, it should be mentioned that using IGRA it is impossible to distinguish between latent and active TB for which no such a method yet exists. However the detection of both latent and active TB has been markedly improved by employing IGRA methods. The factor, that increased the sensitivity and specificity of IGRA was the discovery and use of antigens encoded by Regions of Difference 1 (RD1) in the MTB genome, which is absent in BCG vaccination or NTB. Among the nine antigens encoded by RD1, early secreted antigenic target 6kDa (ESAT-6) and culture filtrate protein 10kDa (CFP-10) are used as a stimulatory antigens. However, ESAT-6 and CFP-10 antigens are also present in NTM, namely M. leprae, wild type M. bovis, M. marium, M. kansasii, M. sulgai, M. flavescens, in NTM endemic areas, IGRA results might be false positive and make it difficult to distinguish MTB between NTM.

3.2.1 QuantiFERON-TB Gold In Tube assay

In comparison to the previous form of QuantiFERON Gold, the QuantiFERON Gold In Tube (QFT-GIT) version enables immediate antigen stimulation of lymphocytes within whole blood. In addition to ESAT-6 and CFP-10, QFT-GIT contains a peptide from the internal section of TB 7.7 (Rv2654), which may increase the sensitivity of the test (Aagaard et al. 2004; Brock et al., 2004), though it is arguable whether specificity is improved. All three antigens are present on the wall surface of the blood collection tubes. Besides the immunity status and the absolute and relative lymphocyte number there are external factors that may influence the QFT results, e.g. drawing an adequate volume of blood, appropriate attachment of lymphocytes to the antigens, sample handling and the ELISA assay procedure. Another important issue is the interpretation of the results. There are two cut-offs given by the manufacture, 0.35 IU/l and 0.1 IU/l. A value of more than 0.35 IU/l seems to be appropriate for good discrimination of truly infected individuals (Harada et al., 2008). On the other hand, the values between 0.35 IU/l and 0.1 IU/l, the intermediate result, should take into account the individual patient`s condition (Harada et al., 2008; Liote H & Liote F, 2011). In Japan, the interpretation criteria differ from those anywhere else. Intermediate results in Japanese people are suspected to be positive and are flagged for follow-up observation (Prevention Committee, Japanese Society of Tuberculosis, 2006). Depending on the MTB infection prevalence, it has been suggested to use different cut-offs (Harada et al., 2008). In areas where the MTB infection prevalence is low, the specificity is probably of great importance. However, in high-risk TB screening situations, identification of LTBI is likely to be more important than the potential side effects of the MTB treatment and a cut-off value of 0.1 IU/l should be employed (Yew & Leung, 2006).

3.2.2 T-SPOT®.TB test (ELISpot)

Using the ELISpot assay it is possible to visualize and count MTB-specific memory T cells producing IFN-γ. The great advantage of this test is that each test well contains the same number of peripheral blood mononuclear cells (PBMCs). Especially in the patients with low T cell counts from HIV or other immune disorders, it enables the objective evaluation by adjusting the designed cell number. While in QFT-GIT all antigens are present in the same tube, in the ELISpot assay ESAT-6 and CFP-10 antigens are added and read separately. The manufacture claims that this assay has very low cross-reactivity with NTM (Oxford

Immunotec, 2011). The important step is the accurate adjustment of the cell count. However, if the cells are not well adjusted and the nil control contains more spots than indicated in the instructions, the test needs to be repeated. What is more, to run the ELISpot assay, a trained professional should be engaged and other special tools such as a plate reader are needed. Exact interpretation of the results is crucial, so the manufacturer prepared a training manual for distinguishing between valid and invalid spots. The ELISpot assay`s intermediate result rate is 3-4% (Dosanjh et al., 2008), which is significantly lower than that for QFT assays (11-21%) (Ferrara et al., 2006; Piana et al., 2006).

QFT-GIT test has recently become routinely used as a diagnostic tool for MTB, but the T-SPOT®.TB test is employed only in few countries, mostly because of the high cost of this assay. In conclusion, IGRA seems to be beneficial tool for TB diagnosis, especially for people with a high-risk of developing active TB.

3.2.3 Other approaches of LTB diagnosis

In addition to ESAT-6 and CFP-10, other antigens have been proposed for ELISpot assay but have not been implemented for commercial use. Addition of the novel antigen Rv3879c increased the diagnostic sensitivity of the standard ELISpot assay and, in combination with TST, reached a sensitivity of 99% (Dosanjh et al., 2008). Other researchers showed that antigen heparin-binding-hemagglutinin was significantly more sensitive than ESAT-6 and more specific than PPD for the detection of LTBI (Hougardy et al., 2007a).

3.2.4 Conditions altering IGRA results

There are various conditions such as oncologic disease, HIV infection, anti-TNF-α, corticoid or other immunomodulatory therapy, diabetes mellitus, renal failure or other immunocompromising conditions that are responsible for intermediate or false negative results (Schoepfer et al., 2008; Matulis et al., 2008; Kim et al., 2009). Particularly, the anti-TNF-α treatment has increased recently, which hampers the activation of the innate immune responses, T cell mediated adaptive immune response and production of protective IFN-γ. Similarly, metabolic diseases such as diabetes mellitus are known to affect chemotaxis, phagocytosis, activation, and antigen presentation by phagocytes in response to MTB, and this defect does not improve with insulin (Moutschen et al., 1992). Importantly, IFN-γ production was found to be impared in hyperglycemia (Yamashiro et al., 2005), but another study showed that both IGRA results were not affected in diabetes mellitus patients (Walsh et al., 2011). Intermediate results have been found to be also associated with lower serum albumin and double immunomodulatory therapy (Papay et al.,2011).

3.3 Role of regulatory T cells in diagnosis of MTB

Since TB is a chronic disease in which bacilli evade the immune system to persist in the host organism, scientists are trying to find and understand the mechanism of MTB immunopathology. It is still unclear what conditions prone to MTB infection, what factors are involved in TB latency, activation or masking of the disease and what causes the imbalance of the immune responses that finally lead to the failure of MTB eradication. The immune system posses a regulatory mechanism in which Treg cells play essential roles in establishing and sustaining self tolerance and immune homeostasis as well as regulate the host response to infection.

3.3.1 Role of Treg in mycobacterium tuberculosis infection

The first demonstration of the suppressive capacity of T cells was performed in 1973 in an animal model of bacillus BCG vaccination. Thymocytes from BCG-injectected rats were harvested and transfected to alive normal recipients. Subsequently, recipients were challenged with the same antigen and the inhibition of their skin reaction was observed (Ha & Waksman, 1973).

The number of CD4+CD25+FoxP3+ Treg cells was found to be increased in the blood or at the site of infection in active tuberculosis patients (Guyot-Revol et al., 2005) and the frequency of CD4+CD25+FoxP3+ T lymphocytes was inversely collated with the local MTB-specific immunity, and both blood and pleural Treg cells were able to suppress IFN-γ and IL-10 production in TB patients (Chen et al., 2007). This mechanism is thought to contribute to the pathogenesis of human TB (Guyot-Revol et al., 2005; Chen et al., 2007). Treg cell expansion is believed to predispose or be a marker of the progression of latent TB to active disease (Hougardy et al., 2007). What is more, it was found that depletion of CD4+CD25+ T cells enhanced the protective IFN-γ production in TB patients (Guyot-Revol et al., 2005) and transiently reduced the bacterial load and granuloma formation (Ozeki et al., 2010).

3.3.2 Objectives of our Treg study

The majority of individuals vaccinated with BCG or infected with MTB develop a delayed-type hypersensitivity which is manifested as a positive response of intradermal injection to a purified protein derivative from MTB. But about 15% of active TB patients show false negative results and are considered to be anergic TB (Bloom & Small,1998). Similarly, in HIV infected individuals, TST results are often found to be false-negative. Concerning the high frequencies of Treg cells in both diseases (Chen et al., 2007; Bi et al., 2009), it is highly probable that Treg cells may play central role in the anergy mechanism. Cutaneus anergy in active TB is associated with the absence of granuloma formation and poor clinical outcome (Boussiotis et al., 2000). Another study showed that, in an anergic patient, sustained MTB stimulation led to enhanced IL-10 production and the generation of anergic MTB-specific T regulatory cells with the Tr-1 phenotype (Boussitis, 2000). In certain closed populations, a high percentage of TB anergy and high prevalence of active TB were observed, which led to the speculation that innate genetic factors may play a role (Delgado & Ganea, 2001). We observed several cases of anergy in health care workers (HCW), who had been in close contact with active TB patients. Therefore, we questioned whether Treg cell may mask latent TB infection.

3.3.3 Materials and methods

Human subjects and samples

According to previously obtained TST results, one TST positive (27 years old) and one TST negative (42 years old) healthy (X-ray and sputum smear negative) health care individuals with no history of previous MTB infection or other chronic disease were recruited in this study. A TST result ≥ 10 mm was considered to be positive. Both individuals were vaccinated with BCG when young. The protocol was approved by the ethical commitee of Tohoku University Medical School. Written informed consent was obtained. Both individuals were HIV, hepatitis B and C virus negative.

From each donor 20 ml of Ethylenediamine tetraacetic acid (EDTA) treated peripheral venous blood was obtained, centrifuged and the peripheral blood mononuclear cells (PBMCs) were isolated by Ficoll separation (Ficoll-Paque PLUS,GE Healthcare Bio-Science AB, Uppsala, Sweden). After washing twice in Phosphate Buffered Saline (PBS), PBMCs were resuspended in complete RPMI 1640 medium (consisting of RPMI 1640 supplemented with 10% heat-inactivated fetal calf serum, 2% glutamine and 1% penicilin/streptomycin) at a concentration $5x10^6$ cells/ml.

Depletion of CD4+CD25+ cells

The cells designed for depletion were centrifuged and resusupended in Running buffer (MACS Separation Buffer, Miltenyi Biotec). To avoid unspecific binding of the antibody, 100 ul of FcR Blocking Reagent (Miltenyi Biotec) was added to the PBMCs which were then incubated for 15 minutes on ice. After adding 25 ul of CD25-Biotin monoclonal antibody (Miltenyi Biotec) and 15 minutes incubation on ice, the cells were washed with Running buffer. To cells resuspended in Running buffer, 25 ul of anti-Biotin Microbeads (Miltenyi Biotec) were added, followed by incubation for 15 minutes on ice. Subsequently, the cells were washed and resuspended in Rising Solution (Miltenyi Biotec) and CD4+CD25+ T cells were depleted by positive selection using a magnetic-activated cell sorter (MACS)-assisted cell sorting system (Miltenyi Biotec, Auburn, CA) according to the manufacturer´s instructions.

Cell phenotype determination

To visualize the biotinylated mAb on CD25+ cells, streptavidin-allophycocyanin (BD PharMingen) was used and the CD4+ cells were stained by anti-CD4 FITC antibody. Flow cytometric analyses were performed with a FACSCalibur flow cytometer (Becton Dickinson) using the CELL quest program (Becton Dickinson). More than 90% of CD4+CD25+ cells were depleted from the PMBCs of both individuals.

Cultivation and cytokine determination

Freshly isolated, undepleted and Treg depleted PBMCs were cultured in triplicate in 96-well plates at a concentration of $2x10^5$ cells per well in 200 ul of complete RPMI 1640 medium and incubated for 24 hours at 37 °C with 5% CO_2. The cells were stimulated with 1 ug/ml of PPD (Statens Serum Institute, Copenhagen, Denmark), 500nM of recombinant CFP-10 and ESAT-6 protein antigen. The cell culture supernatant was harvested from each well for ELISA analysis. IFN-gamma and IL-10 production was determined by using human IFN-gamma and IL-10 BD Opt EIA™ Set according to the manufacturer´s instructions (BD Bioscience). Optical densities were read at 450 nm on an ELISA plate reader (VersaMax-KT, Molecular Devices Corp., CA, USA) and the concentrations were calculated from standard curves using the Soft Max Pro program (Molecular Devices Corp.).

Statistical analysis

Two-sided paired *t*-test was used to analyze the effect of Treg on cytokine production. Differences were considered significant when the p value was less than 0.05.

3.3.4 Results

To investigate the immunosuppressive effect of Treg cells on the anti-TB immune response, CD25+ T cells were depleted from PBMCs of TST positive and TST negative healthy HCW. IFN-γ and IL-10 production upon PPD, CFP-10 and ESAT-6 stimulation was assayed.

The positive response to PPD stimulation in the TST-positive individual agreed with the TST result. Similarly, the low IFN-γ response to PPD in the TST anergic person supported the unresponsiveness of PBMCs to PPD stimulation. Both individuals had low levels of IFN-γ on CFP-10 stimulation, but the TST anergic person, in contrast to the TST positive one, responded to ESAT-6 stimulation, what is suspectious for LTBI. Depletion of Treg cells significantly enhanced the IFN-γ production in the TST anergic person, but in the TST positive person it influenced the IFN-γ level only after PPD stimulation (Fig. 3A). Depletion of Treg cells significantly influenced the IL-10 production only by PPD and CFP-10, but not by ESAT-6 stimulation (Fig. 3B).

3.3.5 Discussion

PPD is the prototypical mycobacterial antigen, which is included also in the Mantoux skin test antigens. The result with PPD stimulation demonstrated a T cell antigen recognition level consistent with TST results. PPD unresponsiveness in anergic TB patients might be due to the inability of their antigen presenting cells to present antigens or to the inability of their T cells to respond to antigen-specific stimulation (Boussiotis et al., 2000). Our results showed that PPD anergy might be due to an impaired T cell response as an effect of the Treg cell activity.

Recombinant antigens such as ESAT-6 and CFP-10 have been reported to be strong IFN-γ inducers. CFP-10 was reported to be less reactive in comparison to ESAT-6 in TB patients as well as in healthy controls (Oliveira et al., 2007), which was also observed in our assay. The anergic subject in our study showed a strong response to ESAT-6 stimulation, which made him highly suspected to be TB infected.

CD4+CD25+FoxP3+ T cells have been found to be increased in MTB infection and to suppress the MTB-specific immunity (Hourgady et al., 2007; Chen et al., 2007). It has been found that elimination of CD4+CD25+ T cells significantly increased the BCG-induced production of IFN-γ and IL-10 by PBMCs from patients with active TB, but not by those from healthy volunteers (Chen et al. 2007), but there is no report of Treg functions in TST anergic LTBI. We have demonstrated for the first time that Treg cell depletion in anergic individual led to enhanced IFN-γ production upon MTB specific ESAT-6 and CFP-10 antigen stimulation, while in the TST positive healthy individual we did not observed such a phenomenon. These results support the argument that CD4+CD25+ T cells suppress the Th1 immune response.

IL-10 is considered a soluble factor that plays a central role in controlling inflammatory processes, suppressing T cell responses, and maintaining immunological tolerance (Moore et al., 2001). In the condition of MTB infection, mycobacteria-induced IL-10 production by macrophages allow mycobacteria-infected cells to elude immune surveillance (Larsen et al., 2007).

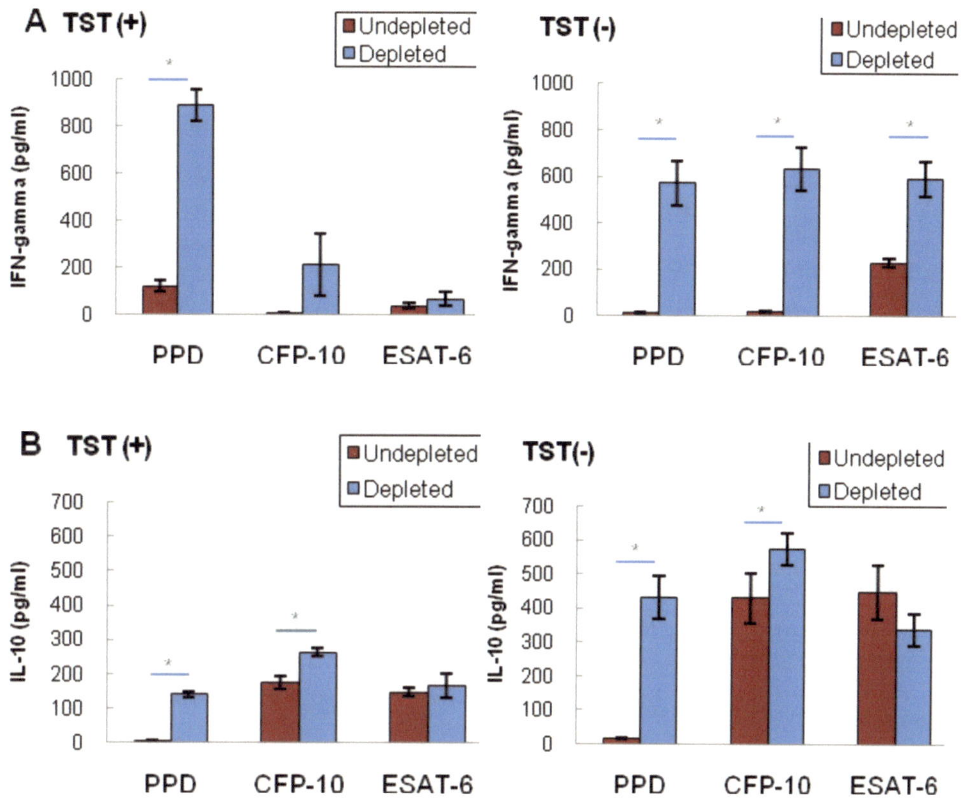

Fig. 3. Immunossuppresive effect of Treg on (A) IFN-γ production and (B) IL-10 production. Statistically significant (*) $p < 0.05$

Antigen presenting cells matured in the presence of BCG are able to instruct naive T cells to develop into cytokine-producing T cells that can be categorized into Th1 (IFN-γ producing), Th2 (IL-4-producing) or Tr1 (IL-10-producing) cells (Larsen et al. 2007). We can speculate that upon first contact with BCG vaccine in early childhood, the naive T cell development may lead to polarization of the immune response in favor of Th2 and Tr1 IL-10-producing cells. An anergic individual, in comparison to a TST positive person, have elevated levels of IL-10 upon MTB antigen stimulation and it might be possible that his immune responses are switched towards an IL-10 immune response. The anergizing effect and antiinflammatory properties of IL-10 might be one of the factors maintaining the anergy and LTBI chronicity.

Even if this is a sporadic finding, we believe that these results enable a better understanding of the immune mechanisms involved in anergy and LTBI in adult, healthy, BCG-vaccinated individuals. It is necessary to confirm these data in larger numbers of volunteers. It might be disputed whether the in vitro conditions mimic MTB infection in vivo.

In summary, Treg cells play a role in masking LTBI by suppressing the specific MTB immune response through altering IFN-γ and IL-10 production.

4. Serological diagnosis of tuberculosis

The diagnosis of tuberculosis infection remain unchanged or with very limited progress for many decades. Until recent years, diagnosis of tuberculosis primarily depends on traditional sputum microscopy for acid fast bacilli (AFB) in low and middle income countries where the disease is heavily concentrated, although the sensitivity of the method is variable (20~60%) (Steingart et al., 2006). In HIV/AIDS infection, frequent occurrence of non-cavitary pulmonary lesion can cause sputum negative tuberculosis disease. Extra-pulmonary involvement is 10-20% of all tuberculosis case and can occur relatively frequently in children than adults and in HIV/AIDS infection than healthy. Since enhancement of B cell immunity and production of antibody along with protective cell-mediated immunity may play an important role in the immunopathogenesis of tuberculosis, detection of specific antibodies against various mycobacterial derived antigens could also play a significant role in the diagnosis of tuberculosis. The value of various mycobacterial native or recombinant protein, lipid or different combinations of purified antigens or commercially available kits as a potential candidate of active tuberculosis sero-marker was evaluated by the ELISA method in many attempts (Abebe et al., 2007; Verma & Jain, 2007; Steingart et al., 2009). Development of a serological test with sufficient diagnostic efficacy for tuberculosis diagnosis could be very much useful tool in resource-limited countries, as the procedures are simple, relatively cost effective and can be performed rapidly.

Characteristics of commonly used antigens have been listed in the following table (Table 2). Until recently, various mycobacterial culture filtrate and surface exposed proteins including 38kDa, Ag85B, MPT51, Ag60 antigens, malate synthase, heat shock protein, RD1 antigens were investigated to determine their diagnostic efficacy.

Target antigen	Type of antigen	Mycobacterial location/Rv region	Biological effects
LAM	Lipoglycan	Cell wall	Immunomodulation, Anti-inflammatory
TDM	Glycolipid	Cell wall	Immunomodulation, Enhance inflammation and granuloma formation
DAT	Glycolipid	Cell wall	Immunmodulation
TAT	Glycolipid	Cell wall	Immunomodulation
SL-I	Glycolipid	Cell wall	Related to MTB virulence
38kDa	Protein	Rv0934	Immunogenic protein
Ag85B	Protein	Rv1886c	Immunogenic protein
Malate synthase	Protein	Rv1837c	Immunogenic protein
MPT51	Protein	3803c	Immunogenic protein
ESAT-6	Protein	3875	Immunogenic protein
CFP-10	Protein	3874	Immunogenic protein
Antigen 60	Glycopeptidolipid		Immunomodulation

Table 2. Characteristic of mycobacterial antigens commonly assessed for the serodiagnosis of tuberculosis.
LAM: lipoarabinomannan; TDM: trehalose 6,6 dimycolate; DAT: 2,3-diacyl trehalose; TAT: 2,3,6-triacyl trehalose; SL-I: 2,3,6,6-tetraacyl trehalose 2′-sulphate (Sulfolipid-I); Ag85B: Antigen85B; ESAT-6: early secreted antigenic target-6; CFP-10: culture filtrate protein-10

4.1 Serodiagnostic markers

38kDa antigen: The 38-kDa antigen (also known as Antigen 5) is a major lipoprotein antigen of M. tuberculosis. As reviewed by Steigart et. al in a meta-analysis, it yielded a sensitivity of 47% and a specificity of 94% in smear positive tuberculosis patients. The increased sensitivity is found to be associated with smear-positive than negative tuberculosis (Wilkinsonson et al. 1997; Julian et al., 2000). Use of native or recombinant protein did not show any difference in term of diagnostic efficacy. But, the sensitivity of IgG detection was relatively higher than that of IgA against 38 kDa antigen (Verma & Jain, 2007). Several commercially available antibody detection kits were also developed using this antigen including Pathozyme Myco (LAM+38kDa), Pathozyme TB complex plus (38kDa+16kDa). The sensitivity varies in both Pathozyme Myco (21-46%) and Pathozyme TB complex plus (29-76%). However, the tests are highly specific (94-100%) for tuberculosis diagnosis (Steingart et al., 2007). The sensitivity was less than 70% and the specificity varies from 70% to 94.9% in different studies for the diagnosis of smear-positive tuberculosis patients co-infected with HIV (Abebe et al., 2007). The sensitivity of Pathozyme Myco and Pathozyme TB complex plus varies from 11% to 51% respectively, although the specificities were more than 90% by both the kits for the diagnosis of extra-pulmonary tuberculosis (Steigart et. al., 2007).

Antigen 85B: It is a member of a family of Ag85 protein complex (Ag85A, Ag85B and Ag85C). It is a major fraction of secreted proteins in the MTB culture filtrate and cell wall. A relatively higher sensitivity in HIV-positive tuberculosis patients (62%) than HIV-negative tuberculosis patients (53%) with a high specificity (>95%) in both groups were reported for Ag85B (Steingart et al., 2009). MPT51 is an antigen also related to the protein family of Ag85 complex. MPT51 provided comparable diagnostic efficacy in both HIV-negative (sensitivity: 59%) and HIV-positive tuberculosis patients (sensitivity: 58%) and the specificities of 94% and 97% respectively (Steingart et al., 2009).

ESAT-6 and CFP-10: These are two low molecular weight secreted proteins, encoded within the RD1 region of M. tuberculosis and highly associated with the virulence of the organism. It is known to induce strong cell mediated immune response. Although the use of ESAT-6 and CFP-10 in IFN-γ based immunological methods for tuberculosis is widely acceptable for the diagnosis of active and latent tuberculosis infection, the potential use of this antigens in antibody-based diagnostic methods were also evaluated. Association of antibody responses against ESAT-6 was described to be related with inactive stage of tuberculosis (Davidow et al., 2005; Doherty et al., 2002), although increased antibody in progressive tuberculosis was also demonstrated in other report (Demissie et al., 2006). In addition, CFP-10 showed a sensitivity of 48% and a specificity of 96% for the diagnosis of active pulmonary tuberculosis. The use of CFP-10/ESAT-6 fusion antigen obtained a relatively higher sensitivity of 60.4% and a specificity of 73.8% in HIV-seronegative tuberculosis patients (Wu et al., 2010).

Antigen 60 (A60): It is a heat-stable component of PPD extracted from BCG that can be recognized by the sera of tuberculosis patients (Abebe et al., 2007). Anda TB (Anda Biologicals, Strasbourg, France), a commercially available ELISA kit was developed using A60 and its diagnostic ability was evaluated by many investigators for the diagnosis of pulmonary and extra-pulmonary tuberculosis. The sensitivity was variable in pulmonary tuberculosis (29%-85%) as well as in extra-pulmonary tuberculosis (0%-100%). However, the specificities ranges 70%-100% for both types of tuberculosis (Steingart et al., 2007).

Non-peptidic antigens from the mycobacterial cell wall grasp the main focus of comprehensive research for the determination of their potential role in the protective immunity or marker of TB disease.

Lipoarabinomannan (LAM): LAM, a complex glycolipid antigen forming is a major part of cell wall of MTB. Evaluation of anti-LAM-IgG against purified LAM from MTB for the serodiagnosis of tuberculosis was reported to have good diagnostic ability (sensitivity: 91%, specificity: 72%) in detection of both pulmonary, pleural and miliary tuberculosis as well as tubercular lymphadenitis (Sada et al., 1990). However, lower rate of sensitivity (50.5%) and comparable specificity (78.3%) for the diagnosis of pulmonary tuberculosis patients were reported by Tessema et al. (2002). In addition, MycoDot, (Genelabs, Switzerland), a commercially available kit for the detection of antibodies against MTB specific LAM was also evaluated in many reports (Steingart et al., 2007; Verma & Jain, 2007). Although the specificities were high (84-100%), low rate of sensitivities (16-56%) were obtained and low sensitivities were mostly related to HIV/TB co-infection (Verma & Jain, 2007)

DAT, TAT and SL-I: Assessment of antibody responses using DAT, TAT, and SL-I antigens in ELISA for serodiagnosis of tuberculosis revealed variable results in terms of diagnostic efficacy. Widely variable ranges of sensitivity of 11 to 88% by DAT antigen were reported in several studies. A similar rate of sensitivity by MTB (44.5%) and M. fortuitum (48.6%) infection were also demonstrated. In addition, the test sensitivities of TAT anigen also vary from 51-93% (Julian et al., 2002). Julian et. al. reported the best performance of IgG (Sensitivity: 81% and specificity: 77.6%) and IgA (sensitivity: 66% and specificity: 87%) antibodies by SL-I among four trehalose contacting glycolipids (DAT, TAT, SL-I, TDM). Although, several reasons including variation in the ELISA protocol, using of different antigen concentrations and population from different subgroups were described as possible reason of such variability, the effectiveness of theses antigens are still uncertain.

TDM (also known as cord factor): It composes a major part of the mycobacterial cell wall, was identified as the most immunogenic glycolipid. Clinical evaluation of serodiagnosis of pulmonary tuberculosis using of TDM purified from Mycobacterium tuberculosis H37Rv, in ELISA reported its sensitivity of 81% and its specificity of 96% (Mizusawa et. al. 2008). Best performance by TDM (sensitivity 69%, specificity: 91%) among other lipid antigens including DAT, TAT, SL-I for the serodiagnosis of tuberculosis were also reviewed by Steingart et al. (2009). IgG antibody against TDM can also recognize mycolic acid sub-classes and highly active against methoxy-mycolic acid in the cord factor of M. tuberculosis than keto-mycolic acid in M. avium complex (Pan et al., 1999). By combining TDM with more hydrophobic glycolipids, a new tuberculous glycolipid (TBGL) antigen was designed and a more sensitive serodiagnostic kit for TB, an anti-TBGL IgG test was developed (Kyowa Medex Co, Japan). Anti-TBGL IgG antibody (TBGL IgG) has been proposed as a useful sero-diagnostic marker of active pulmonary tuberculosis (PTB) (sensitivity: 84% and specificity: 95% in young adults) in Japan (Maekura et al., 2001). Strong association between TBGL IgG and IgA was also revealed in active pulmonary tuberculosis cases and increased TBGL IgG and IgA was found to be associated with CRP and cavity formation indicating their involvement in the disease pathogenesis (Mizusawa et al., 2008). Elevated titers of TBGL IgG were found in aged (>40 yrs) healthy control people (17%) in Japan (Maekura et al., 2001) and high titers of both TBGL IgG (46%) and IgA (36%) in healthy adults was also observed in our recent study in Thailand (Siddiqi et. al.; in press). But, elevated titers of TBGL IgG are not related to BCG vaccination (Nabeshima et al., 2005). Very recently, significant association between the TBGL IgG and Quatiferon-TB Gold IT assay responses in diagnosis of latent tuberculosis infection in healthy healthcare workers was also found (Siddiqi et. al., unpublished data) that represents enhancement of humoral immune responses along with T cell mediated immunity in latent tuberculosis infection. Increased synthesis of TBGL IgA titers that was related to serum IgA were observed in HIV carriers with low CD4+ T cells counts (less than 350/μl) compared to high CD4+ T cells counts (more than 350/μl). However, the sensitivities of TBGL IgG and IgA were very low (10% and 8% respectively) although their specificities were more than 90% for the diagnosis of tuberculosis in pediatric cases (Siddiqi et. al., 2009, unpublished data).

4.2 Discussion

The performance of various purified antigens and commercially available kits for the sero-diagnosis of active pulmonary tuberculosis with or without associated HIV/AIDS co-infection were evaluated in many studies and were reviewed extensively (Abebe et al., 2007; Steingart et al., 2006, 2007, 2009; Varma & Jain, 2007). Protein antigens were reported to have high specificity (>95%) than lipid antigens. In relation to use of single antigen, relatively higher sensitivities can be achieved by using multiple antigens. Cord factor (TDM), among the lipid antigens had the best overall performance. In addition, higher rate of sensitivity can be obtained by evaluation of IgG and/or IgA than IgM. Maes and colleagues has been conceptualized the human immune responses against mycobacteria into four different stages based on BCG vaccination and tuberculosis disease and treatment, initiated from innate response followed by intermingled innate and adaptive response against low molecular weight oligopeptiic and nonpeptidic, as muramyldipeptide and trehalose 6,6 dimycolate and high molecular weight nonpeptidic antigens such as lipoarabinomannan. The final response is directed against protein antigens (Maes et al., 1999). Although it is not clearly understood, enhancement of humoral immune response can be dependent on disease pathogenesis and different stage of infection can influence different subclasses of immunoglobulins. Enhanced IgM expression can usually occur in the early stage of infection that can subsequently be diminished on progression of disease. Therefore, detection of IgM may show limited value in the sero-diagnostic assay. The reason of low sensitivity of IgA antibody is not clear. It is possible that the generation of IgA antibody needs larger amounts of antigens and related with degree of disease pathogenesis than do IgG responses and indicate the heterogeneity of tuberculosis infection.

However, until now, any performance was not successful to show the, stable, consistent and acceptable sero-diagnostic efficacy with a sensitivity of at least more than 85% and a specificity of more than 95% and to replace the traditional sputum microscopy as a reliable diagnostic tool in different groups of tuberculosis patients including HIV-positive, -negative, extra-pulmonary tuberculosis or in pediatric tuberculosis detection. However, extensive study for evaluation of humoral immune responses in different stages of tuberculosis infection and disease and their association with the disease pathogenesis should be consider to clarify the variable antibody responses against different antigens. As most of the investigations for the determination of sero-diagnostic ability of various antigens were carried out in tuberculosis endemic countries, determination of antibody responses in latent tuberculosis infection could be helpful to some extent for explaining the reason of low specificities and the possibility of influence by tuberculosis endemicity in such countries. The immune response in HIV/AIDS patients co-infected with tuberculosis is more complex than single infection. Antibodies against several single or multiple antigens were detected in HIV/AIDS patients with active tuberculosis and even months to year's prior development of tuberculosis related symptoms in some prospective studies. More investigation with diverse antigens for the sero-diagnosis of subclinical and active tuberculosis particularly sputum-negative and extra-pulmonary tuberculosis especially in those with HIV/AIDS co-infection and in pediatric cases is an urgent necessity.

It is generally believed that, T helper immunity and elaboration of IFN-γ offer vital role in protective immunity to clear or containment of the intracellular MTB infection. However, BCG-induced antibodies was shown to potentiate IFN-γ production by mycobacterium-specific CD4+ T cells and also can cause enhancement of mycobacterial phagocytosis probably by inducing opsonization by antibodies and that might be related to mucosal immunity (Abebe & Bjune, 2009). Protective role of antibodies against several TB antigens in mice model was also review by Glatman-Freedman (2009). Therefore, antibody-mediated immunity against diverse mycobacterial antigens in synergy with cell mediated immunity can play a vital role in the protection and immunopathogenesis of tuberculosis infection and disease. Frequent detection of antibodies in latent or progressive stages of latent to active tuberculosis and their relation to immune responses especially with mucosal immunity needs to be clarified further.

5. Acknowledgment

This work is supported the Scientific Research Expenses for Health and Welfare program from the Ministry of Health, Labour and Welfare, Japan (TH) and Science and Technology Research Partnership for Sustainable Development from Japan Science and Technology Agency, Japan (YS). This work was supported by collaborative funding from the Research Centre for Zoonosis Control, Hokkaido University. We are grateful to prof. Ishii N. (Tohoku University) and Dr. Mousavi S.F. (Pasteur Institute of Iran) for the help with Treg depletion experiment. We would like to thank to Mr. Brent Bell for reading the manuscript.

6. References

Aagaard, C.; Brock, I.; Olsen, A.; Ottenhoff, T. H.; Weldingh, K. & Andersen, P. (2004). Mapping immune reactivity toward Rv2653 and Rv2654: two novel low-molecular-mass antigens found specifically in the Mycobacterium tuberculosis complex, *The Journal of infectious disease,* Vol.189, No.5, (March 2004), pp.812-819, ISSN 0022-1899

Abebe, F. & Bjune, G. (2009). The protective role of antibody responses during Mycobacterium tuberculosis infection, *Clinical and experimental immunology,* Vol.157, No.2, (August 2009), pp.235-243, ISSN 1365-2249

Berry, M. P.; Graham, C. M.; McNab, F. W.; Xu, Z.; Bloch, S. A.; Oni, T.; Wilkinson, K. A.; Banchereau, R.; Skinner, J.; Wilkinson, R. J.; Quinn, C.; Blankenship, D.; Dhawan, R.; Cush, J. J.; Mejias, A.; Ramilo, O.; Kon, O. M.; Pascual, V.; Banchereau, J.;

Chaussabel, D. & O'Garra, A. (2010). An Interferon-Inducible Neutrophil-Driven Blood Transcriptional Signature in Human Tuberculosis, *Nature*, Vol.466, No.7309, (August 2010), pp. 973-977, ISSN 1476-4687

Bi, X.; Suzuki, Y.; Gatanaga, H. & Oka, S. (2009). High frequency and proliferation of CD4+ FOXP3+ Treg in HIV-1-infected patients with low CD4 counts, *European journal of immunology*, Vol.39, No.1, (January 2009), pp.301-309, ISSN 1521-4141.

Bloom, B. R. & Small, P. M. (1998). The evolving relation between humans and Mycobacterium tuberculosis, *The New English journal of medicine*, Vol.338, No.10, (March 1998), pp.677-678, ISSN 0028-4793.

Boussiotis, V. A.; Tsai, E. Y.; Yunis, E. J.; Thim, S.; Delgado, J. C.; Dascher, C. C.; Berezovskaya, A.; Rousset, D.; Reynes, J. M. & Goldfeld, A. E. (2000). IL-10-producing T cells suppress immune responses in anergic tuberculosis patients, *The journal of clinical investigation*, Vol.105, No.9, (May 2000), pp.1317-1325, ISSN 0021-9738.

Brock, I.; Weldingh, K.; Leyten, E. M.; Arend, S. M.; Ravn, P. & Andersen, P. (2004). Specific T-cell epitopes for immunoassay-based diagnosis of Mycobacterium tuberculosis infection, *Journal of clinical microbioogy*, Vol.42, No.6, (June 2004), pp.2379-2387, ISSN 0095-1137

Centers for Disease Control and Prevention (CDC). (April 2010). In: *TB Elimination. Tuberculin Skin Testing*. 8.8.2011, Available at: http://www.cdc.gov/tb/publications/factsheets/testing/skintesting.pdf,

Chagan-Yasutan, H.; Saitoh, H.; Ashino, Y.; Arikawa, T.; Hirashima, M.; Li, S.; Usuzawa, M.; Oguma S.; O.Telan, E.F.; Obi, C.L. & Hattori, T. (2009). Persistent Elevation of Plasma Osteopontin Levels in HIV Patients Despite Highly Active Antiretroviral Therapy. *Tohoku Journal of Experimental Medicine*, Vol.218, No.4, pp. 285-292, ISSN 0040-8727

Chen, X.; Zhou, B.; Li, M.; Deng, Q.; Wu, X.; Le, X.; Wu, C.; Larmonier, N.; Zhang, W.; Zhang, H.; Wang, H. and Katsanis, E. (2007). CD4(+)CD25(+)FoxP3(+) regulatory T cells suppress Mycobacterium tuberculosis immunity in patients with active disease, *Clinical immunology*, Vol.123, No.1, (April 2007), pp.50-59, ISSN 521-6616.

Comas, I.; Chakravartti, J.; Small, P. M.; Galagan, J.; Niemann, S.; Kremer, K.; Ernst, J. D. & Gagneux, S. (2010). Human T Cell Epitopes of Mycobacterium Tuberculosis Are Evolutionarily Hyperconserved, *Nature genetics*, Vol.42, No.6, (June 2010), pp.498-503, ISSN 1546-1718

Crowley, T. M.; Haring, V. R. & Moore, R. (2011). Chicken anemia virus: an understanding of the in-vitro host response over time, *Viral immunology*, Vol.24, No.1, (Februry 2011), pp.3-9, ISSN 1557-8976

Davidow, A.; Kanaujia, G. V.; Shi, L.; Kaviar, J.; Guo, X.; Sung, N.; Kaplan, G.; Menzies, D. & Gennaro, M. L. (2005). Antibody profiles characteristic of Mycobacterium tuberculosis infection state, *Infection and immunology*, Vol.73, No.10, (October 2005), pp.6846-6851, ISSN 0019-9567

Day, C. L.; Abrahams, D. A.; Lerumo, L.; Janse van Rensburg, E.; Stone, L.; O'Rie, T.; Pienaar, B.; de Kock, M.; Kaplan, G.; Mahomed, H.; Dheda, K. & Hanekom, W. A. (2011). Functional Capacity of Mycobacterium Tuberculosis-Specific T Cell

Responses in Humans Is Associated with Mycobacterial Load, *Journal of immunology*, (July 2011), ISSN 1550-6606

Delgado, M. & Ganea, D. (2001). VIP and PACAP enhance the in vivo generation of memory TH2 cells by inhibiting peripheral deletion of antigen-specific effectors, *Archives of physiology and biochemistry*, Vol. 109, No.4, (October 2001), pp.372-376, ISSN 1381-3455

Demissie, A.; Leyten, E. M.; Abebe, M.; Wassie, L.; Aseffa, A.; Abate, G.; Fletcher, H.; Owiafe, P.; Hill, P. C.; Brookes, R.; Rook, G.; Zumla, A.; Arend, S. M.; Klein, M.; Ottenhoff, T. H.; Andersen, P. & Doherty, T. M. (2006). Recognition of stage-specific mycobacterial antigens differentiates between acute and latent infections with Mycobacterium tuberculosis, *Clinical and vaccine immunology*, Vol.13, No.2, (February 2006), pp.179-186, ISSN 1556-6811

Diel, R., Loddenkemper, R. & Nienhaus, A. (2010). Evidence-based comparison of commercial interferon-gamma release assays for detecting active TB: a metaanalysis, *Chest*, Vol.137, No.4, (April 2010), pp.952-968, ISSN 1931-3543

Doherty, T. M.; Demissie, A.; Olobo, J.; Wolday, D.; Britton, S.; Eguale, T.; Ravn, P. & Andersen, P. (2002). Immune responses to the Mycobacterium tuberculosis-specific antigen ESAT-6 signal subclinical infection among contacts of tuberculosis patients, *Journal of clinical microbiology*, Vol.40, No.2, (February 2002), pp.704-706, ISSN 0095-1137

Dosanjh, D. P.; Hinks, T. S.; Innes, J. A.; Deeks, J. J.; Pasvol, G.; Hackforth, S.; Varia, H.; Millington, K. A.; Gunatheesan, R.; Guyot-Revol, V. & Lalvani, A. (2008). Improved diagnostic evaluation of suspected tuberculosis, *Annals of internal medicine*, Vol.148, No.5, (March 2008), pp.325-336, ISSN 1539-3704.

Ferrara, G.; Losi, M.; D'Amico, R.; Roversi, P.; Piro, R.; Meacci, M.; Meccugni, B.; Dori, I. M.; Andreani, A.; Bergamini, B. M.; Mussini, C.; Rumpianesi, F.; Fabbri, L. M. & Richeldi, L. (2006). Use in routine clinical practice of two commercial blood tests for diagnosis of infection with Mycobacterium tuberculosis: a prospective study, *Lancet*, Vol. 367, No.9519, (April 2006), pp.1328-1334, ISSN 1474-547X

Glatman-Freedman, A. (2006). The role of antibody-mediated immunity in defense against Mycobacterium tuberculosis: advances toward a novel vaccine strategy, *Tuberculosis*, Vol.86, No.3-4, (May-July), pp.191-197, ISSN 1472-9792

Guyot-Revol, V.; Innes, J. A.; Hackforth, S.; Hinks, T. & Lalvani, A. (2006). Regulatory T cells are expanded in blood and disease sites in patients with tuberculosis, *American journal of respiratory and critical care medicine*, Vol.173, No.7, (April 2006), pp.803-810, ISSN 1073-449X

Ha, T. Y. & Waksman, B. H. (1973). Role of the thymus in tolerance. X. "Suppressor" activity of antigen-stimulated rat thymocytes transferred to normal recipients, *Journal of immunology*, Vol.110, No.5, (May 1973), pp.1290-1299, ISSN 0022-1767

Haddow, L. J.; Dibben, O.; Moosa, M. Y.; Borrow, P. & Easterbrook, P. J. (2011). Circulating Inflammatory Biomarkers Can Predict and Characterize Tuberculosis-Associated Immune Reconstitution Inflammatory Syndrome, *AIDS*, Vol.25, No.9, (June 2011), pp.1163-1174, ISSN 1473-5571

Harada, N.; Higuchi, K.; Yoshiyama, T.; Kawabe, Y.; Fujita, A.; Sasaki, Y.; Horiba, M.; Mitarai, S.; Yonemaru, M.; Ogata, H.; Ariga, H.; Kurashima, A.; Wada, A.;

Takamori, M.; Yamagishi, F.; Suzuki, K.; Mori, T. & Ishikawa, N. (2008). Comparison of the sensitivity and specificity of two whole blood interferon-gamma assays for M. tuberculosis infection, *The Journal of infection,* Vol.56, No.5, (May 2008), pp.348-353, ISSN 1532-2742

Harari, A.; Rozot, V.; Enders, F. B.; Perreau, M.; Stalder, J. M.; Nicod, L. P.; Cavassini, M.; Calandra, T.; Blanchet, C. L.; Jaton, K.; Faouzi, M.; Day, C. L.; Hanekom, W. A.; Bart, P. A. & Pantaleo, G. (2011). Dominant Tnf-Alpha+ Mycobacterium Tuberculosis-Specific Cd4+ T Cell Responses Discriminate between Latent Infection and Active Disease, *Nature medicine,* Vol.17, No.3, (March 2011), pp.372-376, ISSN 1546-170X

He, H.; Nehete, P. N.; Nehete, B.; Wieder, E.; Yang, G.; Buchl, S. & Sastry, K. J. (2011). Functional Impairment of Central Memory Cd4 T Cells Is a Potential Early Prognostic Marker for Changing Viral Load in Shiv-Infected Rhesus Macaques, PloS one, Vol 6, NO. 5, (2011), pp. e19607, ISS 1932-6203

Horsburgh, C. R., Jr. & Rubin, E. J. (2011). Clinical practice. Latent tuberculosis infection in the United States, *The New England journal of medicine,* Vol.364, No.15, (April 2011), pp.1441-1448, ISSN 1533-4406

Hougardy, J. M.; Schepers, K.; Place, S.; Drowart, A.; Lechevin, V.; Verscheure, V.; Debrie, A. S.; Doherty, T. M.; Van Vooren, J. P.; Locht, C. & Mascart, F. (2007a). Heparin-binding-hemagglutinin-induced IFN-gamma release as a diagnostic tool for latent tuberculosis, *PLoS One,* Vol.2, No.10, (October 2007), pp.e926, ISSN 1932-6203

Hougardy, J. M.; Verscheure, V.; Locht, C. & Mascart, F. (2007b). In vitro expansion of CD4+CD25highFOXP3+CD127low/- regulatory T cells from peripheral blood lymphocytes of healthy Mycobacterium tuberculosis-infected humans, *Microbes and infection,* Vol.9, No.11, (September 2007), pp.1325-1332, ISSN 1286-4579

Hua, W.; Jiao, Y.; Zhang, H.; Zhang, T.; Chen, D.; Zhang, Y.; Chen, X. & Wu, H. (2011). Central Memory Cd4 Cells Are an Early Indicator of Immune Reconstitution in Hiv/Aids Patients with Anti-Retroviral Treatment, *Immunological investigations,* (May 2011), ISSN 1532-4311

Jayaraman, P.; Sada-Ovalle, I.; Beladi, S.; Anderson, A.C.; Dardalhon, V.; Hotta, C.; Kuchroo, V.K. & Behar, S.M. (2010). Tim3 binding to galectin-9 stimulates antimicrobial immunity. *Journal of Experimental Medicine,* Vol.207, No.11, (October 2010), pp.2343-2354, ISSN 0022-1007

Julian, E.; Matas, L.; Hernandez, A.; Alcaide, J. & Luquin, M. (2000). Evaluation of a new serodiagnostic tuberculosis test based on immunoglobulin A detection against Kp-90 antigen, *The international journal of tuberculosis and lung disease : the official journal of the International Union against Tuberculosis and Lung Diasease,* Vol.4, No.11, (November 2000), pp.1082-1085, ISSN 1027-3719

Julian, E.; Matas, L.; Perez, A.; Alcaide, J.; Laneelle, M. A. & Luquin, M. (2002). Serodiagnosis of tuberculosis: comparison of immunoglobulin A (IgA) response to sulfolipid I with IgG and IgM responses to 2,3-diacyltrehalose, 2,3,6-triacyltrehalose, and cord factor antigens, *Journal of clinical microbiology,* Vol.40, No.10, (October 2002), pp.3782-3788, ISSN 0095-1137

Kashio, Y.; Nakamura, K. ; Abedin, M.J.; Seki, M.; Nishi, N.; Yoshida, N.; Nakamura, T. & Hirashima, M. (2003). Galectin-9 induces apoptosis through the calcium-calpaincaspase-1 pathway. *Journal of Immunology*, Vol.170, No.7, (April 2003), pp.3631-3636, ISSN 0022-1767

Kim, E. Y.; Lim, J. E.; Jung, J. Y.; Son, J. Y.; Lee, K. J.; Yoon, Y. W.; Park, B. H.; Moon, J. W.; Park, M. S.; Kim, Y. S.; Kim, S. K.; Chang, J. & Kang, Y. A. (2009). Performance of the tuberculin skin test and interferon-gamma release assay for detection of tuberculosis infection in immunocompromised patients in a BCG-vaccinated population, *BMC infection diseases,* Vol.9, (December 2009), p.207, ISSN 1471-2334

Larsen, J. M.; Geisler, C.; Nielsen, M. W.; Boding, L.; Von Essen, M.; Hansen, A. K.; Skov, L. & Bonefeld, C. M. (2007). Cellular dynamics in the draining lymph nodes during sensitization and elicitation phases of contact hypersensitivity, *Contact Dermatitis,* Vol.57, No.5, (November 2007), pp.300-308, ISSN 0105-1873

Liote, H. & Liote, F. (2011). Role for interferon-gamma release assays in latent tuberculosis screening before TNF-alpha antagonist therapy, *Joint Bone Spine,* Vol.78, No.4, (July 2011), pp.352-357, ISSN 1778-7254

Maekura, R.; Okuda, Y.; Nakagawa, M.; Hiraga, T.; Yokota, S.; Ito, M.; Yano, I.; Kohno, H.; Wada, M.; Abe, C.; Toyoda, T.; Kishimoto, T. and Ogura, T. (2001). Clinical evaluation of anti-tuberculous glycolipid immunoglobulin G antibody assay for rapid serodiagnosis of pulmonary tuberculosis, *Journal of clinical microbiology,* Vol.39, No.10, (October 2001), pp.3603-3608, ISSN 0095-1137

Maertzdorf, J.; Repsilber, D.; Parida, S. K.; Stanley, K.; Roberts, T.; Black, G.; Walzl, G. & Kaufmann, S. H. (2011). Human Gene Expression Profiles of Susceptibility and Resistance in Tuberculosis, *Genes and immunity,* Vol.12, No.1, (January 2011), pp.15-22, ISSN 1476-5470

Maes, H. H.; Causse, J. E. & Maes, R. F. (1999). Tuberculosis I: a conceptual frame for the immunopathology of the disease, *Medical hypotheses,* Vol.52, No.6, (June 1999), pp.583-593.

Manosuthi, W.; Kiertiburanakul, S.; Phoorisri, T. & Sungkanuparph, S. (2006). Immune reconstitution inflammatory syndrome of tuberculosis among HIV-infected patients receiving antituberculous and antiretroviral therapy, The *journal of infection, Vol.*53, No.6, (December 2006), pp.357-363, ISSN 1532-2742

Matulis, G.; Juni, P.; Villiger, P. M. & Gadola, S. D. (2008). Detection of latent tuberculosis in immunosuppressed patients with autoimmune diseases: performance of a Mycobacterium tuberculosis antigen-specific interferon gamma assay, *Annals of the rheumatic diseases,* Vol.67, No.1, (January 2008), pp.84-90, ISSN 1468-2060

Middelkoop, K.; Bekker, L. G.; Myer, L.; Johnson, L. F.; Kloos, M.; Morrow, C. & Wood, R. (2011). Antiretroviral Therapy and Tb Notification Rates in a High Hiv Prevalence South African Community, *Journal of acquired immune deficiency syndromes*, Vol.56, No.3, (March 2011), pp.263-269, ISSN 1944-7884

Mizusawa, M.; Kawamura, M.; Takamori, M.; Kashiyama, T.; Fujita, A.; Usuzawa, M.; Saitoh, H.; Ashino, Y.; Yano, I. & Hattori, T. (2008). Increased synthesis of anti-tuberculous glycolipid immunoglobulin G (IgG) and IgA with cavity formation in patients with pulmonary tuberculosis, *Clinical and vaccine immunology,* Vol.15, No.3, (March 2008), pp.544-548, ISSN 1556-679X

Moore, K. W.; de Waal Malefyt, R.; Coffman, R. L. & O'Garra, A. (2001). Interleukin-10 and the interleukin-10 receptor, *Annual review of immunology*, Vol.19, pp.683-765, ISSN 0732-0582

Moutschen, M. P.; Scheen, A. J. & Lefebvre, P. J. (1992). Impaired immune responses in diabetes mellitus: analysis of the factors and mechanisms involved. Relevance to the increased susceptibility of diabetic patients to specific infections, *Diabete & Metabolisme*, Vol.18, No.3, (May-June 1992) pp.187-201, ISSN 0338-1684

Mueller, H.; Detjen, A. K.; Schuck, S. D.; Gutschmidt, A.; Wahn, U.; Magdorf, K.; Kaufmann, S. H. & Jacobsen, M. (2008). Mycobacterium Tuberculosis-Specific Cd4+, Ifngamma+, and Tnfalpha+ Multifunctional Memory T Cells Coexpress Gm-Csf, *Cytokine*, Vol.43, No.2, (August 2008), pp.143-148, ISSN 1096-0023

Murdoch, D. M.; Venter, W. D.; Van Rie, A. & Feldman, C. (2007). Immune reconstitution inflammatory syndrome (IRIS): review of common infectious manifestations and treatment options, *AIDS research and therapy, Vol.*4, pp.9, ISSN 1742-6405

Murphy, K. (2011). *Jenway's Immunobiology*, 8th edition, Garland Science, ISBN 9780815342434, New York, United States.

Nabeshima, S.; Murata, M.; Kashiwagi, K.; Fujita, M.; Furusyo, N. & Hayashi, J. (2005). Serum antibody response to tuberculosis-associated glycolipid antigen after BCG vaccination in adults, *Journal of infection and chemotherapy : official journal of the Japan Society of Chemotherapy*, Vol.11, No.5, (October 2005), pp.256-258, ISSN 1341-321X

Oliveira, J. F.; Henkes, L. E.; Ashley, R. L.; Purcell, S. H.; Smirnova, N. P.; Veeramachaneni, D. N.; Anthony, R. V. & Hansen, T. R. (2008). Expression of interferon (IFN)-stimulated genes in extrauterine tissues during early pregnancy in sheep is the consequence of endocrine IFN-tau release from the uterine vein, *Endocrinology*, Vol.149, No.3, (March 2008), pp.1252-1259, ISSN 0013-7227

Oxford Immunotec. (2011). T-SPOT°,R.TB Get the facts, 6.8.2011, Available from: http://www.oxfordimmunotec.com/getthefacts/

Ozeki, Y.; Sugawara, I.; Udagawa, T.; Aoki, T.; Osada-Oka, M.; Tateishi, Y.; Hisaeda, H.; Nishiuchi, Y.; Harada, N.; Kobayashi, K. & Matsumoto, S. (2010). Transient role of CD4+CD25+ regulatory T cells in mycobacterial infection in mice, *International immunology*, Vol.22, No.3, (March 2010), pp.179-189, ISSN 1460-2377

Pan, J.; Fujiwara, N.; Oka, S.; Maekura, R.; Ogura, T. & Yano, I. (1999). Anti-cord factor (trehalose 6,6'dimycolate) IgG antibody in tuberculosis patients recognizes mycolic acid subclasses, *Microbiology and immunology*, Vol.43, No.9, pp.863-869, ISSN 0385-5600

Papay, P. ; Eser, A. ; Winkler, S. ; Frantal, S. ; Primas, C. ; Miehsler, W. ; Angelberger, S. ; Novacek, G. ; Mikulits, A. ; Vogelsang, H. & Reinisch, W. (2011). Predictors of indeterminate IFN-gamma release assay in screening for latent TB in inflammatory bowel diseases, *European journal of clinical investigation*, (March 2011), ISSN 1365-2362

Piana, F.; Codecasa, L. R.; Cavallerio, P.; Ferrarese, M.; Migliori, G. B.; Barbarano, L.; Morra, E. & Cirillo, D. M. (2006). Use of a T-cell-based test for detection of tuberculosis infection among immunocompromised patients, *The European respiratory journal:official journal of the European Society for Clinical Respiratory Physiology*, Vol.28, No.1, (July 2006), pp.31-34, ISSN 0903-1936

Prevention Commettee, Japanese Society of Tuberculosis: Guidelines for the use of QuantiFERON TB-2G. (2006). *Kekkaku*, Vol.81, No.5, pp.393-397, ISSN 0022-9776

Rueda, C. M.; Marin, N. D.; Garcia, L. F. & Rojas, M. (2010). Characterization of Cd4 and Cd8 T Cells Producing Ifn-Gamma in Human Latent and Active Tuberculosis, *Tuberculosis*, Vol.90, No.6, (Novmenber 2010), pp.346-353, ISSN 1873-281X

Russell, D. G.; VanderVen, B. C.; Lee, W.; Abramovitch, R. B.; Kim, M. J.; Homolka, S.; Niemann, S. & Rohde, K. H. (2010). Mycobacterium Tuberculosis Wears What It Eats, *Cell host & microbe*, Vol.8, No.1, (July 2010), pp.68-76, ISSN 1934-6069

Sada, E.; Brennan, P. J.; Herrera, T. & Torres, M. (1990). Evaluation of lipoarabinomannan for the serological diagnosis of tuberculosis, *Journal of clinical microbiology,* Vol.28, No.12, (December 1990), pp.2587-2590, ISSN 0095-1137

Sant'Anna, F. M.; Velasque, L.; Costa, M. J.; Schmaltz, C. A.; Morgado, M. G.; Lourenco, M. C.; Grinsztejn, B. & Rolla, V. C. (2009). Effectiveness of Highly Active Antiretroviral Therapy (Haart) Used Concomitantly with Rifampicin in Patients with Tuberculosis and Aids, *The Brazilian journal of infectious diseases : an official publication of the Brazilian Society of Infectious Diseases*, Vol.13, No.5, (October 2009), pp.362-366, ISSN 1678-4391

Schoepfer, A. M.; Trummler, M.; Seeholzer, P.; Seibold-Schmid, B. & Seibold, F. (2008). Discriminating IBD from IBS: comparison of the test performance of fecal markers, blood leukocytes, CRP, and IBD antibodies, *Inflammatory Bowel Diseases,* Vol.14, No.1, (January 2008), pp.32-39, ISSN 1078-0998

Science Daily. (2009). In : First Genetic Resistance Factor Against Tuberculosis Infection Identified, 07.08.2011, available from: http://www.sciencedaily.com/releases/2009/12/091201100556.htm

Shelburne, S. A.; Visnegarwala, F.; Darcourt, J.; Graviss, E. A.; Giordano, T. P.; White, A. C., Jr. & Hamill, R. J. (2005). Incidence and Risk Factors for Immune Reconstitution Inflammatory Syndrome During Highly Active Antiretroviral Therapy, *AIDS*, Vol.19, No.4, (March 2005), pp.399-406, ISSN 0269-9370

Siddiqi, U. R.; Warunee, P.; Charoen, P.; Ashino. Y.; Saitoh, H.; Okada, M.; Chotpittayasunondh, T.; & Hattori, T. Elevated anti-tubercular glycolipid antibody titers in healthy adults as well as pulmonary tuberculosis patients in Thailand. *The International Journal of Tuberculosis and Lung Diseases.* in press.

Steingart, K. R.; Dendukuri, N.; Henry, M.; Schiller, I.; Nahid, P.; Hopewell, P. C.; Ramsay, A.; Pai, M. & Laal, S. (2009). Performance of purified antigens for serodiagnosis of pulmonary tuberculosis: a meta-analysis, *Clinical and vaccine immunology,* Vol.16, No.2, (February 2009), pp.260-276, ISSN 1556-679X

Steingart, K. R.; Henry, M.; Laal, S.; Hopewell, P. C.; Ramsay, A.; Menzies, D.; Cunningham, J.; Weldingh, K. & Pai, M. (2007). A systematic review of commercial serological antibody detection tests for the diagnosis of extrapulmonary tuberculosis, *Thorax,* Vol.62, No.10, (October 2007), pp.911-918, ISSN 0040-6376

Steingart, K. R.; Henry, M.; Ng, V.; Hopewell, P. C.; Ramsay, A.; Cunningham, J.; Urbanczik, R.; Perkins, M.; Aziz, M. A. & Pai, M. (2006). Fluorescence versus conventional sputum smear microscopy for tuberculosis: a systematic review, *The Lancet infectious disease* Vol.6, No.9, (September 2006), pp.570-581, ISSN 1473-3099

Streitz, M.; Fuhrmann, S.; Powell, F.; Quassem, A.; Nomura, L.; Maecker, H.; Martus, P.; Volk, H. D. & Kern, F. (2011). Tuberculin-Specific T Cells Are Reduced in Active Pulmonary Tuberculosis Compared to Ltbi or Status Post Bcg Vaccination, *The Journal of infectious diseases*, Vol.203, No.3, (Febrary 2011), pp.378-382, ISSN 1537-6613

Tessema, T. A.; Bjune, G.; Hamasur, B.; Svenson, S.; Syre, H. & Bjorvatn, B. (2002). Circulating antibodies to lipoarabinomannan in relation to sputum microscopy, clinical features and urinary anti-lipoarabinomannan detection in pulmonary tuberculosis, *Scandinavian journal of infectious disease*, Vol.34, No.2, pp.97-103, ISSN 0036-5548

Verma, R. K. & Jain, A. (2007). Antibodies to mycobacterial antigens for diagnosis of tuberculosis, *FEMS immunology and medical microbiology*, Vol.51, No.3, (December 2007), pp.453-461, ISSN 0928-8244

Walsh, M. C.; Camerlin, A. J.; Miles, R.; Pino, P.; Martinez, P.; Mora-Guzman, F.; Crespo-Solis, J. G.; Fisher-Hoch, S. P.; McCormick, J. B. & Restrepo, B. I. (2011). The sensitivity of interferon-gamma release assays is not compromised in tuberculosis patients with diabetes, *The international journal of tuberculosis and lung diseases : the offcial journal of the International Union against Tuberculosis and Lung Diseases*, Vol.15, No.2, (February 2011), pp.179-184, i-iii, ISSN 1815-7920

Walzl, G.; Ronacher, K.; Hanekom, W.; Scriba, T. J. & Zumla, A. (2011). Immunological Biomarkers of Tuberculosis, *Nature reviews. Immunology*, Vol.11, No.5, (May 2011), pp.343-354, ISSN 1474-1741

Wilcke, J. T.; Jensen, B. N.; Ravn, P.; Andersen, A. B. & Haslov, K. (1996). Clinical Evaluation of Mpt-64 and Mpt-59, Two Proteins Secreted from Mycobacterium Tuberculosis, for Skin Test Reagents, *Tubercle and lung disease : the official journal of the International Union against Tuberculosis and Lung Disease*, Vol.77, No.3, (June 1996), pp.250-256, ISSN 0962-8479

Wilkinson, R. J.; Haslov, K.; Rappuoli, R.; Giovannoni, F.; Narayanan, P. R.; Desai, C. R.; Vordermeier, H. M.; Paulsen, J.; Pasvol, G.; Ivanyi, J. & Singh, M. (1997). Evaluation of the recombinant 38-kilodalton antigen of Mycobacterium tuberculosis as a potential immunodiagnostic reagent, *Journal of clinical microbiology*, Vol.35, No.3, (March 1997), pp.553-557, ISSN 0095-1137

Worodria, W.; Massinga-Loembe, M.; Mazakpwe, D.; Luzinda, K.; Menten, J.; Van Leth, F.; Mayanja-Kizza, H.; Kestens, L.; Mugerwa, R.; Reiss, P. & Colebunders, R. (2011). Incidence and Predictors of Mortality and the Effect of Tuberculosis Immune Reconstitution Inflammatory Syndrome in a Cohort of Tb/Hiv Patients Commencing Antiretroviral Therapy, *Journal of acquired immune deficiency syndromes*, (June 2011), ISSN 1944-7884

Wu, B.; Huang, C.; Kato-Maeda, M.; Hopewell, P. C.; Daley, C. L.; Krensky, A. M. & Clayberger, C. (2007). Messenger RNA expression of IL-8, FOXP3, and IL-12beta differentiates latent tuberculosis infection from disease, *Journal of immunology*, Vol.178, No.6 , (March 2007), pp.3688-3694, ISSN 0022-1767

Wu, X.; Yang, Y.; Zhang, J.; Li, B.; Liang, Y.; Zhang, C.; Dong, M.; Cheng, H. & He, J. (2010). Humoral immune responses against the Mycobacterium tuberculosis 38-kilodalton,

MTB48, and CFP-10/ESAT-6 antigens in tuberculosis, *Clinical and vaccine immunology,* Vol.17, No.3, (March 2010), pp.372-375, ISSN 1556-679X

Yamashiro, S.; Kawakami, K.; Uezu, K.; Kinjo, T.; Miyagi, K.; Nakamura, K. & Saito, A. (2005). Lower expression of Th1-related cytokines and inducible nitric oxide synthase in mice with streptozotocin-induced diabetes mellitus infected with Mycobacterium tuberculosis, *Clinical and experimental immunology,* Vol.139, No.1, (January 2005), pp.57-64, ISSN 0009-9104

Yew, W. W. & Leung, C. C. (2006). Antituberculosis drugs and hepatotoxicity, *Respirology,* Vol.11, No.6, (November 2006), pp.699-707, ISSN 1323-7799

Zhu, C.; Anderson, A. C.; Schubart, A.; Xiong, H.; Imitola, J.; Khoury, S. J.; Zheng, X. X.; Strom, T. B. & Kuchroo, V. K. (2005). The Tim-3 ligand galectin-9 negatively regulates T helper type 1 immunity, *Nature immunology,Vol.*6, No.12, (December 2005), pp.1245-1252, ISSN 1529-2908

18

Immune Diagnosis of Tuberculosis Through Novel Technologies

Miguel A. Arroyo-Ornelas[1], Ma. Concepción Arenas-Arrocena[1], Horacio V. Estrada[2], Victor M. Castaño[1] and Luz M. López-Marín[1]

[1]*Centro de Física Aplicada y Tecnología Avanzada, Universidad Nacional Autónoma de México, Querétaro,*
[2]*Centro Nacional de Metrología, Querétaro, México*

1. Introduction

Due to its highly contagious nature, the control of tuberculosis (TB) is strongly dependent on the efficiency of diagnosis. Natural history of TB comprises two main stages: a latent, non-infective form, in which bacilli are efficiently controlled by the human defense system and, active TB disease, whose pulmonary form is the most common and infective variant in humans (Figure 1). Diagnosis of TB is needed at different stages: the detection of latent TB, a condition estimated to be present in one third of the world population (Russell et al 2010), screening tests for active TB in large populations and confirmatory/drug-susceptibility diagnostic tools aimed to select appropriate chemotherapy regimes. In particular, tools to screen active, contagious TB cases are critical to overcome diagnosis delays, transmission and spread of the disease, and represent one of the top priorities for TB control. For more than a century, diagnosis of active TB has been essentially based on sputum smear microscopy (SSM). Simple and rapid, considered a low-cost control tool, SSM fails however to detect about half of active pulmonary cases since its sensitivity is compromised by low bacterial loads: only above 10^4 bacilli per ml of sputum are detectable by SSM (Abebe et al, 2007). Moreover, detection of positive smears needs to be confirmed in three independent samples so that mycobacteria other than *M. tuberculosis*, which may be present as normal flora do not generate false positive diagnosis results. When suspected cases still remain, time-consuming and high-cost *M. tuberculosis* cultures are required. For many decades, a myriad of alternative tools have been explored to replace SSM for screening active TB. After growth of the pathogen inside a body, exposition to bacterial components is followed by the secretion of specific antibodies. Antibodies associated to active TB are not correlated to protective immunity, but their presence may be exploited as biomarker for active TB. In this chapter, the potential of antigen-antibody measurements to screen active TB will be pointed up, with a special emphasis in the need for controlling particular but large populations. The basis, challenges and opportunities of immune diagnosis will be described, putting an emphasis on our work involving novel technologies.

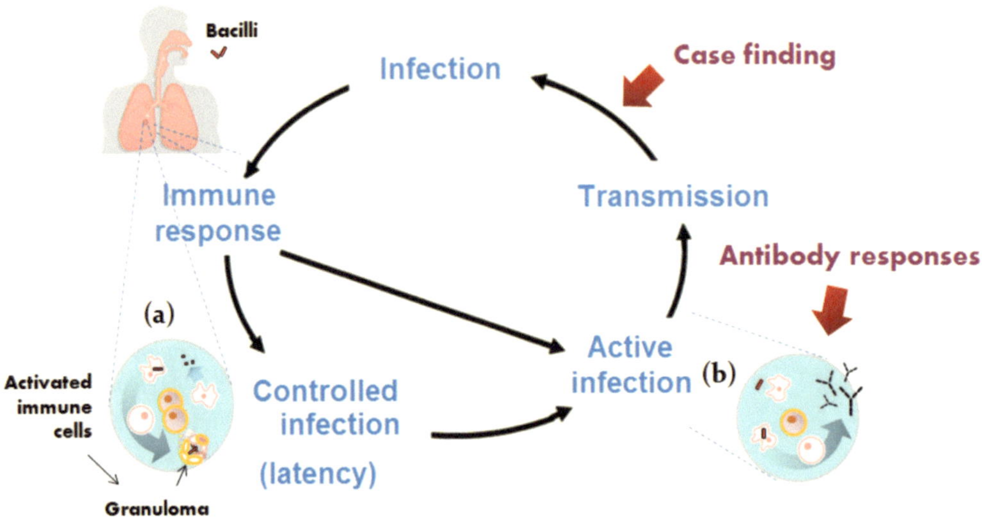

Fig. 1. Natural history of *Mycobacterium tuberculosis* infection. *M. tuberculosis* is an obligate pathogen normally acquired through respiratory tract. After infection, establishment of human response is able to contain microbial growth in 90 - 95% cases; this process is characterized by activation, recruitment and/or proliferation of distinct cells in the infectious foci, growth control and confinement of the pathogen inside a granuloma, a condition called as latent TB (Inlet a). In contrast, immune compromised-associated conditions lead to active disease, characterized by microbial growth, tissue damage and antibody production (Inlet b). Case finding of active cases is critical to stop TB transmission. Antibodies, depicted using the symbol Y, and antigens liberated from bacteria may serve as biomarkers at this infection stage.

2. The need of rapid tests for diagnosing active TB

Efficient treatment is available for most cases of TB. However, thousands of deaths are reported every day due to TB. Due to the fact that healthy immune systems are a condition for TB containment, malnourishment, poverty and a fail in Public Health coverage have been strongly associated to the development of active TB cases. The burdens of TB morbidity and mortality have a tremendous impact in young adults, children and women, and result in the loss of potentially healthy and productive life. It is estimated that active TB cases result in a strong economical impact through loss of work, absence from school and public health expenses. Accentuating this scenario, TB active cases also represent the major cause of death during human immunodeficiency virus (HIV) infection. To deal with this problem, the availability of simple diagnostic tools for the detection of tuberculosis is essential, as it is the basis to treat and control infective cases. During the last years, a set of novel diagnostic methodologies have been developed. Some popular examples are tools based on nucleic acid amplification, such as the polymerase chain reaction (PCR), or the introduction of radioactive probes to speed bacterial culture detection (WHO, 2009). Many new diagnostic technologies had been based on sophisticated equipment and highly specialized training, but up to 90% TB cases occur in low-income settings (WHO 2006), making those methods unaffordable. Thus, novel approaches must be focused in the diagnosis of TB at high-burden settings. A few years ago, the World Health Organization (WHO) has prompted for the development of tests for active TB optimally fulfilling seven requirements, the so-called ASSURED diagnostic tests:

- Affordable by those at risk of infection
- Sensitive (few false-negatives)
- Specific (few false-positives)
- User-friendly (simple to perform and requiring minimal training)
- Rapid (to enable treatment at first visit and Robust (does not require refrigerated storage)
- Equipment-free
- Delivered to those who need them

Currently, the development of ASSURED tests has been considered for the control of a variety of diseases, including TB, malaria, syphilis and dengue. Considering the number of affected people and the feasibility for its development, the availability of an ASSURED test for the screening of active TB would have a tremendous, positive impact in World Public Health (Mabey et al, 2004). Before the emergence of human immune deficiency virus (HIV) epidemy, TB became "invisible to international donors and taken to be a fact of life in the most-affected parts of the world" (Dye & Williams, 2010). Thereby, the search for better vaccines, therapeutic and diagnostic tools was neglected for decades, even for more than a century in some cases (Kaufmann & Parida 2007). At present, this lack of technological developments has made TB control tools virtually inaccessible for most endemic settings. Manipulation of *M. tuberculosis* specimens represents a high level biological risk, requiring high-cost, sophisticated facilities. For these reasons, diagnosis based on the immune response to *M. tuberculosis* represents an alternative to cover the main indications for an ASSURED test, including minimal handling requirements, rapidity and adaptability to close-to- the-patient formats. In this chapter we will describe the biological basis, challenges and opportunities related to immunological tests, with an emphasis on point-of-care (POC) tests. In addition to rapid immunochromatography formats that have been explored by various groups, we herein propose the development of friendly, label-free platforms, using Micro-Electro-Mechanical Systems (MEMS).

3. Human immune response to *Mycobacterium tuberculosis* infection

It is estimated that one third of the World population is currently infected by *M. tuberculosis* (Dye & Williams, 2010). After infection, *M. tuberculosis* is promptly recognized by the innate immune system. Pattern-recognition receptors located at the surface of myeloid cells, such as mannose recognizing receptors located in macrophages or dendritic cells, recognize molecular patterns commonly associated to pathogens and immediately respond through pro-inflammatory signals (Dorhoi et al, 2011). Whether this process is able to control the spread of the bacilli is still controversial. Supporting the hypothesis is the fact that a number of healthy contacts have been reported with no apparent sign of acquired immunity, thus suggesting that innate mediators were able to stop the infection before the establishment of adaptive, memory-derived responses (Dorhoi et al, 2011). In most people, however, the establishment of innate immunity allows a set of specific defence mechanisms to be initiated. This process involves destruction of bacilli by professional phagocytes, and presentation of pathogen molecular fragments (antigens) to lymphocytes, followed by activation and proliferative steps. This response, also known as adaptive immunity, may give rise to either protection via the containment of the bacilli inside a granuloma, or an exacerbated inflammatory process associated to destructive pathology. In both cases, lymphocytes that specifically recognize their cognate antigen are activated, leading to the production of cytokines or antibodies, the destruction of infected cells and, the formation of memory lymphocyte clones. Since these processes involve mechanisms specifically originated during *M. tuberculosis* infection, the associated biomarkers have been largely exploited for diagnostic purposes.

An overview of adaptive, cell-mediated responses to *M. tuberculosis* is schematized in Fig. 2. Adaptive responses take place when lymphocytes recognize mycobacterial molecules as

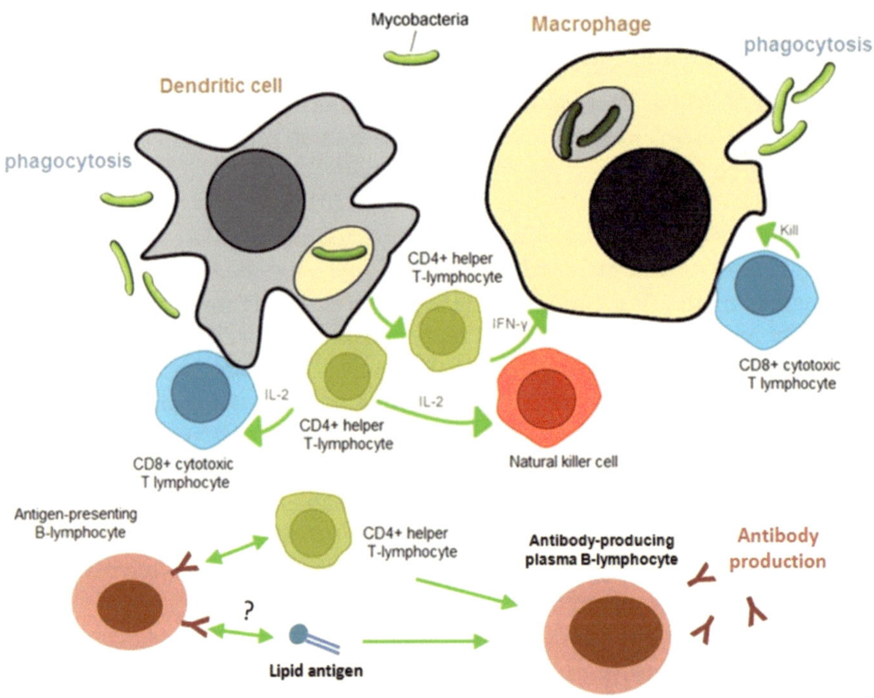

Fig. 2. Cell-mediated immunity against *M. tuberculosis* infection. After recognition and engulfment of the pathogen by phagocytic cells (macrophages, dendritic cells), bacterial components (antigens) are processed into small fragments and presented to lymphocytes. Thymus-derived T-lymphocytes recognize antigens presented by antigen-presenting cells, such as macrophages, dendritic cells and B-lymphocytes. After antigen recognition, T-cells are activated and develop into cytokine-producing (CD4+) cells or cytolytic (CD8+) mediators. B-cells are directly activated by antigens. However, fully activation of B-cells may be coordinated by interactions with CD4+ T-cells, in the case of peptide antigens, or through thymus-independent, poorly described pathways for non-protein antigens, such as lipids. Figure is out of scale.

foreign entities (as antigens). Two lymphocyte families, the T and B-cells, are activated after encountering with their matching antigen, then develop into the effectors of adaptive immunity. For T cells, presentation of foreign entities by antigen-presenting cells is mandatory for recognition. In contrast, B cells recognize their cognate antigens through direct interaction via the B-cell receptor. Once activated, B and T cells trigger a variety of functions, mainly including: (a) secretion of cytokines and chemoattractants by CD4+ helper T-cells, (b) lysis of infected cells via the release of lytic enzymes by CD8+ cytotoxic T-cells, (c) secretion of antibodies by plasma B-cells that have been derived from activated B-lymphocytes, (d) production of a number of long-lived memory T- and B-cells, which last for many years circulating in the bloodstream and monitor for infection (either newly developed or endogenously re-activated).

As depicted in Figure 2, some responses related to cell-mediated immunity are restricted to active infection. One illustrative example is the release of some pro-inflammatory cytokines by T-cells, such as interferon-gamma. The secretion of specific antibodies by plasma B-lymphocytes also occurs during active or newly acquired TB, where antigen-presenting cells are charged with bacterial moieties. Some of the immune responses during active infection are known to be critical for arresting the growth of *M. tuberculosis*. In contrast, antibody secretion has been considered irrelevant, although some recent studies suggest a role for antibodies on the fate of *M. tuberculosis* infection (Glatman-Freedman et al, 2010). Yet, secretion of antibodies during bacterial growth (*i.e.* during active infection) can be exploited to detect infectious cases, thus contributing to stop TB transmission.

Isolated specific antigens have been used for detecting antibodies in human plasma, through the measurement of antigen-antibody reactions *in vitro*. Alternatively, antibodies may be produced in the lab and used to capture mycobacterial antigens that have been secreted to body fluids. Because free mycobacterial antigens are not encountered in many biological fluids, our work has been dedicated to the detection of antibodies. Importantly, antibodies associated to *M. tuberculosis* disease are found in sera from individuals affected by both pulmonary and extra-pulmonary TB, thus allowing the detection of difficult-to-detect TB pathologies (Daniel, 1989). Challenges related to the production of antigens for diagnostic tests will be presented in the following sections.

4. Antigen repertoire of *M. tuberculosis*

Specific activation of immune cells against *M. tuberculosis* occurs after the recognition of bacterial components as foreign entities. With about 4,000 genes (TubercuList web page), *M. tuberculosis* synthesizes a complex array of molecular products, mainly composed of proteins, lipids and carbohydrates. Box 1 summarizes the highlights of different antigens from the bacillus.

5. Immunodiagnosis of TB: From Koch to POC tests

A few years after Robert Koch discovered *M. tuberculosis*, his work was largely dedicated to look for a cure against TB disease, which was the major health threat in Europe by the time. His work allowed the description of *M. tuberculosis* extracts, obtained by glycerol extraction of liquid cultures of the bacilli (Kaufmann & Schaible 2005). Although this material, called tuberculin, was found unable to inhibit the growth of *M. tuberculosis* in guinea pigs or

***M. tuberculosis* is a bacterial pathogen of atypical molecular composition:**

- Protein molecular patterns include stress-inducible proteins of wide distribution within bacteria, enzymes presenting homology with many other human pathogens (bacteria and parasites), and newly described or putative gene products devoid of homology vis-à-vis any other peptide annotated so far (16% of *M. tuberculosis* open reading frames are novel sequences).
- Cellular wall is unusually thick, conferring unique properties of tinction (*M. tuberculosis* is not Gram+ nor Gram-) and atypical antibiotic susceptibility patterns.
- Genes related to lipid metabolism are especially abundant (5-fold more genes in *M. tuberculosis* genome compared to that of *Escherichia coli*). In accordance, the Koch bacillus produces lipids with amazing structural features and sizes (fatty acids up to 80 carbons length). Many of these lipids are recognized as antigens during active TB.
- Carbohydrate products have distinctive structures. Polysaccharides and glycoconjugates (glycolipids, glycoproteins) comprise molecular motifs recognized by innate immune cells and important virulence factors. In contrast to findings in model animals, sera from *M. tuberculosis*-infected humans strongly recognize sugar structures.
- Shared with other bacteria, some small phosphorus-containing compounds, phosphoantigens, constitute a separate group of antigens in *M. tuberculosis*. Phosphoantigens activate a set of unusual T-cells and possess interesting therapeutic effects against specific lymphomas.

Box 1. **Antigens from *Mycobacterium tuberculosis***

humans, Koch reported for the first time that previously-infected individuals developed a local inflammation at the site where tuberculin was injected, whereas healthy controls did not present such a response (Kaufmann & Schaible 2005). This hypersensitivity reaction was later related to the activation of memory T-cells, which are able to recognize tuberculin-containing antigens. Named the delayed-type hypersensitivity (DTH) test, the intradermal reaction to tuberculin constituted the first diagnostic tool based on the immune response against *M. tuberculosis*, and has been used for more than a century to diagnose latent TB (WHO 2006). During latent TB, memory T-lymphocytes may be searched through either DTH tests performed *in-vivo*, or more rapid, *in-vitro* cytokine analyses (Lalvani 2007, Hanekom et al, 2004). In any case, crude mixtures of mycobacterial antigens, such as tuberculin, often produce unspecific, false-positive results. In fact, *M. tuberculosis* shares a number of antigens with other microorganisms, including vaccine strains against TB. To circumvent this problem, the use of single or a small cocktail of antigens has been proposed. Two secreted protein antigens, ESAT-6 and CFP-10, are worth of mention since a high specificity and abundant T-cell responses have been associated to them (Fox et al, 2007). More recently, a non-protein, lipid antigen has also been proposed as a reagent to look for DTH responses (Komori et al 2011). Considering the lack of gene polymorphism of lipid-presenting molecules in humans (De Libero & Mori 2010), introduction of lipid antigens for diagnosing latent TB appears very promising.

In contrast to memory T-cell responses, production of antibodies requires the presence of plasma circulating B-lymphocytes, a phenomenon associated to active infection (see Figure 2). Therefore, the search for antigen-antibody reactions has been largely explored to diagnose active TB. Such a reaction may be measured in a wide set of platforms, from old agglutination and electrophoretic immune precipitation techniques (Zykov et al 1966), to lab-on-chip formats, in which a set of laboratory procedures are automatically performed within a microfluidics technology-based chip (Schulte et al 2002). Contrasting to cell-mediated responses, the assessment of antigen-antibody reactions does not require special conditions, such as regulated temperature or specific environment. In addition, no exposition to high level biological risk bacilli is involved to obtain plasma or serum samples.

The search for antibodies in body fluids may be performed using a variety of technological platforms. Currently, Enzyme-Linked ImmunoSorbent Assay (ELISA) is the most common method for analyzing antigen-antibody reactions. The typical format used for screening antibodies in sera, an indirect ELISA, is schematized in Figure 3. ELISA has been widely used since the late 80's to screen for active TB (Daniel, 1989). Crude bacterial extracts, including tuberculin, represented the first bacterial materials explored as reagents. One of the most popular mixtures was Antigen-5, a preparation composed of various proteins and lipoarabinomannan, a specific cell-wall glycolipid (Daniel, T. M. et al, 1985). As modern Biochemistry tools have been developed, more purified, specific antigens have been obtained. Up to now, many proteins, post-translationally modified peptides, glycolipids and saccharides have been proposed as antigens for immunodiagnosis of active TB (Steingart et al, 2009).

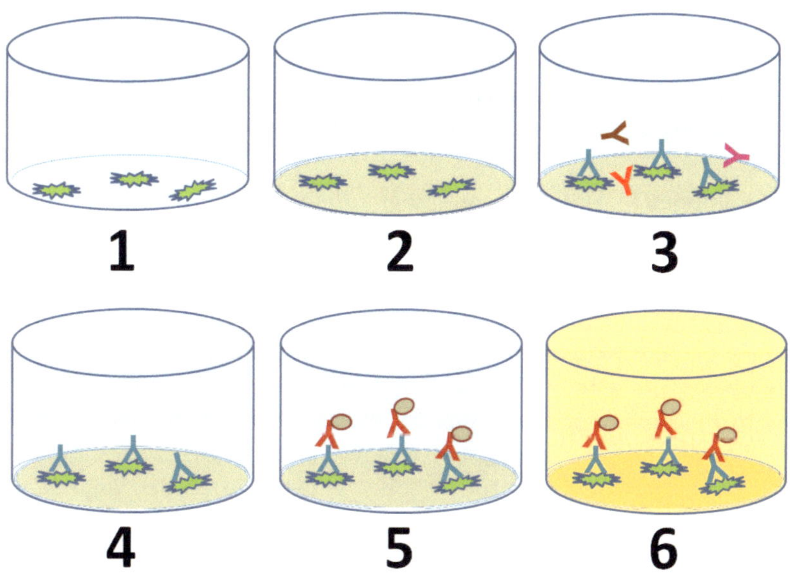

Fig. 3. The Enzyme-Linked ImmunoSorbent Assay for the detection of antibodies. A selected antigen is used to coat a plate surface (1); a solution of non-reacting protein, such as bovine serum albumin, is used to block non-occupied sites at the plate surface, avoiding non-specific binding between serum proteins and the plate (2); serum is added and antibodies bind to matching epitopes of immobilized antigens (3); non-reactive antibodies from sera are eliminated by washings (4); a secondary antibody linked to an enzyme is used to bind the primary, tuberculosis-associated antibody (5); the substrate of the enzyme is added allowing to enzyme-dependent colorimetric changes, which are quantified through spectrophotometry (6).

The development of ELISA represented a breakthrough for the detection of antigen-antibody responses. Before enzyme-linked tests, cumbersome and/or hazardous methods, including radioimmunoassays (RIA), importantly limited the application of immune diagnostic tests for large populations (Lequin, 2005). Yet, an ELISA presents important limitations for large-scale applications. Major drawbacks associated to this technique include: the need of large amounts of samples, a multistep procedure poorly suitable for high throughput scales, and high costs related to the use of enzymatic markers, specialized equipment and trained personnel. Recently, the development of more friendly, equipment-free technologies has been largely explored, importantly including the search for miniaturized analytical devices. In particular, the integration of currently existing detection methods, such as those based on antigen-antibody responses, into microdevices represents a promise for bringing diagnostics closer to those who need it. The introduction of microtechnologies may afford automated systems for the detection of TB at the site of patient care. Such devices have been called Point-Of-Care (POC) tests.

6. Current challenges for the development of POC tests for TB diagnosis

TB is considered one of the most complex diseases ever established in humankind. Active TB has been related to multiple processes but not to any single pathogenic or host factor. Therefore, the demand of technological innovations for the development of POC tests is accompanied by a particular challenge regarding the selection of bioreagents. In the following paragraphs, we enumerate the major current limitations and possible technological solutions for the development of POC tests to diagnose active TB.

6.1 The heterogeneous human response to *M. tuberculosis* antigens

Up to now, few systematic studies to address the antibody response during tuberculosis in humans have been performed. The presence of different antibody secretion patterns in humans has been largely observed. HLA genes encoding for molecules presenting protein antigens, namely the Major Histocompatibility Complex (MHC) molecules, are known to be highly polymorphic in humans, and some data indicate this gene polymorphism as a source of variability to recognize peptide motifs by immune cells (Bothamley et al, 1989). On another side, the spectrum of responses at different stage of the disease may account for important variability. In this way, protein antigens that had proved high sensitivities in some trials, have given unsatisfactory results when tested in a different setting (Gennaro, 2000). The use of species-specific antigens, not present in mycobacteria other than *M. tuberculosis,* is known to be required to avoid false-positive results, and antigens synthesized by vaccine strains are also precluded. According to a meta-analysis reported by Steingart et al. (2009), antibody detection methods could achieve high efficiencies only if a mixture of multiple antigens is used. Most analyzed trials failed, however, to include appropriate healthy controls, thus limiting the results in regard to test specificity. Therefore, in spite of the need to perform better diagnostic trials including appropriate controls, a conclusive remark is the convenience to use a cocktail of antigens. With this in mind, antibodies associated to active TB seem largely elicited by unusual, difficult to obtain mycobacterial antigens.

6.2 The structural nature of various sensitive, specific antigens is not addressable via recombinant technology

According to serodiagnostic analyses performed in TB endemic settings (including ours), antigens able to achieve high diagnostics performances represent mycobacterial components non-addressable by genetic engineering. Some of the highest specificities and sensitivities have been found using glycolipids. These are fatty acyl-containing carbohydrate, secondary genetic products, whose biosynthesis involves multiple enzymatic steps, some of them still undefined. Lipoarabinomannan (LAM), di-*O*-acyl trehalose (DAT) and cord factor (CF) belong to this group of difficult-to-obtain highly performance antigens (Barihuta et al, 1993; Escamilla et al, 1996; López-Marín et al, 2003; Maekura et al, 1993; Julián et al, 2001; Simonney et al, 1996). Besides, some of the best protein antigens to diagnose active TB are post-translationally modified products, namely glycosylated proteins such as the 38-kDa, antigen (Espitia et al, 1989). Worth noting, the best diagnostic performances obtained with this protein have been found when it has been obtained from glycosylating mycobacterial cells. In contrast, a non-glycosylated 38-kDa antigen obtained by recombinant technology in *Escherichia coli* has shown poor efficiencies (Gennaro, 2000).

6.2.1 Surrogate microbial sources of secondary-genetic products

The isolation of glycosylated antigens involves cumbersome steps, making difficult their use in large-scale applications. The involvement of complex, methyl-containing fatty acyl structures in antibody recognition may limit the use of synthetic approaches for these antigens. In view of the structural similarity of glycolipids from *M. tuberculosis* and some other mycobacterial species, we looked for surrogate sources of glycolipids as antigens for TB diagnosis. Structural and serologic studies of glycosylated lipids from mycobacteria allowed the identification of *Mycobacterium fortuitum*, a species of rapidly growing non-tuberculous mycobacteria, as surrogate source for two promising antigens: di-*O*-acyl trehalose (DAT) (Escamilla et al, 1996), and cord factor (López-Marín et al, 2003). Interestingly, *M. fortuitum* synthesizes abundant quantities of DAT and cord factor. The antigens afford specific reactivities vis-à-vis healthy controls and patients infected with other pathogenic actinomycetes (López-Marín et al, 2003). In addition, glycolipids from *M. fortuitum* are not longer recognized by individuals with healed TB and do not present cross-reactivities with vaccinated healthy controls (Escamilla et al, 1996).

6.2.2 Peptide mimicry and combinatorial strategies

Glycosylation has been detected as a critical factor for antibody recognition during active TB. For instance, the ability of antigens from *M. tuberculosis* to bind antibodies in sera from infected people is strongly decreased after periodate treatments, indicating that antibodies predominantly react with carbohydrate determinants (Udaykumar & Saxena, 1991). Sugar antigens in *M. tuberculosis* comprise protein and lipid glycoconjugates. At present, recombinant production of mycobacterial sugars is unfeasible, since biosynthetic pathways are still poorly described. A few decades ago, phage-display based technologies emerged as a powerful method to look for structurally diverse unknown ligands. Through recombinant technology, *E. coli* phages are modified to obtain combinatorial peptides libraries displayed on the virion surface (Smith, 1985). Through this technology, phage displayed peptides with affinity to any ligand can be identified by in-vitro screening (Figure 4). Using a phage displayed dodecapeptide library, we have selected phages with specific binding to a serum directed towards *M. tuberculosis* carbohydrate antigens (Gevorkian et al, 2005). This approach resulted in the identification of peptides that mimic mannose-containing molecules of *M. tuberculosis*. A set of peptides were readily recognized by antibodies raised against mycobacterial sugars. More surprisingly, one of these peptides induced, in rabbits, the production of antibodies recognizing mannan. More recently, Bua and coworkers used this technology to obtain phages as useful reagents for the serodiagnosis of tuberculosis (Bua et al, 2009).

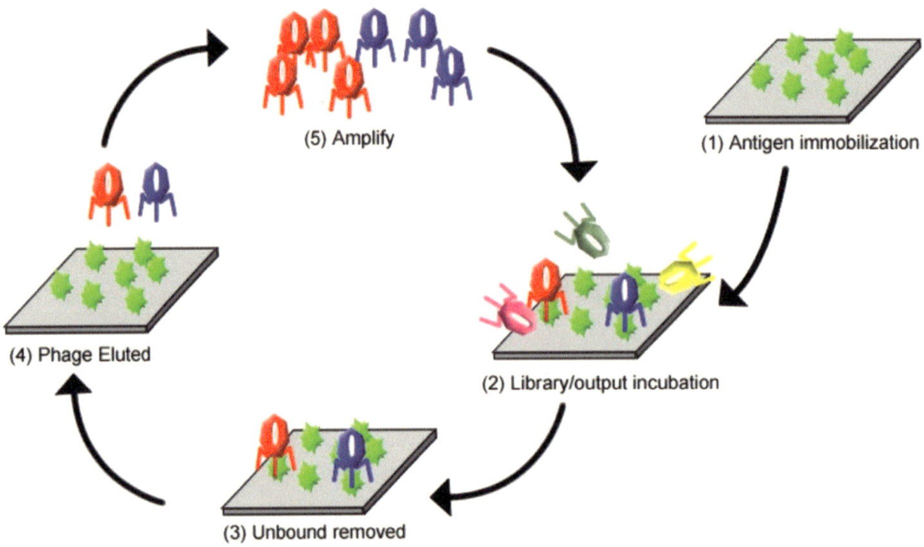

Fig. 4. Phage Display technology for the identification of biological reagents. Combinatorial peptide libraries displayed in virion surfaces can be obtained through genetic engineering. These libraries have proved to be useful for the identification of antibody ligands, even for those associated to poorly defined antigens. In this method, antigens are immobilized on a plate (1) and incubated in the presence of phage suspension (2); non bound phages are removed by washings (3), and selected phage clones are obtained through pH-mediated elution (4); finally, selected clones are amplified (5). The selection cycle is usually repeated 3 times.

Oligopeptides have been found to mimic a set of 3D structures, including sugars, linear and conformational peptide epitopes. Therefore, phage display represents a promising technology for the identification of peptides able to replace difficult-to-obtain or previously unknown antigens. At present, our work is focused to find optimal conditions in order to use peptide mimotopes as immunodiagnostic reagents.

6.2.3 New vectors for the recombinant production of post-translational modified antigens

A different approach to get reagents for diagnosis of TB has been the production of glycosylated proteins of *M. tuberculosis* in novel expression systems. Traditionally, recombinant mycobacterial proteins have been produced in *E. coli*. Mycobacterial glycosyl structures are distinct from mammalian carbohydrates. Thus, expression of *M. tuberculosis* glycoproteins in other actinomycetes, such as rapidly growing *Mycobacterium smegmatis* (Garbe et al, 1993) and *Streptomyces* (Lara et al, 2003) appears as an interesting tool towards the application of serodiagnostics.

6.3 Currently available platforms for POC immunodiagnostics

Screening tests to detect TB are essential to overcome the epidemic. In particular POC tests may be implemented at lower levels of health services, contributing to stop TB transmission. The use of microfluidic technologies seem of special interest since they are associated to small volumes of samples. For instance, POC tests have been already developed to monitor biomarkers in a few blood drops. Two platforms for the study of antigen-antibody interactions are described below, immunochromatography tests and microchip-based devices.

6.3.1 Lateral-flow immunochromatography tests

One of the most advantageous platforms for the study of antigen-antibody reactions is lateral-flow immunochromatography. The basis of this method is schematized in Figure 5. Immunochromatography tests enable added value to antigen-antibody reactions since they allow higher throughput, reduced volume of samples, as well as lower costs than traditional immunoassays, since no specialized equipment or skilled personnel are necessary. Although this format has been used in many endemic settings, antigen evaluations vis-à-vis healthy controls or related pathologies require further studies. To our knowledge, highly specific glycolipid antigens, hydrophobic in nature, have not been included in immunochromatography formats.

6.3.2 Micro-Electro-Mechanical Systems (MEMS)

Based on resistant but flexible silicon platforms constructed through microchip-based technologies, MicroElectroMechanical Systems (MEMS) are micrometric devices which include mechanical parts, such as actuators, sensors or integrated microfluidic systems. MEMS have been widely used in aerospace and automotive industry. Examples of some popular MEMS are microaccelerometers in crash air-bag systems or micromirrors for projection systems. Some of the most attractive features in MEMS are reliability and low-cost, which are associated to their large batch processing. Interestingly, a MEMS is able to perform automated analyses, including transport, separations, chemical reactions and sensing. All necessary instruments can be integrated in a single device, the MEMS, so that new terms, micro Total Analysis Systems (μTAS), and "Lab-On-a-Chip" (LOC) technologies have been coined for such instruments. Over the course of the past fifteen years, MEMS have also been explored for a set of biomedical applications, including metabolite analyses, drug testing, drug discovery, combinatorial assays for DNA screening and, obviously, immunodiagnosis (Hedlund, 2009). Figure 6 shows a scanning electron micrography of a MEMS. A detailed description of MEMS is out of the scope of this chapter. However, we enumerate the key features allowing this technology to be a promising tool for the development of ASSURED tests for diagnosis (Box 2).

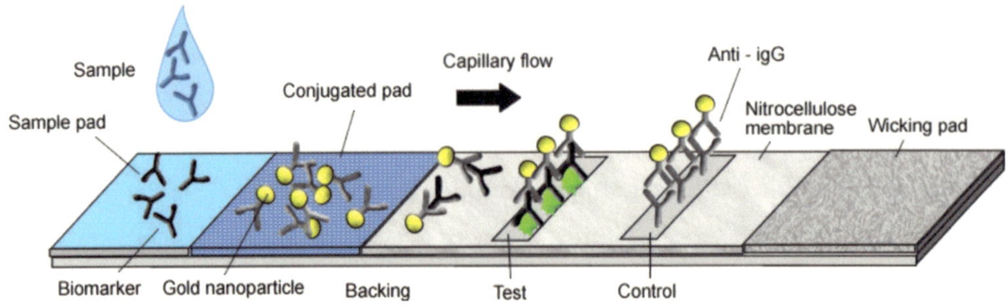

Fig. 5. Immunochromatography platform for assessment of antigen-antibody reactions. Immunochromatography strips contain a sample pad, in which biological fluids are deposited. Capillarity induces a lateral flow of the sample throughout the pad. Frequently, nanocolloidal gold particles are functionalized for conjugation to total antibodies. Antigen immobilized as a line in the nitrocellulose strip captures the antibody-colloidal gold complex. A control line reacting with colloidal gold is also present. After developing, the test can be read since purple lines develop if colloidal gold is hold.

To illustrate the suitability of MEMS technology for clinical POC tests, a good example is the possibility to sense biological markers in a sample using label-free technologies. In MEMS, physical properties, such as conductivity or mass changes, are usually analyzed through electric or optical low-cost systems (Battiston et al, 2001; Fischer, 2011). For immune diagnostic systems, the capture of antibodies by antigen-displaying surfaces will result in changes of mass or conductivity parameters, both of them addressable through MEMS standard technologies (Figure 7).

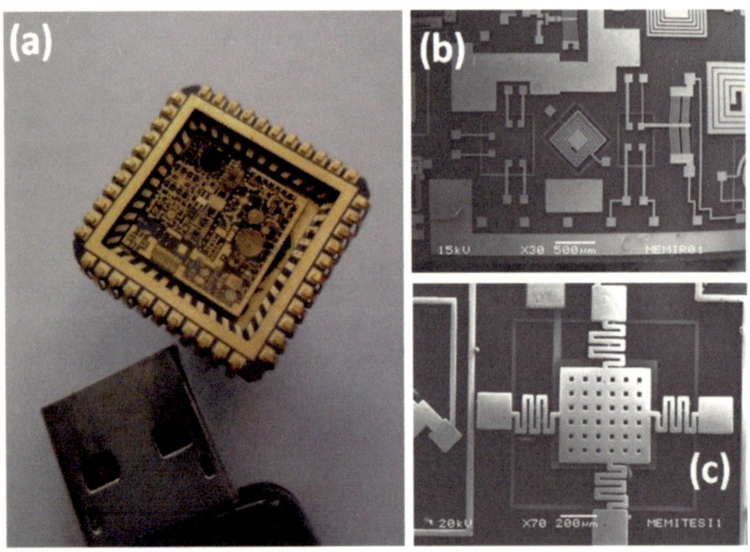

Fig. 6. Panoramic image (a) and scanning electron micrographs (b, c) of a MicroElectroMechanical System (MEMS). Constructed using microchip technology, such as lithography on silica supports, MEMS also contain mechanical components, including beams, gears, diaphragms, grooves, orifices, springs or suspensions and optical systems. Three dimensional fabrication processes allow the design of automated systems able to reproduce any laboratory procedure.

- MEMS are machines with sizes ranging from a micrometer to a few milimetres
- Including mechanical and optical parts, such as actuators, motors or sensors, MEMS are automated Lab-On-Chip machines
- Batch processing determines very low-costs for an individual machine.
- A variety of materials in MEMS technology, including some new advanced materials make possible the application of MEMS in Biomedicine
- Metal surfaces able to immobilize a set of molecules, by keeping bioactivity
- Some developments for biomedical applications already follow clinical tests for their introduction to the market. These include bioMEMS to sense glucose during diabetes or antibodies levels to detect dengue

Box 2. MicroElectroMechanical Systems (MEMS) at a glance

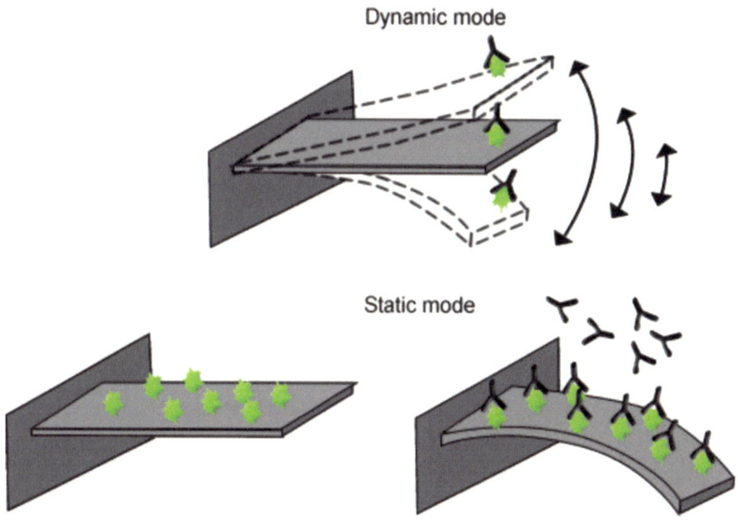

Fig. 7. Label-free measurement systems in MEMS include cantilevers. If antigens are immobilized onto a quartz crystal, fine mass changes, as those produced by antibody capture, will result in measurable alterations in the quartz resonance frequency, an optical property that can be precisely detected combining the use of a laser microbeam and a photodetector

7. Conclusion

A rapid and affordable test for detecting contagious TB patients is the cornerstone of current strategies for TB control. Although a set of clever methods has been proposed for this objective, the search for new tools adaptable to low-resource endemic settings is still a demand. The search of antigen-antibody responses for diagnosing active TB represents a promising alternative, since the associated methods may fulfill the major diagnostic requirements, namely minimal handling, rapidity and adaptability to point-of-care formats. Future success of immunodiagnosis tools for detecting TB will depend on both basic and technological advances: (1) The identification of specific, affordable biological reagents for large scale production (antigens, antibodies or fragments) and (2) The development of immunological tests into low-cost, friendly formats. According to different studies addressing antigen-antibody responses in different populations, the search for antibodies in TB patients must include specific peptides, but also non-protein (lipid) and post-translational modified antigens, such as glycosylated proteins. In this regard, strategies to obtain complex antigens are critical. The development of novel expression systems and phage-display technologies could be the answer. Finally, we herein suggest that, in addition to further improvements of the already explored immunochromatography strips for TB diagnosis, Micro-ElectroMechanical Systems (MEMS) deserve a particular attention to develop better POC tests for diagnosing active, but also to look for tests addressing the detection of inactive, latent TB.

8. Acknowledgments

This work has been supported by Grant IA102611 from Universidad Nacional Autónoma de México (IACOD-DGAPA). We thank the Micro and Nanotechnology Department, ITESI (Guanajuato, Mexico) for providing MEMS devices for Figure 6. Alicia del Real performed SEM analyses of MEMS.

9. References

Abebe, F., Holm-Hansen, C. Wiker, H. G., Bjune, G. (2007). Progress in Serodiagnosis of Mycobacterium tuberculosis Infection. *Scandinavian Journal of Immunology*, Vol.66, No.2-3, (August 2007), pp. 176-191, ISSN 1365-3083.

Barihuta, T., Rigouts, L., Barette, M., Collart, J. P., de Bruyn, J., Kadende, P., Kamamfu, G., Douglas, J. T., Portaels, F. (1993). Rapid, early and specific diagnosis of tuberculosis and other mycobacterial diseases in Burundi. *Annales de la Société Belge de Medicine Tropicale*, Vol.73, Suppl. 1, pp. 41-51, 0365-6527.

Bothamley, G.H., Beck, J.S., Schreuder, G. M., D'Amaro, J., de Vries, R.R., Kardjito, T., Ivanyi, J. (1989). Association of tuberculosis and M. tuberculosis-specific antibody levels with HLA.*The Journal of Infectious Diseases*, Vol.159, No.3, (March 1989), pp. 549-555, ISSN 0022-1899.

Bua, A., Rosu, V., Molicotti, P., das Gupta, S. K., Ahmed, N., Zanetti, S., Sechi, L. A. (2009) Phages specific for mycobacterial arabinomannan help serodiagnosis of tuberculosis. New Microbiologica, Vol.32, No.3, pp. 293-296, ISSN 1121-7138.

Daniel, T.M. (1989). Rapid diagnosis of tuberculosis: Laboratory techniques applicable in developing countries. *Review of Infectious Diseases*, Vol.11, Suppl.2, (April 1989), S471-8, ISSN 0162-088.

Daniel, T.M., Debanne, S.M., van der Kuyp, F. (1985). Enzyme-linked immunosorben assay using Mycobacterium tuberculosis antigen 5 and PPD for the serodiagnosis of tuberculosis, *Chest*, Vol.88, No.3, (September 1985), pp. 388-392, ISSN 1931-3543.

De Libero, G., Mori, L. (2010). How the Immune System Detects Lipid Antigens, *Progress in Lipid Research*, Vol.49, No.2, (October 2009), pp. 120-127, ISSN 0163-7827.

Dorhoi, A., Reece, S.T., Kaufmann, S.H.E. (2011). For better or for worse: the immune response against Mycobacterium tuberculosis balances pathology and protection. *Immunological Reviews*, Vol.240, No.1, (March 2011), pp. 235-251, ISSN 1600-065X.

Dye, C. & Williams, B. G. (2010). The Population Dynamics and Control of Tuberculosis. *Science*, Vol.328, No.5989, (May 2010), pp. 856-861, ISSN 1095-9203.

Escamilla, L., Mancilla, R., Glender, W., López-Marín, L.M. (1996). Mycobacterium fortuitum glycolipids for the serodiagnosis of pulmonary tuberculosis. *American*

Journal of Respiratory and Critical Care Medicine, Vol.154, No.6, (December 1996), pp. 1864-1867, ISSN 0003-0805.

Espitia, C., Cervera, I., González, R., Mancilla, R. (1989). A 38-kD Mycobacterium tuberculosis antigen associated with infection. Its isolation and serologic evaluation. *Clinical and Experimental Immunology*, Vol.77, No.3, (September 1989), pp. 373-377, ISSN 1365-2249.

Fischer, L.M., Pedersen, C., Elkjaer, K., Noeth, N-N, S., Boisen, A., Tenje, M. (2011). Development of a microfabricated electrochemical-cantilever hybrid platform. *Sensors and Actuators, B: Chemical*, Vol.157, No.1, (September 2011), pp. 321-327, ISSN 0925-4005.

Fox, A., Jeffries, D.J., Hill, P.C., Hammond, A.S., Lugos, M.D., et al. (2007). ESAT-6 and CFP-10 can be combined to reduce the cost of testing for Mycobacterium tuberculosis infection, but CFP-10 responses associate with active disease. *Transactions of the Royal Society of Tropical Medicine and Hygiene*, Vol.101, No.7, (July 2007), pp. 691-698, ISSN 0035-9203.

Garbe, T., Harris, D., Vordemeier, M., Lathigra, R., Ivanyi, J., Young, D. (1993). Expression of the Mycobacterium tuberculosis 19-kilodalton antigen in Mycobacterium smegmatis : immunological analysis and evidence of glycosylation. *Infection and Immunity*, Vol. 61, No.1, (January 1993), pp. 260-267, ISSN 1098-5522.

Gevorkian, G., Segura, E., Acero, G., Palma, J.P., Espitia, C., Manoutcharian, K., López-Marín, L.M. (2005). Peptide mimotopes of Mycobacterium tuberculosis carbohydrate immunodeterminants. *Biochemical Journal*, Vol.387, Pt.2, (April 2005), pp. 411-417, ISSN 1470-8728.

Gennaro, M. L. (2000). Immunologic Diagnosis of Tuberculosis. *Clinical Infectious Diseases*, Vol.30, Suppl.3, pp. S243-S246, ISSN 1537-6591.

Glatman-Freedman, A. (2006) The role of antibody-mediated immunity in defense against Mycobacterium tuberculosis: advances toward a novel vaccine strategy. Tuberculosis (Edinb), Vol. 86, No 3-4, pp. 191-197. ISSN 1873-281X.

Hanekom, W.A., Hughes, J., Mavinkurve, M., Mendillo, M., Watkins, M. et al. (2004). Novel application of a whole blood intracellular cytokine detection assay to quantitate specific T-cell frequency in field studies. *Journal of Immunological Methods*, Vol.291, No.1-2, (August 2004), pp. 185-195, ISSN 0022-1759.

Hedlund, J., Lundgren, A., Lundgren, B., Elwing, H. (2009). P13 - A new compact electrochemical method for analyzing complex protein films adsorbed on the surface of modified interdigitated gold electrodes. *Sensors and Actuators, B, Chemical*, Vol.142, No.2, (November 2009), pp. 494–501, ISSN 0925-4005.

Julián, E., Cama, M., Martinez, P., Luquín, M. (2001). An ELISA for five glycolipids from the cell wall of Mycobacterium tuberculosis Tween-20 interference in the assay. *Journal of Immunological Methods*, Vol. 251, No. 1-2, (May 2001), pp. 21-30, ISSN 0022-1759.

Kaufmann, S.H.E., Parida, S.K. (2007). Changing funding patterns in tuberculosis. *Nature Medicine*, Vol.13, No.3, (March 2007), pp. 299-303, ISSN 1078-8956.

Kaufmann, S.H.E., Schaible, U.E. (2005). 100th anniversary of Robert Koch's Nobel Prize for the discovery of the tubercle bacillus. *Trends in Microbiology*, Vol.13, No.10, (October 2005), pp. 469-475. ISSN 0966-842X.

Komori, T., Nakamura, T., Matsunaga, I. et al. (2011). A Microbial Glycolipid Functions as a New Class of Target Antigen for Delayed-type Hypersensitivity. *The Journal of Biological Chemistry*, Vol.286, No.19, (March 2011), pp. 16800-16806, ISSN *0021-9258*.

Lalvani, A. (2007). Diagnosing Tuberculosis Infection in the 21st Century: New Tools to tackle an Old Enemy. *Chest*, Vol.31, No.6, (June 2007), pp. 1898-1906, ISSN 1931-3543.

Lara, M., Servín-González, L., Singh, M., Moreno, C., Cohen, I., Nimtz, M., Espitia, C. (2004). Expression, Secretion, and Glycosylation of the 45- and 47-kDa Glycoprotein of Mycobacterium tuberculosis in Streptomyces lividans. *Applied and Environmental Microbiology*, Vol.70, No.2, (February 2004), pp. 679-685, ISSN 1098-5336.

López-Marín, L.M., Segura, E., Hermida-Escobedo, C., Lemassu, A., Salinas-Carmona, M.C. (2003). 6,6′-dimycoloyl trehalose from a rapidly growing Mycobacterium: an alternative antigen for tuberculosis serodiagnosis. *FEMS Immunology and Medical Microbiology*, Vol.36, No.1-2, (May 2003), pp. 47-54, ISSN 1574-695X.

Mabey, D., Peeling, R.W., Ustianowski, A., Perkins, M.D. (2004). Diagnostics for the Developing World. *Nature Reviews in Microbiology*, Vol.2, No.3, (March 2004), pp. 231-240, ISSN 1740-1526.

Maekura, R., Nakagawa, M., Nakamura, Y., Hiraga, T., Yamamura, Y., Ito, M., Ueda, E., Yano, S., He, H., Oka, S., Kashima, K., Yano, I. (1993). Clinical evaluation of rapid serodiagnosis of pulmonary tuberculosis by ELISA with cord factor (trehalose 6,6′-dimycolate) as antigen purified from Mycobacterium tuberculosis. *American Review of Respiratory Diseases*, Vol.148, Pt.1, (October 1993), pp. 997-1001, ISSN0003-0805

Russell, D.G., Barry, C.E. 3rd, Flynn, J.L. (2010). Tuberculosis: What we don't know can, and does, hurt us. *Science*, Vol.328, No.5980, (May 2010), pp. 852-855, ISSN 1095-9203.

Schulte, T.H., Bardell, R.L., Weigl, B.H. (2002). Microfluidic technologies in clinical diagnostics, *Clinica Chimica Acta*, Vol.321, No.1-2, (July 2002), pp. 1-10, ISSN 0009-8981.

Smith, G. P. (1985).Filamentous fusion phage: novel expression vectors that display cloned antigens on the virion surface. *Science*, Vol.228, No. 4705, (June 1985), pp. 1315-1317, ISSN 1095-9203.

Steingart, K. R., Dendukuri, N., Henry, M., Schiller, I., Nahid, P., Hopewell, P. C., Ramsay, A., Pai, M., Laal, S. (2009). Performance of Purified Antigens for Serodiagnosis of Pulmonary Tuberculosis: a Meta-Analysis. *Clinical and Vaccine Immunology*, Vol.16, No.2, (February 2009), pp. 260-276, ISSN 1556-6811.

Simonney, N., Molina, J.M., Molimard, M., Oksenhendler, E., Lagrange, P.H. (1996). Comparison of A60 and three glycolipid antigens in an ELISA test for tuberculosis. *Clinical Microbiology and Infections*, Vol.2, No.3 (February 1996), pp. 214-222, ISSN 1469-0691.

The New Diagnostics Working Group of the Stop TB Partnership, WHO (2009). *Pathways to better diagnostics for tuberculosis,* WHO, ISBN 9778 92 4 159881 1, Switzerland.

Udaykumar, Saxena, R.K. (1991). Antigenic epitopes on Mycobacterium tuberculosis recognized by antibodies in tuberculosis and mouse antisera. *FEMS Microbiology and Immunology*, Vol.3, No.1, (February 1991), pp. 7-12, ISSN 0920-8534.

World Health Organization/Tropical Diseases (2006). *Diagnostics for Tuberculosis. Global Demand and Market Potential,* WHO, ISBN 978 92 4 156330 7, Switzerland.

Zykov, M.P., Geser, A., Egsmose, T. et al. (1966). A serological test of tuberculosis. A "Blind" Trial of the Kaolin-Agglutination Test (KAT) for Detection of Tuberculosis Antibodies. *Bulletin of the World Health Organization*, Vol.35, No.4, pp. 581-592, ISSN 0042-9686.

19

Exosomes: New Tuberculosis Biomarkers – Prospects From the Bench to the Clinic

Nicole A. Kruh-Garcia[1], Jeff S. Schorey[2] and Karen M. Dobos[1]
[1]*Colorado State University*
[2]*University of Notre Dame*
USA

1. Introduction

Biomarkers, derived from either the host (e.g. immunological markers, such as cytokines) or infectious agent (e.g. exported products, such as lipoarabinomannan), are indicative not only of disease but also of disease stage, severity and drug failure. Discovering new biomarkers from easily attainable bodily fluids is essential if we are to control tuberculosis, a diseases that kills 1.5 to 2 million individuals a year. The ideal biomarker could be used in the diagnosis and prognosis of disease from any suspect patient regardless of age, immune status or vaccination history. One potential biomarker source is exosomes; small membrane-bound vesicles released from cells which can be found circulating in the blood, and can be readily harvested for diagnostic testing. Exosomes shed from *Mycobacterium tuberculosis* (*Mtb*) infected samples (from *in vitro* produced to *in vivo* models and clinical samples) could provide an ideal reservoir of tuberculosis biomarkers. While it is possible to detect and monitor host and other bacterial components on exosomes, the scope of the following experiments are focused specifically on the *Mtb* proteins that are incorporated into exosomes.

1.1 Detection of tuberculosis

New diagnostic measures for the detection of tuberculosis are needed to identify and distinguish individuals with active tuberculosis from those harboring the dormant *Mtb* bacillus. The established method of TB detection for over seventy years is the tuberculin skin test (TST) or Mantoux test. This approach monitors the presence and diameter of induration as an indicator of the delayed-type hypersensitivity reaction to an intradermal injection of purified protein derivative (PPD) of *Mtb*. Despite its worldwide use, there are several fundamental problems with the TST. First, while it can be used as an indicator of both the active disease and the asymptomatic, latent tuberculosis infection (LTBI), the test cannot differentiate between the two. Second, false positive results are frequent, most commonly due to a history of Bacille Calmette Guérin (BCG) vaccination. Similarly, due to the dominance of several conserved heat-shock protein in PPD, and their influence on the antigenicity of PPD (Yang, Troudt et al.), there is frequent cross-reactivity between infections with nontuberculosis mycobacterium (NTM) species (such as *M. avium*). Most disconcerting are false negative readings typically associated with impaired immune function (attributed to infections with HIV or with drug use).

The development of the interferon-gamma release assay (IGRA) has addressed some of the problems associated with the TST. Two types of IGRA test are currently commercially available, QuantiFERON-TB (Cellestis Limited) and T-SPOT-TB (Oxford Immunotec). Both measure the host biomarker, interferon-gamma (INF-γ) in whole-blood after stimulation with the mycobacterial antigens ESAT-6 and CFP10, by either ELISA or ELISpot assay, respectively. The T-SPOT-TB appears to be the most comprehensive diagnostic test to date (Table 1). Lastly, the Xpert MTB/RIF assay (Cephid) is a nucleic acid amplification based diagnostic and has the advantage of identifying resistance to rifampicin. However, since none of the aforementioned tests can distinguish between active and latent infections, sputum collection followed by microscopy (AFB smear) and culture, as well as chest radiography must be performed. The AFB smear test is simple, cost-effective and achieves high specificity; however this test suffers from a lack of sensitivity as on average it only detects 50% of active TB patients and even less in HIV positive patients and children.

Test	**Detects active TB**	**Detects latent TB**	**Distinguishes between active and latent TB**	**Distinguishes between BCG vaccination and *Mtb* infection**	**Distinguishes between *Mtb* and NTM infection**	**Reliable results in immune-compromised patients?**
AFB Smear	Yes	No	Yes	Yes	No	Yes[1]
AFB culture	Yes	No	Yes	Yes	Yes	Yes[1]
TST	Yes	Yes	No	No	No	No
Quanti-FERON	Yes	Yes	No	**Yes**	Yes [2]	[3]
T-SPOT-TB	Yes	Yes	No	**Yes**	Yes [2]	**Yes**
Xpert MTB/RIF	Yes	Yes	[3]	**Yes**	**Yes**	**Yes**
Clearview TB ELISA	Yes	No	Yes		**No**	**Yes**

[1]Provided that sputum can be obtained.
[2]This method can discriminate between most NTM (exceptions are *M. gordonae, M. kansasii, M. szulgai* and *M. marinum*); but it cannot distinguish between other members of the *Mtb* complex (*M. bovis, M. africanum, M. microti* and *M. canetti*).
[3]Data is limited.

Table 1. Comparison of a sampling of tuberculosis detection methods.

The ideal diagnostic would minimize false positives due to BCG vaccination and infections with NTM, eliminate false negatives associated with the immunocompromised and be able to distinguish between active and latent infections while permitting increased case detection via a robust, cheap, fast and sensitive assay for its use in high-burden, low-income countries. According to the World Health Organization (WHO), there were 9.4 million new cases of active tuberculosis (TB) with a prevalence of 14 million cases in 2009, which accounted for about 1.7 million deaths (WHO 2010). A serious issue is the inaccuracy of these estimations, with case detection rates (CDR) of only 63% (even lower in Africa) of pulmonary and other forms of the disease which is primarily due to undiagnosed and unreported cases (WHO 2010). Of those individuals newly infected with *Mtb*, greater than one-tenth involved co-infection with HIV. Uncovering LTBI in at-risk individuals (e.g.. HIV positive, household contacts, those on immunosuppressive drugs) is critical so that the proper medical treatments can be administered to prevent future activation of the disease. Expeditious detection of smear negative cases, of which there were an estimated 2 million instances (WHO 2010), could potentially allow for treatment 4-6 weeks sooner.

1.2 Identifying diagnostic biomarkers of TB

There are two major classes of biomarkers - host response and pathogen generated. The majority of the research being conducted focuses on host biomarkers - including INF-γ (as measured through the IGRA kits), other immunological markers (e.g.. cytokines, like IL-6 and TNF), host protein profiling, as well as, the production of antibodies to dominant *Mtb* antigens (such as, malate synthase and MPT51 (Wanchu, Dong et al. 2008)) (Walzl, Ronacher et al.). One of the primary concerns with using immune response as biomarkers of disease is the variation observed among the patient population due to numerous factors including secondary disease (causing increased/decreased inflammation) and altered response due to drug therapy. Alternatively, products made and released by *Mtb* during infection can also serve as biomarkers. Bacterial molecules including DNA (Cannas, Goletti et al. 2008) and lipoarabinomannan (LAM) (Minion, Leung et al.) can both be detected in urine during infection. Unlike most immunological biomarkers, bacterial products are specific to the tuberculosis. Moreover, identification and quantification of multiple *Mtb* products secreted/released during infection has the potential to be developed into a multiplex assay. Further, by monitoring changes in a panel of biomolecules, one could generate a fingerprint that could be used to indicate the different stages of disease (such as active versus latent).

To identify a combination of novel biomarkers for the generation of a point-of-care diagnostic test, we have begun screening human exosomes as a source of *Mtb* proteins. Preliminary data has proven that these vesicles are an untapped supply of pathogen derived biomarkers. There are several advantages to using exosomes: first, they can be isolated in a facile and expeditious manner. Second, they can be harvested from blood and urine - which is beneficial when sputum collection is not feasible (from children or in MDR cases). Third, our data indicates that *Mtb* proteins are not only contained, but also concentrated in these vesicles - allowing for greater sensitivity than can be achieved using unpurified whole blood or urine.

1.3 Exosomes: Initial discoveries

Exosomes were first described in mid-1980's by Johnstone *et al.* and Stahl *et al.* in reference to the small vesicles that bud from reticulocytes during maturation (Harding, Heuser et al. 1984; Johnstone, Adam et al. 1987). It was hypothesized that this process, was required to remove membrane-bound proteins such as the transferrin receptor from the maturing reticulocyte as these cells lack the lysosomes for protein degradation (Pan and Johnstone 1983). In a series of elegant electron microscopy studies, it was determined that the transferrin receptor (TR) was endocytosed and trafficked to the MVB where it was observed on ~50 nm interluminal vesicles. MVBs containing the TR were shown to fuse with the plasma membrane and release the interluminal vesicles (Pan, Teng et al. 1985). These released vesicles were called exosomes.

Additional studies have shown that exosome release is not specific to maturing reticulocytes, as they are constitutively shed from most mammalian cells types including B-cells, macrophages and dendritic cells (Raposo, Nijman et al. 1996). Exosomes can be readily obtained from most bodily fluids, including but not limited to urine, plasma, breast milk, bronchoalveolar lavage (BAL) fluid and saliva (Admyre, Grunewald et al. 2003; Pisitkun, Shen et al. 2004; Caby, Lankar et al. 2005; Admyre, Johansson et al. 2007; Ogawa, Kanai-Azuma et al. 2008) Exosomes released from antigen presenting cells contain MHC-I and MHC-II as well as CD86 and therefore are capable of antigen presentation (Zitvogel, Fernandez et al. 1999). Interestingly, exosomes derived from tumor cells have also been shown to induce an anti-tumor immune response, implicating a future utility in vaccine development (Zitvogel, Regnault et al. 1998).

1.4 The advent of exosomes in tuberculosis research

The *Mtb* cell wall is composed of a myriad of proteins and lipids, including the highly studied glycolipid, LAM. This molecule has been shown to be readily liberated from the mycobacteria during infection and has been correlated with several immunomodulatory functions (such as interactions with TLRs (Bhatnagar and Schorey 2007)). Beatty et al was the first to recognize LAM accumulation in MVBs and this report is consistent with subsequent exosomal release from infected cells (Beatty, Rhoades et al. 2000). Building upon initial evidence, Schorey et al characterized exosomes released from BCG-infected macrophages. Flow cytometry allowed for the identification of vesicles positive for MHC-II, Hsp70, and LAMP1, as well as mycobacterial pathogen-associated molecular patterns (PAMPs) (Bhatnagar, Shinagawa et al. 2007; Giri and Schorey 2008). They went on to demonstrate the exosomes released from mycobacterial-infected macrophages could activate both the inate and acquired immune responses *in vitro* and *in vivo* (Blood, 2007 and PLoS One 2008). In addition, it was shown that exosomes isolated from the BAL fluid of *M. bovis BCG* infected mice contained LAM and the 19kDa antigen (Bhatnagar, Shinagawa et al. 2007).

1.5 Concentration and siphoning of biomarkers in exosomes

Exosome biology is a relatively new field with roughly 1000 primary journal articles and over 200 reviews (Raimondo, Morosi et al. 2011). Exosomes have been studied with techniques such as western blotting, microscopy, FACS and mass spectrometry. Characterization of exosomal contents, resulted in the identification of a number of host, as well as pathogen derived products, including: lipids (Laulagnier, Motta et al. 2004) and nucleic acids (miRNA and mRNA) (Valadi, Ekstrom et al. 2007), in addition to proteins. However, only a few of these studies utilize proteomics to decipher the contents of these vesicles and their relationship to various diseases, such as cancers, diabetes, prenatal disorders and renal diseases (Ben Ameur, Molina et al. 2010; Diaz, Pinto et al. 2011; Moon, You et al. 2011). Proteomics was performed on purified exosomes as early as 2004 (Bard, Hegmans et al. 2004). Defining the proteomic content of exosomes derived from urine and blood has been key to biomarker discovery in several diseases (Bard, Hegmans et al. 2004; Mears, Craven et al. 2004; Thomas, Sexton et al. 2010). However, the mining of exosome-derived proteins related to infectious diseases has yet to be exploited. The discovery that mycobacterial products could be found in exosomes release from infected animals led to the first full-scale attempt to characterize the *Mtb* exo-proteome (comprehensive collection of proteins capable of being secreted from *Mtb*-infected cells within exosomes) (Giri, Kruh et al. 2010). The objective of this research is to fuel biomarker discovery utilizing mass spectrometry based approaches.

2. The *Mtb* exo-proteome: *in vitro*

Based on the hypothesis that exosomes are a novel source of bacterial components which could be exploited for biomarker identification, we set out to define the mycobacterial proteins contained in exosomes released from *Mtb*-infected macrophages. Exosomes were purified from *Mtb* infected macrophages using differential centrifugation and sucrose gradient (Griffiths, Heesom et al. 2007; Giri, Kruh et al. 2010). The exosomes contained the characteristic size and shape as defined by EM (Figure 1).

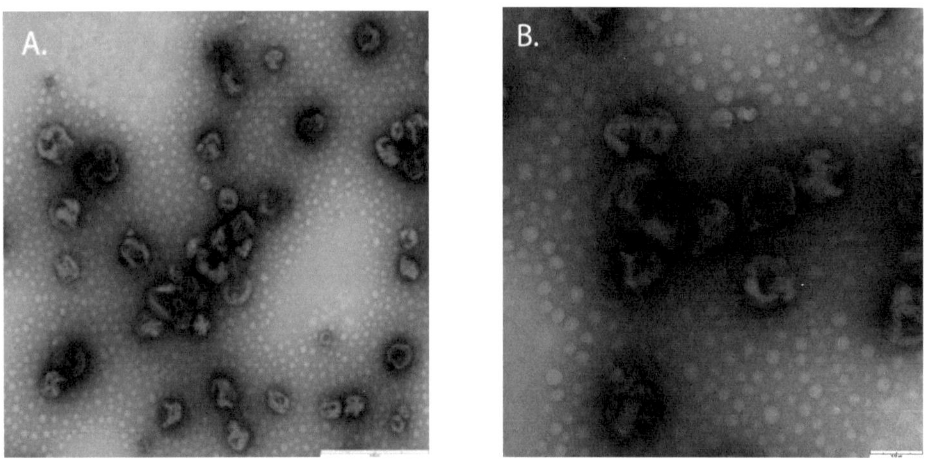

Fig. 1. Electron micrograph of exosomes purified from *Mtb* infected J774a.1 cells at (A) 3000x (bar = 0.5 μm) and (B) 8000x magnification (bar = 0.1 μm). The vesicles showed the size (30 - 100 nm) and spherical or cup-like shape expected of exosomes.

2.1 Proteomics of exosomes released from *Mtb*-infected macrophages

Consistent with previous publications (Bhatnagar, Shinagawa et al. 2007), the host exosomal marker LAMP-1, as well as mycobacterial LAM and 19 kDa antigen (Rv3763) were detected via western blot (data not shown). Several known secreted proteins previously undetected in exosomes, including KatG (Rv1908c), the Ag85 complex (Rv3804c, Rv1886c and Rv0129c), GroES (Rv3418c) and CFP10 (Rv3874), were also demonstrated by western blot analysis (Giri, Kruh et al. 2010). In addition to these proteins, we identified roughly forty mycobacterial proteins by MS, of which 95% were previously defined either experimentally or through predictive algorithms to be secreted (Table 2) (Rosenkrands, King et al. 2000; Malen, Berven et al. 2007; Giri, Kruh et al. 2010). One can hypothesize that the mycobacterial proteins released into the phagosome or cytoplasm are transported to an MVB, incorporated into the interluminal vesicles and released from the infected cell via exosomes into various bodily fluids (Figure 2). As indicated earlier, the exosomes containing both host and mycobacterial components can modulate the host immune response. Similar experiments were performed with irradiated (dead) *Mtb* and only 1 mycobacterial protein was identified. Whether this difference between live and dead *Mtb* was due to differential transport of the mycobacteria within the macrophage or a requirement for mycobacterial metabolic activity requires further investigation.

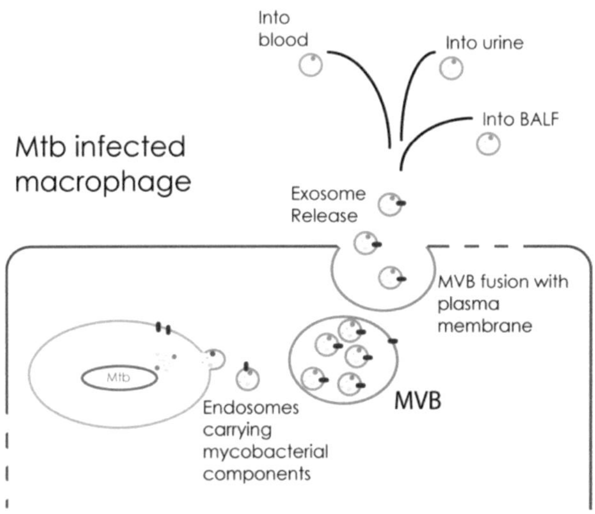

Fig. 2. Hypothesized pathway of exosome secretion in *Mtb*-infected cells. Based on experimental evidence, antigenic proteins are secreted within the *Mtb*-containing host compartment, packaged and shuttled into multivesicular bodies. The MVBs can fuse with the plasma membrane to release the exosomes into the peripheral fluids.

In addition, J774a.1 macrophages were exposed to culture filtrate proteins (CFP), a complex mixture of over 200 proteins secreted from *Mtb* during *in vitro* growth (Sonnenberg and Belisle 1997). Exosomes released during this experiment were collected and analyzed after in-gel digestion. The mycobacterial proteins identified from the CFP-treated exosomes included many well-characterized immunedominant antigens and were remarkably similar (>85%) to those isolated from J774a.1 cells infected with live *Mtb*. As previously mentioned, exosomes are being evaluated as tumor vaccines and the presence of highly antigenic mycobacterial proteins on exosomes from CFP-treated macrophages suggests that they too may be a viable vaccine candidates for TB. This hypothesis is presently under investigtion.

These aforementioned *in vitro* experiments afforded us with enough exosomal material to build our methodology and lay the foundation for the analysis of exosomes isolated from *Mtb*-infected mice, where samples more limited. In prior studies of exosomes, mycobacterial proteins were identified only by western blot. However, mass spectrometry allows for the identification of proteins without the use of antibodies (which are only available to a small subset of proteins). Moreover, while ~8 μg of exosomes is required for each western blot (identifying only one protein per blot), a parallel sample subject to MS analysis, allows for the discrimination of hundreds of proteins of both host and bacterial origin.

Rv #	Protein Name	Relative Abundance (%)
Rv2220	GlnA1	13.05
Rv1860	Mpt32/APA	12.34
Rv1886c	Antigen 85-B	9.58
Rv3804c	Antigen 85-A	8.92
Rv1980c	Mpt64	6.89
Rv1908c	KatG	4.43
Rv3418c	GroES	3.59
Rv0934	PstS1	3.41
Rv3248c	SahH	3.17
Rv0462	LpdC	2.87
Rv1926c	Mpt63	2.46
Rv1355c	MoeY	2.22
Rv2244	AcpM	2.16
Rv2031c	HspX	1.86
Rv1932	Cfp20	1.80

Table 2. Sampling of proteins identified in exosomes from H37Rv-infected J774a.1 cells by LC-MS-MS. See Giri, Kruh et al. 2010, for the extended list. The fifteen most abundant mycobacterial proteins are listed, based on the total number of spectral counts from both in-solution and in-gel processing (compiled in the aforementioned paper plus additional unpublished experiments). Relative abundance was calculated using the following formula: (total # of spectral counts for a given protein/cumulative total # of mycobacterial spectral counts) * 100.

The primary analysis from *in vitro* derived exosomes, provides an extended candidate list for the study of *Mtb* biomarkers. Our next step in the biomarker discovery pipeline is to verify that these results translate to an *in vivo* system.

3. The *Mtb* exo-proteome: *in vivo*

Since tuberculosis is primarily a respiratory affliction, the initial *in vivo* investigation was performed utilizing exosomes isolated from BAL fluid to determine if mycobacterial proteins could be identified from an infected animal model. The hypothesis is that the protein composition of BAL fluid exosomes will reflect the initial *in vitro* findings and the proteins identified will change over the course of the infection. This may provide the starting point for making correlations between exosomal content and stage of infection. The end goal is find "peptide fingerprints" which represent the mycobacterial proteins most commonly present in exosomes of patients with active or latent tuberculosis.

3.1 Proteomics of exosomes released into the bronchoalveolar lavage fluid of *Mtb*-infected mice

BAL fluid was collected from mice infected via aerosol with either wild-type (H37Rv) or a *relA* deficient mutant of *Mtb*. Both the concentration and *Mtb* protein content of the exosomes were monitored over time. To accomplish this, we employed similar MS methodology as in our *in vitro* analysis (Giri, Kruh et al. 2010). MS analysis of BAL fluid derived exosomes from H37Rv *Mtb*-infected mice over the different time points revealed a significant overlap (50%) with the mycobacterial proteins previously identified in the *in vitro* tissue culture experiments (Figure 3). No mycobacterial proteins were identified in exosomes purified from BAL fluid on day 1 post-infection or as expected, in naïve mice. In all other time points, the number of mycobacterial spectral counts (data not shown) as well as the proteins identified changed over time (Figure 4). In exosomes from both H37Rv and the *relA* mutant infections, the largest number of proteins were identified early in the infection (day 14), however the number of proteins identified from the *relA* mutant was half that of the wt strain. Interestingly, during the wt infection, the exosomes that yielded the highest total mycobacterial spectral count was at day 56. Moreover, the exosomes from wt-infected mice showed on average three times as many spectral counts per time point than the *relA* mutant (data not shown). This is likely, at least in part, due to the differences in bacterial load between wt and ΔRelA-infected mice (10 to 100 fold difference in lung colony forming units at different time points). In both wt and ΔRelA-infected mice there were some proteins present on exosomes which were there throughout the course of disease, while others were transiently expressed.

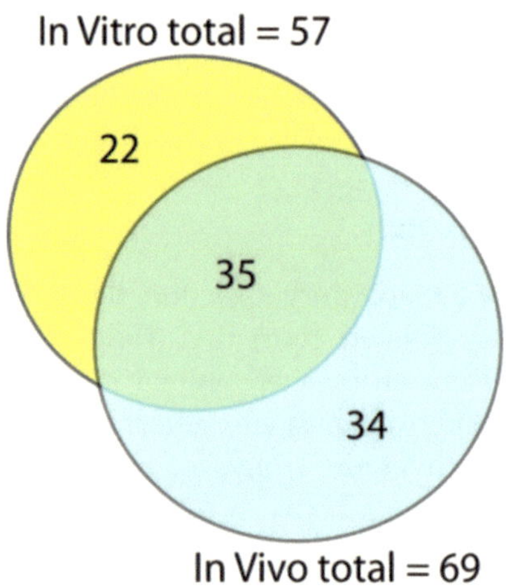

Fig. 3. Venn diagram depicting the number of mycobacterial proteins identified in exosomes from H37Rv-infected macrophages (yellow), the BAL fluid of H37Rv-infected mice (blue), and both (overlap).

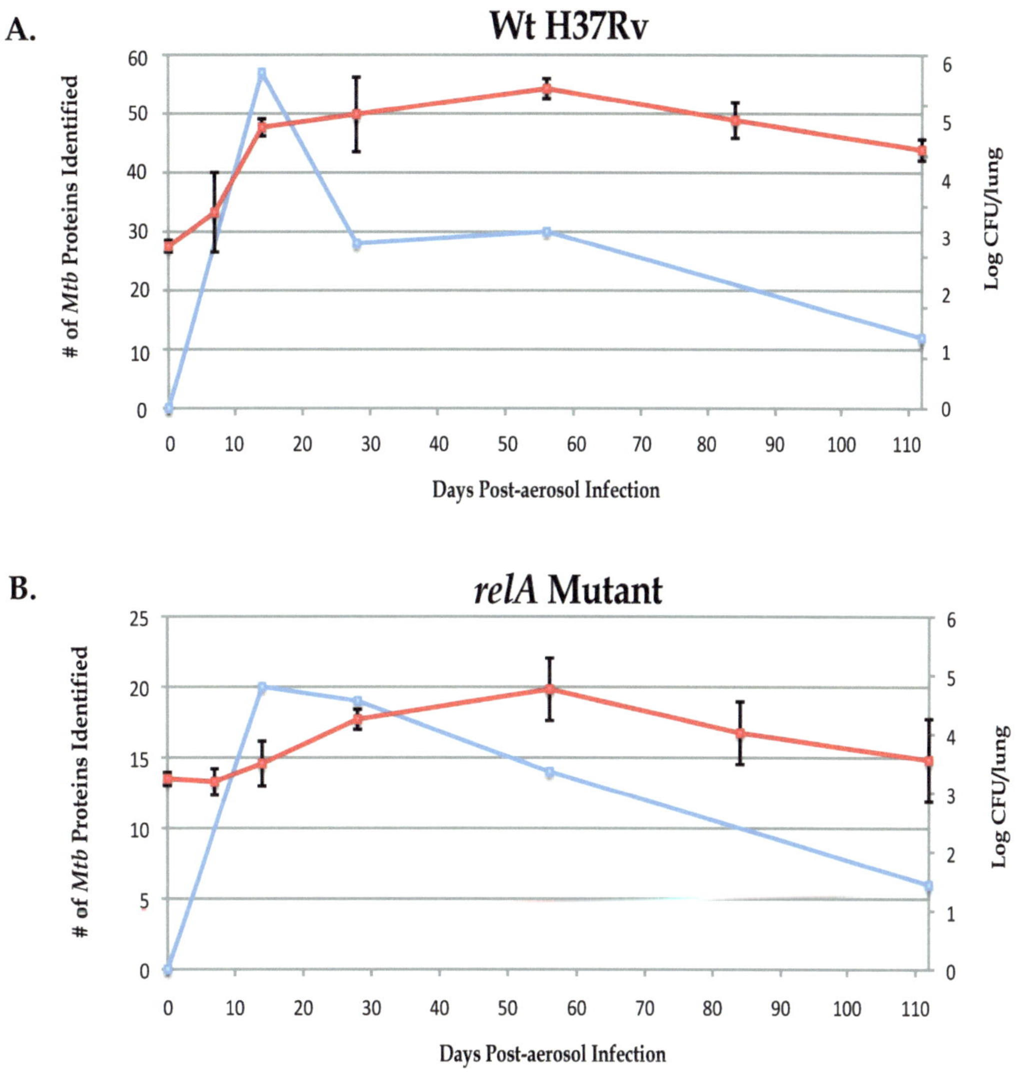

Fig. 4. CFUs versus *Mtb* proteins identified over time in (A) H37Rv *Mtb*-infected mice and (B) ΔRelA-infected mice. The red lines indicate the Log CFU in the lung over time, as indicated on the right y-axius. CFUs are representative of the bacterial load of the lungs of 5 mice per time point. The ble line represents the number of proteins identified by MS over the course of the infection, as measured on the left y-axis.

While majority of the 15 most dominant mycobacterial proteins found in exosomes released from infected J774a.1 cells were seen in the mouse exosomes (Table 3), many of them were less abundant (e.g.. KatG, SahH and Cfp20) and several of these proteins were absent entirely (e.g. LpdC and MoeY). Most interesting are several striking differences in the mycobacterial protein identified on exosomes from BALfluid when mice were infected with wt or *relA* mutant. The *relA* gene is annotated as being a non-essential gene, based on viability of the strain subsequent to the insertion of the *Himar1* transposon (Lamichhane, Zignol et al. 2003). Biochemical characterization of the RelA protein suggests that this enzyme has both 3'-pyrophosphoryltransferase and pyrophosphohydrolase activities. Functional deletion of this protein results in the depletion of hyperphophorylated guanosine ((p)ppGpp), which can decrease protein synthesis leading to effects on long term growth and the ability to transition in and out of dormancy (Avarbock, Salem et al. 1999; Primm, Andersen et al. 2000; Klinkenberg, Lee et al. 2010). Dahl et al. has reported that the gene expression level of several secreted proteins (including the Antigen 85 complex and GroES) are increased in the *relA* mutant (Dahl, Kraus et al. 2003), however, based on spectral counts, the majority of the secreted proteins identified in exosomes display the opposite trend (Figure 5). While a more quantitative approach is necessary to truly hone in on the differences between the wt and *relA* mutant, this preliminary data suggest that there is a qualitative and quantitative difference in proteins targeted to MVB/exosomes when macrophages are infected with wt compared to *relA* mutant *in vivo*. Future experiments, including multiple reaction monitoring (MRM)-MS analysis will allow for the monitoring of the intensity of specific peptides in each sample, while allowing one to ignore the m/z's corresponding to host peptides.

Rv #	Protein Name	Day 14	Day 28	Day 56	Day 112
Rv2220	GlnA1	+	*	*	*
Rv1860	Mpt32/APA	+	*	*	Δ
Rv1886c	Antigen 85-B	+	+	+	+
Rv3804c	Antigen 85-A	+	+	+	+
Rv1980c	Mpt64	+	+	+	*
Rv1908c	KatG	*	*	*	-
Rv3418c	GroES	+	+	*	*
Rv0934	PstS1	+	+	*	-
Rv3248c	SahH	*	+	*	-
Rv0462	LpdC	-	-	-	-
Rv1926c	Mpt63	*	+	*	-
Rv1355c	MoeY	-	-	-	-
Rv2244	AcpM	+	+	+	Δ
Rv2031c	HspX	+	+	+	*
Rv1932	Cfp20	*	*	*	-

Table 3. Comparison of the fifteen most abundant proteins originally identified in exosomes from H37Rv-infected J774a.1 cells (Table 2) to their presence (+) or absence (-) in BAL fluid exosomes at various time-points during the infection of Balc/c mice. + = protein detected in both H37Rv and *relA* mutant exosomes; * = presence in H37Rv exosomes only; Δ = only in *relA* mutant exosomes.

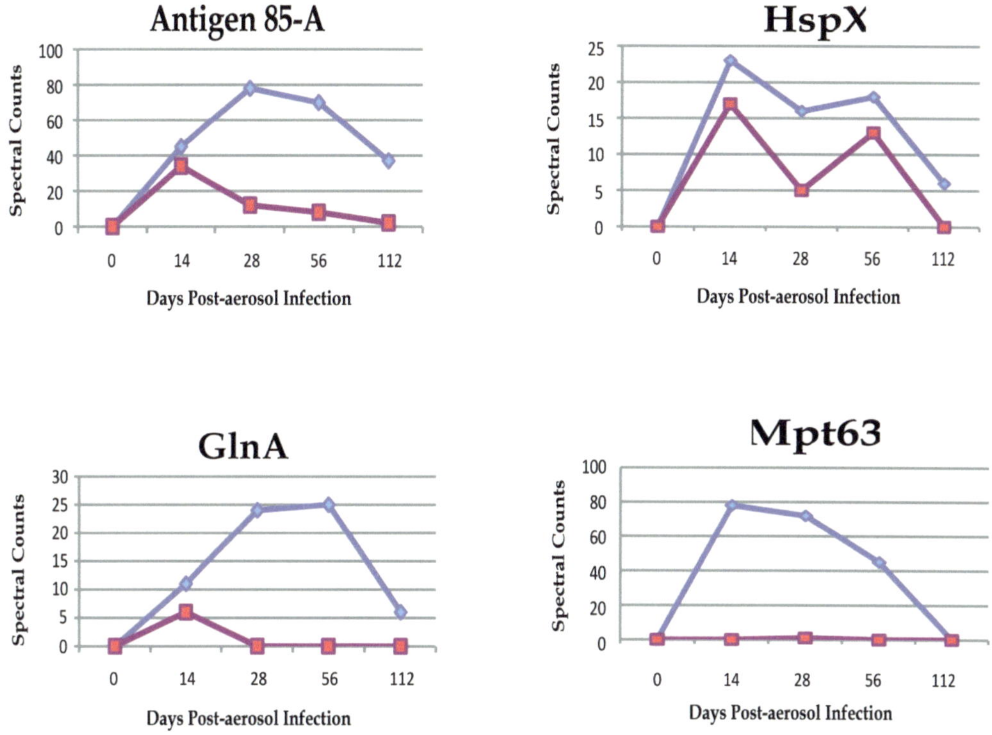

Fig. 5. Kinetics of various proteins during the course of the wild-type H37Rv (blue) compared to the *relA* mutant (red) infection, including GlnA, Antigen 85-A, HspX and Mpt63. These graphs emphasize the range of spectral counts and the pattern of individual protein expression. Transposon mutants effecting the expression of most of these proteins have led to the hypothesis that many of these proteins (HspX, Ag-85a, Mpt63) are "non-essential" (Sassetti, Boyd et al. 2003) - but their presence in exosomes is an indicator that their expression may be triggered during infection (HspX, as seen by transcipts (Hu, Mangan et al. 2000; Dubnau, Fontan et al. 2002) and not in a simple culture.

4. Conclusions: Future of biomarkers in tuberculosis

Tuberculosis research in diagnostics has suffered from a lack of resources for the discovery and down-stream development of a cheap and facile clinical assay for the detection of active TB and to distinguish active from latent infection. This is due in part to the reliance on the TST; which for decades provided a cheap assay for detection of *Mtb* infection, and by our reliance on sputum smear tests to detect active disease. Most would argue that neither are optimal means to detect and diagnose TB nor evaluate drug treatment. However, in the absence of assays that could replace these tests without increases in cost, these remain the gold standard. The *Mtb* proteome has been mined for decades in pursuit of a serodiagnostic or celluar assay for tuberculosis, and the development and use of IGRA tests represent a hallmark of success. The outlook for a serodiagnostic assay appears more dismal, due to the requirement of either a predictable antibody response or high bacterial product shedding into the blood or BAL fluid. Our initial identification of *Mtb* proteins in BAL fluid exosomes was a stepping-stone in the process of novel discovery of resources for development of second-generation diagnostic and prognostic assays. While BAL fluid is not the most ideal fluid to collect from patients, its isolation from mice and the use of it in the discovery phase of biomarker identification is suitable if these *Mtb* exo-proteome findings translate to other bodily fluids. Exosomes can be isolated from urine and serum, both of which are easier to collect than sputum. Harvesting and characterization of sera and urine exosomes are commonplace in diseases such as cancer. Consistent with our findings in the mouse model, our preliminary evidence from a panel of five TB patients and five household contacts suggests that sera analyzed from patients with active disease contain on average over 3000 μg of exosomes per mL, which is over 30 times greater than the concentration of exosomes in the control sera. This makes exosomes an attractive target for pathogen-associated diagnostic biomarkers. Since many diagnostics are unreliable in immune compromised individuals, the allure of an exosome-based diagnostic will be enhanced if the exosomes undergo a similar rise in individuals co-infected with HIV.

Bodily fluids such as urine and blood are highly complex (with an estimate of $>10^6$ protein products in human plasma (Anderson and Hunter 2006)). The purification of exosomes from these samples reduces the amount of biocomponents resulting in a drastic enrichment. Numerous attempts have been made using MS to search for mycobacterial proteins in whole blood or urine. Unfortunately the results from these studies were not encouraging as even immunodepletion (with a MARS column) and various fractionation techniques (e.g. SCX and mRP on an HPLC), did not lead to the identification of a significant number of mycobacterial proteins in blood or urine. One major benefit to isolating exosomes from these fluids prior to proteomic studies is that these vesicles not only serve as a mechanism of concentrating the mycobacterial proteins, but they are also an effective method of removing major contaminants found in bodily fluids.

Urine is an established, readily attainable source of exosomes (Pisitkun, Shen et al. 2004). As previously mentioned, LAM (and mycobacterial DNA) has been found in urine of *Mtb*-infected patients, including those with HIV. One kit currently on the market for the detection of LAM in urine is the Clearview TB ELISA (Inverness Medical Innovations Inc.). How LAM is secreted into the urine is questionable, however one can hypothesize that transport from the site of infection into the urine can occur through exosomes - either by encapsulation or incorporation into the lipid membrane of the vesicle. It is possible that LAM could be an additional marker in combination with *Mtb* proteins in a future clinical assay. Although at this point, like all proteins identified in exosomes, the concentration of LAM per volume of exosome would need to be quantified at various time-points during infection.

The discovery phase of identifying biomarkers from exosomes is in its infancy. While we have the potential to study fluctuations in exosomal host proteins too, deciphering these differences can be tricky due to additional changes in immune response and reactions to secondary infections or inflammatory disease. In the end, the best diagnostic may involve monitoring numerous proteins, perhaps both host and pathogen derived. The content of exosomes has the potential not only for use in diagnostics, but also additional predictive value in the classification of disease status, assessment of therapeutics and overall prognosis.

The use of quantitative proteomics and MRM technology will be key in narrowing down the list of candidates. While this method is not necessarily suitable for the clinical lab (especially those in resource-limited areas) or is it cost effective - it is a mechanism to define biomarkers that can be implemented in a more cost effective diagnostic tool, such as an ELISA, or micro-fluidic "dip-test" that could be performed in a resource poor setting.

Another important consideration is the method used for exosome purification. At present the gold standard calls for differential centrifugation followed by sucrose gradient. Although this results is highly purified exosomes it is not suitable for high throughput analysis of serum/urine samples and cannot be used in the setting where TB diagnostics is most needed. Recently there have been a number of new purification techniques that have been developed include microfiltration using low protein-binding size exclusion filters, size-exclusion chromatography, and microfluidics. ExoQuick™, a recently developed commercial product from *System Biosciences,* allows for rapid isolation of exosomes based on a simple precipitation process and shows promise as a purification technique amenable to a point-of-care diagnostics.

5. Acknowledgements

This work was supported through grants AI056979 and AI052439 (J. S. S.) and HHSN266200400091c (K.M.D) from the National Institute of Allergy and Infectious Diseases (NIAID). We would like to thank Pramod Giri for isolation of exosomes from mouse BAL fluid and EM photos. The antibodies to the various mycobacterial proteins as well as the *Mtb* culture filtrate proteins were provided from Colorado State University as part of NIH, NIAID Contract No. HHSN266200400091C, entitled "Tuberculosis Vaccine Testing and Research Materials". Mouse infections and BAL fluid collection were performed under William Bishai's laboratory at Johns Hopkins School of Medicine and funded under the "Tuberculosis Animal Research and Gene Evaluation Taskforce", NIH/NIAID N01-AI30036. The authors graciously thank Lisa M. Wolfe for critique of this manuscript.

6. References

Admyre, C., J. Grunewald, et al. (2003). "Exosomes with major histocompatibility complex class II and co-stimulatory molecules are present in human BAL fluid." Eur Respir J 22(4): 578-583.

Admyre, C., S. M. Johansson, et al. (2007). "Exosomes with immune modulatory features are present in human breast milk." J Immunol 179(3): 1969-1978.

Anderson, L. and C. L. Hunter (2006). "Quantitative mass spectrometric multiple reaction monitoring assays for major plasma proteins." Mol Cell Proteomics 5(4): 573-588.

Avarbock, D., J. Salem, et al. (1999). "Cloning and characterization of a bifunctional RelA/SpoT homologue from Mycobacterium tuberculosis." Gene 233(1-2): 261-269.

Bard, M. P., J. P. Hegmans, et al. (2004). "Proteomic analysis of exosomes isolated from human malignant pleural effusions." Am J Respir Cell Mol Biol 31(1): 114-121.

Beatty, W. L., E. R. Rhoades, et al. (2000). "Trafficking and release of mycobacterial lipids from infected macrophages." Traffic 1(3): 235-247.

Ben Ameur, R., L. Molina, et al. (2010). "Proteomic approaches for discovering biomarkers of diabetic nephropathy." Nephrol Dial Transplant 25(9): 2866-2875.

Bhatnagar, S. and J. S. Schorey (2007). "Exosomes released from infected macrophages contain Mycobacterium avium glycopeptidolipids and are proinflammatory." J Biol Chem 282(35): 25779-25789.

Bhatnagar, S., K. Shinagawa, et al. (2007). "Exosomes released from macrophages infected with intracellular pathogens stimulate a proinflammatory response in vitro and in vivo." Blood 110(9): 3234-3244.

Caby, M. P., D. Lankar, et al. (2005). "Exosomal-like vesicles are present in human blood plasma." Int Immunol 17(7): 879-887.

Cannas, A., D. Goletti, et al. (2008). "Mycobacterium tuberculosis DNA detection in soluble fraction of urine from pulmonary tuberculosis patients." Int J Tuberc Lung Dis 12(2): 146-151.

Dahl, J. L., C. N. Kraus, et al. (2003). "The role of RelMtb-mediated adaptation to stationary phase in long-term persistence of Mycobacterium tuberculosis in mice." Proc Natl Acad Sci U S A 100(17): 10026-10031.

Diaz, S. O., J. Pinto, et al. (2011). "Metabolic biomarkers of prenatal disorders: an exploratory NMR metabonomics study of 2nd trimester maternal urine and blood plasma." J Proteome Res.

Dubnau, E., P. Fontan, et al. (2002). "Mycobacterium tuberculosis genes induced during infection of human macrophages." Infect Immun 70(6): 2787-2795.

Giri, P. K., N. A. Kruh, et al. (2010). "Proteomic analysis identifies highly antigenic proteins in exosomes from M. tuberculosis-infected and culture filtrate protein-treated macrophages." Proteomics 10(17): 3190-3202.

Giri, P. K. and J. S. Schorey (2008). "Exosomes derived from M. Bovis BCG infected macrophages activate antigen-specific CD4+ and CD8+ T cells in vitro and in vivo." PLoS One 3(6): e2461.

Griffiths, R. E., K. J. Heesom, et al. (2007). "Normal prion protein trafficking in cultured human erythroblasts." Blood 110(13): 4518-4525.

Harding, C., J. Heuser, et al. (1984). "Endocytosis and intracellular processing of transferrin and colloidal gold-transferrin in rat reticulocytes: demonstration of a pathway for receptor shedding." Eur J Cell Biol 35(2): 256-263.

Hu, Y., J. A. Mangan, et al. (2000). "Detection of mRNA transcripts and active transcription in persistent Mycobacterium tuberculosis induced by exposure to rifampin or pyrazinamide." J Bacteriol 182(22): 6358-6365.

Johnstone, R. M., M. Adam, et al. (1987). "Vesicle formation during reticulocyte maturation. Association of plasma membrane activities with released vesicles (exosomes)." J Biol Chem 262(19): 9412-9420.

Klinkenberg, L. G., J. H. Lee, et al. (2010). "The stringent response is required for full virulence of Mycobacterium tuberculosis in guinea pigs." J Infect Dis 202(9): 1397-1404.

Lamichhane, G., M. Zignol, et al. (2003). "A postgenomic method for predicting essential genes at subsaturation levels of mutagenesis: application to Mycobacterium tuberculosis." Proc Natl Acad Sci U S A 100(12): 7213-7218.

Laulagnier, K., C. Motta, et al. (2004). "Mast cell- and dendritic cell-derived exosomes display a specific lipid composition and an unusual membrane organization." Biochem J 380(Pt 1): 161-171.

Malen, H., F. S. Berven, et al. (2007). "Comprehensive analysis of exported proteins from Mycobacterium tuberculosis H37Rv." Proteomics 7(10): 1702-1718.

Mears, R., R. A. Craven, et al. (2004). "Proteomic analysis of melanoma-derived exosomes by two-dimensional polyacrylamide gel electrophoresis and mass spectrometry." Proteomics 4(12): 4019-4031.

Minion, J., E. Leung, et al. "Diagnosing tuberculosis with urine lipoarabinomannan: systematic review and meta-analysis." Eur Respir J.

Moon, P. G., S. You, et al. (2011). "Urinary exosomes and proteomics." Mass Spectrom Rev.

Ogawa, Y., M. Kanai-Azuma, et al. (2008). "Exosome-like vesicles with dipeptidyl peptidase IV in human saliva." Biol Pharm Bull 31(6): 1059-1062.

Pan, B. T. and R. M. Johnstone (1983). "Fate of the transferrin receptor during maturation of sheep reticulocytes in vitro: selective externalization of the receptor." Cell 33(3): 967-978.

Pan, B. T., K. Teng, et al. (1985). "Electron microscopic evidence for externalization of the transferrin receptor in vesicular form in sheep reticulocytes." J Cell Biol 101(3): 942-948.

Pisitkun, T., R. F. Shen, et al. (2004). "Identification and proteomic profiling of exosomes in human urine." Proc Natl Acad Sci U S A 101(36): 13368-13373.

Primm, T. P., S. J. Andersen, et al. (2000). "The stringent response of Mycobacterium tuberculosis is required for long-term survival." J Bacteriol 182(17): 4889-4898.

Raimondo, F., L. Morosi, et al. (2011). "Advances in membranous vesicle and exosome proteomics improving biological understanding and biomarker discovery." Proteomics 11(4): 709-720.

Raposo, G., H. W. Nijman, et al. (1996). "B lymphocytes secrete antigen-presenting vesicles." J Exp Med 183(3): 1161-1172.

Rosenkrands, I., A. King, et al. (2000). "Towards the proteome of Mycobacterium tuberculosis." Electrophoresis 21(17): 3740-3756.

Sassetti, C. M., D. H. Boyd, et al. (2003). "Genes required for mycobacterial growth defined by high density mutagenesis." Mol Microbiol 48(1): 77-84.

Thomas, C. E., W. Sexton, et al. (2010). "Urine collection and processing for protein biomarker discovery and quantification." Cancer Epidemiol Biomarkers Prev 19(4): 953-959.

Valadi, H., K. Ekstrom, et al. (2007). "Exosome-mediated transfer of mRNAs and microRNAs is a novel mechanism of genetic exchange between cells." Nat Cell Biol 9(6): 654-659.

Walzl, G., K. Ronacher, et al. "Immunological biomarkers of tuberculosis." Nat Rev Immunol 11(5): 343-354.

Wanchu, A., Y. Dong, et al. (2008). "Biomarkers for clinical and incipient tuberculosis: performance in a TB-endemic country." PLoS One 3(4): e2071.

WHO (2010). Global Tuberculosis Report, World Health Organization.

Yang, H., J. Troudt, et al. "Three protein cocktails mediate delayed-type hypersensitivity responses indistinguishable from that elicited by purified protein derivative in the guinea pig model of Mycobacterium tuberculosis infection." Infect Immun 79(2): 716-723.

Zitvogel, L., N. Fernandez, et al. (1999). "Dendritic cells or their exosomes are effective biotherapies of cancer." Eur J Cancer 35 Suppl 3: S36-38.

Zitvogel, L., A. Regnault, et al. (1998). "Eradication of established murine tumors using a novel cell-free vaccine: dendritic cell-derived exosomes." Nat Med 4(5): 594-600.

Molecular Techniques for Identification of Species of the *Mycobacterium tuberculosis* Complex: The use of Multiplex PCR and an Adapted HPLC Method for Identification of *Mycobacterium bovis* and Diagnosis of Bovine Tuberculosis

Eduardo Eustáquio de Souza Figueiredo et al.*
Departamento de Alimentos e Nutrição, Universidade Federal de Mato Grosso, Cuiabá/MT, Brasil

1. Introduction

Mycobacterium bovis is a member of the *M. tuberculosis* complex (MTC), a group of species (*Mycobacterium tuberculosis, M. bovis, M. africanum, M. microti*, and *M. canetti*) with a high genetic homology. *M. bovis* is the causative agent of tuberculosis in a range of animal species and humans, with worldwide annual losses to agriculture of $3 billion. The human burden of tuberculosis caused by the bovine tubercle bacillus is still largely unknown. *M. bovis* was also the progenitor for the *M. bovis* bacillus Calmette-Guérin vaccine strain, the most widely used human vaccine. Garnier et al. (2003) described the 4,345,492-bp genome sequence of *M. bovis* AF2122/97 and compared it with the genomes of *Mycobacterium tuberculosis* and *Mycobacterium leprae*. Strikingly, the genome sequence of *M. bovis* is >99.95% identical to that of *M. tuberculosis*, but deletion of genetic information has reduced the genome size.

Bovine tuberculosis (BTB) is a major infectious disease of cattle in many countries. Although cattle are the main host and reservoir of this chronic infection, other mammalian species, including humans, are also susceptible to *Mycobacterium bovis* (Romano et al., 1996). Considering that more than 94% of the world population lives in countries where the

* Carlos Adam Conte Júnior[2], Leone Vinícius Furlanetto[3], Flávia Galindo Silvestre Silva[4], Rafael Silva Duarte[5], Joab Trajano Silva[3], Walter Lilenbaum[6] and Vânia Margaret Flosi Paschoalin[3*]
[1]*Departamento de Alimentos e Nutrição, Universidade Federal de Mato Grosso, Cuiabá/MT, Brasil*
[2]*Faculdade de Veterinária, Universidade Federal Fluminense, Niterói/RJ, Brasil*
[3]*Instituto de Química, Universidade Federal do Rio de Janeiro, Rio de Janeiro/RJ, Brasil*
[4]*Universidade de Cuiabá, Cuiabá/MT, Brasil*
[5]*Instituto de Microbiologia, Universidade Federal do Rio de Janeiro, Rio de Janeiro/RJ, Brasil*
[6]*Instituto Biomédico, Universidade Federal Fluminense, Niterói/RJ, Brasil*

control of bovine tuberculosis is limited or absent (Vordemeier, 2006), there is a consensus about the risks regarding human health.

Humans can develop latent TB infection, active TB or reactivation of latent TB infection. In veterinary medicine, the distinction between latent TB infection and active TB disease is not as important as it is in human beings, since in both cases the animal must be slaughtered. According to the National Control Program implemented in Brazil, treatment of reactive animals is not allowed, and all reactive animals must be slaughtered (Brasil, 2004).

Zoonotic TB is a recognized public health threat in the developing world. In some countries, control measures against bovine tuberculosis are limited or nonexistent (Cosivi, 1998; Thoen, 2006). Human infection by *M. bovis* can occur by the aerogenous route, ingestion of infected milk (WHO, 1994), or, less frequently, by contact with mucous membranes and broken skin. The disease caused by *M. bovis* is clinically, radiologically and pathologically indistinguishable from that caused by *M. tuberculosis*, while, differently from the typical tuberculosis and due to the infection route, the non-pulmonary presentation is most frequent (Grange, 2001). Considering the standard treatment for *M. tuberculosis* infection, the lack of differentiation between *M. bovis* and *M. tuberculosis* is a problem. *M. bovis* is naturally resistant to pyrazinamide, a drug that is frequently used to treat TB in humans. Thus, individuals infected by *M. bovis* may present a treatment failure, which makes them potential transmitters of these resistant strains to other people and animals (Abrahão, 2005).

In industrialized countries, human infection with *M. bovis* has been largely controlled by pasteurization of cow's milk, inspection in slaughterhouses, and culling of cattle reacting to the compulsory diagnosis (Romero et al., 2006). In Brazil, despite the existence of a National Eradication Plan, clandestine meat and milk are marketed without sanitary control, which is a threat to public health; the ingestion of these products is a possible route of infection to humans (Abrahão, 2005). In some developing countries with uncontrolled bovine tuberculosis, most human cases occur in young persons, and result from drinking or handling contaminated milk (Cosivi, 1998).

Zoonotic TB can also be considered a socio-economic disease; it causes direct economic losses in agricultural areas and hampers the commercial exchange of animal products (Zumárraga et al., 1999). Many countries around the world support the control or eradication of bovine tuberculosis by national control programs, based on a test-and-slaughter policy. Brazilian policies regarding the control and eradication of bovine tuberculosis include the National Plan for Control and Eradication of Bovine Brucellosis and Tuberculosis (PNCEBT), written in 2001 and revised in 2004, which is based on the slaughtering of all animals reactive to the tuberculin tests. However, this traditional policy has not been fully successful in many countries, and new tools, including additional diagnostic tests and new vaccines, are urgently required (Pollock et al., 2005).

In cattle, tuberculous lesions are most often found in organs rich in reticuloendothelial tissue, particularly the lungs and associated lymph nodes, and the liver (Corner, 1990). Other studies conducted on naturally and experimentally infected cattle have demonstrated that the lesions are most commonly observed in the lower respiratory tract; however, the upper respiratory tract and associated tissues may also display disease in a significant number of cases. Although tubercles are not a pathognomonic lesion of cattle TB, the presence of clinical signs of the disease is directly associated with their distribution and quantity (Medeiros, 2010).

Airborne infection is the most common transmission route, and more than 15% of cattle with BTB shed the mycobacteria, mainly early in the course of the infection (Cassidy et al., 1998). Studies with molecular markers have shown that infected cattle are a potential source of tuberculosis transmission to humans (Serrano-Moreno et al., 2008). Milk can be an important transmission route, resulting in extra-lung presentation of the illness (Wedlock et al., 2002). This was demonstrated in New York City, where 35 cases of infection by *M. bovis* were reported from 2001 to 2004; when they were traced back, some of the cases were associated with the consumption of cheese made with non-pasteurized milk, imported from an endemic area of BTB (CDC, 2005).

Using bacteriological culture methods, it has been calculated that only about 5% of tuberculin-reacting cattle (TRC) can eliminate *M. bovis* in milk. In such animals, the incidence of visible gross lesions in the mammary gland (MG) or supramammary lymph nodes (LN) is less than 0.5% (Goodchild and Clifton-Hadley, 2001). *M. bovis* has been isolated from milk samples from storage tanks, inadequately pasteurized milk, and milk samples from tuberculin non-reacting cattle (Pardo et al., 2001; Leite et al., 2003). This situation dramatizes the need for sensitive and accurate procedures for rapid identification of the bacteria in milk, to assist in the control of this zoonosis. PCR techniques offer high sensitivity, and have been successfully used for diagnosing BTB in several types of naturally infected organic materials such as tissue, blood and nasal exudates (Figueiredo et al., 2010; Cardoso et al., 2009; Romero et al., 1999). However, PCR techniques have been seldom tested for use in milk, particularly in Brazil (Zanini et al., 1998)

According to OIE, the proportion of zoonotic TB cases in Brazil is unknown (OIE, 2007), since bacteriological culturing for diagnosing TB is not employed routinely for all samples (Sequeira, 2005). The most recently published data estimating the incidence of zoonotic TB in Brazil (Kantor et al., 2008) reported the occurrence of only one occasion in 20 years (1987–2006), where *M. bovis* was confirmed as the etiological agent of human tuberculosis at the Hélio Fraga National Reference Laboratory (NRL) at the Federal University Hospital, Rio de Janeiro. In a two-year study, nearly 8,000 clinical samples were cultured for detection of mycobacteria, and no *M. bovis* isolate was obtained (Sobral, 2009). In the São Paulo laboratory network (Adolfo Lutz Institute), a total of 355,383 cultures were performed in the period 2001–2005, and only two *M. bovis* strains were recovered from two patients, one in 2001 from a lymph-node biopsy, and another in 2002 from a cerebrospinal-fluid sample. At the State Reference Laboratory in Rio Grande do Sul (1997–2005), of approximately 5,000 mycobacterial isolates phenotyped, no *M. bovis* was confirmed (Kantor et al., 2008).

Despite the presence of the disease in Brazil, there is a lack of official data concerning the current prevalence of bovine tuberculosis in the country. From 1989 to 1998, data from official reports indicate a national mean prevalence of 1.3% of infected cows (BRASIL, 2008). Since the implementation of PNCEBT in Brazil, the few studies reporting on the prevalence of the disease have provided estimates ranging from 0.7% to 3.3% (Baptista et al., 2004; Oliveira, 2007; Poletto et al., 2004; Ribeiro et al., 2003). According to the epidemiology of the disease, the higher incidence in dairy than in beef herds will also determine the geographical distribution. Roxo (2005) reported the rate of infection in different areas in

Brazil, and not surprisingly, the region with the lowest rate of infection is the one where beef herds are most predominant. Nevertheless, these data represent only particular regions, and cannot be used for estimates in the national context. It is important to keep in mind the enormous size of the Brazilian herd, which comprises approximately 200 million bovines (PAHO/WHO, 2006).

There is a growing perception that no single method is sufficient for detecting all cattle infected with BTB (Salfinger et al., 1994); therefore, a multidisciplinary approach must be employed, based on currently available methods. Some of the diagnostic methods and combinations of methods that are regularly used for diagnosing BTB are shown in Figure 1.

Bovine tuberculosis infection in cattle is usually diagnosed in the live animal. The diagnosis is based on delayed hypersensitivity reactions (intradermal tuberculin tests), a method that may lack both sensitivity and specificity. However, a definitive diagnosis is still established by isolation and identification of the etiological agent (*M. bovis*) from clinical samples, using a combination of traditional culture and biochemical methods, which is considered the "gold standard". These methods are slow, cumbersome, unreliable, and time-consuming (it may take more than 4 weeks to grow the microorganism, and an additional 2 weeks to identify it). Several alternative approaches have been attempted for the rapid and specific diagnosis of tuberculosis, but molecular methods, especially polymerase chain reaction (PCR) assays, are the most promising for diagnoses in live cattle (Serrano-Moreno et al., 2008; Figueiredo et al., 2010) and direct-detection *post mortem* diagnosis in bovine tissue samples (Cardoso et al., 2009; Liebana et al., 1995; Meickle et al., 2001; Romero et al., 1999; Vitale et al., 1998; Wards et al., 1995; Zanini et al., 1998; Zanini et al., 2001;).

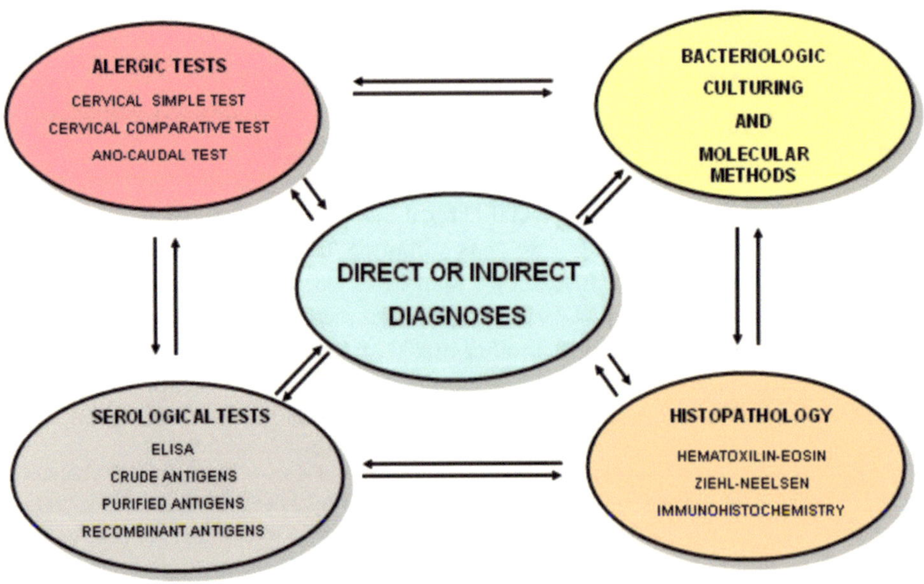

Fig. 1. Methods currently used to diagnose bovine tuberculosis (Medeiros et al., 2010).

The purpose of this chapter is to present new diagnostic approaches for the *Mycobacterium tuberculosis* complex in particular. We focus on discriminating *Mycobacterium bovis* by the use of multiplex PCR and HPLC methods, which have been used to decrease the prevalence of this infection in countries where the disease still occurs.

2. Molecular methods in the diagnosis of bovine tuberculosis: Experiences from the field with a dairy herd in Brazil

Our studies were conducted on a dairy herd comprised of 270 adult crossbred Holstein and Gir cows, located in the Municipality of Macaé, state of Rio de Janeiro in southeast Brazil. Prior to the study, 21 adult cows had positive reactions to a Single Intradermal Tuberculin Test (SITT) and were kept in quarantine for 90 days, awaiting confirmatory tests. After 90 days, a Comparative Intradermal Tuberculin Test (CITT) was performed on these 21 cows (Group A), plus 29 selected cows that were negative for the first SITT test, including those with inconclusive results in the first test (Group B). A total of 34 animals reacted in the CITT (21/21 from Group A and 13/29 from Group B). From all 34 cows, milk samples and nasal swabs were collected and subjected to bacteriological culture, and the isolates were identified by the HPLC method and m-PCR, and also direct detection by m-PCR. All 34 cows were slaughtered 30 days after the injection of PPD, and thorough necropsies were performed. Mediastinal, scapular and retropharyngeal lymph nodes, as well as samples from the lungs were collected and also were analyzed by bacteriological tests, as well as HPLC and m-PCR.

2.1 Identification of *Mycobacterium bovis* isolates by a multiplex PCR (Figueiredo et al., 2009)

Several PCR systems have been developed for the detection of species belonging to the *M. tuberculosis* complex (MTC). The most commonly used system is based on primers that amplify segments of the IS*6110* element, particularly targeting the 123-bp (Eisenach et al., 1990) and 245-bp fragments (Hermans et al., 1990). Another PCR system that has yielded successful identification of *M. bovis* isolates is focused on the amplification of a 500-bp DNA fragment in the RvD1Rv2031c genomic sequence (Rodríguez et al., 1999). A combination of conventional culture and biochemical techniques is the gold-standard method currently used for the identification of *M. bovis*, combining the isolation of the etiological agent and the unequivocal identification of the isolate. Mycobacteria were isolated form suggestive bovine tuberculous lesions, and the pure cultures of acid-fast bacilli (AFB) were identified by molecular analysis. The molecular assay consists of a single-step multiplex PCR (m-PCR), based on two set primers already tested and proved to be reliable, but not yet combined in a single PCR system. The combined PCR assay targets simultaneously the RvD1Rv2031c and IS6110 sequences, aiming to identify bacteria as MTC members as well as to distinguish *M. bovis* isolates from the other members of this complex.

Among the 50 adult cows from this herd that were tested by the intradermal tuberculin test according to official standards (Brasil, 2004), 34 animals were reactive, and were euthanized and necropsied. During the necropsy, a total of 91 samples of lymph nodes and lungs were collected, although not all the animals presented typical lesions. Samples were maintained under refrigeration, and tissues of each animal were processed together as one pooled sample per animal, totaling 34 samples. Samples were decontaminated using the Petroff method, inoculated on slopes of Lowenstein- Jensen medium with sodium pyruvate and incubated for three months at 37ºC. After growth, AFB-positive colonies were screened by m-PCR. Briefly, the mycobacterial DNA was extracted as described previously (Meickle et al., 20073). m-PCR was performed in a reaction mixture (50 µL) containing 5 µl of 10 × PCR buffer (Invitrogen®), 200 µM dNTP (GE Healthcare®), 2.5 U of recombinant *Taq* polymerase (Invitrogen®), 0.2 µM of each primer (Invitrogen®) JB21 (5′-TCGTCCGCTGATGCAAGTGC-3′) and JB22 (5′-CGTCCGCTGACCTCAAGAAAG-3′) (4) and INS1 (5′-CGTGAGGGCATCGAGGTGGC-3′) and INS2 (5′-GCGTAGGCGTCGGTGACAAA-3′) (10), 2.0 mM MgCl2, and 5 µL of purified DNA template. Amplification was carried out in a GeneAmp PCR System 9600 (Applied Biosystems®) with the following cycling parameters: 94ºC for 5 min, followed by 30 cycles of 1 min at 94ºC, 1 min at 68ºC and 1 min at 72ºC, with a final extension at 72ºC for 7 min. PCR products were checked by electrophoresis on 1.5% agarose gels stained with ethidium bromide (10 µg/mL). Negative samples were analyzed by PCR restriction analysis (PRA), using primers Tb11 (5'-ACCAACGATGGTGTGTCCA T-3') and Tb12 (5'-CTTGTCGAACCGCATACCCT-3') targeting for the *hsp*65 gene (Telenti et al., 1993). The amplification products were digested with *Bst*E II and *Hae*III and the resulting fragments were fractionated by agarose gel electrophoresis and stained with ethidium bromide.

Mycobacteria colonies were isolated in Lowenstein-Jensen medium with sodium pyruvate from 17 of 34 (50%) processed samples, therefore confirming the infection. This herd had been TB-free in the last test, performed six months before the study. Therefore, we believe that the reactive cows had a recent infection, where visible lesions are not always present and the bacterial load is low. Considering the decontamination method used, it is not surprising that not all cultures yielded *M. bovis*. Nevertheless, it is noteworthy that the presence of some positive cultures is sufficient to characterize the outbreak of TB in this herd.

In these 17 isolates, m-PCR successfully amplified both target regions (the 500-bp fragment specific for *M. bovis* and the 245-bp fragment diagnostic for MTBC) in 15 of them (88.24%) (Figure 2, lanes 1-15). The two (11.76%) m-PCR-negative isolates (Figure 2, lanes 16 and 17) were confirmed by PCR-restriction analysis as *Mycobacterium* sp., but were not included in the *Mycobacterium tuberculosis* complex (results not shown).

PCR assays using primers JB21/JB22 have been considered to be highly reliable in identifying *M. bovis* isolates, showing 100% concordance with the conventional microbiological method (Rodríguez et al., 1999). However, the absolute specificity of JB21/JB22 primers for *M.* bovis has been disputed by another study, which reported that 13.3% (4/30) of *M. bovis* isolates failed to produce the 500-bp fragment (Sechi et al., 2000). Using specific primers for the IS6110 sequence, the 500-bp negative isolates were identified as belonging to the MTC, leading the authors to suggest that these isolates may lack the genomic target for JB21/JB22 primers. As this genotypic characteristic may not be infrequent, the use of a single primer pair can produce false negative results. On the other hand, an additional primer pair targeting for a different sequence, as in m-PCR, minimizes the occurrence of such false-negative results. The two sets of primers, although already described in the literature (Hermans et al., 1990; Rodríguez et al., 1999), as explained before, for the first time were combined to optimize a mPCR assay able to identify unequivocally *M. bovis* among mycobacterial isolates. The mPCR method was fast, reproducible and useful for the study of slow-growing mycobacteria, particularly in cultures where the small number of bacilli hinders identification by classical methods. It also can be a valuable tool for the rapid identification of acid-fast bacilli isolated from suggestive bovine TB lesions.

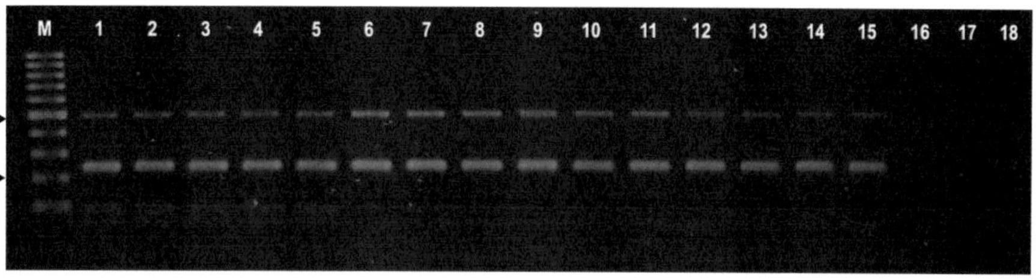

Fig. 2. **Identification of ABF isolates by m-PCR.** DNA extracted from 17 different acid-fast bacilli isolates was used as a template for m-PCR amplification of the RvD1Rv2031c and the IS6110 sequences. Amplification products were separated by electrophoresis on 1.5% agarose gel and stained with ethidium bromide (10 µg/mL). Lane M: 100-bp DNA ladder (Fermentas®); lanes 1-17: m-PCR products of acid-fast bacilli isolated from suggestive BT lesions; lane 18: negative control. Arrows indicate the positions of the fragments of 500 bp (diagnostic for *M. bovis*) and 245 bp (diagnostic for MTBC members).

2.2 Detection of *Mycobacterium bovis* DNA in nasal swabs from tuberculous cattle by a multiplex PCR (Figueiredo et al., 2010)

The multiplex PCR-based method for the simultaneous detection of mycobacteria belonging to MTC and the specific identification of *M. bovis* was adapted to screen nasal swabs collected from live cows, suspected to be tuberculous. A total of 50 adult cows from a dairy herd with a previous history of bovine tuberculosis, including clinical cases, from Macaé were tested by the cervical comparative intradermal tuberculin test (ITT) with PPD (purified protein derivative) according to official standards (Brasil, 2004). In parallel, samples of nasal mucus were collected using sterile swabs and submitted to both microbiological culture and m-PCR. All 34 ITT-reactive animals (68% of the total of cows examined) were slaughtered; the lungs and lymph nodes were removed and processed for bacteriology according to the OIE Terrestrial Manual (OIE, 2009). Briefly, after decontamination by the Petroff method, samples from lungs, lymph nodes and nasal swabs were inoculated on Lowenstein-Jensen and Stonebrink agar slopes and the tubes were incubated at 37ºC for up to 12 weeks. The presence of *M. bovis* and other mycobacteria belonging to MTC in nasal mucus was investigated by a single-step multiplex PCR (m-PCR) using two sets of primers, as previously described (Figueiredo et al., 2009), that targets simultaneously the *RvD1-Rv2031c* (specific for *M. bovis*) and IS*6110* (present in all MTC species) genomic sequences, but that to date had not yet been combined together in a single m-PCR assay. DNA was extracted from nasal swabs by a modification of a QIAamp Blood and Tissue Kit (Qiagen). The bacterial pellet was suspended in 180 µl of 20 mg/mL lysozyme in 20 mM Tris·HCl, pH 8.0; 2 mM EDTA; 1.2% Triton and incubated for 30 min at 37°C prior to the proteinase K treatment, in order to improve the process of bacterial lysis. DNA eluted from the QIAamp Mini spin columns was concentrated by precipitation with absolute ethanol at -80ºC. m-PCR was performed in a reaction mix (50 µL) as described by Figueiredo et al. (2009). No mycobacterial growth was observed on agar slopes inoculated with nasal swab samples collected either from ITT-reactive or ITT-negative cows. On the other hand, mycobacterial colonies were observed in cultures from lung or lymph-node samples isolated from 17 of 34

PPD-positive cows (50% of the total of positive cows). In parallel, nasal swabs were examined for the presence of mycobacteria by m-PCR. DNA was extracted from nasal swabs collected from 34 ITT-reactive and 16 ITT-negative cows, using a modification of a QIAamp blood and tissue kit (Qiagen) that was devised to improve bacterial lysis and concentrate DNA. The nucleic acids isolated from all samples using the above-modified procedure showed high quality in terms of integrity and purity, and were suitable for use as templates in the m-PCR. The 500-bp fragment specific for *M. bovis* and the 245-bp fragment diagnostic for MTC were simultaneously observed in 2 of 34 (5.9%) of m-PCR reactions performed using nasal-swab DNA from ITT-reactive cows. Importantly, neither the 500-bp band nor the 245-bp band was found as m-PCR reaction products when swabs from ITT-negative cows were tested (results not shown).

M. bovis has been recovered from nasal exudates collected from cattle in naturally infected herds by using conventional culture techniques (de Kantor & Roswurm, 1978; McIlroy et al., 1986; Meickle et al., 2007). In these reports, recovery efficiencies varied from 8.7 (4) to 28.5%, when solely ITT-reactive animals were assessed (Meickle et al., 2007), regardless of the difficulty of the procedure, since it requires the presence of 10-100 viable organisms in the sample for a positive result, a condition attained only in advanced stages of the disease (Barry et al., 1993). Using PCR-based methods, the presence of species of the MTC group in nasal exudates of ITT-reactive animals was detected in 26% of the tested samples (Tejada et al., 2006), with some studies reporting detection rates of 50 or 58% (13,23), even though some PCR techniques may detect *M. bovis* using as little as 5 fg of DNA, which is equivalent to the amount of nucleic acid in a single mycobacterial genome (Estrada-Chávez et al., 2004).

The number of positive animals was smaller than expected, which was probably caused by limitations in the current PCR protocols for detection of mycobacteria in nasal exudates, such as intermittent shedding, inefficient DNA extraction, or the presence of PCR inhibitors in the samples (de la Rua-Domenech et al., 2006). None of the nasal-exudate samples from 34 ITT-reactive cows were found to be positive for the growth of *M. bovis*. Furthermore, 2 of 34 nasal-exudate samples (5.9%) were positive by m-PCR, a more sensitive and specific method than culturing (Meickle et al., 2007; Zanini et al., 1998; Zumárraga et al., 2005). These figures are lower than those previously obtained by using culture- or PCR-based methods to evaluate the presence of *M. bovis* in nasal exudates (de la Rua-Domenech et al., 2006; Meickle et al., 2007; Tejada et al., 2006; Vitale et al., 1998). The low rate of positive results may possibly be a consequence of the small numbers of viable bacteria present in nasal-swab samples, because the growth of the etiological agent was observed in cultures of lung and lymph-node samples from 17 of these cows, using the same procedure.

It has been well documented that in cattle experimentally infected with *M. bovis*, after each infection there is a lag period during which the etiological agent cannot be isolated from nasal mucus (Neill et al., 1998; McCorry et al., 2005; Kao et al., 2007). In a previously reported study, all experimentally infected animals shed *M. bovis* in the nasal mucus (Neill et al., 1998); but failure of some experimental animals to shed mycobacteria has also been reported (McCorry et al., 2005; Kao et al., 2007). Importantly, differences in the shedding profiles were observed, where those animals shedding *M. bovis* in nasal exudates were classified as either intermittent or as persistent shedders. It also appears that the overall level of shedding increases during the first four weeks after exposure and then begins to decline (Kao et al., 2007), although shedding can still be detected for many weeks, and in some cases for several months. In conclusion, we have successfully used m-PCR assay to detect *M. bovis* in nasal exudates of naturally infected cattle, as previously reported (Meickle et al., 2007; Tejada et al., 2006; Vitale et al.,1998). Indeed, Vitale et al. (1998) reported high specificity and positive predictive value in the detection of MTC in nasal swabs by PCR, and Romero et al. (1999) demonstrated that nasal-mucus samples work better for the *in vivo* PCR-based detection of the microorganism than other fluids such as blood or milk. However, all these previous reports utilized primers to detect MTC species, and the identification of *M. bovis* was presumptive. The mPCR used here has the advantage of being specific for *M. bovis,* but simultaneously identifies the presence of *M. bovis* and other non-*M. bovis* mycobacterial species belonging to MTC. Although limited by the natural evolution of the infection, since shedding of mycobacteria in nasal mucus is required, the use of m-PCR for detecting live tuberculous animals by testing the nasal mucus could be an effective and highly specific *ante-mortem* ancillary method for surveillance of bovine tuberculosis in herds, if a periodic sampling scheme is followed; or as a confirmatory method for animals with inconclusive intradermal testing, thus assisting the bovine tuberculosis control and eradication program.

2.3 Detection of *Mycobacterium bovis* DNA in milk by m-PCR

Another valuable tool in confirming tuberculous cows is the identification of *M. bovis* in milk produced by the suspected animals. A PCR assay was developed for direct detection of *M. bovis* DNA in artificially and naturally contaminated milk. The assay used a pair of primers that were previously tested and proved reliable in targeting putative gene RvD1-Rv2031c.

Milk previously seeded with *M. bovis* was used as the starting material. The procedure involved DNA extraction by enzymatic lysing (proteinase K and lysozyme) and phenol:chloroform:isoamyl alcohol, followed by ethanol precipitation and m-PCR. The m-PCR was performed according to Figueiredo et al. (2010), and allowed us to detect *M. bovis* DNA in artificially contaminated milk, with a detection limit of 100 CFU/mL.

The use of the PCR method in spiked milk samples does not guarantee that it would perform equally effectively in the analysis of naturally infected samples. One could expect that in the latter, the interaction between the bacilli and the milk matrix could be more complex, and even that bacilli in milk might have already been killed by mammary macrophages (Zumarraga et al., 2005) and the DNA partially degraded. Therefore, the mPCR described here was evaluated for detection of *M. bovis* DNA in fresh unprocessed milk from CITT-reactive cows. A total of 50 adult cows from a dairy herd with a previous history of bovine tuberculosis, including clinical cases, from Macaé were tested by the cervical comparative intradermal tuberculin test (CITT) with PPD (purified protein derivative) according to official standards (Brasil, 2004). Thirty-four animals were CITT-reactive, and from all 50 cows, milk samples were collected (on the day that PPD was injected) and were subjected to bacteriological culture and m-PCR assay.

No mycobacterium growth was observed in CITT-negative cows (0/16). but in five milk samples collected from CITT-reactive cows (5/34) mycobacterial growth was observed. Only one isolate was confirmed as *M. bovis* by m-PCR (Figure 1, lane 1). Mycobacterial colonies were also observed in cultures from lung or lymph-node samples isolated from 17 of the 34 PPD-positive cows, and were confirmed as *M. bovis* by m-PCR (Figueiredo et al., 2009). In parallel, milk samples were tested for the presence of mycobacterium DNA using the m-PCR. The 500-bp fragment specific for *M. bovis* and the 245-bp fragment diagnostic for MTC were simultaneously observed in 4 of 34 (12%) m-PCR reactions performed with milk DNA templates from CITT-reactive cows (Figure 4). Importantly, neither the 500-bp nor the 245-bp amplicons were found when milk from CITT-negative cows was tested.

Similarly, in analyzing milk samples of cows from infected herds, previous studies have not detected any positive animal (Perez et al., 2002), while others targeting for the RvD1-Rv2031c, IS6110 sequence and MPB70 gene have reported amplifications from 2% to 28% of the cows (Romero et al., 1999; Zumárraga et al., 2005). Other studies using nested PCR (Serrano-Moreno et al., 2008; Vitale et al., 1998) also showed that the presence of *M. bovis* in milk is heterogeneous. The variable PCR results can be explained since the bacilli shed may be associated with cell-mediated immunity (CMI) in tuberculous cows (Pollock et al., 2001; Romero et al., 2006), as well as with epidemiological factors such as viral immunosuppression, metabolic imbalance, corticosteroids and peripartum (Doherth et al., 1995, 1996; Sordillo et al., 1997; Piccinini et al., 2006).

Thirty of the milk samples from CIIT-reactive cows were negative by PCR. This suggests that some periods of bacterial excretion might have been missed, due to the design of the study, which included only one sampling. The intermittent character of bacilli secretion after a short constant post-infection period was documented by Menzies and Neill (2000). Another important point is that the 500-bp band was not found as a PCR product when milk from CITT-negative cows was tested, and mycobacterial colonies could not be isolated by culturing. The lack of recovery of *Mycobacterium* sp. could be due to the small number of excreted bacteria, or to the presence of dead or non-viable bacilli due to the action of macrophages, or even to the use of the Petroff decontamination method and reduced sensitivity of culturing compared with PCR (Zumárraga et al., 2005).

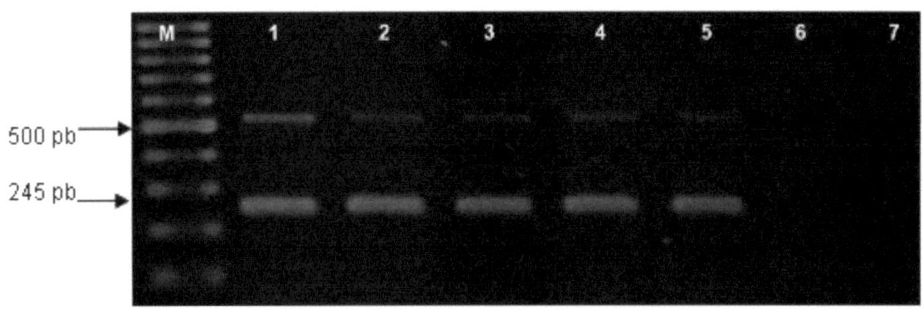

Fig. 3. **Direct Detection of** *M. bovis* **DNA in milk samples from CITT-reactive cows.** DNA templates obtained from 1 mL of milk samples were amplified by m-PCR of the RvD1Rv2031c and the IS6110 sequences. Amplicons were resolved on a 1.5% agarose gel stained with ethidium bromide. Lane M: 100-bp DNA ladder (Promega®); lane 1: positive control, *M. bovis* IP; lanes 2-5: milk samples from CITT-reactive cows; lane 6: negative control (water); lane 7: negative control (DNA template from *M. fortuitum* ATCC 6841). From each cow, three samples were analyzed and three independent experiments were performed.

The PCR assay allowed us to detect *M. bovis* DNA in artificially contaminated milk, with a detection limit of 100 CFU/mL, and also proved to be able to detect the bacilli in naturally infected milk. This method could be useful to assist the *in vivo* diagnosis for BTB, complementing the serological or microbiological tests, and is an alternative option in cases of mammary tuberculosis where the efficiency of serological diagnosis is nil. The method will be useful in epidemiological studies of BTB transmission and in quality control for the dairy industry, to prevent contaminated milk from entering the food supply.

2.4 Detection of *Mycobacterium bovis* DNA in bovine tissues by m-PCR

We adapted the m-PCR assay targeting the RvD1Rv2031c and IS6110 sequences, which are specific for *M. bovis* and MTC respectively, to identify *M. bovis* DNA in tissues from slaughtered positive-skin-test animals. The results are compared with those from the skin test and conventional culture for *M. bovis*.

Of 270 adult crossbred Holstein and Gir cows in a herd located in Macaé, 34 cows were considered CITT-reactive and also infected, by IFN assay (Marasi et al., 2010). At 30 days after CIIT, all 34 reactive animals were slaughtered and necropsied. Tissue samples were collected and analyzed by bacteriological methodology and m-PCR. DNA was extracted from lymph nodes, lung and udder tissues taken from the slaughtered animals, by a modification of a QIAamp Blood and Tissue Kit (Qiagen). One sample was selected per animal. A small piece of tissue (1-2 g) was macerated and an aliquot of 1 mL was taken. The pellet was suspended in 180 µl of 20 mg/mL lysozyme in 20 mM Tris·HCl, pH 8.0; 2 mM EDTA; and 1.2% Triton, and incubated for 1 h at 37°C prior to proteinase K treatment, in order to improve the process of bacterial lysis. DNA eluted from the QIAamp mini spin columns was concentrated by precipitation with absolute ethanol at -80ºC and eluted with 200 µL of the buffer.

The m-PCR was performed according to Figueiredo et al. (2010). In 17/34 (50%) samples *Mycobacterium* sp. isolates were obtained, and 15/17 were confirmed as *M. bovis* by m-PCR (Figueiredo et al., 2009). Direct m-PCR on tissue samples from CITT-reactive cows was positive for *M. bovis* DNA in 25/34 (73.5%) of the samples. All positive-culture specimens were also positive for m-PCR; and 10 (59%) samples that were negative by culturing yielded a positive result after m-PCR assay. It should be mentioned that the PCR was sensitive enough to detect *M. bovis* in a large proportion (59%) of those samples that failed to grow in culture, as also reported by Liebana et al. (1995), Zanini et al. (2001) and Araújo et al. (2005). The efficiency of the culture method used as a first criterion for *M. bovis* identification is low, because of the small number of live bacilli present in some tissues. Small numbers of live bacilli may be a consequence of a short delay in getting tissues to the laboratory, or may be due to the sensitivity of mycobacteria to the NaOH used in the Petroff method.

The improved identification shown here can be attributed to the removal of unwanted inhibitors. Ward et al. (1995) and Liebana et al. (1995) stated that "mycobacteria are difficult organisms from which to extract DNA and because they often exist as intracellular pathogens, may also be difficult organisms to purify from clinical samples, particularly tissues". Some compounds present in tissues, such as eukaryotic DNA or blood-originated inhibitory substances such as hemoglobin, lactoferrin and undegraded nucleic-acid samples from inflamed tissue can inhibit DNA amplification (Cardoso et al., 2009). On the other hand, the use of the QIAamp Blood and Tissue Kit (Qiagen) circumvented those problems and supplied DNA templates suitable for amplification.

The nine remaining CITT-reactive cows were negative by both the culturing and m-PCR assays. Those results could be attributed to an inhibitory effect in the PCR assay (Al-Soud and Radstrom, 2001; Cardoso et al., 2009), and additional inquires are needed with regard to DNA extraction methods. In addition, it should be considered that the tissue samples collected from those animals contained a low pathogen load, characterizing paucibacillary lesions that are commonly observed in recent infections occurring intra-herd. Two previous studies (Zanini et al., 2001; Cardoso et al., 2009) also reported a decreased efficiency in detecting mycobacteria in paucibacillary tissue samples. It is generally accepted that the CITT is a correlate of *M. bovis* infection and not necessarily of disease (Neill et al. 1994). In this study, CIIT-reactive animals developed disease, as demonstrated by the presence of lesions.

The results presented here indicate that m-PCR can detect *M. bovis* DNA in tissue samples, and represents a valid additional tool for the *post-mortem* diagnosis of BTB. Multiplex PCR is faster than culture-based detection, reducing diagnosis time from 120 to approximately 2 days, even when automated culturing with broth medium is used. Moreover, m-PCR is useful when the bacilli are non-viable and cannot be detected by culture methods. It can be of valuable help during sanitary inspection at slaughterhouses for condemnation of carcasses that show suspected lesions, or slaughtered animals suspected of having the disease. It is also important to note that a detailed inspection of bovine organs performed during necropsy in the field is more efficient than a rapid inspection at the slaughterhouse, because in the latter situation small lesions may be not detected.

2.5 Identification of species of the *Mycobacterium tuberculosis* complex by adapted High-Performance Liquid Chromatography (HPLC)

Complex high-molecular-weight β-hydroxyl fatty acids with a 22- or 24-carbon alkyl chain at the α-position are structural characteristics of mycolic acids, a fatty acid found in the *Mycobacterium* cell wall. By using several methods of fatty acid analysis, mycolic acids have been considered to be species- or group-specific (Butler et al., 1991). High-performance liquid chromatography (HPLC) analysis of mycolic acids has emerged as a reliable method for the diagnosis of mycobacteria, due to its rapid and reproducible nature, and because the mycolic-acid elution pattern observed for each mycobacterial species has generally been found to be unique, except for a few species that share the same pattern profile (Hagen & Thompson, 1995). The HPLC method has been considered a standard test for chemotaxonomic classification and rapid identification of *Mycobacterium* species by the Centers for Disease Control and Prevention (CDC) (http://www.cdc.gov), since 1990, and has been reported to achieve accuracy above 96% compared with DNA probe tests (Butler & Guthertz, 2001). A dedicated database, using adapted local protocols, must be developed in order to obtain chromatogram profiles from reference strains in the new analytic conditions, accrediting the local methodology and allowing for the correct analysis of clinical samples.

An HPLC method to identify *Mycobacterium* species, originally developed on a short column (CDC, 1996), was transferred to a longer column with similar stationary phase properties, but with a length of at most 33% of the initial one. Protocol modifications improved the separation capabilities and the methodology specificity. Mycolic acids from 35 different reference *Mycobacterium* strains were saponified, extracted, derivatized, analyzed and successfully identified by the adapted HPLC method. The identification of mycobacteria was based on the relative retention times (RRT) of the chromatograms, comparing the profile obtained from the reference strains with profiles available in external databases. Although an internal standard was not used to align the chromatograms, the method showed good reproducibility and standardization, using the range of the relative standard deviation (RSD) of absolute retention time (ART) and the RRT, which varied from 0.68% to 0.97% and from 0.39% to 0.72%, respectively. The adapted method improved the identification of *Mycobacterium* species of clinical and veterinary interest, by comparing the new isolates with a database of mycolic acid chromatogram patterns from 35 reference mycobacteria strains, and comparing those profiles with those previously reported in the literature to enable identification of MTC species.

A suspension of acid-fast bacteria grown in LJ medium was removed with a swab and saponified with 2 ml KOH 25% in methanol:H_2O (v:v) autoclaved for 1 h at 121°C, 15 psi, to cleave the mycolic acids bound to the cell wall (Butler et al., 1991). Mycolic acids were then separated by acidification with HCl:H_2O (v:v) and extraction in chloroform. After conversion to ultraviolet (UV)-absorbing *p*-bromophenacyl esters (Pircen®) (Butler & Guthertz, 2001) and clearing with HCl:H_2O:Methanol (1:1:2, v:v:v), the mycolic acids were analyzed on a reverse-phase C18 100 x 4.6 mm column (Kromasil®) using high-performance liquid chromatography (Cage, 1994; Duffey et al., 1996). A gradient of methanol and dichloromethane (methylene chloride) generated by microprocessor-controlled pumps was used to separate the mycolic acid esters (Butler et al., 1991, Viader-Salvadó et al., 2007), which were detected with a UV detector at 260 nm (Du et al., 2008). Reproducible chromatographic patterns containing combinations of different diagnostic peaks (Butler et al., 1991, Glickman et al., 1994) were obtained by using reference strains (*M. abscessus* ATCC 19977, *M. africanum* ATCC 25420, *M. agri* ATCC 27406, *M. aichiense* ATCC 27280, *M. asiaticum* ATCC 25276, *M. aurum* ATCC 23366, *M. avium* ATCC 25291, *M. bovis* ATCC 19210, *M. bovis* BCG INCQS 00062, *M. chelonae* ATCC 35752, *M. flavescens* ATCC 14474, *M. fortuitum* ATCC 6841, *M. gastri* ATCC 15754, *M. godornae* ATCC 141470, *M. intracellulare* ATCC 13950, *M. malmoense* ATCC 29571, *M. mucogenicum* ATCC 49650, *M. scrofulaceum* ATCC 19981, *M. simiae* ATCC 25275, *M. terrae* ATCC 15755, *M. tuberculosis* ATCC 25177, *M. vaccae* ATCC15483 and *M. triviale* ATCC23292). Pattern recognition was done by visual comparison of the results for the reference strains with mycolic acid patterns from species of known mycobacteria (CDC, 1996, 1999). Identification of mycobacterial species by mycolic acid analysis was performed by visually comparing the UV patterns obtained from the samples with UV patterns from reference species, following recommendations of Butler and collaborators (Butler et al., 1991; Butler and Guthertz, 2001). Chromatographic patterns for each strain were examined for differences in the heights for pairs of peaks. HPLC patterns were grouped according to species, and the calculated values for each ratio were combined, sorted in numerical order, and examined for their ability to discriminate species, using the range of the relative standard deviation (RSD) of absolute retention time (ART) and the relative retention time (RRT). The 35 species were grouped into three general patterns (single, double and triple clusters) and divided accordingly into subgroups, according to Butler and Guthertz (2001).

A total of 21 *M. bovis* isolates from tissue, milk and nasal-swab samples from a dairy herd comprised of 270 adult crossbred Holstein and Gir cows, located in Macaé were confirmed by multiplex PCR (m-PCR) targeting for RvD1Rv2031c and IS6110 sequences, which are specific for the *M. bovis* and *M. tuberculosis* complexes, respectively (Figueiredo et al., 2009). Spoligotyping (Kamerbeek et al., 1997) was used to validate the HPLC methodology.

It has been reported that BCG-attenuated strains of *M. bovis* could be successfully differentiated from the MTC by HPLC (Floyd et al., 1992). This observation was confirmed in the present study, by comparing the chromatograms obtained from reference strains (Fig. 4). Other members of the complex, such as *M. bovis* and *M. tuberculosis,* were known to produce very similar chromatogram patterns, making it impossible to discriminate between them by this methodology. However, although requiring further work, the chromatogram profiles generated by the adapted elution protocol showed discrete and consistent differences in their chromatograms that could be used to discriminate them (Fig. 5-A). The simple and late-emerging single-cluster peak pattern group also included *M. asiaticum*, *M. gordonae* chromotype I (Fig. 5-B) and *M. kansasii* (Fig. 5-B). *M. triviale* was the only mycobacterium species present in this group, and it can be easily recognized (Fig. 5-B).

In these 21 isolates, m-PCR successfully amplified both target regions (the 500-bp fragment specific for *M. bovis* and the 245-bp fragment diagnostic for MTBC) in all isolates. A total of four spoligotypes were identified among the 21 *M. bovis* isolates. Two spoligotypes (SB0120 and SB0833) were described in the *M. bovis* spoligotype database (Brudey et al., 2006; www.mbovis.org). The other two represent novel, previously undescribed spoligotypes. The HPLC assay also identified the clinical *M. bovis* isolates as members of the *Mycobacterium tuberculosis* complex (Figure 6).

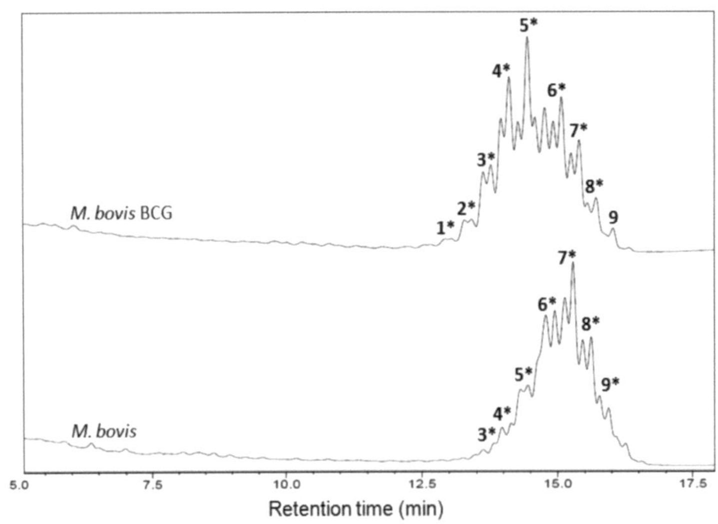

Fig. 4. Mycolic acid chromatograms from *M. bovis* BCG (INCQS0062) and *M. bovis* (ATCC 19210). * peaks showing a high degree of separation (appearing as a "double peak"), named according to Butler et al. (1991).

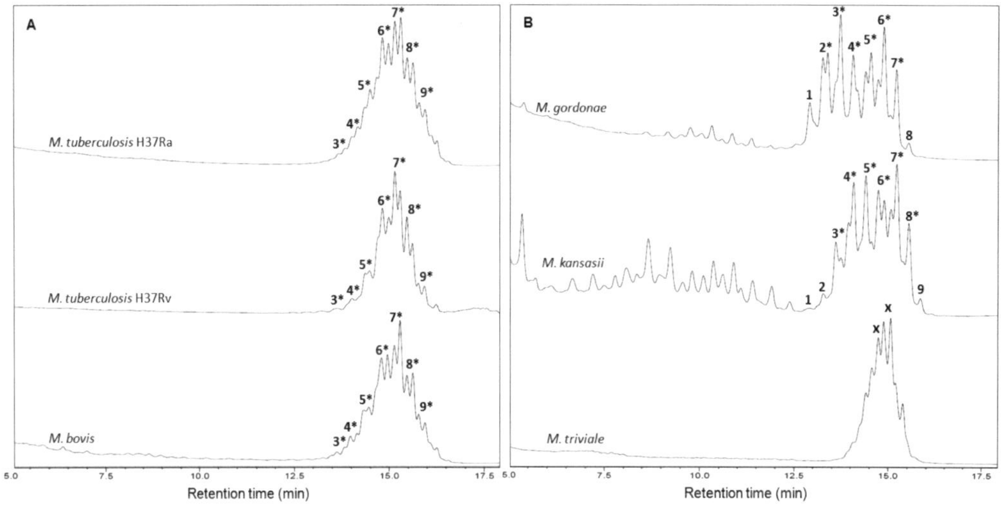

Fig. 5. Characteristic HPLC chromatograms of *Mycobacterium* species with late-emerging, simple, single-cluster peak patterns. **A**) *M. tuberculosis* H37Ra (ATCC 25177) and H37Rv (ATCC 27294) and *M. bovis* (ATCC 19210). **B**) *M. gordonae* chromotype I (ATCC 14470), *M. kansasii* (ATCC 12478) and *M. triviale* (ATCC 23292). *peaks showing a high degree of separation (appearing as a "double peak"), named according to Butler et al. (1991). *M. triviale* strain: ˣpeaks showing a high degree of separation (appearing as a "double peak"), compared to the chromatogram profile described by Butler & Guthertz (2001).

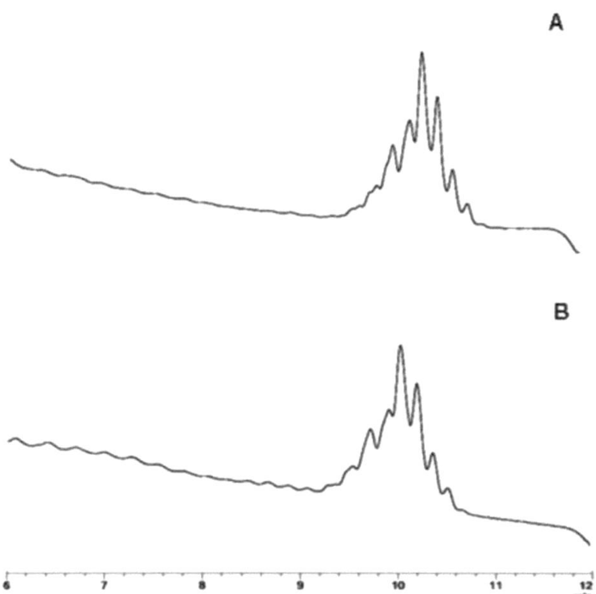

Fig. 6. Representative reverse-phase HPLC chromatograms of mycolic acid methylesters from reference strains and isolates: (A) *M. bovis* ATCC 19210; (B) 21 clinical *M. bovis* isolates from dairy herds in Brazil.

Identification of mycobacterium species using HPLC for mycolic acid analysis has proven to be rapid, reproducible and easily executed by several laboratories, making this approach one of the most appropriate methods to distinguish among the species. The separation capability using the modified method was superior to CDC patterns, and could be an alternative to allow discrimination between species with homologous HPLC chromatogram profiles.

3. Conclusion

Despite all efforts to control BTB, the disease persists, with serious implications for human health and the economy, particularly in the context of global trade. Because of the particular and complex characteristics of BTB, there is a growing realization that no single method by itself is sufficient to detect all the reactive animals in every stage of infection. Therefore, a multidisciplinary approach must be employed, using various categories of currently available methods. In a modern approach to the diagnosis and control of BTB, bacteriological, molecular, histopathological, and immunological assays must be employed, considering the indications, advantages, and disadvantages of each method. In this study we found that molecular diagnosis, combined with *ante mortem* and *post mortem* inspection, appeared to be a promising technique to improve the surveillance of BTB in herds, slaughterhouses, and the dairy industry, contributing to the success of the bovine tuberculosis eradication program.

4. References

Abrahão, R.M.C.M.; Nogueira, P.A. & Malucelli, M.I.C. O comércio clandestino de carne e leite no Brasil e o risco da transmissão da tuberculose bovina e outras doenças ao homem: Um problema de saúde pública (Meat and milk black market - Bovine tuberculosis). *Archives of Veterinary Science*. v. 10, n. 2, p. 1-17, 2005.

Araújo, C.P., Leite, C.Q.F.; Prince, K.A. Jorge, K.S.G. & Osorio, A.L.R. (2005). *Mycobacterium bovis* identification by a molecular method from post-mortem inspected cattle obtained in abattoirs of Mato Grosso do Sul, Brazil. *Mem. Inst. Oswaldo Cruz* 100, 749–752.

Al-Soud, W.A., & P. Radstrom. (2001). Purification and characterization of PCR-inhibitory components in blood cells. *J. Clin. Microbiol.* 39, 485–493.

Baptista, F; Moreira, E. C; Santos, W. L. M & Naveda, L. A. B. (2004). Prevalência da tuberculose em bovinos abatidos em Minas Gerais/ Prevalence of tuberculosis among bovines slaughtered in Minas Gerais, Brazil. *Arq. bras. med. vet. zootec*; 56(5): 577-580.

Barry, T.; Glennon, M.; Smith, T. & Gannon, F. (1993). Detection of Mycobacterium bovis in bovine blood by combined PCR and DNA probe methods. *Vet Rec.* 132 (3), 66–67.

Brasil. PNCEBT-Ministério da Agricultura Pecuária e Abastecimento do Brasil. Manual técnico, 2004.

Brasil. MAPA-Ministério da Agricultura Pecuária e Abastecimento do Brasil. www.agricultura.gov.br. Acessed 03 Sept 2008.

Butler, W. R.; Jost. K. C.; Kilburn, J. O. Identification of mycobacteria by high-performance liquid chromatography. *J. Clin. Microbiol.* 29:2468–2472, 1991.

Butler, W.R.; Guthertz, L.S. Mycolic acid analysis by high-performance liquid chromatography for identification of Mycobacterium species. *Clin. Microbiol. Rev.* 14:704-726, 2001.

Brudey, K., Driscoll, J. R., Rigouts, L., Prodinger, W., Gori, A., Al-Hajoj, S. A. M., Allix, C., Aristimun˜o, L., Arora, J., Baumanis, V., Binder, L., Cafrune, P., Cataldi, A., Cheong, S., Diel, R., Ellermeier, C., Evans, J. T., Fauville, M., Ferdinand, S., Garcia de Viedma, D., Garzelli, C., Gazzola, L., Gomes, H. M., Guttierez, M. C., Hawkey, P. M., van Helden, P. D., Kadival, G. V., Kreiswirth, B. N., Kremer, K., Kubin, M., Kulkarni, S. P., Liens, B., Lillebaek, T., Ly, H. M., Martin, C., Martin, C., Mokrousov, I., Narvskaı¨a, O., Ngeow, Y. F., Naumann, L., Niemann, S., Parwati, I., Rahim, M. Z., Rasolofo-Razanamparany, V., Rasolonavalona, T., Rossetti, M. L., Ru¨sch-Gerdes, S., Sajduda, A., Samper, S., Seth, P., Shemyakin, I., Singh, U. B., Somoskovi, A., Skuce, R., van Soolingen, D., Streicher, E. M., Suffys, P. N., Tortoli, E., Tracevska, T., Vincent, V., Victor, T. C., Warren, R., Yap, S. F., Zaman, K., Portaels, F., Rastogi, N. and Sola, C., 2006. *Mycobacterium tuberculosis* complex genetic diversity: mining the fourth international spoligotyping database (SpolDB4) for classification, population genetics and epidemiology. *BMC Microbiol.* 6, 23–39.

Cage, G.D. (1994). Direct identification of *Mycobacterium* species in BACTEC 7H12B medium by high-performance liquid chromatography. *J. Clin. Microbiol.* 32: 521-524.

Corner, L.A.; Melville, L.; McCubbin, K.; Small, K.J.; McCormick, B.S.; Rothel, J.S. (1990). Efficiency of inspection procedures for detection of tuberculous lesions in cattle. *Aust. Vet. J.* 67 (11), 389-392

Cardoso, M. A.; Cardoso, R. F.; Hirata, R. D. C.; Hirata, M. H.; Leite, C. Q. F.; Santos, A. C. B.; Siqueira, V. L. D.; Okano, W.; Rocha, N. S. and Lonardoni, M. V. C. Direct Detection of Mycobacterium bovis in Bovine Lymph Nodes by PCR. (2009). *Zoonoses Public Health.*

CDC. Human tuberculosis caused by *Mycobacterium bovis*. New York City, 2001-2004. MMWR, 54, 605-608, 2005.

CDC. Centers for Disease Control and Prevention. Mycolic Acid Pattern Standards for HPLC Identification of Mycobacteria. U.S. Department of Health and Human Services, Public Health Service. Atlanta, 1999. 86 p.

CDC. Centers for Disease Control and Prevention. Standardized Method for HPLC Identification of Mycobacteria. U.S. Department of Health and Human Services, Public Health Service. Atlanta, 1996. 99 p.

Cosivi, O., ET AL, Zoonotic Tuberculosis due to *Mycobacterium bovis* in Developing Countries, Emerging Infectious Diseases; Vol. 4 Number1.

Corner, L.A., Melville, L., McCubbin, K., Small, K.J., McCormick, B.S., Rothel, J.S.. Efficiency of inspection procedures for detection of tuberculous lesions in cattle. Australian Veterinary Journal, Vol.67, n°11, November, 1990.

Cassidy, J. P.; Bryson D. G; And Neill, S. D. Tonsillar lesions in cattle naturally infected with *Mycobacterium bovis*. *Vet. Rec.* 144, 139–142, 1999.

De Kantor, I.N.; Roswurm, J.D. (1978). Mycobacteria isolated from nasal secretions of tuberculin test reactor cattle. *Am. J. Vet. Res.* 39 (7), 1233-1234.

de la Rua-Domenech, R.; Goodchild, A.T.; Vordermeier, H.M.; Hewinson, R.G.; Christiansen, K.H.; Clifton-Hadley, R.S. (2006). Ante mortem diagnosis of tuberculosis in cattle: a review of the tuberculin tests, gamma-interferon assay and other ancillary diagnostic techniques. *Res. Vet. Sci.* 81 (2), 190-210.

Doherty, M. L., M. L. Monaghan, H. F. Bassett, P. J. Quinn, And W. C. Davis. Effect of dietary restriction on cellmediated immune responses in cattle infected with *Mycobacterium bovis*. Vet. Immunol. Immunopathol. 49, 307–320, 1996.

Du Rong, Chen B., Guo L., Li Y., Xie J, Wang G. & Zhou H. (2008). Identification of Mycobacterium species using reversed-phase high performance liquid chromatographic analysis of mycolic acid. *Chin J Chromatogr*, , 26(5): 534–539.

Duffey, P.S., Guthertz, L.S. & Evans, G.C. (1996). Improved rapid detection of mycobacteria by combining solid-phase extraction with high-performance liquid chromatography analysis of BACTEC cultures. *J. Clin. Microbiol.* 34: 1939-1943.

Estrada-Chávez, C.; Otero, F.D.; Díaz, C.A.; Villegas-Sepúlveda, N.; González, R.P.; Salazar, D.G. (2004). Concordancia de la PCR y métodos rutinarios para el diagnóstico de tuberculosis bovina. *Vet. Mex.* 35, 225-236.

Figueiredo, E.E.S.; Silvestre, F.G.; Campos, W.N.; Furlanetto, L.V.; Medeiros, L.; Lilenbaum, W.; Fonseca, L.S.; Silva, J.T.; Paschoalin, V.M.F. Detection of *Mycobacterium bovis* DNA in nasal swabs from tuberculous cattle by a multiplex PCR. *Brazilian Journal of Microbiology*, v. 41, n.2, 2010.

Figueiredo, E.E.S.; Silvestre, F.G.; Campos, W.N.; Furlanetto,L.V.,Medeiros, L.; Lilenbaum, W.; Fonseca, L. S.; Silva, J.T.; Paschoalin, V. Identification of *Mycobacterium bovis* Isolates by a multiplex PCR. *Braz. J. Microbiol.*, v.40: 231-233, 2009.

Floyd, M. M.; Silcox, V. A.; Jones, W. D.; Butler, W. R.; Kilburn, J. O. Separation of Mycobacterium bovis BCG from Mycobacterium tuberculosis and Mycobacterium bovis by using high-performance liquid chromatograph of mycolic acids. J. Clin. Microbiol. 30:1327-1330, 1992.

Garnier T, Eiglmeier K, Camus JC, Medina N, Mansoor H, Pryor M, Duthoy S, Grondin S, Lacroix C, Monsempe C, Simon S, Harris B, Atkin R, Doggett J, Mayes R, Keating L, Wheeler PR, Parkhill J, Barrell BG, Cole ST, Gordon SV, Hewinson RG. The complete genome sequence of *Mycobacterium bovis*. Proc Natl Acad Sci U S A. 2003 Jun 24;100(13):7877-82.

Goodchild, A.V.; Clifton-Hadley, R. S. Cattle-tocattle transmission of *Mycobacterium bovis*. *Tuberculosis* 81, 23–41, 2001

Glickman, S.E., Kilburn, J.O., Butler, W.R. & Ramos, L.S. (1994). Rapid identification of mycolic acid patterns of mycobacteria by high-performance liquid chromatography using pattern recognition software and a *Mycobacterium* library. *J Clin Microbiol* 32: 740-745.

Grange, J.M. *Mycobacterium bovis* infection in human beings Tuberculosis, 81 (1-2), February 2001, Pages 71-77

Hagen, S.R.; Thompson , J.D. Analysis of mycolic acids by high-performance liquid chromatography and fluorimetric detection Implications for the identification of mycobacteria in clinical samples. J. Chromatogr. A. 692:167-172, 1995

Kamerbeek, J., Schouls, L., Kolk, A., vanAgterveld, M., vanSoolingen, D., Kuijper, S., Bunschoten, A., Molhuizen, H., Shaw, R., Goyal, M., vanEmbden, J., 1997. Simultaneous detection and strain differentiation of *Mycobacterium tuberculosis* for diagnosis and epidemiology. J. Clin. Microbiol. 35, 907–914.

Kantor, I.N.; Ambroggi, M.; Poggi, S.; Morcillo, N.; Telles, M.A.S.; Ribeiro, M.O., Torres, M.C.G.; Polo, C.L.; Ribón, W.; García, V.; Kuffo, D.; Asencios, L.; Campos, L.M.V.; Rivas, C.; Waard , J.H. Human *Mycobacterium bovis* infection in ten Latin American countries. Tuberculosis, Volume 88, Issue 4, July 2008, Pages 358-365 Kao, R.R.; Gravenor, M.B.; Charleston, B.; Hope, J.C.; Martin, M.; Howard, C.J. (2007). Mycobacterium bovis shedding patterns from experimentally infected calves and the effect of concurrent infection with bovine viral diarrhoea virus. *J. R. Soc. Interface* 4, 545-551.

Leite, C. Q. F.; Anno, I.S.; Leite, S. R.; Roxo, E.; Morlock, G. P.; Cooksey, R. C. Isolation and identification of mycobacteria from livestock specimens and milk obtained in Brazil. *Mem. Inst. Oswaldo Cruz* 98, 319–323, 2003.

Liebana E, Arana A, Mateos A, Vilafranca M, Gomez-Mampaso E, Tercero JC, Alemany J, Suarez G, Domingo M & Dominguez L (1995). Simple and rapid detection of *Mycobacterium tuberculosis* complex organisms in bovine tissue samples by PCR. *J Clin Microbiol 33*: 33-36.

Marassi, C.D.; Medeiros, L.; Lilenbaum, W. The use of a Gamma-Interferon assay to confirm a diagnosis of bovine tuberculosis in Brazil. (2010). Acta Tropica 113, 199–201.

McCorry, T.; Whelan, A.O.; Welsh, M.D.; McNair, J.; Walton, E.; Bryson, D.G.; Hewinson, R.G.; Vordermeier, H.M.; Pollock, J.M. (2005). Shedding of Mycobacterium bovis in the nasal mucus of cattle infected experimentally with tuberculosis by the intranasal and intratracheal routes. *Vet. Rec.* 157, 613-618.

McIlroy, S.G.; Neill, S.D.; McCracken, R.M. (1986). Pulmonary lesions and Mycobacterium bovis excretion from the respiratory tract of tuberculin reacting cattle. *Vet. Rec.* 118, 718-721.

Meikle, V.; Schneider, M., Azenzo, G.; Zumarraga, M.; Magnano, G. and Cataldı A. Individual Animals of a Cattle Herd Infected with the Same Mycobacterium bovis Genotype Shows Important Variations in Bacteriological, Histopathological and Immune Response Parameters. Zoonoses Public Health. 54 (2007) 86–93.

Medeiros, L.S.; Marassi, C.D.; Figueiredo, E.E.S.; Lilenbaum, W. Potential Aplication of New Diagnostic Methods for Controlling Bovine Tuberculosis in Brazil. Brazilian Journal Microbiology, v.1, 531-541, 2010.

Menzies, F. D., & Neill, S. D. Cattle-to-cattle transmission of bovine tuberculosis. *Vet. J.* 160, 92–106, 2000.

Neill, S.D.; Cassidy, J.; Hanna, J.; Mackie, D.P.; Pollock, J.A.; Clements, A.; Walton, E. & Bryson, D.G. (1994). Detection of *Mycobacterium bovis* infection in skin test-negative cattle with an assay for bovine interferon-gamma. *Vet. Rec.* 135 (6), 134-135.

Neill, S.D.; Hanna, J.; O'Brien, J.J.; McCracken, R.M. (1998). Excretion of Mycobacterium bovis by experimentally infected cattle. *Vet. Rec.* 123, 340-343.

Oliveira, I., Melo, H., Câmara, A., Dias, R, Soto-Blanco, B., Prevalência de tuberculose no rebanho bovino de Mossoró, Rio Grande do Norte. Braz. J. vet. Res. anim. Sci., São Paulo, v. 44, n. 6, p. 395-400, 2007.

OIE, 2007; http://www.oie.int/wahid-prod/public.php. WAHID Interface Acessed 12 Aug 2008.

OIE, Terrestrial Manual (2008). Captured January 2009. http://www.oie.int/eng/normes/mmanual/2008/pdf/2.04.07_bovinetb.pdf.

Perez, A.; A. Reniero, A.; Forteis, S.; Meregalli, B.; Lopez, And V. Ritacco. Study of *Mycobacterium bovis* in milk using bacteriological methods and the polymerase chain reaction. *Rev. Argent. Microbiol.* 34, 45–51, 2002.

PAHO/WHO, 2006. http://bvs.panaftosa.org.br/docs/level2. Acessed 22 Jan 2009.

Pardo, R.B.; H. Langoni, L.J.P.; Mendoca, & K. D. Chi. Isolation of *Mycobacterium* spp. In milk from cows suspected or positive to tuberculosis. *J. Vet. Res. Anim. Sci.* 38, 284–287. 2001.

Piccinini, R.; C., Luzzago, M.; Frigerio, V.; Dapra, E.; Liandris, And Zecconi, A. Comparison of blood non-specific immune parameters in Bovine virus diarrhea virus (BVDV) persistently infected and in immune heifers. *J. Vet. Med. B. Infect. Dis. Vet. Public. Health* 53, 62–77, 2006.

Poletto, R.; Kreutz, L.C.; Gonzales, J.C.; Barcellos, L.J.G. Prevalência de tuberculose, brucelose e infecções víricas em bovinos leiteiros do município de Passo Fundo, RS/ Prevalence of tuberculosis, brucelosis and viral infections in dairy cattle from the county of Passo Fundo, RS, Brazil. *Ciência Rural*; 34(2): 595-598, mar.-abr. 2004.

Pollock, J.M., Welsh, M.D., McNair, J.. Immune Response in bovine tuberculosis: Towards new strategies for the diagnosis and control of disease. *Veterinary Immunology and Immunopathology* 108 (2005), 37-43.

Pollock, J. M., J.; Mcnair, M. D.; Welsh, R. M.; Girvin, H. E.; Kennedy, D. P.; Mackie, & Neill, S. D. Immune responses in bovine tuberculosis. *Tuberculosis* 81, 103–107, 2001.

Ribeiro, A. R. P; Lobato, F. C. F; Abreu, V. L. V; Faria, E. S; Silva, J. A. Prevalência de tuberculose e brucelose bovina no município de Ilhéus/ Prevalence of bovine tuberculosis and brucellosis in Ilhéus, Bahia - Brazil. *Arq. bras. med. vet. zootec*; 55(1): 120-122, fev. 2003.

Romano, M.I., Alito, A., Fisanotti, J.C., Bigi, F., Kantor, I., Cicuta, M.E., Cataldi, A. Comparision of different genetic markers for molecular epidemilogy of bovine tuberculosis. Veterinary Microbiology 50 (1996), 59-71.

Romero, B., Aranaz, A., Juan, L., Álvarez, J., Bezos, J., Mateos, A., Mampaso, E.G., Domínguez, L. Molecular Epidemiology of Multidrug-Resistant *Mycobacterium bovis* Isolates with the Same Spoligotyping Profile as Isolates from Animals. J Clin Microbiol. 2006 September; 44(9): 3405–3408.

Romero, R. E.; Garzon, D. L.; Mejia, G. A.; Monroy, W.; Patarroyo, M. E.; Murillo, L. A. Identification of *Mycobacterium bovis* in bovine clinical samples by PCR species-specific primers. Can. J. Vet. Res. 63, 101–106, 1999.

Romero, T. A., C. Arriaga, V. J. Guevara, S. J. A. Garci´A, L. R. A. Torres, & C. Estrada-Chavez. (2006). Confirmacio n de la Excreción de *Mycobacterium bovis* en Exudados Nasales Mediante PCR Anidada en un Hato Lechero. *Vet. Méx.* 37, 137–142.

Salfinger, M.; Pfyffer, G.E. (1994). The new diagnostic mycobacteriology laboratory. *Eur. J. Clin. Microbiol. Infect. Dis.* 13(11), 961–979.

Sequeira, M.D., Ritacco, V., Kantor, I.N., 2005. In: Thoen, O., Gilsdorf, M.J., Steele, J. (Eds.), Mycobacterium bovis Infection in Animals and Humans. Blackwell Publishing, Ames, IA.

Serrano-Moreno, B. A.; Romero, T. A.; Arriaga, C.; Torres R. A.; Pereira-Suarez, A. L.; Garcia-Salazar, J. A.; Estrada-Chavez, C. High Frequency of *Mycobacterium bovis* DNA in Colostra from Tuberculous Cattle Detected by Nested PCR. *Zoonoses Public Health.* 55, 258–266, 2008.

Sobral, L.F. Pesquisa de Mycobacterium bovis entre cepas de micobactérias isoladas no Complexo Hospitalar HUCFF/IDT-UFRJ no período de 2005-2006; 2009. Dissertação (Mestrado) - Programa de Pós-Graduação em Clínica Médica Programa acadêmico de tuberculose, Universidade Federal do Rio de Janeiro.

Sordillo, L. M., K.; Shafer-Weaver, And D. Derosa. Immunobiology of the mammary gland. *J. Dairy Sci.* 80, 1851–1865, 1997.

Viader-Salvadó, J.M., Molina-Torres, C.A. & Guerrero-Olazarán, M. (2007). Detection and identification of mycobacteria by mycolic acid analysis of sputum specimens and young cultures. *J. Microbiol. Methods,* 70(3): 479-483.

Vitale F, Capra G, Maxia L, Reale S, Vesco G, Caracappa S 1998. Detection of *Mycobacterium tuberculosis* complex in cattle by PCR using milk, lymph node aspirates, and nasal swabs. *J Clin Microbiol 36*: 1050-1055.

Vordermeier, H.M., Chambers, M.A., Buddle, B.M., Pollock, Hewinson, R.G.. Progress in the development of vaccines and diagnostic reagents to control tuberculosis in cattle. *Veterinary Journal* 171 (2006), 229-244.

Tejada, A.R.; Diaz, C.A.; Vivero, J.G.; Salazar, J.A.G.; Leon, R.A.T.; Estrada-Chavez, C. (2006) Confirmation of Mycobacterium bovis excretion in nasal exudates by means of nested PCR in a dairy cattle herd. *Vet. Mex.* 37, 137-146.

Thoen, C.; LoBue, P.; de Kantor, I. The importance of *Mycobacterium bovis* as a zoonosis. *Veterinary Microbiology,* 112 (2-4), 2006, 339-345.

Wards BJ, Collins DM, Lisle GW 1995. Detection of *Mycobacterium bovis* in tissues by polymerase chain reaction. *Vet Microbiol 43*: 227-240.

Wedlock, D. N.; M. A. Skinner, G. W.; De Lisle, And B. M. Buddle. Control of *Mycobacterium bovis* infections and the risk to human populations. *Microbes Infect.* 4, 471–480, 2002.

Zumárraga, M. J., Martin, C., Samper, S., Alito, A., Latini, O., Bigi, F., Roxo, E., Cicuta, M.E., Errico, F., Ramos, M.C., Cataldi, A., Soolingen, D & Romano, A.A. (1999). Usefulness of Spoligotyping in Molecular Epidemiology of *Mycobacterium bovis*-Related Infectious in South America. *Journal of Clinical Microbiology*. p.296-303.

Zanini, M.S, Moreira E.C, Lopes, M.T.P., Oliveira, R.S, Leão, S.C., Fioravanti, R.L., Roxo, E , Zumarraga, M , Romano, M.I , Cataldi, A & Salas, C.E. (2001). Mycobacterium bovis: Polymerase Chain Reaction Identification in Bovine Lymphonode Biopsies and Genotyping in Isolates from Southeast Brazil by Spolygotyping and Restriction Fragment Length Polymorphism. Mem Inst Oswaldo Cruz, Rio de Janeiro, Vol. 96.

Zanini, M.S.; Moreira, E.C.; Lopes, M.T.P. & Salas, C.E. (1998). Detection of *Mycobacterium bovis* in milk by polymerase chain reaction. *J. Vet Med* 45, 1129-1132, 1998.

Zumarraga, M.J.; Meickle, V.; Bernardelli, A.; Abdala, A.; Tarabla, H.; Romano, M. I. & Cataldi, A. (2005). Use of touch-down polymerase chain reaction to enhance the sensitivity of Mycobacterium bovis detection. *J.Vet. Diagn. Invest.* 17, 232-238.

Part 3

Improving Detection and Control of Resistances

21

Survey and Molecular Characterization of Drug-Resistant *M. tuberculosis* Clinical Isolates from Zunyi, Guizhou Province of China

Ling Chen[1*], Hong Zhang[1,2*], Jian-Yong Zhang[1], Na-Na Li[1], Mei Liu[1], Zhao-Jing Zong[1], Jian-Hua Wang[1] and Sheng-Lan Wang[1]

[1] Laboratory of Respiratory Medicine, Department of Respiratory Medicine Affiliated Hospital of Zunyi Medical College,

[2]Z-BioMed, Inc.,

[1]China

[2]USA

1. Introduction

Tuberculosis (TB) is one of the leading infectious disease killers in the world, especially in developing countries. The increasing frequency of human-to-human transmission of multidrug-resistant (MDR) and extensively drug-resistant (XDR) strains of *Mycobacterium tuberculosis* poses challenges for effective therapeutic options and infection control. MDR-TB is defined as a form of TB that is resistant to at least isoniazid and rifampin, which are used to treat all TB patients. XDR-TB is a form of TB that is resistant to at least rifampicin and isoniazid in addition to any fluoroquinolone, and at least one of the three injectable second-line anti-TB drugs (amikacin, capreomycin and kanamycin). Based on the WHO Report 2010, China was ranked number one among high burden countries in terms of the estimated number of MDR-TB cases in 2008, and number two in terms of total numbers of TB cases in the world with the incidence rate per capita of 99 per 100,000 populations (WHO, 2011). Guizhou province is one of the highest-incidence-rate areas in China, and its prevalence of drug-resistant TB is higher than most of other provinces of China (Chen et al., 2011). The Affiliated Hospital of Zunyi Medical College is one of the specialized centers in Guizhou certified by the provincial government for the treatment of MDR-TB patients. In 2010, more than 15,000 TB patients were treated at the hospital. In order to determine the molecular characteristics of drug-resistant TB and assist in making informed TB treatment decisions for TB patients in the Zunyi area of Guizhou province, hundreds of *M. tuberculosis* clinical isolates were collected at the Affiliated Hospital of Zunyi Medical College and used for the systematic surveillance and other studies. We have made some progresses in the detection and molecular characterization of drug-resistant *M. tuberculosis* clinical isolates using different research methods such as *M. tuberculosis* culture, spoligotyping, gene sequencing, proteomics and drug susceptibility testing against first-line and second-line anti-tuberculosis drugs.

---

* Corresponding authors

In this chapter, we will briefly review the recent advances in the area of MDR-TB research; provide detailed descriptions about our research methods and the summary of our current research progresses. This chapter is written for researchers, scientists and physicians in academic institutions, clinical laboratories, pharmaceutical companies and research hospitals. This chapter will also be suitable for readers such as undergraduate, graduate and medical students who wish to learn more about the drug-resistant *M. tuberculosis*, especially MDR/XDR-TB, and some of the current research methods used for the determination of the genetic diversity and anti-tuberculosis drug susceptibility profile of *M. tuberculosis* clinical isolates, and the detection of drug-resistant *M. tuberculosis*.

2. Survey of drug-resistant *M. tuberculosis* clinical isolates

Mycobacteria are aerobes and grow most successfully in tissues with high oxygen content. The suitable growth temperature for mycobacteria is 37°C. Mycobacteria are "acid-fast bacilli" (AFB) because of their lipid-rich cell walls, which are relatively impermeable to various basic dyes unless the dyes are combined with phenol. Once stained, mycobacteria are resistant to decolorization with acidified organic solvents. *M. tuberculosis* is an intracellular pathogen usually infecting mononuclear phagocytes, and slow-growing with a generation time of 18 to 22 hours. The diagnosis of tuberculosis usually requires the detection of acid-fast bacilli in sputum via the acid-fast staining method (Ziehl-Neelsen method), which uses carbolfuchsin as the stain, acid-alcohol as the destaining solution and methylene blue as the counterstain. The culture confirmation of *M. tuberculosis* is the gold standard for diagnosis of tuberculosis and the drug susceptibility testing (DST) provides the basis for surveillance of drug-resistant TB and for physicians to adjust chemotherapy.

Even though TB laboratory services formed an essential part of the DOTS (Directly Observed Treatment Short course) strategy for National Tuberculosis Programs, it was often the most neglected component of these programs because of the absence of standardized techniques which complicated the activities of new laboratory services. Based on those considerations, WHO prepared guidelines in 1998 for laboratory services for the framework of National Tuberculosis Programs (WHO, 1998). The guidelines included three detailed manuals, two of which focused on the technical aspects of TB microscopy and culture, and a third one dealt with laboratory management including lab safety and proficiency testing. These manuals were specifically developed for use in low- and middle-income countries with high TB prevalence and incidence rates (WHO, 1998). Most of the methods used in our laboratory at the Affiliated Hospital of Zunyi Medical College and described in this chapter are based on these three manuals.

2.1 Collection of sputum specimens from patients

M. tuberculosis may be isolated from various clinical specimens, including respiratory specimens such as sputum, body fluids and body tissues (Goodwin, 2007). TB clinical strains from sputum of patients with active pulmonary tuberculosis were collected at the Affiliated Hospital of Zunyi Medical College. Sputum specimens were collected into a sterile single-collection Universal container (28ml) with a tightly fitted lid. A good sputum specimen is considered to be recently-discharged materials from the bronchial tree of the patient, with a minimum amount of oral or nasal materials (WHO, 1998). In an ideal situation, a sputum specimen produced by a deep cough of the patient should have a volume of 5 to 10 ml, although less volumes are acceptable if the quality is good. All sputum specimens should be transported to the laboratory and processed as soon as possible after collection. If delay is unavoidable, the sputum specimens should be refrigerated to inhibit the growth of unwanted microorganisms.

2.1.1 Solutions for acid-fast staining

Staining solution: 0.8% carbolfuchsin solution

Destaining solution: 3% hydrochloric acid- alcohol solution

Counterstaining solution: 0.3‰ methylene blue solution

2.1.2 Acid-fast staining procedure

The procedures for acid-fast staining were based on the modified method described by Hu et al. (Hu et al., 2008). To prepare a smear for AFB, appropriate specimens were spread uniformly on a microscope slide, which was then fixed at 80°C for 15 minutes. Smears were stained with a carbolfuchsin stain and were examined using a 100× oil immersion objective on a light microscope. In smears stained with carbolfuchsin, AFB typically appear as purple to red slightly curved, short or long rods (2-8μM). They may also appear beaded or banded. Following is the acid-fast staining procedure:

1. Turn on the thermostat-controlled water-bath and set up the temperature to 56°C.
2. Air dry smear on the slide, flame fix, and transfer it to the water-bath.
3. Add carbolfuchsin dye to the heat-fixed smear on slide for 15min, and take out the slide.
4. Allow the slide to cool to room temperature, then, decolorize slide by adding the fresh destaining solution, and wait until red color disappears.
5. Add counterstaining solution for 1 min, wash, and dry.
6. Examine the slide by a 100× oil immersion objective on a light microscope.
7. Interpret acid-fast staining results

Smears should be carefully examined with a minimum of 300 fields, and three horizontal sweeps of a smear should be performed (Goodwin, 2007). The positive smear requires the cut-off of at least 5000 bacilli/ml. The overall sensitivity of the acid-fast staining method varies from 20% to 80% (Goodwin, 2007).

2.2 Drug susceptibility testing against different drugs

WHO has endorsed commercial liquid culture systems and molecular line-probe assays as gold standards for rapid detection of MDR-TB; however, because of technical complexity, cost and the requirement of sophisticated lab infrastructure, their uses have been limited in many resource-constrained settings (WHO, 2010). Several noncommercial culture and DST methods have been developed for those resource-constrained settings, and assessed by WHO. Based on the testing results, WHO recently recommended MODS (microscopic observation of drug susceptibility) and NRA (nitrate reductase assay) under certain conditions for direct testing of sputum speciments (WHO, 2010).

M. tuberculosis drug susceptibility testing methods using solid media include proportional, resistance ratio and absolute concentration, which are inexpensive and highly standardized for testing susceptibility to many drugs (WHO, 2009). The proportion method is the most commonly used worldwide. Sputum specimens were digested, decontaminated and used to inoculate egg-based media such as L-J slants for DST. The instructions for the preparation of the egg-based media such as L-J, and detailed protocols for performing standardized bacteriological services for detecting infectious cases of pulmonary tuberculosis, monitoring treatment progress and documenting cure at the end of treatment by means of microscopic examination were well described by WHO in Part III (Culture) of the Laboratory Services in Tuberculosis Control (WHO, 1998) and should be followed strictly.

2.2.1 Preparation of culture media

The recommended TB diagnostic laboratory procedures (WHO, 1998; Chinese Antituberculosis Association, 2006) were followed for the preparation of media and suspension, inoculation and mycobacterium culture in a biologic safety cabinet. Löwenstein-Jensen (L-J) solid media were prepared in the laboratory of the Affiliated Hospital of Zunyi Medical College. All the samples were cultured on L-J solid media and grown colonies were identified to the species level using TCH (2-thiophene carboxylic acid) and PNB (paranitrobenzoicacid) selective media or by standard biochemical procedures.

2.2.1.1 Procedure for preparation of L-J culture medium (for 1632 ml)

1. Dissolve salts from the following ingredients in order in about 300ml of distilled water by heating (WHO, 1998):

Potassium dihydrogen phosphate anhydrous (KH_2PO_4)	2.4g
Magnesium sulfate ($MgSO_4 \cdot 7H_2O$)	0.24g
Magnesium citrate	0.6g
Sodium glutamate	7.2g
Glycerol (reagent grade)	12ml
Malachite green (2% solution)	20ml
Distilled water	600ml

2. Add glycerol, malachite green solution and make up to 600ml with distilled water.
3. Sterilize the solution by autoclaving at 121°C for 30 minutes.
4. Cool the solution to room temperature.
5. Rinse fresh hen's eggs (not more than 7 days old) thoroughly in running water and soak them in 70% ethanol for 15 minutes.
6. Crack the eggs with the edge of the beaker and pour into a sterile beaker.
7. Stir them with an old-fashioned sterile egg beater until completely blended.
8. Mix the sterilized solution containing all the ingredients (600ml) with homogenized eggs (1000ml) in a large sterile beaker (2 L capacity) and let it stand at room temperature for 1 hour.

2.2.1.2 Preparation of drug-containing solid media

Drug stock solutions at recommended concentrations (Table 1) were made in distilled water. To make media containing the end concentration of different drugs (Table 1), 0.4ml of stock solution for each drug was diluted separately with 400ml of L-J mixture mentioned above.

Media containing different drugs were distributed to sterile universal screw-cap centrifuge tubes (7ml medium per tube); tubes were labeled and caps were tightened. The labeled tubes were placed in an oven at a slanted position (30° angle) and baked at 85°C for 50 min. Baked tubes were cooled down to room temperature and stored at 4°C refrigerator until use. Since the medium was prepared with sterile precautions, this heating process was to solidify the medium instead of sterilizing it. The quality of the egg-based media deteriorates when the baking temperature is too high or the baking time is too long. The L-J medium should be dated and stored in the refrigerator for up to 4 weeks if the caps are tightened to prevent drying of the medium (WHO, 1998).

Drug	Dissolvent	Diluent	Concentration (µg/ml)	
			Stock solution	Drug Medium
Capreomycin	dH_2O	dH_2O	40000	40
Ciprofloxacin	dH_2O	dH_2O	2000	2
Ethambutol	dH_2O	dH_2O	2000	2
Isoniazid	dH_2O	dH_2O	200	0.2
Levofloxacin	dH_2O	dH_2O	2000	2
Rifampicin	DMF	dH_2O	40000	40
Streptomycin	dH_2O	dH_2O	4000	4

Table 1. Recommended concentrations of anti-TB drugs used in the drug susceptibility testing (WHO, 2009). dH_2O, distilled water; DMF, dimethylformamide.

2.2.1.3 Digestion and decontamination

M. tuberculosis grows slowly and takes four to eight weeks or longer to give visible colonies. Cultures are usually made in bottles because of the long incubation time required. The bottles are tightly capped to prevent drying of the cultures. The majority of clinical specimens submitted to the clinical laboratory are contaminated to varying degrees by more rapidly growing normal flora. These would rapidly overgrow the entire surface of the medium before the *M. tuberculosis* start to grow (Goodwin, 2007). Therefore, specimens must be subjected to digestion and decontamination that liquefies the organic debris and eliminates the unwanted normal flora. All currently available digesting and decontaminating methods are to some extent toxic to *M. tuberculosis*. Therefore, to ensure the survival of the maximum number of *M. tuberculosis* in the specimen, the digestion and decontamination procedure must be precisely followed (WHO, 1998).

2.2.2 Drug susceptibility testing

We have collected hundreds of TB culture samples from TB patients, and used them for the DNA extraction and drug-susceptibility testing against seven anti-TB drugs: rifampicin (RIF), isoniazid (INH), streptomycin (STR), ethambutol (EMB), capreomycin (CPM), ciprofloxacin (CIP) and levofloxacin (LVF). The proportion method on L-J media was used to perform the DST against different drugs in most of clinical *M. tuberculosis* isolates. The following drug concentrations in L-J media were used for the DST: RIF, 40µg/ml; INH, 0.2µg/ml; STR, 4µg/ml; EMB, 2µg/ml; CPM, 40µg/ml; CIP, 2µg/ml; and LVF, 2µg/ml.

2.2.3 Quality control

After coagulation, 5% of the slopes were picked up randomly and continued for incubation for 2 days at 37 °C to check for sterility. If no colony was grown on the solid medium after 48 hours of incubation at 37°C, the whole media batch should be good for DST.

2.2.4 Results criteria

The proportion testing results can be recorded at 28 days and again at 42 days as 3+ for confluent growth; 2+ for more than 100 colonies; and 1-99 colonies for the actual number of colonies. The percentage of drug resistance can be expressed as: Number of colonies on drug-containing medium/Number of colonies on L-J medium × 100%. If the percentage >1, the tested bacterium is considered to be drug resistant.

2.2.5 Results and discussion

We analyzed 316 clinical *M. tuberculosis* isolates for DST against four drugs (RIF, INH, STR and EMB). Results showed that 51.3% of isolates were resistant to one or more drugs, 19.0% were MDR, 20.9% were resistant to any single drug, 12.0% were resistant to any two drugs, 10.8% were resistant to any three drugs, and 7.6% were resistant to four drugs (Table 2). The prevalence of single drug-resistance was STR>RIF>EMB>INH in combined cases. There were 209 isolates in the first-treated (new TB cases) group, in which 42.1% were resistant to at least one drug, and 23.9% were resistant to any single drug. In addition, there were 107 isolates in the previously treated group, in which 69.2% were resistant to at least one drug, and 15.0% were resistant to any single drug. Our results indicated that the prevalence of drug-resistance in new tuberculosis cases was very high in the Zunyi area of Guizhou province, with 42.1% of the isolates resistant to at least one drug, and there were obvious differences in the drug susceptibility profiles between new and previously treated TB cases. These results also highlight the importance of surveillance of drug-resistant TB in order to improve the treatment outcomes of TB patients.

Drug Susceptibility*	PT (107 isolates)		FT (209 isolates)		Combined (316 isolates)	
	No. of cases	%	No. of cases	%	No. of cases	%
Resistant to any single drug	16	15.0	50	23.9	66	20.9
Resistant to any 2 drugs	23	21.5	15	7.2	38	12.0
Resistant to any 3 drugs	22	20.6	12	5.7	34	10.8
Resistant to 4 drugs	13	12.1	11	5.3	24	7.6
Total	74	69.2	88	42.1	162	51.3

*Drugs tested: isoniazid, rifampincin, ethambutol and streptomycin; PT, previously treated; FT, First-time treated (new cases).

Table 2. Drug susceptibility profiles of 316 clinical *M. tuberculosis* isolates.

3. Molecular characterization of drug-resistant *M. tuberculosis*

The recommended standard or first-line treatment of tuberculosis includes a combination of four drugs, rifampicin, isoniazid, ethambutol and pyrazinamide, with or without streptomycin. Resistance to the first-line anti-TB drugs has been linked to mutations in at least 13 genes: *rpoB* for rifampicin resistance, *katG, inhA, kasA, ahpC, ndh, furA*, and *oxyR* for isoniazid resistance, *embCAB* for ethambutol resistance, *pncA* for pyrazinamide resistance, and *rpsL, rrs,* and *gidB* for streptomycin resistance. Resistance to the second-line anti-TB drugs has been linked to mutations in at least 10 genes (Banerjee, et al., 2008). For the detection of mutations in genes linked to rifampicin and isoniazid resistance, we amplified *rpoB* and *KatG* gene fragments from many drug-resistant *M. tuberculosis* clinical isolations and performed DNA sequencing analyses. We also detected mutations in 5 other genes associated with drug-resistance (*inhA, rpsl, rrs, gyrA and gyrB*). Nucleotide sequences of primers used for PCR amplification and DNA sequencing were listed in Table 3.

Gene	Primer Sequence (5'→3')	Product Size (bp)
rpoB	Forward, TCAGACCACGATGACCGTTCC Reverse, GTCCATGTAGTCCACCTCAGACG Sequencing, TCGGCATGTCGCGGATGGAG	688
katG	Forward, GCTCGGCGATGAGCGTTAC Reverse, CTCGTAGCCGTACAGGATCTCG Sequencing, GCTCGGCGATGAGCGTTAC	409
inhA	Forward, TCGCAGCCACGTTACGCTC Reverse, CCAGCCGCTGTGCGATC Sequencing, TCGCAGCCACGTTACGCTC	175
rpsl	Forward, GGCAGCCCGCAGCGTCGTG Reverse, TGTAGCGCACACCAGGCAGGT Sequencing, GGCAGCCCGCAGCGTCGTG	211
rrs	Forward, TCAGGAGGAACACCGGTGGCG Reverse, AATCCACATGCTCCGCCGCTTG Sequencing, TCAGGAGGAACACCGGTGGCG	253
gyrA	Forward, CAGCTACATCGACTATGCGA Reverse, GGGCTTCGGTGTACCTCAT Sequencing, CAGCTACATCGACTATGCGA	320
gyrB	Forward, CGCAAGTCCGAACTGTATGTCGTAG Reverse, GTTGTGCCAAAAACACATGC Sequencing, CGCAAGTCCGAACTGTATGTCGTAG	346

Table 3. Primers used in this study for PCR amplification and DNA sequencing

3.1 Determination of mutation profiles in drug-related genes

3.1.1 DNA isolation and PCR amplification

The genomic DNA was extracted from *M. tuberculosis* clinical isolates using a Bacterial DNA Kit (Tiangen, China) following the manufacturer's instruction. DNA fragments for 7 drug-related genes were amplified by PCR using synthetic oligonucleotide primers listed in Table 3. The following thermocycler parameters were applied with initial denaturation at 94°C for 5 min; 35-42 cycles of denaturation at 94°C for 30 sec; primer annealing at 58-62°C for 30 sec; extension at 72°C for 30-60 sec; and a final extension at 72°C for 7 min. The obtained DNA fragments were analyzed by electrophoresis in 2.0% agarose gel and were visualized under UV light on a transilluminator.

3.1.2 DNA sequencing analysis

In order to determine mutation profiles of 7 drug-related genes (*rpoB, katG, inhA, rpsl, rrs, gyrA* and *gyrB*), we purified PCR-amplified gene fragments and sent them to Shanghai Invitrogen for DNA sequencing using primers listed in Table 3. The FinchTV program was downloaded from Geospiza's website and used to view the original sequencing data. Sequence alignment analysis was conducted using the BLAST program at the NCBI website (http://blast.ncbi.nlm.nih.gov/Blast.cgi) to compare our sequencing results with those wild-type *M. tuberculosis* genes listed in the GenBank.

3.1.3 Results and discussion

In 32 rifampicin-resistant strains, we identified 13 different types of missense mutations at codons 509, 511, 516, 522, 526, 531, 533, 550 and 572 of *rpoB* gene, and compared the mutation profile with those of rifampicin-resistant *M. Tuberculosis* isolates from different geographical regions of the world. Comparison of the results showed that the *rpoB* gene mutation profile in rifampicin-resistant *M. Tuberculosis* clinical isolates from Guizhou province differed not only from other provinces of China but also from other countries of Asia, Europe and America (Chen et al., 2010). Two new mutations (Val550Leu and Ser509Arg) were identified and deposited in GenBank (GQ250580 and GQ250581). We concluded that mutation profiles of rifampicin-resistant *M. Tuberculosis* isolates were variable depending on the geographical locations, and further studies would be needed to determine the molecular basis for such variations (Chen et al., 2010).

In 30 isoniazid-resistant strains, 18 (60%) of them had mutations in *katG* and/or *inhA* genes and two newly identified mutations in *katG* gene (Val230Met and Pro232Gln) were deposited to GenBank (GQ250582 and GQ250583). Results from this study further confirmed that mutations in *katG* and *inhA* genes are related to the isoniazid resistance in *M. tuberculosis* (Chen Y et al., 2010).

To better compare drug resistance and mutation profiles of clinical *M. Tuberculosis* isolates collected at our hospital, we selected 23 representative isolates and combined the DST results against 4 drugs with mutation profiles in 7 genes related to drug resistance in the same table (Table 4). It is clear that the relationship between drug resistance and mutations in specific genes may be more complex than we expected. For example, no mutations were found in 6 of the 7 drug-related genes for isolate number 2, which was resistant to all 4 drugs tested, suggesting that there must be changes in other regions of the genes or other genes. Further studies will be needed to determine the molecular mechanism underlining the resistance of this kind of isolates to different anti-TB drugs. In another example, two mutations were identified in isolate number 17, one in *rpoB* gene (TCG531TTG) and another in *katG* gene (AGC315ACC). However, isolate number 17 was resistant only to rifampicin but sensitive to 3 other drugs. It will be necessary for us to repeat the DST for this isolate to confirm whether this isolate does have a mutation in *katG* gene but still sensitive to isoniazid. In summary, more studies are need to identify new genes related to MDR-TB.

No.	R	H	S	E	Mutations in specific resistant genes						
					rpoB	*katG*	*inhA*	*rpsL*	*rrs*	*gyrA*	*gyrB*
1	r	r	r	r	TCG531TTG	AGC315ACC CCG232CAG GGC237GAG GAG340AAG	CGT16GGT GGA23CGA	WT	WT	NA	WT
2	r	r	r	r	WT	WT	WT	WT	WT	NA	WT
3	r	r	r	r	CTG533CCG	AGC315ACC	WT	AAG43AGG	WT	NA	WT
4	r	r	r	r	CAC526TAC	WT	WT	WT	WT	NA	WT
5	r	r	r	r	CAC526GAC	WT	WT	WT	WT	GCG90GTG AGC95ACC	NA
6	r	r	r	s	WT	WT	GCC5TCC	WT	WT	AGC95ACC	WT
7	r	r	r	s	GAC516GTC	AGC315ACC	GCC5TCC ACT6AGT	NA	WT	GCG90GTG AGC95ACC	WT
8	r	r	r	r	CTG533CCG	GTG230ATG	GCC5TCC	NA	NA	NA	NA
9	r	r	r	r	WT	WT	GCC5TCC	WT	WT	AGC95ACC	WT
10	r	r	r	s	TCG531TTG	AGC315ACC	GCC5TCC GAA7GCA GGG8GCT	WT	WT	NA	WT
11	r	r	r	r	TCG531TTG	WT	GCC5TCC	WT	WT	NA	WT
12	r	r	r	s	CAC526GAC	WT	WT	AAG43AGG	WT	GCG90GTG AGC95ACC	WT

No.	R	H	S	E	Mutations in specific resistant genes						
					rpoB	*katG*	*inhA*	*rpsL*	*rrs*	*gyrA*	*gyrB*
13	r	r	r	r	CAC526TAC	AGC315ACC	WT	WT	WT	GAC94GGC AGC95ACC	GAG528GCG
14	r	r	s	r	TCG522TTG GTG550TTG	AGC315ACC	WT	WT	WT	ACC80ATC AGC95ACC	WT
15	r	r	r	r	TCG531TTG	AGC315ACC	WT	WT	WT	AGC95ACC	WT
16	r	r	r	r	TCG531TTG	AGC315ACC	WT	AAG43AGG	WT	GAC94GGC AGC95ACC	ACC539CCC
17	r	s	s	s	TCG531TTG	AGC315ACC	WT	NA	NA	NA	NA
18	r	r	r	r	TCG531TTG	AGC315ACC	WT	WT	WT	AGC95ACC	WT
19	r	r	r	s	CTG511CCG GAC516AAC	WT	WT	AAG43AGG	WT	AGC95ACC	WT
20	s	r	r	s	CTG533CCG	AGC315ACC	WT	NA	NA	NA	NA
21	r	r	r	r	TCG522TTG GTG550TTG	AGC315ACC	WT	WT	WT	AGC95ACC	WT
22	r	r	r	r	TCG531TTG	AGC315ACC	WT	AAG43AGG	WT	AGC95ACC	WT
23	r	r	s	r	AGC509AGG CTG511CCG GAC516GTC	Gene loss	WT	NA	WT	NA	WT

Abbreviations: R, rifampicin; H, isoniazid; S, streptomycin; E, ethambutol; s, susceptible; r, resistant; WT, wild type; and NA, data not available.

Table 4. Drug susceptibility profiles and mutational patterns of 23 representative clinical isolates

3.2 Genotyping

3.2.1 Spoligotyping and its application in surveillance

Spacer oligonucleotide typing (Spoligotyping) is a molecular method used to differentiate *M. Tuberculosis Complex (MTC)* isolates. This method is based on PCR analysis of polymorphisms in the MTC direct repeat (DR) chromosomal region containing multiple 36bp DR loci. Each DR is interspersed by a unique spacer sequence of 35 to 41 bp. After PCR amplification, the fragment containing the whole DR region was hybridized to specific oligonucleotide probes designed according to the different spacer sequences, and genotypes were determined depending on the hybridization patterns. The most widely used 43 sites were developed in 1997 by Kamerbeek et al, including 37 derived from the reference strain H37Rv and 6 spacers derived from *M. bovis* BCG (Kamerbeek et al., 1997). This method is more rapid and easier to perform than the standard genotyping technique based on IS6110 profiling.

Member of M. TB complex	Characterization of Spoligotyping (Missing Spacers)
Mycobacterium tuberculosis	33~36 (Viana-Niero et al., 2001)
Mycobacterium bovis	39~43 (Soini et al., 2000; Filliol et al., 2003)
Mycobacterium africanum	8, 9, 39 (Viana-Niero et al., 2001; Filliol et al., 2003)
Mycobacterium microti	37, 38 (Niemann et al., 2000)

Table 5. Characterization of *M. tuberculosis complex* by Spoligotyping

MTC includes *M. tuberculosis*, *M. bovis*, *M. voles* and *Africa mycobacterium*. *M. tuberculosis* is one of the leading pathogens to human and animal, followed by *M. bovis*. *M. tuberculosis* and *M. bovis* can be distinguished from MTC by using L-J agar slants, PNB and TCH. *M. bovis* can be quickly identified by spoligotyping. Considering the difficulties in determining *M. vole* and *Africa mycobacterium* by traditional methods of bacteriology, Soolingen et al. developed the spoligotyping method to distinguish the *M. vole* from MTC (van Soolinger et al. 1998). Results from Niemann et al. proved that *M. bovis* could be differentiated from *M. Africa* by spoligotyping (Niemann et al., 2000). In addition, Viana-Niero et al. also indicated that the spoligotyping fingerprint of *M. Africa* was between *M. tuberculosis* and *M. bovis* (Viana-Niero et al., 2001). Spoligotyping can be used to distinguish MTC members based on their characteristic spoligotypes (Table 5). Until now, IS6110-RFLP has been the gold standard for genotyping of *M. tuberculosis* (Majeed et al., 2004). However, a comparison study using IS6110-RFLP and spoligotyping indicated that the genotyping capacity of spoligotyping was better than IS6110-RFLP to strains containing low-copy numbers of IS6110 (Bauer et al., 1999).

To study the genotypic diversity, we choose spoligotyping for molecular typing of 100 clinical *M. tuberculosis* isolates collected at the Affiliated Hospital of Zunyi Medical College from 2008 to 2009. Bacterial growth and chromosomal DNA isolation were carried out by the method of Soolingen et al. (van Soolinger et al., 1991). The extracted DNA was used as a template for PCR amplification of the DR region of the genome with the biotinylated forward primer, 5′-GGTTTTGGGTCTGACGAC-3′ and the reverse primer 5′-CCGAGAGGG GACGGAAAC-3′. The following thermocycler parameters were applied with initial denaturation at 94°C for 5 min; 35 cycles of denaturation at 94°C for 30 s; primer annealing at 56°C for 30 s; extension at

72°C for 30 s; and a final extension at 72°C for 8 min. The PCR amplified products were hybridized to a membrane containing a set of 43 immobilized oligonucleotides, each corresponding to one of the unique spacer DNA sequences within the DR locus. DNAs isolated from *M. tuberculosis* H37Rv and *M. bovis* BCG were used as controls. The hybridized PCR products were incubated with 1:4000-diluted streptavidin-peroxidase conjugate (Boehringer) for 30min at 42°C. Detection of hybridizing DNA was done by using the chemiluminescent ECL (Amersham) detection system followed by exposure to X-ray film (Hyperfilm ECL; Amersham) in accordance with the manufacturer's instructions.

Spoligotypes in binary format were entered in the SITVIT database (Pasteur Institute of Guadeloupe). Twenty-nine distinct spoligotyping patterns were observed. In total, 20 orphan patterns were identified and the remaining 77 were contained within 9 superfamilies: Beijing, T1, T3, T2, MANU2, Beijing-like, U, H3 and H3-T3. Results showed that almost half of the isolates were clustered to the Beijing lineage, and 13 isolates were clustered to the T1 lineage.

To analyze the MTC population structure, evaluate the complicacy of the global TB transmission and provisional evolution of the TB genetic landscape, Institute Pasteur had built a genetic diversity database for the MTC DR locus in 1999. This database was updated to SpolDB4 (Spoligotyping Database 4) in 2006. The updated database contained 1939 shared-types (STs) of 39,295 strains from 122 countries, which were temporarily classified into 62 clades/lineages (Brudey et al., 2006). In this database, the 10 most prevalent clades are ST1 (Beijing family), ST53 (T1), ST190 (Beijing family), ST52 (T2), ST50 (H3), ST54 (MANU2), ST37 (T3), ST742 (H3), ST265 (Beijing family) and ST127 (H4).

The Beijing genotype family was originally identified in China (Brudey et al., 2006) and defined as strains that presence of at least three spacers 35-43 and absence of spacers 1-34 (van Soolinger et al., 1995). Beijing family strains represent at least 13% of strains worldwide and about half of strains in the East Asia. A total of 2,346 *M. tuberculosis* isolates from 13 provinces, excluding Guizhou province, in China were genotyped by spoligotyping, and results showed that 74.08% of the isolates belonged to the Beijing family (Dong et al., 2010). Other studies also examined the relationship of Beijing genotype with drug resistance, however, the association between them was still not clear. The possible reasons for this uncertainty might be: 1) the diversity of treatment programs; 2) compliance to treatment; 3) different quality of anti-TB drugs; and 4) spread of different and not yet distinguished sublineages of the Beijing strains (Parwati et al., 2010).

The "T" families were the most prevalent following Beijing family, belonged to modern TB strains, and ill-defined with more than 600 unclassified STs. The "T" families were further divided into 5 subclades (T1-T5) based on single spacer-differences (Brudey et al. 2006). The numbers of T1 and T2 families were ranked the second and third respectively after Beijing family in the updated SpolDB4.

4. Application of proteomics in drug-resistant *M. tuberculosis*

4.1 Proteomics and its application in tuberculosis research

Proteomics is defined as the large-scale study of proteins, their post-translational modifications, and their structures and functions underlying different biological processes.

Proteomics enables the qualitative and quantitative analyses of proteins in complex biological systems, such as cells, tissues, and body fluids under specific conditions or in response to different stimuli (Graham et al., 2011; Lim & Elenitoba-Johnson, 2004; List et al., 2008; Wu & Liu, 2009). Proteomics is an effective means to rapidly identify new proteins as diagnostic or prognostic markers and as therapeutic targets for various diseases including cancers, genetic diseases, and infectious diseases such as tuberculosis (Chung et al., 2007; Kavallaris & Marshall, 2005; Drake et al., 2005; Stulik & Butaye, 2011).

Proteomics has been applied to the research area of *M. tuberculosis* (Bahk et al., 2004; He et al., 2003; Kumar et al., 2010; Lee et al. 1999; Mattow et al. 2001; Mustafa, 2005; Pheiffer et al., 2005; Sharma et al., 2010; Wang et al., 2007; Zhu et al., 2003) and become an important tool to study functional genomics of the bacterium (Mattow et al., 2003; Jiang et al., 2006; Rison et al., 2007; Xie et al., 2009; Jungblut et al., 2001). Proteins from *M. tuberculosis* missing in attenuated *M. bovis* BCG strains were identified by using proteomics (Mattow et al., 2001). Comparative proteome analyses of culture supernatant proteins from virulent *M. tuberculosis* H37Rv and attenuated *M. bovis* BCG (Mattow et al., 2003) or H37Ra (He et al., 2003) were performed to identify new virulent factors. Proteomics was also used for genome-wide analysis of the host intracellular network regulating survival of *M. tuberculosis* (Kumar et al., 2010). It was demonstrated that protein expression by a Beijing strain was different from that of another clinical isolate and *M. tuberculosis* H37Rv (Pheiffer et al., 2005). The major membrane protein of virulent *M. tuberculosis* was characterized using proteomics technology (Lee et al., 1999). Xie et al. used proteomics to compare proteins of MDR-TB isolate with drug-sensitive isolate (Xie et al. 2009). Additionally, proteomics has been successfully used for vaccine design to improve protection against tuberculosis (Mollenkopf et al., 2004).

The development of proteomic profiles for *M. tuberculosis* is needed to identify proteins that are differentially expressed in clinical strains with different drug susceptibility profiles such as MDR-TB and XDR-TB comparing to the standard strain, which can provide insights into the mechanisms by which the mycobacteria resistant to anti-TB drugs and the selection of suitable biomarkers for new diagnostics, new virulent factors and/targets for the development of potential therapeutics and new vaccines.

The most commonly used method for proteomic analysis is the two-dimensional polyacrylamide gel electrophoresis (2-DE), which allows the separation and display of thousands of proteins from a complex mixture by their charges (pI) and relative molecular mass (Mr). Gel-separated proteins can be identified rapidly by mass spectrometry (MS), and such analyses permit the systematic identification of the proteome if genomic information is available. In this preliminary study, we used 2-DE and mass spectrometry to compare protein expression profiles among different clinical *M. tuberculosis* strains such as MDR-TB, XDR-TB and the reference strain H37Rv, and identified some up-regulated, down-regulated genes which might be associated with MDR or XDR.

4.2 Sample preparation for MDR/XDR-TB isolates

The sensitive strain used in this study was the standard *M. tuberculosis* strain H37Rv, which was obtained as a gift from the Chinese Centre for Disease Control and Prevention. Both MDR-TB and XDR-TB strains were clinical isolates collected at the Affiliated

Hospital of Zunyi Medical College. Five to six inoculating loops of *M. tuberculosis* colonies were scraped from improved L-J culture media and transferred to 4 ml of purified water in a screw-top centrifuge tube. The mycobacterium suspension was heated at 80°C for 30 min in a water bath to inactivate *M. tuberculosis*, and centrifuged at 4000*g* for 10min for removing the supernatant. The precipitation was resuspended in the phosphate-buffered saline (pH7.4), and centrifuged at 4000*g* for 10min to remove the supernatant. The inactivated *M. tuberculosis* sample was resuspended in 0.3ml of lysis buffer, and 10μl of proteinase inhibitors were added to the suspension followed by incubation at 4°C for 20 min. The suspension was then sonicated (200W, 1min×30 times), and centrifuged at 4000*g* for 30min at 4°C. Four-fold volume of cold dimethyl ketone were added to the suspension and the mixture was kept at -20°C overnight for precipitating proteins. The protein precipitates were centrifuged at 10000*g* for 5min at 4°C, and resuspended in 7M carbamide and 2M sulfourea solution to dissolve proteins followed by centrifugation at 4000*g* for 30min at 4°C. Concentration of protein samples was measured by the NanoDrop-1000 (Thermo, Germany) and protein samples were stored at -20°C until use.

4.3 Two-dimensional electrophoresis (2-DE)

Protein samples (200-300 μg) were resuspended in 480 μl of rehydration buffer and applied to pH 4-7 IPG strips (Amersham Biosciences) for rehydration. When IPG strips were rehydrated with the protein samples, isoelectric focusing (IEF) was performed in the following voltage mode: 0V 1h, 50V 10h fast voltage, 500V 1.5h linear voltage, 2000V 1.5h linear voltage, 5000V 1.5h linear voltage, 8000V 1.5h linear voltage, 8000V 70000VH fast voltage, and 500V 16h fast voltage.

Equilibration was performed immediately prior to the second-dimension run, in which step IPG strips should be laid in the strip equilibrium solution buffer I (6 mol/L Urea, 2% SDS, 0.375mol/L pH 8.8 Tris-HCl, 20%Glycerol, and 2% DTT), then strip equilibrium solution buffer II (mol/L Urea, 2% SDS, 0.375mol/L pH8.8 Tris-HCl, 20% Glycerol, and 2.5% Iodoacetamide) each for 14 minutes. The equilibrated IPG strip was located into prepared 13% SDS-PAGE with low-melting point agarose smother. Following electrophoresis, proteins were visualized by either silver staining (analytical gels) or Coomassie Brilliant Blue G-250 staining (preparative gels).

The pI and Mr gradient of the 2-DE gels were determined using an iterative calibration method after 2-DE gel images transferred to computer by means of the image scanner. Spot detection and image analysis were performed and compared using the program Progenesis SameSpots (Nonlinear Dynamics, UK) for 2-DE database construction. Images of MDR-TB and XDR-TB were compared to the gel image of the standard strain H37Rv, and protein spots showing differential expression levels of more than two-fold were analyzed.

4.4 MALDI-MS and database

Twenty protein spots of interest (5 spots from H37Rv, 10 spots from XDR-TB, and 5 up-regulated protein spots from MDR-TB) were excised from Coomassie Brilliant Blue G-250 stained two dimensional gels (2-DE) and digested in gel using trypsin for 18h at 37°C. Masses of the peptides extracted from gel slices were applied to the sample plate of a matrix-assisted laser desorption ionization–time-of-flight MS (MALDI-TOF-MS). Peptide mass fingerprint data were searched using the Mascot search (www.matrixscience.com) of the National Center for Biotechnology Information (NCBI) database.

4.5 Comparison of XDR and MDR patterns

The comparison was repeated at least three times, and only those differences confirmed in all comparisons were accepted as strain specific. This study compared the proteome of XDR-TB clinical isolate to those of MDR-TB clinical isolate and the standard strain H37Rv, and demonstrated that the 2-DE protein expression patterns of XDR-TB and MDR-TB clinical isolates were highly correlated, but there were some visible differences between drug-resistant strains and the reference H37Rv strain. Results also showed that more basic proteins were expressed in drug-resistant *M. tuberculosis* isolates than in the standard H37Rv stain. Figure 1 shows differences among three different mycobacterium strains.

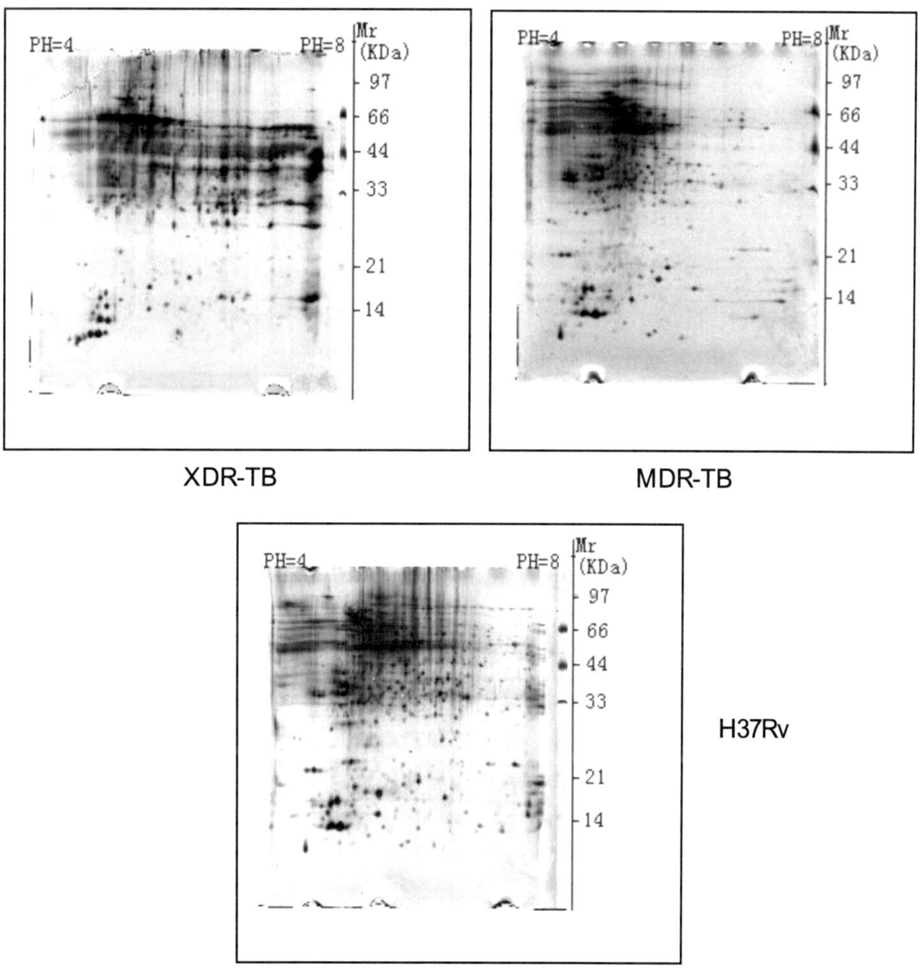

Fig. 1. Protein expression patterns of XDR-TB and MDR-TB clinical isolates compared to the standard strain H37Rv in two-dimensional electrophoresis

Spot No.	XDR-TB	MDR-TB	H37Rv	Spot No.	XDR-TB	MDR-TB	H37Rv
2984	156.1	20.42	10.68	1328	36.14	3.39	6.39
1622	145.0	11.43	30.65	2418	31.63	3.22	3.04
2980	99.99	9.90	3.91	1440	31.49	3.43	3.28
1692	85.41	4.34	6.95	2679	26.51	5.71	3.25
1813	78.84	6.39	5.42	1600	26.19	1.36	3.61
1805	67.34	3.31	5.65	2379	13.16	1.821	1.12
2978	49.75	5.09	2.44	2787	11.91	1.79	0.85
1839	46.13	5.60	3.89	1994	9.77	0.90	2.11
1245	38.84	2.79	3.15	2449	5.37	0.72	0.74
2726	36.46	3.16	3.07				

Table 6. Expression levels of 19 proteins specifically overexpressed in the XDR-TB (protein expression level=number in the tablex10^4)

There were 19 proteins specifically overexpressed in XDR-TB (Table 6), 3 proteins up-regulated (Table 7), 13 proteins down-regulated (Table 8) and 10 proteins disappeared in the XDR-TB clinical isolate compared to the reference H37Rv strain.

Spot No.	XDR- TB	MDR-TB	H37Rv
2561	22.26	29.82	14.69
1228	46.98	4.657	20.38
2378	37.97	9.587	4.238

Table 7. Expression levels of 3 up-regulated proteins in XDR-TB (protein expression level=number in the tablex10^4)

Out of these forty-five protein spots, twenty were selected for the mass spectrometry analysis, and only three proteins were identified by the MALDI-TOF-MS (Table 9). The differential expression of the ribosomal protein S3 and 19 kda major membrane protein in the XDR-TB strain was validated by the real-time RT-PCR (data not shown). It is not clear how differential expression of these three proteins contributes to the drug resistance of the XDR-TB. Further function analysis of these three proteins will be conducted in our laboratory to determine their relationship with drug resistance of XDR-TB.

Spot No.	XDR-TB	MDR-TB	H37Rv	Spot No.	XDR-TB	MDR-TB	H37Rv
2394	58.18	159.8	122.2	2695	5.16	17.13	13.47
2994	43.26	11.03	92.87	2365	4.76	44.01	48.32
2991	26.93	41.37	65.52	2989	4.56	23.36	13.34
2499	18.92	49.45	49.02	2436	2.67	7.96	13.41
2637	16.45	84.32	53.78	1627	1.87	1.70	11.67
1279	11.77	18.13	36.18	2174	1.40	8.94	16.15
1616	7.60	22.65	12.33				

Table 8. Expression levels of 13 down-regulated proteins in XDR-TB (protein expression quantity=number in the tablex10^4).

Spot No.	Protein Name	Function
2994	MMP=19 kda major membrane protein	Lipomannan, overlapping peptide sequences
1994	Ribosomal protein S3	Ribonucleoprotein, binding and positioning mRNA for translation
1813	YclD	Unknown

Table 9. Description of three proteins identified by MALDI-TOF-MS

5. Conclusion

In this chapter, we have provided the detailed description about our current progresses in the field of survey and molecular characterization of drug-resistant *M. tuberculosis* clinical isolates using different research methods such as *M. tuberculosis* culture, spoligotyping, gene sequencing, proteomics and drug susceptibility testing against first-line and second-line anti-tuberculosis drugs. We hope this chapter will be useful for researchers, scientists and physicians in academic institutions, clinical laboratories, pharmaceutical companies and research hospitals who have interest in the research related to drug-resistant *M. tuberculosis*, especially MDR/XDR-TB.

6. Acknowledgments

This project was funded in part with federal funds from the CDC, Department of Health and Human Services, under the contract no. 200-2007-M-22792, and by grants of International Cooperation Project from Guizhou Province of China [Qian Science co-G (2009) No. 700120], the Guizhou Science and Technology Fund Project [Qian Science co-J (2007) no. 2223] and Scientific Research Start Foundation from Zunyi Medical College in (F-327). The following people in the Affiliated Hospital of Zunyi Medical College made contributions to the research reported in this chapter: Xin Gan, Yang Chen, Kai-Lun Li, Yuan-Bo Lan, Zhen-Yong Chen, Lin-Mei Zhou, and Yi He. We would like to thank all health care staff in the Affiliated Hospital of Zunyi Medical College who participated in the research. We are also grateful to Professor Kanglin Wan, Zhiguang Liu, and Bing Lv in the Chinese Center for Disease Control and Prevention for their support with the spoligotyping analyses.

7. References

Bahk, Y.Y.; Kim, S.A.; Kim, J.S.; Euh, H.J.; Bai, G.H.; Cho, S.N. & Kim, Y.S. (2004). Antigens secreted from Mycobacterium tuberculosis: identification by proteomics approach and test for diagnostic marker. *Proteomics* 4(11): 3299-307.

Banerjee, R.; Schecter, G.F.; Flood, J. & Porco, T.C. (2008). Extensively drug-resistant tuberculosis: new strains, new challenges. *Expert Rev Anti Infect Ther* 6(5): 713-24.

Bauer, J.; Andersen, A.B.; Kremer, K. & Miörner, H. (1999). Usefulness of spoligotyping To discriminate IS6110 low-copy-number Mycobacterium tuberculosis complex strains cultured in Denmark. *J Clin Microbiol* 37(8): 2602-6.

Borile, C.; Labarre, M.; Franz, S.; Sola, C. & Refrégier, G. (2011). Using affinity propagation for identifying subspecies among clonal organisms: lessons from M. tuberculosis. *BMC Bioinformatics* 12: 224.

Brudey, K.; Driscoll, J.R.; Rigouts, L.; Prodinger, W.M.; Gori, A. et al. (2006) Mycobacterium tuberculosis complex genetic diversity: mining the fourth international spoligotyping database (SpolDB4) for classification, population genetics and epidemiology. *BMC Microbiol* 6: 23.

Chen, L.; Gan, X.; Li, N.N.; Wang, J.H.; Li, K.L. & Zhang, H. (2010). rpoB gene mutation profile in rifampicin-resistant Mycobacterium tuberculosis clinical isolates from Guizhou, one of the highest incidence rate regions in China. *J Antimicrob Chemother* 65: 1299-301.

Chen, L.; Li, N.; Liu, M.; Zhang, J. & Zhang, H. (2011). High prevalence of multidrug-resistant tuberculosis in Zunyi, Guizhou Province of China. *J Antimicrob Chemother* 66: 2435-7. DOI:10.1093/jac/DKR319.

Chen, Y.; Chen, L.; Zhang, H.; Wang, J.H.; Li, N.N.; Li, K.L. & Zhang, J.Y. (2010). Study of the relationship between resistant to isoniazid and mutation of KatG and inhA in Mycobacterium tuberculosis isolates. *Chin J Antibiotics* 35: 788-92.

Chinese Antituberculosis Association. (2006). TB diagnostic laboratory procedures. SBN 988-98193-1-7/ G.360.

Chung, C.H.; Levy, S.; Chaurand, P. & Carbone, D.P. (2007). Genomics and proteomics: emerging technologies in clinical cancer research. *Crit Rev Oncol Hematol* 61(1): 1-25.

Dong, H.; Liu, Z.; Lv, B.; Zhang, Y.; Liu, J.; Zhao, X.; Liu, J. & Wan, K. (2010). Spoligotypes of Mycobacterium tuberculosis from different Provinces of China. *J Clin Microbiol* 148(11): 4102-6.

Drake, R.R.; Deng, Y.; Schwegler, E.E. & Gravenstein, S. (2005). Proteomics for biodefense applications: progress and opportunities. *Expert Rev Proteomics* 2(2): 203-13.

Filliol, I.; Driscoll, J.R. & van Soolingen, D. (2003). Snapshot of moving and expanding clones of *Mycobacterium tuberculosis* and their global distribution assessed by spoligotyping in an international study. *J Clin Microbiol* 41(5): 1963-70.

Goodwin, A. (2007). *Mycobacterium tuberculosis* and other nontuberculous mycobacteria, p.683-717. *In* Mahon, C.R.; Lehman, D.C. & Manuselis, G. (Eds.) *Textbook of Diagnostic Microbiology* (Third Edition). SAUDERS ELSEVIER Press, ISBN-13: 978-1-4160-2581-8, Missouri, USA.

Graham, C.; McMullan, G. & Graham, R.L. (2011). Proteomics in the microbial sciences. Bioeng Bugs 2(1): 17-30.

He, X.Y.; Zhuang, Y.H.; Zhang, X.G. & Li, G.L. (2003). Comparative proteome analysis of culture supernatant proteins of Mycobacterium tuberculosis H37Rv and H37Ra. *Microbes Infect* 5(10): 851-6.

Hu, Y.L.; Zhang, J.; Pan, J.; Min, X.; Fu, S.N. & He, Y.Z. (2008). Steam heated water bath for acid-fast staining alternative flame heating. *Clin Lab Science* 26(1):19.

Jiang, X.; Zhang, W.; Gao, F.; Huang, Y.; Lv, C. & Wang, H. (2006). Comparison of the proteome of isoniazid-resistant and -susceptible strains of Mycobacterium tuberculosis. *Microb Drug Resist* 12(4): 231-8.

Jungblut, P.R.; Müller, E.C.; Mattow, J. & Kaufmann, S.H. (2001). Proteomics reveals open reading frames in Mycobacterium tuberculosis H37Rv not predicted by genomics. *Infect Immun* 69(9): 5905-7.

Kamerbeek, J.; Schouls, L.; Kolk, A.; Kuijper, S.; Bunschoten, A.; Molhuizen, H.; Shaw, R. & Goyal, M. (1997). Simultaneous detection and strain differentiation of Mycobacterium tuberculosis for diagnosis and epidemiology. *J Clin Microbiol* 35(4): 907-14.

Kavallaris, M. & Marshall, G.M. (2005). Proteomics and disease: opportunities and challenges. *Med J Aust* 182(11): 575-9.

Kremer, K.; Glynn, J.R.; Lillebaek, T.; Niemann, S.; Kurepina, N.E.; Kreiswirth, B.N.; Bifani, P.J. & van Soolingen, D. (2004). Definition of the Beijing/W lineage of Mycobacterium tuberculosis on the basis of genetic markers. *J Clin Microbiol* 42(9): 4040-9.

Kumar, D.; Nath, L.; Kamal, M.A.; Varshney, A.; Jain, A.; Singh, S. & Rao, K.V. (2010). Genome-wide analysis of the host intracellular network that regulates survival of Mycobacterium tuberculosis. *Cell* 140(5): 731-43.

Lee, B.Y.; Hefta, S.A. & Brennan, P.J. (1999). Characterization of the major membrane protein of virulent Mycobacterium tuberculosis. *Infect Immun* 60(5): 2066-74.

Lim, M.S. & Elenitoba-Johnson, K.S. (2004). Proteomics in pathology research. *Lab Invest* 84(10): 1227-44.

List E.O.; Berryman, D.E.; Bower, B., Sackmann-Sala, L.; Gosney, E.; Ding, J.; Okada, S. Kopchick, J.J. (2008). The use of proteomics to study infectious diseases. *Infect Disord Drug Targets* 8(1): 31-45.

Majeed, A.A.; Ahmed, N.; Rao, K.R.; Ghousunnissa, S.; Kauser, F.; Bose, B.; Nagarajaram, H.A.; Katoch, V.M.; Cousins, D.V.; Sechi, L.A.; Gilman, R.H. & Hasnain, S.E. (2004). AmpliBASE MT: a Mycobacterium tuberculosis diversity knowledgebase. *Bioinformatics* 20(6): 989-92.

Mattow, J.; Jungblut, P.R.; Schaible, U.E.; Mollenkopf, H.J.; Lamer, S.; Zimny-Arndt, U.; Hagens, K.; Müller, E.C. & Kaufmann, S.H. (2001). Identification of proteins from Mycobacterium tuberculosis missing in attenuated Mycobacterium bovis BCG strains. *Electrophoresis* 22(14): 2936-46.

Mattow, J.; Schaible, U.E.; Schmidt, F.; Hagens, K.; Siejak, F.; Brestrich, G.; Haeselbarth, G.; Müller, E.C.; Jungblut, P.R. & Kaufmann, S.H. (2003). Comparative proteome analysis of culture supernatant proteins from virulent Mycobacterium tuberculosis H37Rv and attenuated M. bovis BCG Copenhagen. *Electrophoresis* 24(19-20): 3405-20.

Mollenkopf, H.J.; Grode, L.; Mattow, J.; Stein, M.; Mann, P.; Knapp, B.; Ulmer, J. & Kaufmann, S.H. (2004). Application of mycobacterial proteomics to vaccine design: improved protection by Mycobacterium bovis BCG prime-Rv3407 DNA boost vaccination against tuberculosis. *Infect Immun* 72(11): 6471-9.

Mustafa, A.S. (2005). Mycobacterial gene cloning and expression, comparative genomics, bioinformatics and proteomics in relation to the development of new vaccines and diagnostic reagents. *Med Princ Pract* 14 Suppl 1:27-34.

Niemann, S.; Richter, E. & Rusch-Gerdes, S. (2000). Differentiation among members of the Mycobacterium tuberculosis complex by molecular and biochemical features: evidence for two pyrazinamide-susceptible subtypes of M. bovis. *J Clin Microbiol* 38(1): 152-7.

Parwati, I.; van Crevel. R. & van Soolingen. D. (2010). Possible underlying mechanisms for successful emergence of the Mycobacterium tuberculosis Beijing genotype strains. *Lancet Infect Dis* 10(2): 103-11.

Pheiffer, C.; Betts, J.C.; Flynn, H.R.; Lukey, P.T. & van Helden, P. (2005). Protein expression by a Beijing strain differs from that of another clinical isolate and Mycobacterium tuberculosis H37Rv. *Microbiology* 151(Pt 4): 1139-50.

Rison, S.C.; Mattow, J.; Jungblut, P.R. & Stoker, N.G. (2007). Experimental determination of translational starts using peptide mass mapping and tandem mass spectrometry within the proteome of Mycobacterium tuberculosis. *Microbiology* 153(Pt 2): 521-8.

Sharma, P.; Kumar, B.; Singhal, N.; Katoch, V.M.; Venkatesan, K.; Chauhan, D.S. & Bisht, D. (2010). Streptomycin induced protein expression analysis in Mycobacterium tuberculosis by two-dimensional gel electrophoresis & mass spectrometry. *Indian J Med Res* 132:400-8.

Soini, H.; Pan, X. ; Amin, A. ; Graviss, E.A. ; Siddiqui, A. & Musser, J.M. (2000). Characterization of Mycobacterium tuberculosis isolates from patients in Houston, Texas, by spoligotyping. *J Clin Microbiol* 38(2): 669-76.

Stulik, J. & Butaye, P. (2011). Introduction: application of proteomic technologies for the analysis of microbial infections. *In BSL3 and BSL4 Agents: Proteomics, Glycomics, and Antigenicity*, First Edition. Edited by Jiri Stulik, Rudolf Toman, Patrick Butaye, Robert G. Ulrich. 2011 Wiley-VCH Verlag GmbH & Co. KGaA.

van Soolingen, D.; Hermans, P.W.; de Haas, P.E.; Soll, D.R.; & van Embden, J.D. (1991). Occurrence and stability of insertion sequences in Mycobacterium tuberculosis complex strains: evaluation of an insertion sequence-dependent DNA polymorphism as a tool in the epidemiology of tuberculosis. *J Clin Microbiol* 29(11): 2578-86.

van Soolingen, D.; Qian, L.; de Haas, P.E.; Douqlas, J.T.; Traore, H.; Portaels, F.; Qing, H.Z.; Enkhsaikan, D.; Nymadawa, P. & van Embden, J.D. (1995). Predominance of a single genotype of Mycobacterium tuberculosis in countries of east Asia. *J Clin Microbiol* 33(12): 3234-8.

van Soolingen, D.; van der Zanden, A.G.; de Haas, P.E.; Noordhoek, G.T.; Kiers, A.; Foudraine, N.A.; Portaels, F.; Kolk, A.H. & Kremer, K. (1998). Diagnosis of Mycobacterium microti infections among humans by using novel genetic markers. *J Clin Microbiol* 36(7): 1840-5.

Viana-Niero, C.; Gutierrez, C.; Sola, C.; Filliol, L.; Boulahbal, F.; Vincent, V. & Rastoqi, N. (2001). Genetic diversity of Mycobacterium africanum clinical isolates based on IS6110-restriction fragment length polymorphism analysis, spoligotyping, and variable number of tandem DNA repeats. *J Clin Microbiol* 39(1): 57-65.

Wang, Q.; Yue, J.; Zhang, L.; Xu, Y.; Chen, J.; Zhang, M.; Zhu, B.; Wang, H. & Wang, H. (2007). A newly identified 191A/C mutation in the Rv2629 gene that was significantly associated with rifampin resistance in Mycobacterium tuberculosis. *J Proteome Res* 6(12): 4564-71.

World Health Organization. (1998). Laboratory services in tuberculosis control. Part III: Culture. Geneva, WHO (document WHO/TB/98.258).

World Health Organization. (2009). Guidelines for surveillance of drug resistance in tuberculosis. 4th Ed. who.int/tb/publications/mdr_surveillance/en/index.html.

World Health Organization. (2010). Noncommercial culture and drug-susceptibility testing methods for screening patients at risk for multidrug-resistant tuberculosis. www.who.int/tb/laboratory/whopolicy_noncommercialculture_and_dst_methods_mar2011.pdf

World Health Organization. WHO Report 2010. (2011). Global Tuberculosis Control 2010. http://www.who.int/tb/publications/global_report/2010/en/index.html.

Wu, X.Q. & Liu, Y.N. (2009). Advances in Mycobacterium tuberculosis proteomics. *Zhonghua Jie He He Hu Xi Za Zhi* 32(7): 527-9.

Xie, Y.E.; Ren. B.X.; Hu, W.M.; Tang, E.J. & Jing, B.Q. (2009). Comparison of proteins of multi-drug-resistant Mycobacterium tuberculosis isolate with drug-sensitive isolate. *Chin J Public Health* 25(5): 515-6.

Zhu, N.X.; Zheng, S.; Xu, R.Z. & Yu, R.X. (2003). Overexpression of S3 ribosomal protein gene is involved in drug resistance in K562/DOX cells. *Zhonghua Xue Ye Xue Za Zhi* 24(3): 141-3.

22

Molecular Biological Techniques for Detection of Multidrug Resistant Tuberculosis (MDR) and Extremely Drug Resistant Tuberculosis (XDR) in Clinical Isolates of *Mycobacterium tuberculosis*

K.L. Therese, R. Gayathri and H.N. Madhavan
L&T Microbiology Research Centre, Vision Research Foundation, Chennai, India

1. Introduction

Tuberculosis (TB) is a contagious disease caused by *Mycobacterium tuberculosis* (*M. tuberculosis*). When people infected with tuberculosis cough, sneeze, talk or spit, the bacilli are propelled into the air. Each person with active TB disease will infect on average between 10 and 15 people every year. But people infected with TB bacilli will not necessarily become sick with the disease. The immune system "walls off" the TB bacilli which, protected by a thick waxy coat, can lie dormant for years. When the immune system is weakened, the chances of the infection progressing to disease are higher.

Overall, one-third of the world's population is currently infected with the TB bacillus. 5 - 10% of people who are infected with TB bacilli (but who are not infected with HIV) become sick or infectious at some time during their life. People with HIV and TB infection are much more likely to develop TB [WHO, 2010].

Globally, there were an estimated 14 million prevalent cases of TB in 2009, equivalent to 200 cases per 100 000 population. Most of the estimated number of cases in 2009 occurred in Asia (55%) and Africa (30%); 3 smaller proportions of cases occurred in the Eastern Mediterranean Region (7%), the European Region (4%) and the Region of the Americas (3%) [WHO, 2010]. In 2009, an estimated 1.3 million deaths (range: 1.2 - 1.5 million) occurred among HIV-negative cases of TB, including 0.38 million deaths (range: 0.3–0.5 million) among women. This is equivalent to 20 deaths per 100 000 population [WHO, 2010].

Until 50 years ago, there were no medicines to cure TB. Now, strains that are resistant to a single drug have been documented in every country surveyed and strains of TB resistant to all major anti-TB drugs have emerged. Drug-resistant TB is caused by inconsistent or partial treatment, when patients do not take all their medicines regularly for the required period because they start to feel better, or the doctors and health workers prescribe the wrong treatment regimens, or the drug supply is unreliable. A particularly dangerous form of drug-resistant TB is multidrug-resistant TB (MDR-TB), which is defined as the disease caused by TB bacilli resistant to isoniazid and rifampicin, the two most powerful anti-TB drugs. Rates of MDR-TB are high in some countries, especially in the former Soviet Union, and threaten TB control efforts [WHO, 2010].

While drug-resistant TB is generally treatable, it requires extensive chemotherapy (up to two years of treatment) with second-line anti-TB drugs which are more costly than first-line drugs, and which produce adverse drug reactions that are more severe, though manageable. Quality assured second-line anti-TB drugs are available at reduced prices for projects approved by the Green Light Committee [WHO, 2010].

The emergence of extensively drug-resistant (XDR) TB, particularly in settings where many TB patients are also infected with HIV, poses a serious threat to TB control, and confirms the urgent need to strengthen basic TB control and to apply the new WHO guidelines for the programmatic management of drug-resistant TB.

The important ramifications in the laboratory diagnosis of tuberculosis and drug resistant tuberculosis are: the delay in the isolation of the bacilli in culture, low sensitivity/detection limit of the direct smears and lack of technically trained personnel. Identification of tuberculosis using molecular techniques namely, polymerase chain reaction (PCR), PCR based restriction fragment length polymorphism (PCR-RFLP) and PCR based DNA sequencing are very rapid, more sensitive and reliable when compared to the conventional culture. There are several in house nested PCR (nPCR) standardized for the detection of *M. tuberculosis* from clinical specimens targeting MPB64 [Therese KL et al, 2005], IS6110 [Wang et al, 2004] and 16S rRNA [Ninet et al, 1996] genes. MPB64 is an immunogenic protein produced by *M. tuberculosis* and a few strains of *M. bovis* and BCG strain. IS6110 is an insertion element present in single or multiple copies in *M. tuberculosis* complex isolates. There are studies which reported on the lack of IS6110 insertion element in strains isolated from Asian population. Also there are strain variations among the *M. tuberculosis* isolates. Thus multiplex PCR or nPCR targeting more than one gene target will be a better tool for the detection of *M. tuberculosis* from direct clinical specimens.

Drug resistance in *M. tuberculosis* is caused by mutations in relatively restricted regions of the genome. Mutations associated with drug resistance occur in *rpoB* for rifampicin (RIF) *katG* and the promoter region of the *mabA (fabG1)-inhA* operon for Isoniazid (INH), *embB* for ethambutol (EMB), *pncA* for pyrazinamide (PZA), *rpsL* and *rrs* for streptomycin (STR) and *gyrA, gyrB* for fluoroquinolones (FQs) such as ofloxacin (OFX) and levofloxacin (LVX) [Musser et al, 1995; Zhang et al, 2000].

2. MDR-TB

2.1 Worldwide reports on MDR-TB

In 2008, there were an estimated 440,000 (range, 390 000-510 000) MDR-TB cases emerging worldwide. About 250,000 of these cases (range: 230 000–270 000) should have been reported to WHO, if countries had tested all the TB patients that they notified for drug resistance. However, only just over 30,000 MDR-TB cases (12%) were actually notified globally in 2009 [WHO, November 2010].

Almost 50% of MDR-TB cases worldwide are estimated to occur in China and India. In 2008, MDR-TB caused an estimated 150,000 deaths. Since 1994, 114 countries have reported surveillance data on MDR-TB: 42 perform continuous surveillance of anti-TB drug resistance based on routine testing of all TB patients; 72 rely on periodic surveys of representative samples of TB patients. The Russian Federation, which was able to provide high-quality continuous surveillance data from 12 of its oblasts and republics, reported proportions of 23.8–28.3% MDRTB among new TB cases in three of its oblasts in the northwest part of the country. Other Russian oblasts were found to have proportions of MDR-TB as low as 5.4% among new TB cases. Tajikistan, in its first ever survey, found proportions of 16.5% MDR-TB among new TB cases and 61.6% MDR-TB among previously treated TB patients in Dushanbe city and Rudaki district, the highest proportion ever reported among previously treated TB patients. To date, 12 countries have reported nationwide or subnational proportions of MDR-TB of 6% or more among new TB cases [WHO, November 2010].

Five of these countries also report MDR-TB proportions of 50% or more among previously treated cases. All of these settings are located in the eastern part of Europe or in Central Asia.

2.2 Recently developed molecular techniques for the detection of drug resistance in tuberculosis

2.2.1 Solid-phase Hybridization techniques

There are currently two commercially available solid-phase hybridization techniques: the Line Probe Assay (INNO-LiPA Rif TB Assay; Innogenetics, Ghent, Belgium) for the detection of rifampicin resistance and the GenoType MTBDR assay (Hain Lifesciences, Nehren, Germany) for the simultaneous detection of isoniazid and rifampicin resistance. The LiPA assay was introduced several years ago and is based on the hybridization of amplified DNA from cultured strains or clinical samples to 10 probes covering the core region of the *rpoB* gene of *M. tuberculosis*, immobilized on a nitrocellulose strip. The GenoType MTBDR on the other hand, detects resistance to isoniazid and rifampicin in culture samples based on the detection of the most common mutations in the *katG* and *rpoB* genes respectively. Both assays have now been evaluated in different settings, giving encouraging results. In a recent study Hillemann *et al* evaluated the GenoType MTBDR assay and found that 99% of MDR strains with mutations in the *rpoB* gene and 88.4% of strains with mutations in the codon 315 of the *katG* gene were correctly identified. Correlation with DNA sequencing was 100% and compared with conventional tests good sensitivity and specificity were also obtained. Both solid hybridization methods have shown to be relatively simple to perform although basic expertise in molecular biology and PCR techniques is required. As with other genotypic methods the sensitivity of the test depends on the amount of DNA present in the sample and also the presence of inhibitors could cause false-negative results.

INNOLiPA Rif. TB kit: INNOLiPA Rif. TB kit simultaneously detects the *M. tuberculosis* complex and the presence of mutations in the *rpoB* gene associated with resistance to rifampicin which is considered a marker for MDR-TB strains. The strip contains 5 probes for detection of sensitive genotypes (S1-S5) [Morgan et al, 2005; Makinen et al, 2006] and 4 probes for detection of resistance genotypes (R2,R4a, R4b and R5). Rifampicin resistance is indicated by the absence of one or more sensitive probes, possible accompanied by the appearance of one or more mutant probes.

The **GenoType MTBDR** test is able to detect mutations in the *rpoB* gene for RIF resistance, and the most frequent mutation at codon 315 of the *katG* gene for INH resistance, either in isolates or clinical specimens. The specificity and sensitivity of the assay for RIF resistance were nearly 100%; for INH-resistance, despite a high specificity (approximately 100%), the sensitivity of the test ranged from 70% to 90%, depending on the prevalence of the particular mutation at the *katG* locus [Hilleman et al, 2007].

GenoType MTBDRplus (Hain Lifescience, Germany), an advanced version of the assay, includes probes for the identification of other mutations in the hotspot region of the *rpoB* gene for RIF resistance, and probes to detect mutations in the promoter region of the *inhA* gene involved in INH resistance. These improvements facilitate the detection of another 10% to 20% of INH-resistant cases, with an enhancement in rapid MDR-TB diagnosis.

The line probe assays are accurate and useful for rapid detection of drug resistance directly in clinical specimens. However, the number of genes that can be analyzed remains limited and the test fails to distinguish insertion mutations. Furthermore, they retain a lower sensitivity among acid fast bacilli-negative samples. In general, line probe assays are expensive and require sophisticated laboratory infrastructure. Their role and utility in low-income, high-burden countries needs to be evaluated in field studies.

2.2.2 Real-time Polymerase Chain Reaction techniques

Real-time PCR techniques have also been introduced for rapid detection of drug resistance. Different probes have been used like the TaqMan probe, fluorescence resonance energy transfer (FRET) probes, molecular beacons and bioprobes. The main advantages of real-time PCR techniques are the speed of the test and a lower risk of contamination. The main disadvantages would be the requirement for expensive equipment and reagents, and the need for skilled technical personnel. Real-time PCR was initially applied to *M. tuberculosis* strains but more recently it has been successfully applied directly in clinical samples. Results could be obtained in an average of 1.5-2.0 h after DNA extraction. Real-time PCR could eventually be implemented in reference laboratories with the required capacity to properly set up the technique and in settings where it can contribute to the management of TB patients.

Detection of antitubercular drug resistance is vital to effective patient management. Real-time PCR offers the potential to detect gene mutations responsible for drug resistance within hours from patient specimens compared with the average of 2 weeks required for traditional susceptibility test methods. The *rpoB* and *katG* genes are the most common *M. tuberculosis* targets utilized in real-time PCR methods and well-known mutations in these genes correlate with resistance to rifampin and isoniazid, respectively [Edwards et al, 2001; El-Hajj et al, 2001; Garcia de Viedma et al, 2002; O'Mahony et al, 2002; Piatek et al, 2002; Torres et al, 2000; Torres et al, 2003; van Doorn et al, 2003]. The significance of other gene targets such as *kasA*, *ahpC-oxyR*, and *inhA* for the prediction of isoniazid resistance is somewhat controversial [Piatek et al, 2000]. Torres et al used two sets of FRET hybridization probes to detect *rpoB* mutations in 24 rifampin-resistant strains *of M. tuberculosis* and another set of FRET hybridization probes to detect *katG* mutations in 15 isoniazid-resistant *M. tuberculosis* strains [Torres et al, 2000]. Additionally, Garcia de Viedma et al. used two sets of *rpoB* probes and one set of *katG* probes to detect *rpoB* and *katG* mutations, but in a single tube, for

29 resistant *M. tuberculosis* isolates [Garcia de Viedma et al, 2002]. Since not all gene mutations conferring drug resistance are well characterized and are thus not amenable to PCR assay development, traditional culture-based susceptibility testing methods are still required. However, the ability to predict rifampin and isoniazid resistance up to 2 weeks sooner than current methods for some isolates should have significant benefit for patient care.

2.2.3 Microarray

An array is an orderly arrangement of samples where matching of known and unknown DNA samples is done based on base pairing rules [Heyman et al, 1999]. An array experiment makes use of common assay systems such as microplates or standard blotting membranes. The sample spot sizes are typically less than 200 microns in diameter usually contain thousands of spots. Thousands of spotted samples known as probes (with known identity) are immobilized on a solid support (a microscope glass slides or silicon chips or nylon membrane [Heyman et al, 1999]. The spots can be DNA, cDNA, or oligonucleotides. These are used to determine complementary binding of the unknown sequences thus allowing parallel analysis for gene expression and gene discovery. An experiment with a single DNA chip can provide information on thousands of genes simultaneously. An orderly arrangement of the probes on the support is important as the location of each spot on the array is used for the identification of a gene [Heyman et al, 1999].

Microarray technology is used in the detection of drug resistant *M. tuberculosis* rather than the detection of *M. tuberculosis* from clinical specimens. The TB Biochip oligonucleotide microarray is the most widely used Microarray for the detection of isoniazid and rifampicin resistance simultaneously [Garcia de Viedma D et al, 2003].

TB-Biochip oligonucleotide microarray for the detection of rifampicin resistant *M. tuberculosis*

The TB-Biochip oligonucleotide microarray system is designed to detect and identify 29 codon substitutions and 1 codon deletion distributed over 10 codon positions (507, 511, 512, 513, 515, 516, 522, 526, 532, 533) within the rifampicin resistant determining region (RRDR). Each element of the microarray contains an immobilized oligonucleotide whose sequence matches that of either a wild-type or mutated segment of the RRDR. The use of acrylamide gel pads increases the robustness of the hybridization reaction. Hybridization of the microarray with fluorescently labeled target DNA produces a spatial pattern of fluorescence intensities corresponding to the efficiencies of hybridization of the labeled target DNA to the various oligonucleotide probes.

In the TB-Biochip system, the fluorescence intensities are recorded using a charge-coupled device camera, and the relative intensities of fluorescence for the elements representing wildtype sequences and mutant sequences for each codon are compared using imaging software and automated computer-assisted interpretation of hybridization results [Garcia de Viedma D et al, 2003; Cavusoglu et al, 2004]. The isolate is designated **RIF susceptible** if the fluorescence of each of the wild-type elements is greater than the fluorescence of any of the corresponding mutant elements. The isolate is designated **RIF resistant** if the fluorescence of any one of the mutant elements is greater than the fluorescence of its corresponding wild-type element.

Advantange and disadvantage of TB- biochip system

The complete TB-Biochip system may be suitable for use in clinical laboratories with molecular biology expertise because it requires relatively little hands-on time for experimental manipulations or data analysis, tests can be run individually or in batches, and specialized training is not required. The observed discrepancies between the results of conventional DST and the TB-Biochip system (all were falsely called susceptible with the TB-Biochip system) likely result from the large number of mutations found in RIF-resistant isolates and the limited range of mutations included on the biochip.

Although technically a solid-phase-type hybridization assay, microarrays, also known as biochips, have been proposed as new molecular methods for detecting drug resistance in *M. tuberculosis*. They are based on the hybridization of DNA obtained from clinical samples to oligonucleotides immobilized in a solid support, such as miniaturized glass slides. They have been mainly used to detect resistance to rifampicin. In a recent evaluation using oligonucleotide microarrays for analysis of drug resistance, Gryadunov *et al.* detected over 95% rifampicin resistant and almost 80% isoniazid resistant *M. tuberculosis* isolates within 12 h in a sample of drug-resistant isolates and clinical samples. For the time being and due to the high cost involved, the use of microarrays for detecting drug resistance in TB is still beyond the reach of most clinical mycobacteriology laboratories.

2.3 DNA sequencing

Sequencing DNA of PCR amplified products has been the most widely used method; it is accurate and reliable and it has become the gold standard for mutation detection. It has been performed by manual and automated procedures although the latter is now the most commonly used. It has been widely used for characterizing mutations in the *rpoB* gene in rifampicin-resistant strains and to detect mutations responsible for resistance to other anti-tuberculosis drugs. It would be rather difficult, however, to implement it routinely for detection of drug resistance mutations for several drugs since it would involve several reactions for each isolate, making the cost high.

2.3.1 DNA extraction

DNA from clinical *M. tuberculosis* isolates can be extracted by using Qiagen kit (Germany) and also by keeping the MGIT suspension at 80°C for 10 minutes. After 10 minutes, centrifuged at 3000 rpm and the supernatant can be used as template DNA for PCR. The procedure for extraction of DNA using Qiagen kit is mentioned below.

Reagents and other accessories required

a. Proteinase K
b. Lysis buffer (AL buffer)
c. Ethanol
d. Washing buffer-1 (AW1 buffer)
e. Washing buffer-2 (AW 2 Buffer)
f. Elution buffer (AE Buffer)
g. Minispin (eppendorff)
h. Sterile 1.5ml vials

i. Micropipettes (20-200µl)
j. Filter barriers tips (20-200µl)

Procedure

- Pipette 20µl QIAGEN Proteinase k into the bottom of a 1.5ml microfuge tube.
- Add 200µl of the sample to the microfuge tube. Use up to 200µl whole blood, plasma, serum, Buffy coat upto 5 X 10^6 lymphocytes in 200µl PBS
- Add 200µl of AL buffer to the sample. Mix by pulse vortexing for 15 seconds
- Incubate at 56° C for 10 minutes.
- Briefly centrifuge the micro centrifuge tube to remove drops from inside of the lid.
- Add 200µl of ethanol (96-100%) to the sample, mix by pulse vortexing for 15 seconds. After mixing, briefly centrifuge the 1.5ml microfuge tube to remove drops from inside of the lid.
- Carefully apply the mixture from step 6 to the QIAamp mini spin column (in a 2ml collecting tube) without wetting the rim. Close the cap, and centrifuge at 8000 rpm for 1 min. Place the QIAamp mini spin column in a clean 2 ml collecting tube and discard the tube containing the filtrate.
- Carefully open the QIAamp mini spin column and add 500µl buffer AW1 without wetting the rim. Close the cap and centrifuge at 8000 rpm for 1min. Place the QIAamp mini spin column in a clean 2ml collecting tube and discard the tube containing filtrate.
- Carefully open the QIAamp mini spin column and add 500µl buffer AW2 without wetting the rim. Close the cap and centrifuge at 14,000 rpm for 3min, followed by an empty spin at 14,000 rpm for 1min.
- Place the QIAamp mini spin column in a clean 1.5 ml microfuge tube and discard the tube containing filtrate. Carefully open the QIAamp mini spin column and add 200µl AE Buffer. Incubate at room temperature for 1min, and then centrifuge at 8,000 rpm for 1min. Discard the column and store the DNA at -20°C.

2.3.2 PCR protocol

Reagents and other accessories required:

- Stock dNTPs dilution: 100 mM concentration of dNTPs- dATP, dCTP, dTTP and dGTP
- Working standard dNTP (200µM): 2 µl of each of the stock dNTP made up to 400 µl using MilliQ water.
- Forward and reverse primers
- *Taq* DNA polymerase (3 units)
- PCR Thermal cycler
- Cyclomixer
- Sterile 0.5 ml or 0.2 ml vials
- Micropipettes (20-200µl, 0.5- 10µl)
- Filter barrier tips (20-200µl)
- Gel casting tray/trough
- Gel combs
- Electrophoresis tank
- Powerpack
- Gel documentation system

The PCR cocktail contained the following:

dNTP	8 µl
10X buffer (15mM Mg2+,Tris, Kcl(500 mM)-pH 8.3)	5 µl
Forward Primer (1 pM)	1 µl
Reverse Primer (1 pM)	1 µl
MilliQ water	30 µl
Taq polymerase	0.3 µl

2.3.3 PCR protocol for amplification of *embB* gene using primers targeting 640-1577 region

PCR targeting *embB* gene was standardized with a specialized Taq DNA polymerase enzyme called "Z Taq" enzyme (Takara Bio, Ohtsu, Shiga, Japan). The *Z-Taq* polymerase offers unmatched PCR productivity, with a processing speed five times faster than those of other commercially available *Taq* polymerases. The total PCR cycle takes only 29 minutes. All the reagents for PCR (dNTP, 10X, Z Taq) will be provided along with the buffer. Each 50 µl reaction contained 2.5mM dNTP, 10X, 1pM of forward and reverse primers and 2.5 Units of Z taq enzyme. The details of primer targeting drug resistance genes, their thermal profile used and the expected amplicon size are given in the Table2.

Detection Of Amplified Products: The amplified product is subjected to electrophoresis on 2% agarose gel incorporated with 0.5 µg/ml ethidium bromide for visualization by UV transilluminator (Vilber Lourmat - France).

2.3.4 DNA sequencing of amplified products

The term **DNA sequencing** refers to sequencing methods for determining the order of the nucleotide bases—adenine, guanine, cytosine, and thymine—in a molecule of DNA. DNA sequencing enables us to perform a thorough analysis of DNA because it provides us with the most basic information of all: the sequence of nucleotides. The classical chain-termination method requires a single-stranded DNA template, a DNA primer, a DNA polymerase, radioactively or fluorescently labeled nucleotides, and modified nucleotides that terminate DNA strand elongation. *Dye-terminator sequencing* utilizes labelling of the chain terminator ddNTPs, which permits sequencing in a single reaction, rather than four reactions as in the labelled-primer method. In dye-terminator sequencing, each of the four dideoxynucleotide chain terminators is labelled with fluorescent dyes, each of which with different wavelengths of fluorescence and emission. Owing to its greater expediency and speed, dye-terminator sequencing is now the mainstay in automated sequencing. Its limitations include dye effects due to differences in the incorporation of the dye-labelled chain terminators into the DNA fragment, resulting in unequal peak heights and shapes in the electronic DNA sequence trace chromatogram after capillary electrophoresis. This problem has been addressed with the use of modified DNA polymerase enzyme systems and dyes that minimize incorporation variability, as well as methods for eliminating "dye

Target genes / Primer sequence (5′-3′ Direction)	**Thermal profile**	**No. of Cycles**	**Expected Amplicon Size (bp)**
rpoB for rifampicin CCACCCAGGACGTGGAGGCGATCACAC AGTGCGACGGGTGCACGTCGCGGACCT	95 °C-5 min 95°C-30sec 72°C-1min 72°C -5 min	35	286
katG1 for isoniazid GCCCGAGCAACACCC ATGTCCCGCGTCAGG	94°C - 1min 58°C -1min 72°C -2 min	35	237
katG2 for isoniazid CGAGGAATTGGCCGACGAGTT CGGCGCCGCGGAGTTGAATGA	94°C - 1min 55°C -1min 72°C -2 min	35	414
katG3 (targeting 138 codon) for isoniazid CCGGCACCTACCGCATCCAC GCCCCAATAGACCTCATCGG	95°C - 1min 60°C -30sec 72°C -1 min	30	269
katG4 (targeting 315 codon) for isoniazid GAAACAGCGGCGCTGGATCGT GTTGTCCCATTTCGTCGGGG	Same as above		209
inhA for isoniazid CCTCGCTGCCCAGAAAGG A ATCCCCCGGTTTCCTCCGGT	94°C - 5min 94°C - 1min 64°C -1min 72°C -2 min	40	248
oxyR-ahpC for isoniazid GCTTGATGTCCGAGAGCAT GGTCGCGTAGGCAGTGCCCC	94°C - 2min 94°C - 1min 60°C -1min 72°C -2 min	35	701
rpsL for streptomycin GGCCGACAAACAGAACGT GTTCACCAACTGGGTGAC	94°C - 1min 94°C - 1min 56°C -1min 72°C -1 min 72°C - 7 min	35	505
rrs for streptomycin TTGGCCATGCTCTTGATGCCC TGCACACAGGCCACAAGGGA	94°C - 1min 94°C - 1min 56°C -1min 72°C -1 min 72°C - 7 min	35	1140
pncA for pyrazinamide GGCGTCATGGACCCTATATC CAACAGTTCATCCCGGTTC	94°C - 30 sec 60°C - 30 sec 72°C - 30 sec	35	670
embB for ethambutol CCGACCACGCTGAAACTGCTGGCGAT GGTGGGCAGGATGAGGTAGT	95°C - 5 sec 55°C - 10 sec 72°C - 10 sec	35	937

Table 2. Primer sets used in the study to sequence the different loci of target genes with their thermal profile and expected amplicon sizes[Sekiguchi et al, 2007; Siddiqi et al, 2002; Sreevatsan et al 1997]

blobs". The dye-terminator sequencing method, along with automated high-throughput DNA sequence analyzers, is now being used for the vast majority of sequencing projects.

DNA sequencing involves the following steps,

- Amplification of specific sequence from DNA
- Electrophoresis of amplified products in 2% agarose gel
- Elution of amplified products
- Cycle sequencing
- Purification of extension products
- Sequence analysis

Gel elution (Qiagen DNA Elution kit)

1. The amplified product (30 µl) is run on 2% agarose gel
2. Excise the DNA fragment from the agarose gel with a clean, sharp scalpel.
3. Weigh the gel slice in a colorless tube. Add 3 volumes of Buffer QG to 1 volume of gel (100 mg is approximately 100 µl).
4. Incubate at 50ºC for 10 mins in thermal cycler (or until the gel slice has completely dissolved with intermittent vortexing).
5. After the gel slice has dissolved completely, check that the color of the mixture is yellow (similar to buffer QG without dissolved agarose).
6. NOTE: If the color of the mixture is orange or violet, add 10µl of 3 M Sodium acetate, pH 5.0, and mix. The color of the mixture will turn yellow.
7. Add one gel volume of Isopropanol to the sample and mix by repeated pipetting.
8. Place a MinElute column in a 2ml collection tube provided in a suitable rack.
9. Apply the sample to MinElute column, and centrifuge at 13,000 rpm for 1 minute.
10. Discard the flow through and place the MinElute column back in the same collection tube.
11. Add 500µl of buffer QG to the spin column and centrifuge at 13,000 rpm for 1 minute.
12. Discard the flow through, and place the MinElute column back in the same collection tube.
13. To wash, add 750µl of buffer PE to the MinElute column and centrifuge at 13,000 rpm for 1 minute.
14. Discard the flow through, and place the MinElute column for an additional 1 minute at 13,000 rpm.
15. Place the MinElute column into a clean 1.5ml micro centrifuge tube.
16. To elute DNA, add 10µl of buffer EB (10mM Tris.Cl, pH 8.5) or water (pH 7.0-8.5) to the centre of the membrane, let the column stand for 1 minute, and centrifuge at 13,000 rpm for 1 minute.
17. Store the eluted products at -20 ºC.

2.3.4 Cycle sequencing

Cycle sequencing combines amplification and enzymatic DNA sequencing using 5′ dye labeled terminators.

Requirements for Cycle Sequencing

- Forward primer or Reverse primer at the concentration of 1 picomole/µl each.

- Big Dye Terminator cycle sequencing Ready reaction kit (ABI prism, USA)

Reaction Protocol

- Ready reaction mix (2.5X RR mix)	- 2.0μl
- 5x sequencing buffer	- 1.0μl
- Forward/Reverse primer (1pmol/μl)	- 2.0 μl
- Milli Q water	- 2.0 μl
- Amplified PCR product (eluted)	- 2.0 μl

Reaction Condition for Cycle Sequencing

Initial Denaturation	- 96°C for 1 minute.	
Denaturation	- 96°C for 10 seconds.	25 cycles
Annealing	- 50°C for 5 seconds.	25 cycles
Extension	- 60°C for 4 minutes.	25 cycles
Holding Temp	- 4°C	

Purification of Cycle Sequenced Product

The cycle sequenced products are purified to remove the unincorporated dye terminators before the samples are analyzed.

Reagents Required

- 500 mM EDTA
- 3M sodium acetate
- Chilled ethanol
- 70% ethanol

Procedure

- Take 0.5ml sterile PCR vial and add 10 μl of Milli Q water.
- Then add 2 μl of 125mM EDTA, followed by 10 μl of cycle sequenced product, 2 μl of 3M-sodium acetate (pH 4.6) and 50 μl of chilled ethanol. Vortex well and incubate at room temperature (22-28°C) for 15 minutes
- Centrifuge at 12,000 rpm for 20 minutes.
- Pipette out the supernatant and wash the pellet twice with 250 μl of 70% ethanol at 12,000 rpm for 10 minutes. Care should be taken not to touch the sides of the eppendorf vial during pipetting.
- The vials are then dried at 37°C (incubator) until ethanol completely evaporates. Presence of ethanol will prevent complete dissolving of DNA in formamaide.

2.3.5 Loading into DNA sequencer

Once the ethanol is completely dried, add 10 μl of formamide. This is denatured at 95°C (Thermal cycler) for 3 minutes and immediately snap cooled in ice. The sequence of the PCR amplified DNA is deduced with the help of the ABI Prism 3100 AVANT (Applied Biosystems, USA) genetic analyzer that works based on the principle of Sanger dideoxy sequencing. The amplified products with the dye at the terminated 3'end is subjected to capillary electrophoresis by an automated sample injection. The emitted flurorescence from the dye labels on crossing the laser area are collected in the rate of one per second by cooled, charge-coupled device (CCD) camera at particular wavelength bands (virtual filters) and stored as digital signals on the computer for processing.

2.3.6 Basic Local Alignment Search Tool (BLAST) analysis

The sequences are analysed by sequence analysis softwares such as Bio Edit sequence alignment software or Chromas software. BLAST analysis, using pubmed, http://www.ncbi.nlm.nih.gov/BLAST is done to confirm the sequenced data with the standard strains and to determine the percentage homology.

2.3.7 Multalin analysis

Multalin analysis (http://multalin.toulouse.inra.fr/multalin/) to be done to identify the presence of polymorphism or mutation by comparing with the reference strain from genbank (Accession No. L27989 for *rpoB*, U41314 for *katG*, MTU16243 for *inhA* and *oxyR-ahpC*, X70995 for *rrs* and *rpsL*, AY743320 for *pncA* and MTU68480 for *embB*). An example of multalin analysis targeting *rpoB* and *katG* are shown in the figure 1&2.

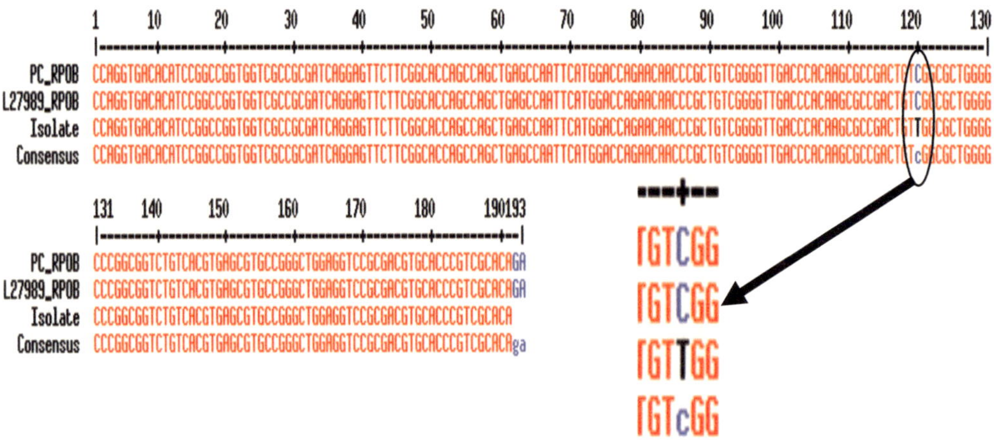

Fig. 1. An example of multalin result targeting *rpoB* gene using forward primer showing the presence of most commonly reported mutation TCG→TTG (Ser531Leu). Inset enlarged view of the mutation.

2.3.8 PCR based DNA sequencing for XDR-TB strains

If an MDR-TB strain has the above-mentioned mutations, it should be screened for resistance to Amikacin, capreomycin, kanamycin and the fluoroquinolones by PCR based DNA sequencing targeting *rrs, tlyA, thyA, gyrA* and *gyrB*. The details of primer targeting drug resistance genes, their thermal profile used and the expected amplicon size are given in the Table 3.

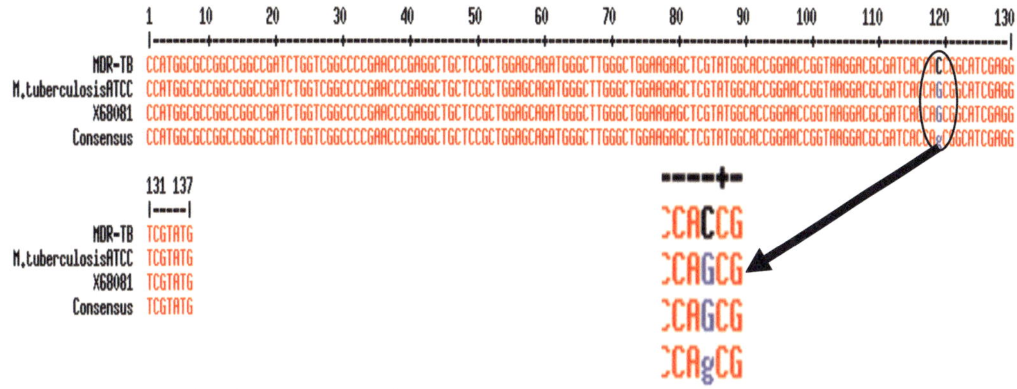

Fig. 2. An example of multalin result targeting *katG* gene using forward primer showing the presence of most commonly reported mutation A**GC**→ACC (Ser315Thr). Inset enlarged view of the mutation.

Target genes / Primer sequence (5′-3′ Direction)	Thermal Profile	No. of Cycles
thyA (Amikacin, capreomycin, kanamycin) ATCGTGTGCCCCATGGTGATCT CTCGGTGTATTCCCGTCGACT	95°C – 1 min 60°C – 1 min 72°C – 1 min	30
tlyA(Amikacin, capreomycin, kanamycin) CATCGCACGTCGTCTTTC AATACTTTTTCTACGCGCCG	95°C – 1 min 60°C – 1 min 72°C – 1 min	30
gyrA for Moxifloxacin,Ofloxacin, Ciprofloxacin CAGCTACATCGACTATGCGA GGGCTTCGGTGTTACCTCAT	94°C – 1 min 52°C – 1 min 72°C – 1 min	40
gyrB for Moxifloxacin,Ofloxacin, Ciprofloxacin CCACCGACATCGGTGGATT CTGCCACTTGAGTTTGTACA	94°C – 1 min 57°C – 1 min 72°C – 1 min	40

Table 3. Primer sets used in the study to sequence the different loci of target genes with their thermal profile and expected amplicon sizes [Sekiguchi et al, 2007; Siddiqi et al, 2002; Sreevatsan et al 1997]

For PCR protocol and DNA sequencing protocol, please refer to procedures 2.3.1 to 2.3.7.

3. Conclusion

The expectation that molecular techniques would surpass conventional methods for diagnosis of TB or phenotypic susceptibility testing has not yet been realized. The genetic basis of resistance must be understood before achieving such a goal. However, the clinician now has a variety of new tools to improve the diagnosis of TB and drug resistance. Most of them still require detailed and systematic evaluations using standard techniques as references before their widespread application in clinical settings. Most of these techniques require trained personnel and specialized equipment, hindering their application in field conditions, but they can be used in reference laboratories as part of the TB control programs.

The physician must be cautious when using results obtained by these techniques, especially when diagnosing drug resistance. Although it is not recommended, these molecular methods might be used as a complement to the standard methods in situation of difficult diagnosis, but never should be used solely to base such decisions.

4. Acknowledgement

The authors gratefully acknowledge the infrastructure facility and support provided by Vision Research Foundation, Chennai and for the financial support through a research grant by Chennai Willingdon Corporate Foundation, Chennai, India.

5. References

Cavusoglu C, Karaca-Derici Y, Bilgic A. (2004). In-vitro activity of rifabutin against rifampicin-resistant *Mycobacterium tuberculosis* isolates with known *rpoB* mutations. *Clin Microbiol Infect*, Vol. 10, No. 7, pp. 662–665.

Edwards K J, Metherell LA, Yates M and Saunders NA. (2001). Detection of *rpoB* mutations in *Mycobacterium tuberculosis* by biprobe analysis. *J Clin Microbiol*, Vol. 39, No. 9, pp. 3350–3352.

El-Hajj HH, Marras SA, Tyagi S, Kramer FR and Alland D. (2001). Detection of rifampin resistance in *Mycobacterium tuberculosis* in a single tube with molecular beacons. *J Clin Microbiol*, Vol. 39, No. 11, pp. 4131–4137.

Garcia de Viedma D, del Sol Diaz Infantes M, Lasala F, Chave F, Alcala L and Bouza E. (2002). New real-time PCR able to detect in a single tube multiple rifampin resistance mutations and high-level isoniazid resistance mutations in *Mycobacterium tuberculosis*. *J Clin Microbiol*, Vol. 40, No. 3, pp. 988–995.

Garcia de Viedma D. (2003). Rapid detection of resistance in *Mycobacterium tuberculosis*: review discussing molecular approaches. *Clin Microbiol Infect*,Vol. 9,No.5,pp349–59.

Gryadunov D, Mikhailovich V, Lapa S, Roudinskii N, Donnikov M, Pan'kov S, et al (2005). Evaluation of hybridisation on oligonucleotide microarrays for analysis of drug-resistant *Mycobacterium tuberculosis*. *Clinical Microbiology and Infection*, Vol. 11, No.7, pp. 531–539.

Heyman SJ, Brewer TF, Wilson ME. (1999). The need for global action against multidrug-resistant tuberculosis. JAMA , Vol. 281, No. 1, pp. 2138–2140.

Hillemann D, Rüsch-Gerdes S, Richter E. (2006). Application of the Genotype MTBDR assay directly on sputum specimens. *Int J Tuberc Lung Dis*, Vol. 10, No. 9, pp. 1057-9.

Hillemann D, Rüsch-Gerdes S, Richter E. (2007). Evaluation of the GenoType MTBDRplus assay for rifampin and isoniazid susceptibility testing of *Mycobacterium tuberculosis* strains and clinical specimens. *J Clin Microbiol*, Vol. 45, No. 8, pp. 2635-40.

Morgan M, Kalantri S, Flores L, Pai M. (2005). A commercial line probe assay for the rapid detection of rifampicin resistance in *Mycobacterium tuberculosis*: A systematic review and meta-analysis. *BMC Infect Dis*, Vol. 5, No. 62,pp. 62-65.

Mäkinen J, Marttila HJ, Marjamäki M, Viljanen MK, Soini H. (2006). Comparison of two commercially available DNA line probe assays for detection of multidrug-resistant *Mycobacterium tuberculosis*. *J Clin Microbiol*. Vol. 44, No. 2, pp.350-2.

Musser JM. (1995). Antimicrobial agent resistance in mycobacteria: molecular genetic insights. *Clin Microbiol Rev*, Vol. 8, No. 4, pp. 496–514.

Ninet B, Monod M, Emler S, Pawlowski J, Metral C, Rohner P, et al. (1996). Two different 16S rRNA genes in mycobacterial strains. J Clin Microbiol. Vol. 34, No. 10, pp. 2531-1536.

O'Mahony J and Hill C. (2002). A real time PCR assay for the detection and quantitation of *Mycobacterium avium subsp. paratuberculosis* using SYBR Green and the Light Cycler. *J Microbiol Methods*, Vol. 51, No. 3, pp. 283–293.

Palomino JC. (2006). Newer Diagnostics for Tuberculosis and Multi-Drug Resistant Tuberculosis. Curr Opin Pulm Med. Vol. 12, No. 3, pp. 172-178.

Piatek AS, Tyagi S, Pol AC, Telenti A, Miller LP, Kramer FP and Alland D. (1998). Molecular beacon sequence analysis for detecting drug resistance in *Mycobacterium tuberculosis*. *Nat Biotechnol*, Vol. 16, No. 3, pp.359–363.

Piatek AS, Telenti A, Murray MR, El-Hajj H, Jacobs WR, KrameR FR and D. Alland. (2000). Genotypic analysis of *Mycobacterium tuberculosis* in two distinct populations using molecular beacons: implications for rapid susceptibility testing. Antimicrob. Agents Chemother. Vol. 44, No. 1, pp. 103–110.

Sekiguchi J, Miyoshi-Akiyama T, Augustynowicz-Kopeć E, Zwolska Z, Kirikae F, Toyota E, et al. (2007). Detection of multidrug resistance in *Mycobacterium tuberculosis*. *J Clin Microbiol*, Vol. 45, No. 1, pp.179-192.

Siddiqi N, Shamim M, Hussain S, Choudhary RK, Ahmed N, Prachee et al. (2002). Molecular characterization of multidrug resistant isolates of *Mycobacterium tuberculosis* from patients in North India. *Antimicrob. Agents Chemother*. 2002; Vol. 46, No. 2, pp. 443-450.

Sreevatsan S, Pan X, Zhang Y, Deretic V and Musser JM. (1997). Analysis of the *oxyR-ahpC* Region in Isoniazid-resistant and susceptible *Mycobacterium tuberculosis* complex organisms recovered from diseased humans and animals in diverse localities. *Antimicrob Agents Chemother*, Vol. 41, No. 3, pp. 600-606.

TB India 2010. RNTCP status report. Central TB Division. Directorate General of Health Services. Ministry of Health and Family Welfare . Nirman Bhawan, New Delhi - 110001. This can be obtained from the webste http://www.tbcindia.org. ISBN 81-902652-5-3

Therese KL, Jayanthi U, Madhavan HN. (2005). Application of nested Polymerase Chain Reaction (nPCR) using MPB64 gene primers to detect M. tuberculosis DNA in clinical specimens from extrapulmonary tuberculosis patients. Indian J Med Res, Vol.122, No. 2, pp.165-170

Torres M J, Criado A, Palomares JC and Aznar J. (2000). Use of real-time PCR and fluorimetry for rapid detection of rifampin and isoniazid resistance-associated mutations in *Mycobacterium tuberculosis*. *J Clin Microbiol*, Vol. 38, No. 9, pp. 3194–3199.

van Doorn HR., Claas EC, Templeton KE, van der Zanden AG, te Koppele Vije A, de Jong MD, Dankert J and Kuijper EJ. (2003). Detection of a point mutation associated with high-level isoniazid resistance in *Mycobacterium tuberculosis* by using real-time PCR technology with 3'-minor groove binder-DNA probes. *J Clin Microbiol*, Vol. 41, No. 10, pp. 4630–4635.

Wang JY, Lee LN, Chou CS, Huang CY, Wang SK, Lai HC, Hsueh PR, Luh KT. (2004). Performance assessment of a nested-PCR assay (the RAPID BAP-MTB) and the BD

ProbeTec ET system for detection of Mycobacterium tuberculosis in clinical specimens. J Clin Microbiol. Vol. 42, No. 10, pp.4599-603.

WHO Library Cataloguing-in-Publication Data. Multidrug and extensively drug-resistant TB (M/XDR-TB): 2010 global report on surveillance and response. WHO/HTM/TB/2010.3. ISBN 978 92 4 159919 1

Zhang Y, Heym B, Young AD and Cole S. (1992). The catalase-peroxidase gene and isoniazid resistance of *Mycobacterium tuberculosis*. *Nature*, Vol. 358, No. 6387, pp. 591-593.

23

Detection of *Mycobacterium tuberculosis* and Drug Resistance: Opportunies and Challenges in Morocco

I. Chaoui[1], M. Abid[2], My. D. El Messaoudi[2] and M. El Mzibri[1]
[1]*Unité de Biologie et Recherche Médicale, Centre National de l'Energie, des Sciences et Techniques Nucléaires (CNESTEN), Rabat, Maroc*
[2]*Institut Pasteur du Maroc*
Morocco

1. Introduction

Tuberculosis (TB) was responsible for millions of human deaths in the past, when there were no adequate treatment methods for infected patients. Introduction of chemotherapy and prophylactic measures led to drastic death reduction, which was maintained for various decades. However, "the good times" waned, as this disease became worldwide recognized as the one responsible for most human deaths caused by a single infectious agent: *Mycobacterium tuberculosis* (MTB). TB resumption is basically a consequence of anthropic factors, such as the recent HIV/AIDS pandemic and the development of drug resistant strains (stemmed from inappropriate treatments and/or patient non-compliance).

International attention has turned toward the evolving burden of multi-drug resistant tuberculosis (MDR TB) that has emerged in epidemic proportions in the wake of widespread HIV infection in the world's poorest populations, including sub-Saharan Africa. Extensively drug-resistant TB (XDR TB) was first reported in 2006 but has now been documented on six continents [WHO the global laboratory initiative]. These trends are critically important for global health, since drug-resistant TB mortality rates are high and second-line agents for the treatment of drug-resistant TB are less potent and less tolerable than first-line therapies.

Global control of tuberculosis is hampered by slow, insensitive diagnostic methods, particularly for the detection of drug-resistant forms and in patients with human immunodeficiency virus infection. Failure to quickly and effectively recognize and treat patients with drug-resistant tuberculosis (TB), particularly MDR and XDR tuberculosis, leads to increased mortality, nosocomial outbreaks and resistance to additional antituberculosis drugs. We believe that early detection is essential to reduce the death rate and interrupt transmission, but the complexity and infrastructure needs of sensitive methods limit their accessibility and effect.

Therefore, there's a critical need for methods that can rapidly detect *M. tuberculosis* and identify drug-resistant cases to optimize TB treatment with appropriate drugs.

The present review describes the main techniques used to detect TB and related resistant strains as well as the issues and challenges associated with implementing molecular techniques in Morocco to enhance the National Program against Tuberculosis.

2. History of tuberculosis

2.1 Looking at past: Before the discovery of BCG

First reference of a disease similar to TB in humans dates back to ancient Egypt. Examinations of mummies and tomb paintings reveal that tuberculosis was present at that time (around 5000 BC). The ancient Egyptian paintings portray spinal tuberculosis, indicating the presence of the disease. The reference of a disease called "phthisis" is found in ancient Greek literature by Hippocrates. In 1680, F. Sylvius carried out anatomic-pathologic studies in pulmonary nodules from TB patients, which he named as "tubercula", observing their evolution to lung ulcers (cavities). However, most of the great pathologists of his time believed that these knots were some type of tumor or abnormal gland, rejecting any probable infectious origin. The first credible speculation of the infectious nature of TB was performed by B. Marten, who proposed in 1722 that TB could be caused by micro-organisms. R. Morton used the term "consumption" to specifically denote TB, and finally, in 1819, the inventor of the stethoscope, R. Laennec identified for the first time the TB manifestation unit. As the disease became completely established among every European social level, afflicting many of the intellectual and artists of the continent by the half of the XIX century, TB was romanticized, as typical symptoms like thin and pale faces of the infected ones became signs of beauty.

In 1865, JA Villemin demonstrated formally that TB is a contagious disease; although his experimentation could be effectively reproduced in rabbits, the finding was ignored by his contemporaries for a long time.

2.2 BCG as prophylactic strategy

One of the greatest works on TB was performed in 1882 by Robert Koch, who isolated and cultured *M. tuberculosis* from crushed tubercles. His experimental work identified the bacterium as the TB etiological agent (Bloom & Murray 1992, Daniel 1997). In August of 1890, during The First Ordinary Session of the International Medical Congress, in Berlin, he announced the discovery of a TB therapeutic drug. Three months later, M. Wochenschkift published a new statement of Koch, revealing that although interested in the therapeutic properties of his findings, he observed that the referred liquid, named tuberculin, could be useful as a diagnostic tool to detect the disease due to the intensified reaction developed by sick animals inoculated with this drug, as no measurable effect was ever observed in healthy ones. This concept was perpetuated for several years, until it was observed that even healthy animals could react to the drug. The veterinarians clarified the fact by demonstrating that the healthy ones could be simply infected, although not ill. As a result, it was established that *M. tuberculosis*-infected animals will react to tuberculin infusion, whereas the non-infected ones will not. This drug, the first industrialised one, was called old tuberculin; subsequently, other tuberculins were produced, such as purified protein derivate (PPD), PPD-S, and PPD RT23, among others (Vaccarezza 1965, Ruffino- Netto 1970). The tuberculin skin test became the principal tool for infection diagnosis. In the same period, Koch developed staining methods for the identification of the bacillus; these techniques were subsequently improved by the bacteriologist "Paul Ehrlich", whose method for detection of the bacillus provided the basis for the development of the Ziehl-Nielsen staining, which still is an important tool to diagnose TB. Koch's discovery allowed researchers to focus their efforts on the development of new and more efficient therapies to treat TB patients. One of the first attempts to fight the disease in 1884 was the introduction for TB patients of "sanatorium cure" concept, where the patients were isolated and taken care of, the treatment was based on rest, fresh air and a healthy diet.

In 1896, the bacteriologist T. Smith demonstrated that bovine TB was not caused by *M. tuberculosis*, but rather by another species, *M. bovis*. Twelve years later, the scientist-couple A. Calmette and C. Guérin isolated the bovine variant from its host and grew the bacilli in dispersed culture. By the 39th passage they observed a morphological variant that was avirulent in several animal models and which conferred immunological protection against subsequent challenges with virulent *M. tuberculosis*. Thirteen years of experimentation led to the obtaining of the 231st passage, the variant that was administered for the first time in humans (orally), as an attempt to immunize a child whose mother died in childbirth victim of TB. Currently known as BCG (Bacille Calmette-Guérin), the "intradermal" vaccine has become widely used to combat TB; it relies on a prophylactic administration of live attenuated bacilli to children.

2.3 Tuberculosis chemotherapy

Significant progress has been made in TB chemotherapy. In the pre-antibiotic era, before 1940, there were no drugs against the disease. The tuberculosis treatment at the time consisted mainly of cod liver oils (which by the way, include vitamin D), bed rest and fresh air.

The first TB drug, Streptomycin (SM), was discovered in 1944. It was followed by Para-aminosalicylic acid (PAS), which was discovered in 1946. Then, in 1952, two important first-line TB drugs were discovered, Isoniazid (INH) and Pyrazinamide (PZA). The last TB drug discovered was Rifampin, in 1963.

Hence, the introduction of TB chemotherapy in 1950's led to a significant decline in the incidence of the disease, particularly in developed countries. This reduction has prompted some public health professionals, mainly in the US, to claim that tuberculosis no longer poses a problem in developed countries. They have even eliminated many TB control programmes in the country. However, in the late 1980's, a major outbreak of MDR-TB occurred in New York City, which has cost USD 1 billion to control. This outbreak has led to a renaissance in TB research.

2.4 Drug combinations

It is noteworthy that the current TB therapy is based on the principle of drug combination. The first advantage of using drug combinations is that it reduces drug resistance. A second advantage of drug combinations is that they can enhance the efficacy of the therapy. This point is illustrated by the Mitchison hypothesis, also referred to as the Special Bacterial

Populations Theory. According to this theory, TB bacteria found in the lesions consist of four different sub-populations. Population A, which is actively growing, is killed by Isoniazid. In case of Isoniazid resistance, it is killed by Rifampicin, Streptomycin, or Ethambutol. Population B, which has a slower metabolism, is killed by Rifampicin. Population C, which resides in an acidic environment, is killed by PZA. Finally, population D is a dormant population, and there are currently no drugs that can effectively kill this population (Paramasivan, 2005).

2.5 Directly Observed Treatment Short course strategy

TB persists as a global public health problem and the main focus for the twentieth century is firstly to cure the individual patient and secondly to minimise the transmission of *M. tuberculosis* to other persons (WHO, 2003; Blumberg, 2003). The ongoing TB problem has been due to the neglect of TB control by governments, inadequate access and infrastructure, poor patient adherence to medication, poor management of TB control programs, poverty, population growth and migration, and a significant rise in the number of TB cases in HIV infected individuals. Treatment of patients with TB is done according to the following five key components of the Directly Observed Treatment Short course (DOTS) strategy recommended by World Health Organization (WHO) (Walley, 1997):

- Government commitment
- Case detection by sputum smear microscopy
- Standardised treatment regimen of six to eight months
- A regular, uninterrupted supply of all essential anti-TB drugs
- A standard recording and reporting system.

Since the introduction of the DOTS strategy in the early '90s by the WHO, considerable progress has been made in global TB control (Sterling, 2003). In 1997, the estimated average treatment success rate worldwide was almost 80%. However, less than 25% of people who are sick with TB are treated through the DOTS strategy (Bastian, 2000). A total of 180 countries (including both developed and developing countries) had adopted and implemented the DOTS strategy by the end of 2002 and 69% of the global population are living in areas covered by the DOTS strategy (Blumberg, 2003). However, even though DOTS programs are in place, treatment success rates are very low in low income countries due to poor management of TB control programs and patient non-compliance (Lienhardt and Ogden, 2004; Bastian, 2003). Furthermore, the effectiveness of DOTS is facing new challenges with respect to the spread and increase of MDR-TB and the co-epidemic of TB/HIV (WHO, 2003). Since 1999, WHO and partners have addressed these new challenges and have developed DOTS-Plus strategy which prevent further development and spread of MDR-TB and help to manage MDR-TB using second line drugs in low- and middle-income countries within DOTS strategy. Morocco joined the global project in 2004 and carried out its first simultaneous survey on primary and acquired drug resistance in tuberculosis patients exactly according WHO/IUATLD recommendations.

Subsequently, 41 million of TB patients have been successfully treated in DOTS programs and up to 6 million lives saved since 1995. Moreover, 5 million more lives could be saved up to 2015 by fully funding and implementing The Global Plan to Stop TB 2011-2015.

3. Epidemiology of tuberculosis

3.1 Tuberculosis throughout the world: A catastrophic situation

More than two billion people, equal to one third of the world's total population, are infected with TB bacilli. A total of 1.7 million people died from TB in 2009 (including 380 000 people with HIV), equal to about 4700 deaths a day. TB is a disease of poverty, affecting mostly young adults in their most productive years. The vast majority of TB deaths are in the developing world, with more than half occurring in Asia. There were 9.4 million new TB cases in 2009, of which 80% were in just 22 countries. Per capita, the global TB incidence rate is falling, but the rate of decline is very slow (less than 1%) (Wilson, 2011).

TB is a worldwide pandemic. Among the 15 countries with the highest estimated TB incidence rates, 13 are in Africa, while a third of all new cases are in India and China. There were an estimated 440 000 new MDR-TB cases in 2008 with three countries accounting for over 50% of all cases globally: China, India and the Russian Federation (WHO, 2010). Extensively drug-resistant TB (XDR-TB) occurs when resistance to second-line drugs develops. It is extremely difficult to treat and cases have been confirmed in more than 58 countries. The world is on track to achieve two TB targets set for 2015:

- The Millennium Development Goal, which aims to halt and reverse global incidence (in comparison with 1990);
- The Stop TB Partnership target of halving deaths from TB (also in comparison with 1990).

3.2 Tuberculosis status in Morocco

During last years, the incidence of TB has stagnated and is reported to be 81 per 100,000 overall. However, the incidence was significantly higher in several urban areas, or "hot spots": Casablanca, Tangier and Rabat (together 43% of all notified cases in 2010). Statistical data show that 59% of TB patients are male and 65% are 15-34 years old. Of the roughly 28,000 new TB cases reported annually, 12% are re-treatment cases. Moreover, the prevalence of tubeculosis in HIV individuals is 1.7% in 2008 (Dooley, 2010, WHO, 2010). The prevalence of MDR TB is 0.5% within new cases and reaches 12.2% among previously treated patients with failure treatment, relapse or chronical cases (Othmani, 2003; WHO, 2010).

National TB treatment guidelines in 2007 and 2008 recommended a Category I treatment regimen - 2 months of INH, RIF, PZA, and SM followed by 4 months of RIF and INH (2SHRZ/4RH) - for new smear-positive cases and a Category II regimen - 2HRZES/1RHEZ/5RHE (E = Ethambutol) - for re-treatment cases. By the beginning of 2009, ethambutol has replaced streptomycin in Category I regimen.

The follow up of tuberculosis which lasts from 6 to 18 months is done in specialised centres of TB diagnosis of the ministry for Health. The late consultations and the no observance of treatments are responsible for TB resistance in Morocco. To strengthen its efforts, the ministry for Health is planning to carry a national plan of acceleration of the fight against tuberculosis.

4. Drug resistance

4.1 Drug resistance and global surveillance: History

Shortly, after the first anti-tuberculosis (TB) drugs were introduced, streptomycin (STR), para-aminosalicylic acid (PAS) and isoniazid (INH), resistance to these drugs was observed in clinical isolates of *Mycobacterium tuberculosis* (Crofton and Mitchison, 1948). This led to the need to measure resistance accurately and easily. The Pasteur Institute introduced the critical proportion method in 1961 for drug susceptibility testing in TB and this method became the standard method of use (Espinal, 2000; 2003). Studies on drug resistance in various countries in the 1960s showed that developing countries had a much higher incidence of drug resistance than developed countries (Espinal, 2000; 2003). By the end of the 1960s rifampicin (RIF) was introduced and with the use of combination therapy, there was a decline in drug resistant and drug susceptible TB in developed countries. This led to a decline in funding and interest in TB control programs. As a result, no concrete monitoring of drug resistance was carried out for the following 20 years (Espinal, 2000; 2003). The arrival of HIV/AIDS in the 1980s resulted in an increase in transmission of TB associated with outbreaks of multidrug- resistant TB (MDR-TB) (Edlin, 1992; Fischl, 1992). In the early 1990s drug resistance surveillance was resumed in developed countries, but the true incidence remained unclear in the developing world (Cohn, 1997).

The emergence of MDR TB is the third epidemic, complicating the epidemics of acquired immune deficiency syndrome (AIDS) and tuberculosis, and is requiring urgent attention to achieve more rapid diagnosis, to develop new therapeutic regimens and to address the social and hospital environment to care for these patients (Neville, 1994).

4.2 Primary and acquired resistance: Definition and data

WHO estimated that 50 million people were infected with drug resistant MTB. Single-drug resistance is defined as resistance to only one antituberculous agent.

MDR-TB, or multidrug-resistant TB, is a specific form of drug-resistant TB. It occurs when the TB bacteria are resistant to at least isoniazid and rifampicin, the two most powerful anti-TB drugs. XDR-TB is an MDR TB strain that is resistant to any fluoroquinolone, and at least one of three injectable second-line drugs (capreomycin, kanamycin or amikacin).

Traditionally, patients with drug-resistant tuberculosis are classified as having primary or acquired drug resistance on the basis of a history of previous treatment. WHO criteria define acquired drug resistance as the isolation of drug-resistant *M. tuberculosis* from a patient with a record of previous treatment for 1 month, and primary drug resistance as the isolation of a drug-resistant strain from a patient without a history of previous treatment.

The classification of drug resistance as primary or acquired is used as an indicator of the efficiency of national tuberculosis programs and in the adjustment and development of these programs. The rate of primary drug resistance is interpreted as an epidemiological indicator for long-term surveillance of the quality of tuberculosis treatment in the community. The rate of acquired drug resistance reflects the efficacy of management of individual patients.

5. Molecular mechanisms of drug resistance

As a consequence of the increase in DR TB and the relatively restricted number of therapeutic agents, there has been a renewed effort during the 2 past decades to define the molecular basis of drug resistance in MTB.

MTB acquires drug resistance by antibiotic selection of mutations that occur randomly at chromosomal loci. No plasmids or transposable elements (horizontal gene transfer) are involved in this process. Individual nucleotide changes (point mutations) confer resistance to single drugs, and the stepwise accumulation of these mutations leads to MDR TB. drug resistance strains emerge when chemotherapy is intermittent or otherwise inadequate (Ducati, 2006; Zhang and Yew, 2009).

5.1 First line drugs

First-line drugs are mainly bactericidal and combine a high degree of efficacy with a relative toxicity to the patient during treatment.

Currently, a five-drug regimen is used consisting of INH, RIF, SM, PZA and EMB. Resistance to first line anti-TB drugs has been linked to mutations in at least 10 genes; *katG, inhA, ahpC, kasA* and *ndh* for INH resistance; *rpoB* for RIF resistance, *embB* for EMB resistance, *pncA* for PZA resistance and *rpsL* and *rrs* for STR resistance.

5.1.1 Isoniazid

***katG* gene alterations**. INH or isonicotinic acid hydrazide, was synthesized in the early 1900s but its anti-TB action was first detected in 1951 (Heym, 1999; Slayden and Barry, 2000; Rattan, 1998). INH enters the cell as a prodrug that is activated by a catalase peroxidase encoded by *katG*. The peroxidase activity of the enzyme is necessary to activate INH to a toxic substance in the bacterial cell (Zhang, 1992). This toxic substance subsequently affects intracellular targets such as mycolic acid biosynthesis which are an important component of the cell wall. A lack of mycolic acid synthesis eventually results in loss of cellular integrity and the bacteria die (Barry, 1998). Middlebrook *et al.* (1954) initially demonstrated that a loss of catalase activity can result in INH resistance. Subsequently, genetic studies demonstrated that transformation of INH-resistant *Mycobacterium smegmatis* and *M. tuberculosis* strains with a functional *katG* gene restored INH susceptibility and that *katG* deletions give rise to INH resistance (Zhang, 1992; Zhang, 1993). However, mutations in this gene are more frequent than deletions in clinical isolates and these can lower the activity of the enzyme.

Most mutations are found between codons 138 and 328 with the most commonly observed gene alteration being at codon 315 of the *katG* gene (Slayden and Barry, 2000). The Ser315Thr substitution is estimated to occur in 30–60% of INH resistant isolates (Ramaswamy and Musser, 1998; Musser, 1996; Slayden and Barry, 2000). The *katG* 463 (CGG-CTG / Arg-Leu) amino acid substitution is the most common polymorphism found in the *katG* gene and is not associated with INH resistance.

Resistance to INH could be also due to mutations in the promoter region of the *ahpC* gene. Indeed, it has been observed that a loss of *katG* activity due to the S315T amino acid substitution is often accompanied by an increase in expression of an alkyl hydroperoxide reductase (*ahpC*) protein that is capable of detoxifying damaging organic peroxides (Sherman, 1996). Five different nucleotide alterations have been identified in the promoter region of the *ahpC* gene, which lead to over expression of *ahpC* and INH resistance (Ramaswamy and Musser, 1998). *AhpC* overexpression exerts a detoxifying effect on organic peroxides within the cell and protects the bacteria against oxidative damage but does not provide protection against INH. *KatG* expression can also be up regulated under conditions of oxidative stress. The correlation between polymorphic sites in the *ahpC* regulatory region with INH resistance in *M. tuberculosis* requires further examination.

***inhA* gene alterations**. One of the targets for activated INH is the protein encoded by the *inhA* locus. *InhA* is an enoyl-acyl carrier protein (ACP) reductase which is proposed to be the primary target for resistance to INH and ethionamide (ETH) (Banerjee, 1994). ETH, a second line drug, is a structural analogue of INH that is also thought to inhibit mycolic acid biosynthesis and several studies have suggested that low-level INH resistance is correlated with resistance to ETH. Activated INH binds to the InhA-NADH complex to form a ternary complex that results in inhibition of mycolic acid biosynthesis. Six point mutations associated with INH resistance within the structural *inhA* gene have been identified (Ile16Thr, Ile21Thr, Ile21Val, Ile47Thr, Val78Ala and Ile95Pro) (Ramaswamy and Musser, 1998; Basso and Blanchard, 1998). A Ser94Ala substitution results in a decreased binding affinity of *inhA* for NADH, resulting in mycolic acid synthesis inhibition. Although these mutations in the structural *InhA* gene are associated with INH resistance, it is not frequently reported in clinical isolates. *InhA* promoter mutations are more frequently seen and are present at positions -24(GT), -16(A-G), or -8(T-G/A) and -15(C-T). These promoter mutations result in over expression of *inhA* leading to low level INH resistance. To date approximately 70–80% of INH resistance in clinical isolates of *M. tuberculosis* can be attributed to mutations in the *katG* and *inhA* genes (Ramaswamy and Musser, 1998).

***kasA* gene alterations**. There seems to be considerable contreverse within the literature as to the role of *kasA* as a possible target for INH resistance (Sherman, 1996). This gene encodes a β-ketoacyl-ACP synthase involved in the synthesis of mycolic acids. Mutations have been described in this gene that confer low levels of INH resistance. Genotypic analysis of the *kas*A gene reveals 4 different amino acid substitutions involving codon 66 (GAT-AAT), codon 269 (GGT-AGT), codon 312 (GGC-AGC) and codon 413 (TTC-TTA) (Ramaswamy and Musser, 1998; Mdluli, 1998). However, similar mutations were also found in INH susceptible isolates (Lee, 1999; Piatek, 2000). Nevertheless, the possibility of *kasA* constituting an additional resistance mechanism should not be completely excluded.

***Ndh* gene alterations**. In 1998 another mechanism for INH resistance in *M. smegmatis* was described by Miesel *et al.* (1998). The *ndh* gene encodes NADH dehydrogenase that is bound to the active site of *inhA* to form the ternary complex with activated INH. Structural studies have shown that a reactive form of INH attacks the NAD(H) co-factor and generates a covalent INH-NAD adduct. Mutations in the *ndh* gene, encoding NADH dehydrogenase, cause defects in the enzymatic activity. Thus, defects in the oxidation of NADH to NAD result in NADH accumulation and NAD depletion (Lee, 2001). These high levels of NADH can then inhibit the binding of the INH-NAD adduct to the active site of the InhA enzyme (Rozwarski, 1998; Miesel, 1998). Prominent point mutations in the *ndh* gene at codons 110 and 268 (T110A and R268H) were detected in 9.5% of INH resistant samples. These similar mutations were not detected in the INH susceptible group (Lee, 2001).

5.1.2 Rifampicin

Rifampicin (RIF) is a major compound of anti-tuberculosis chemotherapy. A resistance to RIF is rarely found without associated resistance to other tuberculostatics. RIF resistance is a good marker for MDR-TB. Moreover, RIF resistance is a good predictor of poor treatment outcome. The mode of action of RIF is based on the inhibition of the elongation of transcripts by RNA polymerase in MTB, by covalent binding to the Beta sub-unit of RNA polymerase, thus leading to cell death. The RNA polymerase Beta sub-unit is encoded by the rpoB gene. RIF resistance is associated with a hotspot (codon 507 to 533) core region called RRDR, for "rifampicine resistance determining region" (81 bp) of the *rpoB* gene. More than 95% of RIF^R *M. tuberculosis* has a mutation in this specific region (Telenti, 1993; Telenti, 1997).

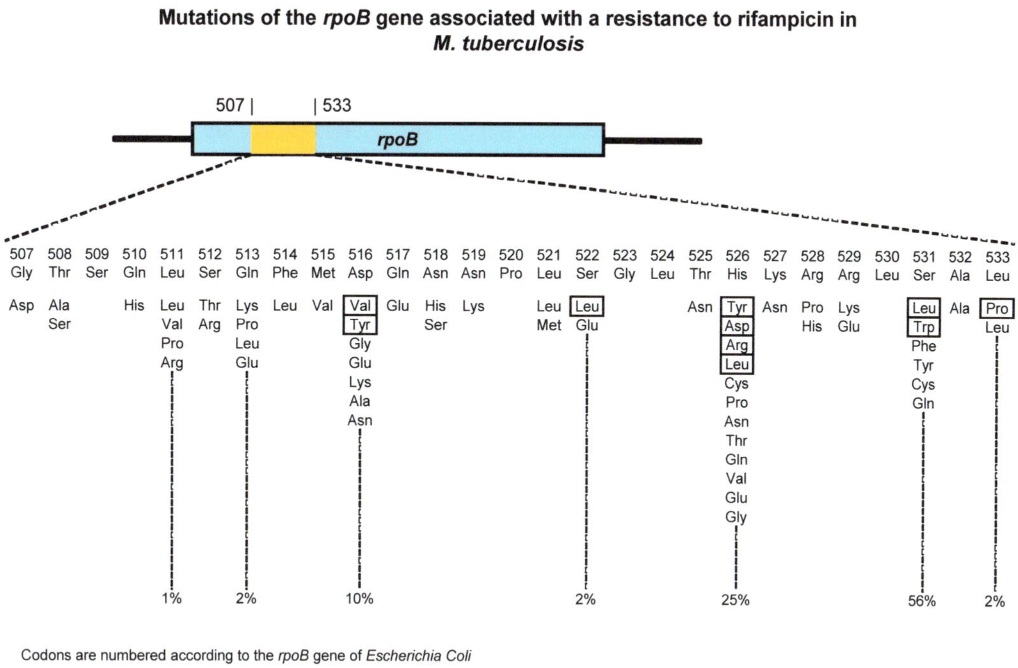

Fig. 1. Mutations of the *rpoB* gene associated with a resistance to rifampicin in *M. tuberculosis*

Resistance to RIF occurs at a frequency of 1 out of 10^7 to 10^8 bacterial cells. Most RIF-resistant strains show one mutation in the gene. Two to four mutations are rarely reported (Mani, 2001; Sekiguchi, 2007). The most prevalent mutations (81%) affect codons 531 and 526 and usually lead to a high level of phenotypical resistance (MIC > 64 µg/ml) as well as cross resistance to other rifamycins (Riska, 2000; Zhang, 2005). Mutations at codons 511, 516, 518 and 522 result in a low-level resistance to RIF and rifapentine; and some susceptibility to rifabutin (Zhang, 2005).

At the same time, mutations in this hotspot region seem to confer low phenotypical resistance (deletion of codon 508-509, mutation at 515) (Taniguchi, 1996) or variable resistance (L533P) (Kim, 1997), which could lead to an overly hasty interpretation of resistance. The latest observations of Asian strains suggest a geographic variability that can influence the accuracy of genotypic tests (Riska, 2000).

Silent mutations (Leu511 and Leu521) have been reported in resistant strains. Interestingly, the L511L mutation is always associated with other mutations that confer resistance (Siddiqi, 2002). In rare cases, double mutations appear to have an additive effect on the degree of resistance. The role of mutations, combined with those known to confer resistance, is uncertain, as in the case of S509R described with H526R (Sekiguchi, 2007).

Finally, less than 5% of resistant strains do not show a mutation in the *rpoB* resistance region (Riska, 2000; Mani, 2001). Rare loci found outside the hotspot region of *rpoB* are associated with resistance without associated mutation known for conferring resistance (Taniguchi, 1996; Fang, 1999; Schilke, 1999; Yuen, 1999; Heep, 2001; Zhang, 2005; Rigouts, 2007; Prammananan, 2008).

Mutated strains in Val146Phe (Heep, 2001; Rigouts, 2007; Prammananan, 2008) show a low-level resistance (MIC 4 µg/ml) (Rigouts, 2007). The Ala381Val mutation (Taniguchi, 1996) is described on a strain of MIC 200, with no other mutation on the *rpoB* gene.

Most susceptible strains show no mutation, except for a few: seven susceptible Japanese strains are mutated in TCG Ser 450 Leu TTG, ATG Met511 Val GTG, CTG Leu 521 Pro CCG, CTG Leu 533 Pro CCG, GCC Ala 679 Ser TCC (two strains) and CGC Arg 687 Pro CCC (Taniguchi, 1996; Yang, 1998). The CTG Leu 533 Pro CCG mutation has been shown on two strains of low-level resistance (MIC 12.5 µg/ml) and on a strain that is susceptible according to phenotypic tests, yet clinically resistant (Riska, 2000). Other studies describe some sensitive strains with mutations as Ser 450 Leu (Sekiguchi, 2007), Leu 511 Arg or Ser 512 Thr (Moghazeh, 1996) or Gln CAA 513 Gln CAG (Kim, 1997). Genotypic detections would therefore be more sensitive in certain circumstances.

5.1.3 Streptomycin

SM is an aminocyclitol antibiotic that is one of the first drug used to treat TB, SM binds to 16S rRNA, inhibits translational initiation and detrimentally affects translation fidelity. Mutations associated with SM resistance in MTB have been identified mainly in *rpsL* gene encoding ribosomal protein S12 and in the 16S rRNA gene (*rrs*) in 65–67% of STR resistant isolates (Ramaswamy and Musser, 1998).

In the *rrs* gene a C-T transition at positions 491, 512 and 516, and a A-C/T transversion at position 513 were observed in the highly conserved 530 loop. The 530 loop region is part of the aminoacyl-tRNA binding site and is involved in the decoding process (Carter, 2000). The C-T transition at codon 491 is not responsible for resistance to STR as it occurs in both STR resistant and susceptible isolates but is strongly associated with the global spread of *M. tuberculosis* with a Western Cape F11 genotype (van Rie, 2001; Victor, 2001). Other mutations in the 915 loop [903 (C-A/G) and 904 (A-G)] have also been reported to have an association with STR resistance (Carter, 2000). Mutations in the *rpsL* gene at codon 43 (AAG-AGG/ACG) (Lys-Arg/Thr) and codon 88 (AAGAGG/ CAG) (Lys-Arg/Gln) are associated with STR resistance. MIC analysis of STR resistant isolates indicate that amino acid replacements in the *rpsL* genes correlate with a high level of resistance, whereas mutations in the *rrs* gene correlate with an intermediate level of resistance (Cooksey, 1996; Meier, 1996). In addition, it has been suggested that low levels of STR resistance are also associated with altered cell permeability or rare mutations which lie outside of the *rrs* and *rpsL* genes.

5.1.4 Pyrazinamide

Pyrazinamide (PZA) is a structural analog of nicotinamide that is used as a first -line TB drug. PZA kills semi-dormant tubercle bacilli under acidic conditions. PZA targets an enzyme involved in fatty-acid synthesis and is responsible for killing persistent tubercle bacilli in the initial intensive phase of chemotherapy (Somoskovi, 2001). However, during the first two days of treatment, PZA has no bactericidal activity against rapidly growing bacilli (Zhang and Mitchison, 2003). PZA on the other hand has effective sterilizing activity and shortens the chemotherapeutic regiment from 12 to 6 months. PZA is a prodrug which is converted to its active form, pyrazinoic acid (POA) by the pyrazinamidase (PZase) encoded by *pncA*. The activity of PZA is highly specific for *M. tuberculosis,* as it has no effect on other mycobacteria. *Mycobacterium bovis* is naturally resistant to PZA due to a unique C-G point mutation in codon 169 of the *pncA* gene. PZA is only active against *M. tuberculosis* at acidic pH where POA accumulates in the cytoplasm due to an ineffective efflux pump. Accumulation of POA results in the lowering of intracellular pH to a level that inactivates a vital fatty acid synthase (Zimhony, 2004). Cloning and characterization of the *M. tuberculosis pncA* gene by Scorpio *et al.* (1997) showed that some *pncA* mutations conferred PZA resistance. Various *pncA* mutations have been identified in more than 70% of PZA resistant clinical isolates scattered throughout the *pncA* gene but thus far no mutational hot spot has been identified (Scorpio and Zhang, 1996; Sreevatsan, 1997b; Scorpio, 1997). PZA susceptibility testing is not done routinely in many countries due to technical difficulties. Thus the extent of PZA resistance globally is largely unknown. PZA resistant isolates had diverse nucleotide changes scattered throughout the *pncA* gene. However, PZA resistant isolates without *pncA* mutations were also observed suggesting that another mechanism may be involved in conferring PZA resistance in these isolates. In addition, not all mutations (e.g. Thr114Met) were associated with PZA resistance. In summary, the complexity of PZA resistance makes the development of molecular methods for rapid diagnosis difficult.

5.1.5 Ethambutol

Ethambutol (EMB) is a very specific and effective drug that is used in combination with INH to treat *M. tuberculosis* infection (Ramaswamy and Musser, 1998). EMB inhibits an arabinosyl transferase (*embB*) involved in cell wall biosynthesis (Takayama and Kilburn, 1989).Three genes designated *emb*C, A and B (Telenti, 1997) encode homologous arabinosyl transferase enzymes involved in EMB resistance. Various studies have identified five mutations in codon 306 of *embB* gene [(ATG-GTG), (ATG-CTG), (ATG-ATA), (ATG-ATC) and (ATG-ATT)] which result in three different amino acid substitutions (Val, Leu and Ile) in EMB-resistant isolates (Lee, 2002; Sreevatsan, 1997c; Mokrousov, 2002b; Ramaswamy, 2000). These five mutations are associated with 70–90% of all EMB resistant isolates (Ramaswamy and Musser, 1998). Missense mutations were identified in three additional codons: Phe285leu, Phe330Val and Thr630Ile in EMB resistant isolates. MIC's were generally higher for strains with Met306Leu, Met306Val, and Phe330Val and Thr630Ile substitutions than those organisms with Met306Ile substitutions. Mutations outside of codon 306 are present but quite rare. However a number of EMB phenotypic resistant isolates (about 30%) still lack an identified mutation in *embB*. There is therefore a need to fully understand the mechanism of EMB resistance in clinical isolates.

5.2 Second line drugs

5.2.1 Fluoroquinolones

Ciproflaxin (CIP) and ofloxacin (OFL) are the two fluoroquinolones (FQs) used as second-line drugs in MDR-TB treatment (WHO, 2001). These FQs are bactericidal against MTB. Their target is the DNA gyrase, an ATP-dependent type II DNA topoisomerase that catalyses negative supercoiling of DNA. DNA gyrase is a tetrameric protein composed of two A and two B subunits encoded by the gyrA and gyrB genes, respectively. FQs bing to gyrase and inhibit supercoiling of DNA, thereby disrupting cellular processes dependent on DNA topology (Ramaswamy and Musser, 1998).

The quinolone resistance-determining region (QRDR) is a conserved region in the *gyrA* (320bp) and *gyrB* (375bp) genes (Ginsburg, 2003) which is the point of interaction of FQ and gyrase (Ginsburg, 2003). Missense mutations in codon 90, 91, and 94 of *gyrA* are associated with resistance to FQs (Takiff, 1994; Xu, 1996). A 16-fold increase in resistance was observed for isolates with a Ala90Val substitution, a 30-fold increase for Asp94Asn or His94Tyr and a 60-fold increase for Asp94Gly (Xu, 1996). A polymorphism at *gyrA* codon 95 is not associated with FQ resistance, and is used, with the *katG*463 polymorphism, to classify *M. tuberculosis* into 3 phylogenetic groups (Sreevatsan, 1997a).

5.2.2 Ethionamide

Ethionamide (ETH) is a derivative of isonicotinic acid with potent activity against MTB and other mycobacteria. Like INH, ETH is also thought to be a prodrug that is activated by bacterial metabolism. The activated drug then disrupts cell wall biosynthesis by inhibiting mycolic acid synthesis. Mutations in the promoter of the *inhA* gene are associated with resistance to INH and ETH (Morlock, 2003). *EthA* catalyses a two step activation of ETH and gene alterations leading to reduced EthA activity lead to ETH resistance (Engohang- Ndong, 2004; Morlock, 2003; Vannelli, 2002). The expression of *ethA* is under the control of the neighbouring *ethR* gene encoding a repressor. *EthR* negatively regulates the expression of *ethA*, by binding upstream of *ethA* to suppress *ethA* expression (Engohang-Ndong, 2004).

5.2.3 Kanamycine and amykacine

KAN and AMY are aminoglycoside antibiotics that inhibits protein synthesis by inhibiting the normal function of ribosomes (Taniguchi, 1997; Ramaswamy and Musser, 1998). These drugs are used as second line anti-TB agents. Nucleotide substitutions in the region of *rrs* especially at position 1400 (between the *rrs* gene and 23S rRNA gene) are a major cause of resistance to KAN and AMY in *M.tuberculosis*. It seems that nucleotide substitutions at rrs position 1400 is implicated in high-level resistance to KAN and AMY (Taniguchi, 1997).

5.2.4 D-Cycloserine

D-cycloserine (DCS) is a cyclic analog of D-alanine which is one of the central molecules of the cross linking step of peptidoglycan assembly (Ramaswamy and Musser, 1998; Feng and Barletta, 2003). DCS inhibits cell wall synthesis by competing with D-Alanine for the enzymes D-alanyl-D-alanine synthetase (Ddl) and D-alanine racemase (Alr) and also inhibiting the synthesis of these proteins. Overexpression of *alr* causes DCS resistance. The

G→T transversion in the *alr* promoter may lead to the overexpression of *alr* (Feng and Barletta, 2003; Ramaswamy and Musser, 1998).

5.2.5 Peptides

Viomycin (VIO) and capreomycin (CAP) are basic peptide antibiotics that inhibit prokaryotic protein synthesis and have shown that resistance to VIO in *M. smegmatis* is caused by alterations in the 30S or 50S ribosomal subunits (Taniguchi, 1997). Mutations in the *rrs* gene that encodes the 16S rRNA is associated with resistance to VIO and CAP, specifically a G→A or G→T nucleotide change at codon 1473 (Taniguchi, 1997).

6. Availables tests for tuberculosis diagnosis

6.1 History

Since the 1880s with the development of the sputum smear microscopy, the most commonly used for TB diagnostic, several new and established methods were developed and implemented in many laboratory services worldwide to enhance MTB diagnosis and tuberculosis management.

The sputum smear microscopy has remained largely unchanged and is often described as a simple technology. However, it requires a high level of training and diligence.

Because microscopy is both cumbersome to implement and inherently insensitive, many patients remain undiagnosed and many non-TB patients are incorrectly treated with TB drugs on the basis of clinical suspicion alone. In endemic countries, simply obtaining an accurate diagnosis often takes weeks or months from the time a patient first visits a health centre. This delay prevents prompt treatment of TB and leads to continued disease transmission, at substantial cost to the individual and at huge cost to society.

Mounting drug resistance, including MDR-TB and extensively drug-resistant (XDR) TB, coupled with a growing number of people co-infected with TB and HIV, have highlighted the urgent need for more accurate and rapid diagnostic tests. Many patients are never diagnosed and contribute to the astonishing number of yearly deaths from TB worldwide.

The global control of tuberculosis remains a challenge from the standpoint of diagnosis, detection of drug resistance, and treatment. Thus, there recently has been a marked increase in the development and testing of novel assays designed to detect MTB complex and/or MDR MTB based either on conventional techniques or on molecular approaches. The Figure 2 summarise the main techniques used and under development for TB diagnosis.

Recently, the WHO has endorsed some of these novel methods, and they have been made available at discounted prices for procurement by the public health sector of high-burden countries. In addition, international and national laboratory partners and donors are currently evaluating other new diagnostics that will allow further and more rapid testing in point-of-care settings. While some techniques are simple, others have complex requirements, and therefore, it is important to carefully determine how to link these new tests and incorporate them within a country's national diagnostic algorithm. Finally, the successful implementation of these methods is dependent on key partnerships in the international laboratory community and ensuring that adequate quality assurance programs are inherent in each country's laboratory network. Moreover, it's widely accepted that if left untreated, each person with active TB infects an average of 10 to 15 people each year. Interrupting disease transmission will require early and accurate detection paired with appropriate treatment.

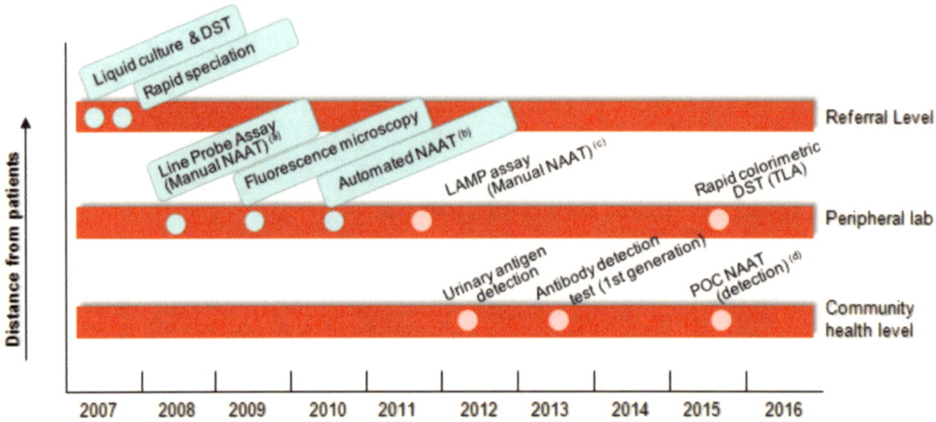

Fig. 2. Tuberculosis product deliverables 2007 2016

6.2 Conventional tests

Tuberculosis is generally diagnosed by traditional laboratory procedures, including microscopic examination of samples for the presence of acid-fast bacilli (AFB) and/ or isolation by culture followed by identification using biochemical tets.

6.2.1 Microscopic examination

The etiological diagnosis of tuberculosis is based on the appearance of bacilli in clinical samples (sputum). Direct sample examination according to Ziehl-Neelsen staining is used to screen for positive bacilli results. For pulmonary tuberculosis, direct examination of sputum is fast and reveals the quantity of acid-fast bacillus, and thus the risk of contagiousness. However, direct examination has a low susceptibility of 22% to 78% and can only detect a concentration of 103 bacilli / ml or more in the sample. In addition, it is not species specific. As a result, false-positives occur, particularly in heavily colonized samples from children patients with other chronic pulmonary infections and paucibacillary cases common among HIV-infected individuals. Nevertheless, many countries use direct examination of samples as a quick test for diagnosing tuberculosis. Early diagnosis can improve patient survival and reduces the spread of the *M. tuberculosis* strain.

Because of the limitations of conventional light microscopy using stains such as Ziehl-Neelsen, fluorochrome stains such as auramine were introduced that improve the sensitivity of the test and take less time to perform. However, fluorescence microscopy has the limitations of requiring a fluorescent microscope, a dark room, and an expensive light source.

Mercury vapor light sources used for this type of microscopy can also pose a hazard if bulbs are broken. To overcome these limitations, light emitting diode (LED) microscopy was developed. This type of microscopy uses LED technology as a light source but still allows for the advantages of using a fluorescent stain while eliminating most of the disadvantages of fluorescent microscopy. LED microscopy is more sensitive and equally specific, compared with either conventional light or fluorescent microscopy.

The World Health Organization (WHO) recommends that conventional fluorescence microscopy could be replaced by LED microscopy, and that LED microscopy should be "phased in as an alternative for conventional light microscopy".

6.2.2 Culture

It's widely accepted that TB culture is substantially more sensitive, but is very slow, and results often do not get back to the health care workers until too late to be clinically useful.

Culture is needed to screen for bacilli either on solid (Lowenstein-Jensen [LJ]) or liquid (mycobacterial growth indicator tube [MGIT 960]) media.

In Morocco, as it's the case in many countries worldwide, culture on solid media using Lowenstein-Jensen is the main technique used to detect TB in samples. The culture-dependent laboratory procedures may take 4 to 6 weeks to have MTB cultures both for TB diagnosis and for further analyses e.g. Drug susceptibility testing (Eing, 1998).

The liquid culture (LC) gives an alternative opportunity to enhance TB diagnosis by conventional techniques. In fact, LC is significantly faster: the average time-to-growth detection with liquid culture is 10 to 14 days. Controlled trials have demonstrated that the performance of liquid media culture (LMC) is superior to that of solid media culture for diagnosis of MTB (Srisuwanvilai, 2008), but there is limited evidence about its performance in resource-limited settings.

TB culture on liquid media uses the Mycobacterium Growth Indicator Tube (MGIT). The MGIT is a commercial liquid culture system and the leading rapid culture method in the developed world. MGIT is manufactured in unbreakable plastic tubes containing enriched culture media. At the bottom of the tube is a silicone plug containing chemicals that become fluorescent when bacteria consume oxygen during the process of growth, making detection possible using either manual or automated systems. MGIT was approved by the World Health Organisation in 2007 and is already in use in high income countries and in the private sector. Its implementation in endemic countries is ongoing.

The roll-out of MGIT for case detection is especially important for patients with low numbers of TB bacteria in their sputum, such as children and individuals infected with HIV.

6.3 Molecular tests for diagnosis and identification of mycobacterial species

Because traditional techniques have several limitations, considerable progress has recently been made in developing novel approaches and tools, especially molecular methods (commercial and 'in-house'), for direct detection and identification of *M. tuberculosis* in clinical specimens within a single day after sputum collection. The potential advantages of molecular assays are the ability to (1) design assays that are highly sensitive and specific; (2) manufacture some assays in large quantities, allowing for decreased cost and ease of standardization in field use; (3) yield rapid results; and (4) be used more widely, because they require less training and infrastructure than do conventional mycobacterial cultures and AST.

These potential advantages must be weighed against the disadvantages of these assays, some of which are common to all molecular techniques and others specific to particular assays. Among the disadvantages of molecular assays are (1) a need for laboratory infrastructure that can accommodate molecular testing; (2) cost; (3) a continued need of cultures for AST; and (4) most work better with smear-positive than with smear-negative specimens.

These methods, based on nucleic acid amplification (NAA) of different targets, aim to identify the M. tuberculosis complex, and eventually drug resistant strains. In general, commercial methods are recommended since they have a better level of standardization, reproducibility and automation. Although some aspects such as cost-efficiency and the appropriate setting for the implementation of these techniques are not yet well established, organizations such as the WHO are strongly supporting the implementation and universal use of these new molecular methods (Moure, 2010).

The available molecular methods for direct detection of MTB from clinical samples include in house polymerase chain (PCR) using essentially IS6110, hsp65 and 16SrRNA as target. Two Commercial nucleic acid amplification (NAA) tests for MTB detection in clinical specimens are available: the Enhanced MTB Direct Test (E-MTD), the Amplicor MTB test and its automated version the Cobas Amplicor MTB test, the BDProbe tec ET test, GeneXpert MTB/RIF Assay and the INNO-LiPA-Rif (Innogenetics, Ghent, Belgium).

6.3.1 Classical PCR using essentially IS6110, Hsp 65 and 16SrRNA as targets

The polymerase chain reaction (PCR) has been most widely used for the detection of *M. tuberculosis* in clinical specimens including sputum, blood, bone marrow, and biopsy samples.

The MTB Complex-specific insertion sequence 6110 is commonly used as a target for detecting MTB. The overall sensitivity and specificity of the assay range from 84.2-100% and 83-100%, respectively, for respiratory specimens (Shamputa, 2004).

The performance of the in house IS6110 PCR in direct detection of MTB on sputum has been evaluated in Morocco and showed promising results (under publication).

However, in non-respiratory samples, lower sensitivities were recorded in most studies with the exception of successful detection in pleural biopsy specimens in one study, and even in blood samples in another study.

The main advantage of the IS6110 targeted NAATs is the fact that most MTBC isolates carry more than five copies of this transposon, thereby increasing the sensitivity of the test. However, in some Asian regions MTBC isolates with no or few IS6110 copies are more prevalent.

The 16S rRNA and the Hsp65 genes have also been used to detect MTBC in respiratory and non-respiratory clinical specimens with high sensitivity and specificity values. In Morocco, the use of *hsp656* gene as a PCR target was evaluated as a direct method for the diagnosis of MTB in 70 clinical specimens (62 sputum, 6 cerebrospinal fluids, and 2 biopsies). Results showed a sensitivity of 81.13 % with specificity of 88, 24 % as compared with conventional techniques. Moreover, the positive and negative predictive values were 95.56 %, 60% respectively (Zakham, 2011).

6.3.2 The amplicor MTB test and its automated version the Cobas Amplicor MTB test

The amplicor test is based on the PCR. In this assay, mycobacterial DNA is amplified with genus-specific primers formulated on the basis of the 16S rRNA gene. After denaturation, the amplicons are added to a microtiter plate containing a bound, *M tuberculosis* complex-specific oligonucleotide probe. An avidin-horseradish peroxidase conjugate then binds to the bound, biotin labelled amplicons. The conjugate then reacts with with peroxide and 3,39,5,59-tetramethylbenzidine in dimethylformamide to form a color complex. The results are measured with a photometer (D'Amato, 1995; Soini and Musser, 2001; Ozkutuk, 2006).

The Amplicor results are available in 6.5 h. An automated version of this test is available (Cobas Amplicor).The overall sensitivity of the Amplicor test (compared with culture) for respiratory specimens is 79.4 -91.9%, the specificity is 99.6 -99.8%. However, the sensitivity for smear negative specimens is somewhat lower, 40.0–73.1% (Bergmann, 1996; Stauffer, 1995; Tevere, 1996; Eing, 1998). Therefore, the Amplicor test has been approved by the Food and Drug Administration (FDA) only for direct detection of *M. tuberculosis* in AFB smear-positive respiratory specimens. Chin *et al.* (Chin, 1995) reported that the sensitivity of the Amplicor test was similar to that of culture (58% vs 56%) for detecting *M. tuberculosis* from respiratory specimens when the clinical case definition of TB was used as the reference standard. However, Al Zahrani *et al.* (2000) reported that although the Amplicor test had excellent specificity (100%), it was less sensitive than culture (42% vs 73%) for diagnosis of minimal active pulmonary TB (patients suspected of having TB but without spontaneous sputum or with AFB-negative smears).

6.3.3 Enhanced MTB direct test (E-MTD)

The E-MTD test is based on the transcription-mediated amplification system developed by Kwoh *et al.* (1989). In this assay, rRNA is released from the target cells by sonication, and a promoter-primer binds to the rRNA target. Reverse transcriptase is then used to copy rRNA to a cDNA-RNA hybrid. The initial RNA strand is degraded, and a second primer binds to the cDNA and is extended, leading to the formation of double-stranded cDNA, which is then transcribed by DNA-directed RNA polymerase to produce more rRNA molecules. The new transcripts serve as templates for reverse transcription and further amplification. The RNA amplicons are detected with an acridinium ester-labeled DNA probe in a solution hybridization assay. Importantly, the amplification procedure is isothermal and the reaction is performed in a single tube, which helps to reduce carryover contamination. After standard decontamination of the clinical specimen, the E-MTD test can be completed in 3.5 h.

The E-MTD test is FDA-approved for detection of *M. tuberculosis* in both AFB smear-positive and smear-negative specimens. The overall sensitivity (compared with culture) for respiratory specimens is 90.9 -95.2%, the specificity 98.8–100% (Bergmann, 1999; Gamboa, 1998; Smith, 1999).The performance of the E-MTD and the Cobas Amplicor is the same (Scarparo, 2000). However, it was noted that although the turnaround time is shorter for the

E-MTD test, the Amplicor test can be fully automated and has an internal control for monitoring amplification inhibitors.

6.3.4 BDProbeTec ET test

The BDProbeTec ET system allows amplification and detection of *M. tuberculosis* complex (MTBC) DNA in 1 h and simultaneously detects the presence of inhibitors as well. The target of the BDProbeTec ET system is a 95-bp region of IS*6110*, a highly specific insertion element in the MTBC DNA where it is present in multiple copies. Nucleic acid amplification is isothermal and is based on homogeneous strand displacement amplification (SDA) (Spargo, 1993), while detection is based on real-time fluorescent energy transfer (Little, 1999). An internal amplification control (IAC) is run with each sample to confirm the validity of the amplification reaction and to identify potential inhibitory factors from the processed specimen.

Of the published studies on the BDProbeTec system, sensitivities and specificities for respiratory samples were ranging from 82.7% to 100% and from 96.5% to 99.8% respectively (Mazzarelli, 2003). The extrapulmonary specimens represent a major diagnostic problem, mainly as they are often paucibacillary and at times contain inhibitors. With such samples, the resolved sensitivity of the BDProbeTec ET system is lower (77.8%) than with pulmonary specimens (91.5%), but nevertheless higher than with microscopy (63.1%) (Mazzarelli, 2003; Cho, 2007).

Other tests, Xpert MTB/RIF Assay (Cepheid) and INNO-LiPA-Rif (Innogenetics, Ghent, Belgium), used both for TB diagnosis and TB drug resistance screening will be discussed in later.

7. Diagnosis of drug resistant tuberculosis

7.1 Conventional tests

7.1.1 Microscopic Observation Drug Susceptibility (MODS) assay

The MODS assay is a broth microtiter method designed to detect *M. tuberculosis* complex and to detect resistance to isoniazid and rifampin (Moore, 2006; Mello, 2007; Ha, 2010). The method uses standard microtiter plates and other materials that are readily available in larger diagnostic laboratories. The method is straightforward: microtiter plates are prepared that contain Middlebrook 7H9 broth medium, growth supplements, and antimicrobial agents to prevent overgrowth of bacterial contaminants. Anti-TB drugs, at different concentrations, are added to some of the wells (Wilson, 2011).

The performance characteristics of the MODS assay were summarized in a recent meta-analysis. For detecting lowlevel resistance to isoniazid the pooled sensitivity of the assay is 97.7% and specificity is 95.8%. For detecting high-level isoniazid resistance, the sensitivity decreases to 90.0%, but the specificity increases to 98.6%. For detection of rifampin resistance, the pooled sensitivity is 98.0% and the specificity is 99.4%. This meta-analysis did not summarize the ability of the assay to identify the presence of *M. tuberculosis* in sputum specimens (Ha, 2010; Minion, 2010).

The published sensitivity of the assay varies from 87.4% to 97.8%, although the assay was compared with different gold standards in these studies. The contamination rate for the MODS assay, although lower than that of solid media, is higher than that of liquid media (Minion, 2010).

7.1.2 Drug susceptibility testing

The standard methods using the Lowenstein-Jensen (LJ) or agar proportion method (PM) (Canetti 1963, 1969, Kent & Kubica 1985) and the radiometric method in BACTEC TB-460 system (Becton-Dickinson) (Roberts 1983) are the current standard methods recommended to perform susceptibility testing of *M. tuberculosis*. The absolute concentration method is also commonly used on account of its technical simplicity for inoculums preparation and for reading results.

In order to shorten the turnaround time and make it more convenient for case management, numerous new techniques have appeared, aiming to detect growth inhibition as early as possible. The most commonly used systems are detection of CO_2 production, such as BACTEC 460 (Hawkins, 1991) or MB/Bact (Diaz-Infantes, 2000), and oxygen consumption, such as Mycobacteria Growth Indicator Tube (Bemer, 2002); there are others in developmental stage. However, many of those new techniques are difficult to implement in the developing countries where they are needed the most, because of high costs, technical complexity and absence of appropriately trained human resources.

7.1.3 DST on liquid medium

MGIT can also be used to perform drug susceptibility testing (DST), which is done by comparing the growth of mycobacteria with and without the addition of drugs used to treat TB. The combined use of MGIT for both TB detection and DST can shave months off the conventional process of identifying multidrug-resistant (MDR) TB (Hanna, 1999; Rusch-Gerdes, 1999).

Despite having been developed over a decade ago, the advantages of MGIT for TB detection were not reaching most endemic settings for several reasons. This was primarily due to the cost of the test, the lack of a simple means to confirm the growth of *M. tuberculosis* species in positive tubes, and the lack of data demonstrating that the use of liquid culture was feasible in resource-constrained settings. FIND has partnered with BD to overcome these obstacles and introduce MGIT as a solution for case detection and DST in developing countries.

7.1.4 Colorimetric assays

A colorimetric method for detecting microbial growth in drug-resistant strains was described in 1998 and subsequently evaluated in a limited number of clinical trials (Martin, 2005; Abate, 2004; Montoro, 2005). The assay is based on the observation that growing tubercle bacilli convert a yellow dye [3-(4,5-dimethylthiazol-2-yl)-2,5- diphenyl tetrazolium bromide or MTT] to a purple color that can be detected visually or by use of a spectrophotometer. In field trials, the method has been shown to have a high degree of concordance with conventional AST (Martin, 2005; Abate, 2004; Montoro, 2005). The method has been compared with a nitrate reduction assay and a resazurin assay for detecting resistance to isoniazid, rifampin, ethambutol, and streptomycin; similar results were obtained for isoniazid and rifampin, but only the nitrate reduction assay showed a high level of concordance with all of the first-line drugs. Although these methods are conceptually straightforward, they are likely to be useful primarily in larger laboratories with the capacity to perform more complex assays (Montoro, 2005; Wilson, 2011).

7.2 Molecular tests

Several molecular detection methods for drug resistance are of great value; all these methods are based on the observation that resistance to anti-TB drugs develops through the sequential accumulation of mutations in mycobacterial genes targeted by different drugs. Mutations in specific codons can therefore be used to rapidly detect drug resistance, since drug susceptible samples lack the corresponding gene mutation. These Molecular methods are fast and reliable and can potentially reduce the diagnosis time from weeks to days, These methods include PCR-based sequencing, PCR-Restriction Fragment Length Polymorphism, PCR-Single Strand Conformation Polymorphism (PCR-SSCP), Heteroduplex Analysis, DNA Microarrays and Probe methods. Moreover, a commercially available DNA strip assay (Genotype MTBDR; Hain Lifescience, Nehren, Germany) for detection of mutations conferring resistance to Rifampin (RMP) and Isoniazid (INH) in clinical *Mycobacterium tubercu*losis isolates is now widely used. GeneXpert MTB/RIF Assay and the INNO-LiPA-Rif (Innogenetics, Ghent, Belgium), are two rapid assays for simultaneous detection of MTBC and determination of the rifampicin (RIF) resistance profile (a marker for multidrug resistance).

7.2.1 PCR-based sequencing

PCR-based sequencing is the main technique used to elucidate the genetic mechanisms of drug resistance in *M. tuberculosis*. It is the most direct and reliable method for studying mutations and allows for detection of both previously recognized and unrecognized mutations. Unfortunately, the method is not as readily applicable for routine identification of drug resistance mutations as it is for identification of mycobacterial species because many different genes may be involved, as is the case in INH resistance, or the mutations may be scattered in a large segment of the gene. This means that several sequencing reactions need to be performed for each isolate. However, for targets such as *rpoB*, where mutations associated with RIF resistance are concentrated in a very short segment of the gene, PCR-based sequencing is a useful technique (Soini, 2001; Johnson, 2006; Kourout, 2009).

A previous study was done in Morocco to characterize mutations in rpoB gene associated with rifampicin (RMP) resistance in 47 RMP-resistant and 147 RMP-susceptible clinical strains of *Mycobacterium tuberculosis* by DNA sequencing. RMP-resistant mutations were identified in 85% of RMP-resistant isolates. Sequence analysis identified 10 alleles, including two deletions not previously reported: 514-515 Δ (Phe-Met → Leu) and 519-520 Δ (Asn-Pro). Nucleotide changes at codons 531, 526 and 516 were the most prominent, accounting for 74.4% of our RMP-resistant strains. These results demonstrate that DNA sequencing is an efficient tool for rapid detection of RMP resistance (Kourout, 2009).

7.2.2 Probe based hybridization methods

DOT BLOT strategy

It is a technique which can detect any known or newly described mutations and which can fulfil the criteria of accuracy, speed and simplicity. The hybridization with wild type probes can be used to efficiently screen for all mutations conferring drug resistance. The method includes:

- PCR amplification for target genes
- Confirmation of PCR amplification by gel electrophoresis
- Blotting PCR product on a filter using dot blot apparatus
- Labelling of probes for region of interest: the probes are 5′ end-labelled by phosphorylation with [∂^{32}P]-ATP or 3′ end-labelled with digoxigenin by terminal transferase.
- Dot Blot hybridization
- Autoradiography.

Although radioactive and non-radioactive detection procedures gave similar results, the radioactive procedure was favoured to empirically evaluate stringent hybridization washes during the development phase of this strategy.

The dot -blot procedure may be specifically useful in countries with a high incidence of TBand where procedures such as automated DNA sequencing are not readily available. As the predictive value of any test is dependent on prevalence, a mutational screening strategy should initially focus on the mutations most frequently diagnosed in the geographic area studied.

Codons 315 (KatG), 516,526 and 531 (rpoB), 43 (rpsL), 491,513 (rrs) and 306 (emb) are frequently altered in clinical isolates from many studies (Victor, 1999, Sabouni, 2008; Kourout, 2009; Chaoui, 2009). Such methods are needed to determine the most important mutations associated with drug resistance in different geographical regions, since it is known that drug resistant mutations may vary with the geographical origin of the sample.

The wild type probe strategy is unable to provide a precise understanding of the different mutations occurring at a specific codon, however, it is known that 99% of mutations within these loci confer resistance and therefore the absence of a hybridization signal has been interpreted to directly reflect drug resistance. The application of specific mutant probes allows the identification or the confirmation of the nature of this mutational event. The method is reproducible, not technically demanding and it takes about two normal working days to obtain results. This technique could be adapted to amplify and detect drug resistant mutations directly from sputum samples or microscopy stained slides.

7.2.3 Reverse line probe assay

This approach involves a combination of DNA amplification and reverse-line blot hybridisation. This home made and low cost test was first developed to detect RIF resistant isolates (RIFO): in this test , the DNA of *rpoB* gene of MTB is amplified by PCR using specific primers. Then, the PCR products are hybridized to oligonucleotides on a DNA membrane, encoding the consecutive parts of of the *rpoB* gene sequence and the consecutive parts of of the *rpoB* gene sequence with the most frequently occurring mutations in rifampicin-resistant strains. The rpoB PCR products of in rifampicin-resistant strains will fail to hybridize to one or more of the wild type oligonucleotides, and will in most case show affinity to a mutant oligonucleotide. With this method, rifampicin resistance in MTB isolates can be detected within a few hours. In principle, the method can also be applied directly to clinical material and Ziehl-Neelsen (ZN) slides containing sufficient numbers of acid -fast bacilli, as has been demonstrated for spoligotyping, a PCR reverse-line blot assay to detect and type *M.tuberculosis.*

The accuracy, the high positive predictive value and the high sensitivity of the RIFO assay make it a useful tool for the early detection of MDR-TB cases (Morcillo, 2002; Senna, 2006). Even starting from early primary cultures, several important weeks can be saved with the application of the RIFO assay in comparaison with conventional laboratory methods.

The cost of the RIFO assay is 10 times lower than that of the commercially available kit to determine the RIF resistance of M.tuberculosis complex bacteria.

Later on, Mokrousov *et al* (1994) developed a home made reverse line blot (RLB) assay targeting a wide range of mutations in six genes (*rpoB*, *inhA*, *ahpC*, *rpsL*, *rrs*, *emb*B) associated with resistance to four first line anti-TB drugs (RIF, INH, SM and EMB).this macroarray based technique presnts in fact a rapid alternative to sequencing and may be recommended for use in TB reference laboratories. Its implementation can start with detection of RIF resistance as MDR marker and shoud focus on locallypredominant rpoB mutations. It is open to further development and it permits easy incorporation of new probes targeting mutations related either to newly uncovered mechanisms of resistance to the first-line anti-TB drugs, or to the second line drugs and newer anti-TB compounds. Analysis of the additional genes, such as, *gyrA* and *gyrB* (FQ resistance), other *rrs* mutations in the 530 and 912 regions (SM resistance), and *rpoB* mutations outside RRDR, eventually using a multiple co-amplification/co-hubridisation approach, seems promising.

7.2.4 PCR-Single Strand Conformation Polymorphism (PCR-SSCP)

SSCP is a gel based method that can detect short stretches of DNA approximately 175–250bp in size. Small changes in a nucleotide sequence result in differences in secondary structures as well as measurable DNA mobility shifts that are detected on a non-denaturing polyacrylamide gel.

PCR-SSCP analysis is increasingly useful. To date various studies have applied PCR-SSCP to identify mutational changes associated with drug resistance in *M. tuberculosis* for frontline drugs like, RIF and INH (Kim, 2004; Cardoso, 2004; Fang, 1999; Heym, 1995; Pretorius, 1995) In particular, the development of nonisotopic PCR-SSCP analysis has simplified the procedure, enhancing its utility in routine laboratories (Kalia, 1997; Lee, 2003). However, PCR-SSCP analysis has been found to be technically demanding and not sufficiently sensitive. Furthermore SSCP conditions must be carefully evaluated since not all mutations will be detected under the same conditions. Also, results obtained with SSCP analysis should be interpreted with caution as the technique only detects mutations and gives no information on the nature of associated mutation. For example, silent mutations in the *rpo*B gene have been identified that give altered mobility patterns on SSCP analysis but have no association with RIF resistance, which underlines the need for caution in interpreting results and phenotypic or genotypic correlation (Kim, 1997).

7.2.5 PCR-Restriction Fragment Length Polymorphism

Mutations associated with resistance can be identified by digestion of amplified PCR products with a restriction enzyme that cuts at the specific polymorphic DNA sequence followed by gel electrophoresis. Since not all mutations result in the gain or loss of a restriction site, general use of RFLP to screen for mutations associated with drug resistance is limited (Victor *et al.*, 2002).

7.2.6 Microarrays

Although technically a solid-phase-type hybridization assay, microarrays, also known as biochips, have been proposed as new molecular methods for detecting drug resistance in *M. tuberculosis*. They are based on the hybridization of DNA obtained from clinical samples to oligonucleotides immobilized in a solid support, such as miniaturized glass slides. They have been mainly used to detect resistance to rifampicin. In a recent evaluation using oligonucleotide microarrays for analysis of drug resistance, Gryadunov et al. (2005) has detected over 95% rifampicin resistant and almost 80% isoniazid resistant *M. tuberculosis* isolates within 12 h in a sample of drug-resistant isolates and clinical samples. For the time being and due to the high cost involved, the use of microarrays for detecting drug resistance in TB is still beyond the reach of most clinical mycobacteriology laboratories.

7.2.7 Line-probe assays

This technology involves a series of steps including extraction of DNA from mycobacterial isolates or directly from clinical specimens, polymerase chain reaction (PCR) amplification of nucleic acid sequences, hybridization of labeled PCR products with oligonucleotide probes immobilized on a strip, and colorimetric development that allows for lines to be seen where the probes are located (hence, the term "line-probe" assay) .

In 2008, the WHO issued a policy statement regarding the molecular line-probe assays for use in detection on *M. tuberculosis* and for detection of drug resistance.

The first line-probe assay was the INNO-LiPA Rif TB (Innogenetics NV) (Rossau, 1997). The results of clinical evaluations of the assay indicated that it accurately detects resistance to rifampin, but some of the evaluations showed that the assay was less sensitive for the detection of *M. tuberculosis* complex. A meta-analysis performed in 2005 showed that 12 of 14 published studies showed 95% of sensitivity with a specificity of 100% but that, in studies in which the assay was applied to clinical specimens, the sensitivity ranged from 80% to 100%. One study showed that the assay could be used successfully in a resource-poor setting, compared with reference laboratories (Wilson, 2011).

The second line-probe assay was the GenoType MTBDR® developed by Hain Lifescience. Initially, this assay was developed as the GenoType MTBDR assay, but early evaluations showed that the assay did not detect drug resistance to a satisfactory degree, detecting only 90%-95% of isolates with rifampin or low-level isoniazid resistance. The assay was eventually modified to include detection of more rpoB and inhA mutations under the name

GenoType MTBDRplus®. Although 2 evaluations of the new assay showed improvement of the detection of isoniazid resistance (Hillemann, 2007), 3 other evaluations showed that detection of isoniazid resistance remained suboptimal (particularly for strains with low-level resistance) (Helb, 2010).

GenoType MTBDRplus® is a DNA strip test that allows simultaneous molecular identification of tuberculosis and the most common genetic mutations causing resistance to rifampicin and isoniazid. This technology can diagnose MDR-TB directly from smear-positive sputum samples, providing results in just five hours - an enormous improvement on the 1 to 2 months needed for conventional DST (Figure 3).

A meta-analysis performed in 2008 confirmed these findings; the assay shows high sensitivity and specificity for detecting resistance to rifampin but variable results for detecting resistance to isoniazid (Barnard, 2008, Ling, 2008). A second meta-analysis performed the subsequent year showed similar results, although in this analysis, the pooled sensitivity of the GenoType MTBDRplus assay showed better sensitivity for detecting isoniazid resistance (Wilson, 2011). Overall, this genotyping kit is a rapid, manual nucleic acid amplification test (NAAT) and capable of both detecting *M. tuberculosis* and carrying out drug susceptibility testing (DST), however, results of studies' evaluations indicate that the assay is of limited use with smear-negative specimens and that detection of isoniazid resistance is more variable but generally lower than detection of rifampin resistance (Barnard, 2008).

More recently, another version, named GenoType MTBDRsl®, was developed to detect resistance to fluoroquinolones, ethambutol, kanamycin, amikacin and capreomycin. Two evaluations of this assay have shown promising but variable results for detection of resistance to the second-line drugs (Brossier, 2010).

As with any new diagnostic test, the impact of GenoType MTBDRplus® Assay will depend on the reproducibility of the results under actual field conditions, the manner and extent of their introduction, the strength of the laboratories and the degree to which access to appropriate therapy follows access to diagnosis.

LPA is now being rolled out by FIND and partners in 27 high MDR-TB burden countries under the EXPANDx-TB programme, supported by UNITAID.

Currently, the implementation of the GenoType MTBDRplus® as a tool for detection of MDR / XDR strains is under evaluation in two regions of Morocco and is supported by WHO under EMRO - COMSTECH projects. The first assay concerned Rabat and neighbours cities which is the highest rate of pulmonary tuberculosis in Morocco and containing the major and the reference hospital of pulmonary diseases. In fact, this hospital receives patients from hall the country and concentrate patients infected with MDR and XDR TB strains

The second assay concerned Tangier and neighbours cities, with a high prevalence of tuberculosis. Moreover, Tangier area has been the theater of a new phenomenon that can affect the epidemiology of tuberculosis in this region; immigration from the sub-Saharan region to attend Europe.

We believe that the implementation of the GenoType MTBDRplus® will be of a great interest to enhance drug resistant TB diagnosis and therefore to improve TB management in Morocco.

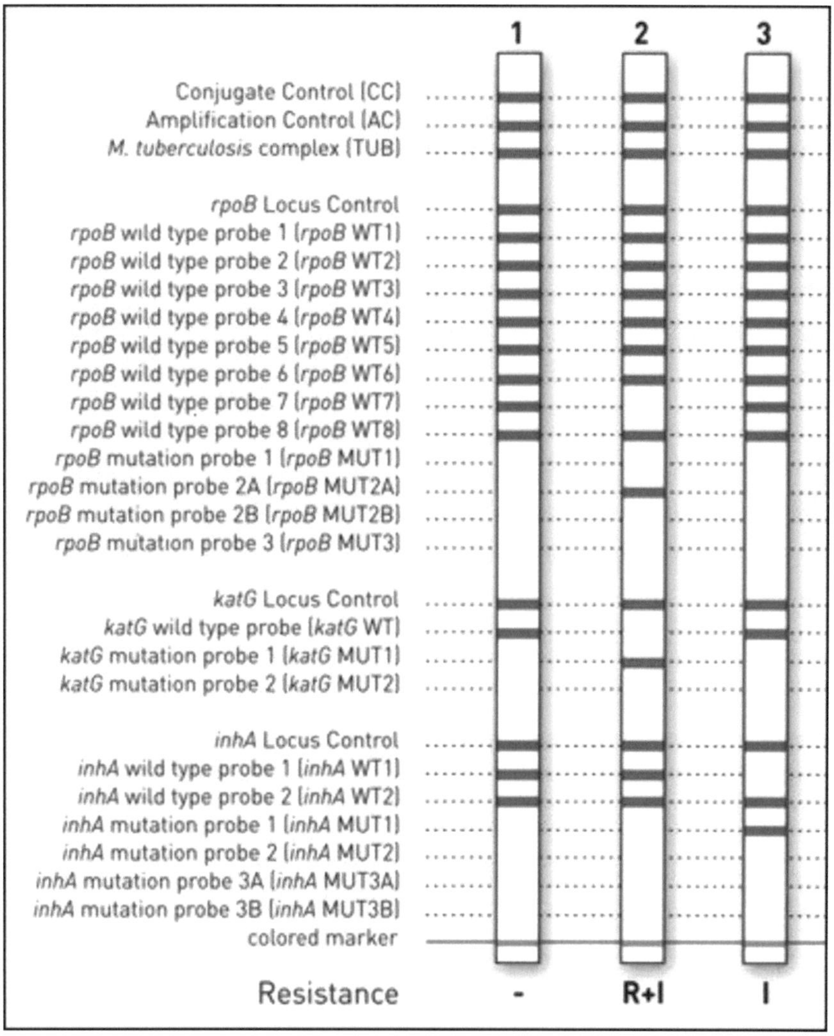

Fig. 3. Schematic representation of results obtained with the GenoType MTBDRplus® test
- : Sensitive strain
R+I: Strain resistant for both rifampicin and isoniazid,
I: Strain resistant only for isoniazid

7.2.8 Cartridge-based automated NAAT

This assay, usually called Xpert MTB/RIF, is a self-contained and fully automated technological platform that integrates sputum processing, DNA extraction and amplification, TB and MDR-TB diagnosis. This assay, which was CE (Conformité Européenne) marked in 2009, avoids many of the pitfalls of conventional nucleic acid amplification tests (Blakemore, 2010; Helb, 2010; Boehme, 2010; Hillemann, 2011). This is largely because the device is self-enclosed and, therefore, requires less sophisticated infrastructure in terms of laboratory facilities, user training, and supply chain management.

The assay has recently undergone performance evaluation to detect TB and rifampicin resistant strains on respiratory specimens (Wilson, 2011; Helb, 2010; Boehm, 2010; Rachow, 2011) as well as on non-respiratory samples (Rachow, 2011). The sensitivity of the test to detect smear-positive isolates reached 100%. However, the sensitivity for the identification of smear-negative culture positive isolates ranged from 71 to 72.5%. Xpert MTB/RIF test was shown to be specific in 99.2% of patients without TB. Moreover, its usefulness in detecting sputum smear and culture negative patients needs further studies (Helb, 2010; Marlowe, 2011).

On the other hand, and as compared with phenotypic drug-susceptibility testing, Xpert® MTB/RIF test was shown to be highly sensitive for detecting rifampin resistance, correctly identifying 97.6% of rifampicin-resistant isolates and 98.1% of rifampicin susceptible isolates (Boehme, 2010).

The main disadvantage of this system is the inability to test for and detect isoniazid resistance. Other potential disadvantages are related to the cost and a continued need for adequate laboratory infrastructure and training of personnel.

As for GenoType MTBDRplus® test, the Xpert MTB/RIF Assay will depend on the reproducibility of the results, the manner and extent of their introduction, the strength of the laboratories and the degree to which access to appropriate therapy follows access to diagnosis.

Thus, due to its high sensitivity and specificity, time consuming and the facility to use, the Wold Health Organisation endorsed in December 2010 Xpert® MTB/RIF technology and released a roadmap to guide its rapid adoption in endemic countries. In this context, the Xpert® MTB/RIF technology will be implemented in different cities of Morocco and should be used as the initial diagnostic test in individuals suspected of having MDR-TB or HIV-associated TB and may be considered as a follow-on test to microscopy in settings where MDR-TB or HIV is of lesser concern, especially in further testing of smear-negative specimens.

8. The place of molecular approaches in the TB management policy in Morocco

Guidelines for the use of nucleic acid amplification (NAA) tests for the diagnosis of tuberculosis (TB) were published in 1996 (CDC, 1996) and updated in 2000 (CDC, 2000). Since then, NAA testing has become a routine procedure in many institutions for the diagnosis of TB, because NAA tests can rapidly and reliably detect *Mycobacterium tuberculosis* bacteria directly in a specimen one or more weeks earlier than culture. Earlier laboratory confirmation of TB can lead to earlier treatment initiation, better patient care and outcomes, greater opportunities to interrupt transmission and improved public health interventions.

Guidelines for the use of nucleic acid amplification (NAA) tests for the diagnosis of tuberculosis (TB) were published in 1996 (CDC, 1996) and updated in 2000 (CDC, 2000). Since then, NAA testing has become a routine procedure in many institutions for the diagnosis of TB, because NAA tests can rapidly and reliably detect *Mycobacterium tuberculosis* bacteria directly in a specimen one or more weeks earlier than culture. Earlier laboratory confirmation of TB can lead to earlier treatment initiation, better patient care and outcomes, greater opportunities to interrupt transmission and improved public health interventions.

In Morocco, TB biological diagnosis is mainly limited to conventional techniques. These techniques (AFB smear, bacterial culture on solid and liquid media) are well established across the network of tuberculosis control laboratories. However, 2 laboratories, considered as reference laboratories, are authorized to perform drug susceptibility tests to antibiotics. According to WHO guidelines, the tested antibiotics are: INH, RIF, SM and EMB.

In some cases, molecular techniques based on PCR amplification are used to detect TB especially in extra-pulmonary tuberculosis.

Moreover, molecular techniques are well used in research and epidemiology (RFLP, spoligotyping, MIRUs,...). Currently, manual and automated techniques based on molecular approaches are achievable in some well-equipped laboratories in major centrs in Casablanca, Rabat and Tangier.

As in many developing countries, where the incidence of tuberculosis is declining slowly, molecular based tests should be introduced in the national program of Morocco; or at least tested for a period to verify the impact of such tests on the annual incidence of tuberculosis. In response to a request from many researchers in the field of tuberculosis, an advisory council should be set up to evaluate the place of NAA tests in the national program; against tuberculosis in Morocco. This committee must include TB clinicians, TB control officials; laboratory directors or supervisors from small, medium and large public health laboratories, hospital laboratories, and commercial laboratories and representatives from the Regional Training and Medical Consultation Centres. This suggestion is based on general observations for the use of NAA test to diagnose tuberculosis infections and drug resistance of *Mycobacterium tuberculosis* (CDC, 2009).

NAA testing has significant potential added value for clinicians and TB control officials.

a. Earlier diagnosis leads to earlier initiation of treatment, a reduced period of infectiousness and improved patient outcomes.
b. Earlier notification of TB cases to public health authorities should permit public health interventions sooner and may engage a TB expert sooner in the care of the TB patient.
c. Earlier detection of *M. tuberculosis* bacteria in sputum specimens can facilitate earlier infection control (respiratory isolation) decisions.
d. Earlier differentiation of AFB-smear positive specimens containing *M. tuberculosis* from those containing other Mycobacteria can eliminate unnecessary contact investigations.

NAA tests can provide substantial savings

i. for the patient (earlier diagnosis, improved outcomes, reduced health-care costs);
ii. for the health care provider (definitive diagnosis earlier, focused diagnostic testing, optimum patient care);
iii. for the hospital (less potential for nosocomial transmission, briefer period of respiratory isolation if TB is excluded);
iv. for the public health program (interrupt transmission earlier, abbreviated period for transmission, focused contact investigations).

For achieving this Implementation, that we believe will have benefic on the national program for TB in Morocco, research projects are needed to:

1. Conduct operational, translational, and implementation research for developing, evaluating, and selecting the most effective and efficient NAA testing algorithms for routine use and for specific scenarios.
2. Develop and evaluate suitable tests for use with non-respiratory specimens (e.g., cerebrospinal fluid, gastric aspirates, or biopsies).
3. Develop and evaluate tests that will enhance the diagnosis of TB in children.
4. Develop and evaluate optimal specimen collection, transport, and processing methods.
5. Determine the influences of specimen quality and quantity on NAA test performance.
6. Characterize the ability of NAA tests to detect *M. tuberculosis* bacteria in mixed infections, specimens and cultures.
7. Develop, evaluate and deploy NAA tests with improved performance and ease-of-use.

9. Conclusion

Truly rapid results for drug susceptibility tests are particularly important in the management of drug-resistant tuberculosis. Thus, the improvements made by molecular biology suggest that effective diagnostic strategies could be used to identify patients with or without MDR and even XDR TB strains. However, these techniques suffer from the problem that the genetic basis of resistance is not fully understood for any TB drug for all *M. tuberculosis* isolates.

Conventional techniques will yet be considered as a gold and reference methods. The currently available molecular methods may aid in rapid detection of mutations associated with drug resistance, but the test results must always be confirmed by phenotypic methods.

10. References

Abate G., A. Aseffa, A. Selassie, S. Goshu, B. Fekade, D. WoldeMeskal and H. Miörner. 2004. Direct colorimetric assay for rapid detection of rifampin-resistant Mycobacterium tuberculosis. J Clin Microbiol. 42: 871–873.

Al Zahrani K., H. Al Jahdali, L. Poirier, P. René, M.L. Gennaro and D. Menzies. 2000. Accuracy and utility of commercially available amplification and serologic tests for the diagnosis of minimal pulmonary tuberculosis. Am J Respir Crit Care Med. 162: 1323-1329

Banerjee A., E. Dubnau, A. Quemard, V. Balasubramanian, K.S, UM, T. Wilson, D. Collins, G. de Lisle and W.R., Jr Jacobs. 1994. inhA, a gene encoding a target for isoniazid and ethionamide in *Mycobacterium tuberculosis*. Science. 263: 227–230.

Barnard M, H. Albert, G. Coetzee, R. O'Brien, M.E. Bosman. 2008. Rapid molecular screening for multidrug-resistant tuberculosis in a highvolume public health laboratory in South Africa. Am J Respir Crit Care Med. 177: 787–92.

Barry. C.E, III, R.E. Lee, K. Mdluli, A.E. Sampson, B.G. Schroeder, R.A. Slayden, and Y. Yuan. 1998. Mycolic acids: structure, biosynthesis and physiological functions. Prog. Lipid Res. 37: 143–179.

Basso, L.A. and J.S. Blanchard. 1998. Resistance to antitubercular drugs. Adv. Exp. Med. Biol. 456: 115–144.

Bastian I., L. Rigouts, A. Van Deun and F. Portaels, F. 2000. Directly observed treatment, short-course strategy and multidrug-resistant tuberculosis: are any modifications required? Bull. World Health Organ. 78: 238–251.

Bastian I., R. Stapledon and R. Colebunders. 2003. Current thinking on the management of tuberculosis. Curr. Opin. Pulm. Med. 9, 186–192.

Bemer P., F.R. Palicova, S. Rusch-Gerdes, H.B. Drugeon, G.E. Pfyffer. 2002. Multicenter evaluation of fully automated BACTEC Mycobacteria Growth Indicator Tube 960 system for susceptibility testing of Mycobacterium tuberculosis. J Clin Microbiol. 40: 150–154.

Bergmann J.S. and G.L. Woods. 1996. Clinical evaluation of the Roche Amplicor PCR *Mycobacterium tuberculosis* test for detection of *M.* tuberculosis in respiratory specimens J Clin Microbiol. 34: 1083-1085.

Bergmann J.S., G. Yuoh, G. Fish and G.L. Woods. 1999. Clinical evaluation of the enhanced Gen-Probe amplified Mycobacterium tuberculosis direct test for rapid diagnosis of tuberculosis in prison inmates. J Clin Microbiol. 37: 1419-1425.

Bloom B.R. and C.J.L. Murray. 1992. Tuberculosis: commentary on a reemergent killer. *Science 257*: 1055-1064.

Blumberg, H.M., W.J. Burman, R.E. Chaisson, C.L. Daley, S.C. Etkind, L.N. Friedman, P. Fujiwara, M. Grzemska, P.C. Hopewell, M.D. Iseman, R.M. Jasmer, V. Koppaka, R.I. Menzies, R.J. O'Brien, R.R. Reves, L.B. Reichman, P.M. Simone, J.R. Starke and A.A. Vernon, 2003. American Thoracic Society/ Centers for Disease Control and Prevention/Infectious Diseases Society of America: treatment of tuberculosis. Am. J. Respir. Crit Care Med. 167, 603–662.

Boehme C.C., P. Nabeta, D. Hillemann, M.P. Nicol, S. Shenai, F. Krapp, J. Allen, R. Tahirli, R. Blakemore, R. Rustomjee, A. Milovic, M. Jones, S.M. O'Brien, D.H. Persing, S. Ruesch-Gerdes, E. Gotuzzo, C. Rodrigues, D. Alland and M.D. Perkins. 2010. Rapid molecular detection of tuberculosis and rifampin resistance. N Engl J Med. 363: 1005-1015

Brossier F., N. Veziris, A. Aubry, V. Jarlier and W. Sougakoff. 2010. Detection by GenoType MTBDRsl test of complex mechanisms of resistance to second-line drugs and ethambutol in multidrug-resistant Mycobacterium tuberculosis complex isolates. J Clin Microbiol. 48: 1683–1689.

Canetti G, Fox W, Khomenko A, Mahler HT, Menon NK, Mitchison DA, Rist N, Smelev NA. 1969. Advances in techniques of testing mycobacterial drug sensitivity, and the use of sensitivity tests in tuberculosis control programmes. Bull WHO 41: 21-43.

Canetti G., F. Froman, J. Grosset, P. Hauduroy, M. Langerova, H.T. Mahler, G. Meissner, D.A. Mitchison and L. Sula. 1963. Mycobacteria: laboratory methods for testing drug sensitivity and resistance. Bull WHO. 29: 565-578.

Carter A.P, W.M. Clemons, D.E. Brodersen, R.J. Morgan- Warren, B.T. Wimberly, and V. Ramakrishnan. 2000. Functional insights from the structure of the 30S ribosomal subunit and its interactions with antibiotics. Nature. 407: 340–348.

Caviedes, L., T.S. Lee, R.H. Gilman, P. Sheen, E. Spellman, E.H. Lee, D.E. Berg, S. Montenegro-James and the Tuberculosis Working Group in Peru. 2000. Rapid, efficient detection and drug susceptibility testing of Mycobacterium tuberculosis in sputum by microscopic observation of broth cultures. J. Clin. Microbiol. 38:1203–1208.

CDC. 1996. Nucleic acid amplification tests for tuberculosis. MMWR. 45: 950-951.

CDC. 2000. Update: nucleic acid amplification tests for tuberculosis. MMWR. 49:593-594.

CDC. 2009. Updated Guidelines for the Use of Nucleic Acid Amplification Tests in the Diagnosis of Tuberculosis. MMWR. 58: 7-10.

Chaoui I, R. Sabouni, M. Kourout, A.M. Jordaan, O. Lahlou, R. Elouad, M. Akrim, T.C. Victor and M. El Mzibri. 2009. Analysis of isoniazid, streptomycin and ethambutol resistance in Mycobacterium tuberculosis isolates from Morocco. J Infect Dev Ctries. 3: 278-284.

Chin D.P., D.M. Yajko, W.K. Hadley, C.A. Sanders, P.S. Nassos, J.J?. Mandej and P.C. Hopewell. 1995. Clinical utility of a commercial test based on the polymerase chain reaction for detecting *Mycobacterium tuberculosis* in respiratory specimens. Am J Respir Crit Care Med. 151: 1872-1877.

Cho SN. 2007. Current issues on molecular and immunological diagnosis of tuberculosis. Yonsei Med J. 48 : 347-59.

Cohn D.L., F. Bustreo and M.C. Raviglione. 1997. Drug-resistant tuberculosis: review of the worldwide situation and the WHO/IUATLD Global Surveillance Project. International Union Against Tuberculosis and Lung Disease. Clin. Infect. Dis. 24 Suppl 1, S121- S130.

Cooksey R.C, G.P. Morlock, A. McQueen, S.E. Glickman, and J.T. Crawford. 1996. Characterization of streptomycin resistance mechanisms among *Mycobacterium tuberculosis* isolates from patients in New York City. Antimicrob. Agents Chemother. 40: 1186–1188.

Crofton J. and D.A. Mitchison. 1948. Streptomycin resistance in pulmonary tuberculosis. Br Med J. 2: 1009-1015.

D'Amato, R. F., A. A. Wallman, L. H. Hochstein, P. M. Colaninno, M. Scardamaglia, E. Ardila, M. Ghouri, K. Kim, R. C. Patel, and A. Miller. 1995. Rapid diagnosis of pulmonary tuberculosis by using Roche AMPLICOR Mycobacterium tuberculosis PCR test. J. Clin. Microbiol. 33:1832–1834

Daniel T.M. 1997. Captain of Death: the Story of Tuberculosis, University of Rochester Press, New York.

Diaz-Infantes M.S., M.J. Ruiz-Serrano, L. Martinez-Sanchez, A. Ortega and E. Bouza. 2000. Evaluation of the MB/BacT mycobacterium detection system for susceptibility testing of Mycobacterium tuberculosis. J Clin Microbiol. 38: 1988–1989.

Dooley K.E., O. Lahlou, I. Ghali, J. Knudsen, M.D. Elmessaoudi, I. Cherkaoui and R. El Aouad. 2011. Risk factors for tuberculosis treatment failure, default, or relapse and outcomes of retreatment in Morocco. BMC Public Health. 11: 140-146.

Ducati RG., AR. Netto, LA. Basso, DS. Santos. 2006. The resumption of consumption. A review on tuberculosis. *Mem Inst Oswaldo Cruz,* Rio de Janeiro. 101: 697-714.

Edlin B.R., J.I. Tokars, M.H. Grieco, J.T. Crawford, J. Williams, E.M. Sordillo, K.R. Ong, J.O. Kilburn, S.W. Dooley and K.G. Castro. 1992. An outbreak of multidrug-resistant tuberculosis among hospitalized patients with the acquired immunodeficiency syndrome. N. Engl. J. Med. 326: 1514–1521.

Eing B.R., A. Becker, A. Sohns and R. Ringelmann. 1998. Comparison of Roche Cobas Amplicor Mycobacterium tuberculosis assay with in-house PCR and culture for detection of M. tuberculosis. J. Clin. Microbiol. 36: 2023–2029.

Engohang-Ndong J, D. Baillat, M. Aumercier, F. Bellefontaine, G.S. Besra, C. Locht and A.R. Baulard. 2004. EthR, a repressor of the TetR/CamR family implicated in ethionamide resistance in mycobacteria, octamerizes cooperatively on its operator. Mol. Microbiol. 51: 175–188.

Espinal M.A. 2003. The global situation of MDR-TB. Tuberculosis. (Edinb.). 83: 44–51.

Espinal M.A., S.J. Kim, P.G. Suarez, K.M. Kam, A.G. Khomenko, G.B. Migliori, J. Baez, A. Kochi, C. Dye and M.C. Raviglione. 2000. Standard short-course chemotherapy for drug-resistant tuberculosis: treatment outcomes in 6 countries. JAMA 283: 2537–2545

Fang Z, C. Doig, A. Rayner, D.T. Kenna, B. Watt, and K.J Forbes. 1999. Molecular evidence for heterogeneity of the multiple-drug-resistant *Mycobacterium tuberculosis* population in Scotland (1990 to 1997). J. Clin. Microbiol. 37: 998–1003.

Feng Z. and R.G. Barletta. 2003. Roles of Mycobacterium smegmatis D-Alanine:D-Alanine Ligase and D-Alanine Racemase in the Mechanisms of Action of and Resistance to the Peptidoglycan Inhibitor DCycloserine. Antimicrob. Agents Chemother. 47, 283–291.

Fischl M.A., R.B. Uttamchandani, G.L. Daikos, R.B. Poblete, J.N. Moreno, R.R. Reyes, A.M. Boota, L.M. Thompson, T.J. Cleary and S. Lai. 1992. An outbreak of tuberculosis caused by multiple-drug-resistant tubercle bacilli among patients with HIV infection. Ann. Intern. Med. 117: 177–183.

Gamboa F., G. Fernandez, E. Padilla, J.M. Manterola, J. Lonca, P.J. Cardona, L. Matas and V. Ausina. 1998. Comparative evaluation of initial and new versions of the Gen-Probe amplified Mycobacterium tuberculosis direct test for direct detection of *Mycobacterium tuberculosis* in respiratory and nonrespiratory specimens. J Clin Microbiol. 36: 684-689.

Ginsburg A.S, J.H. Grossetand W.R. Bishai. 2003. Fluoroquinolones, tuberculosis, and resistance. Lancet Infect. Dis. 3: 432–442.

Gryadunov D., V. Mikhailovich, S. Lapa, N. Roudinskii, M. Donnikov, S. Pan'kov, O. Markova, A. Kuz'min, L. Chernousova, O. Skotnikova, A. Moroz, A. Zasedatelev and A. Mirzabekov. 2005. Evaluation of hybridisation on oligonucleotide microarrays for analysis of drug-resistant Mycobacterium tuberculosis. Clin Microbiol Infect. 11: 531-539.

Ha D.T., N.T. Lan, V.S. Kiet, M. Wolbers, H.T. Hang, J. Day, N. Hien, N. Tien, P.T. An, T.T. Anh, T.T. Oanh do, C. Hoa, N.T. Chau, N. Hai, N.T. Binh, H. Ngoc le, D.T. Phuong, T.V. Quyet, N.T. Tuyen, V.T. Ha, N.T. Nho, D.V. Hoa, P?T. Anh, N.H. Dung, J. Farrar and M. Caws. 2010. Diagnosis of pulmonary tuberculosis in HIV-positive patients by microscopic observation drug susceptibility assay. J Clin Microbiol. 48: 4573-4579.

Hanna B.A., A. Ebrahimzadeh, L.B. Elliott, M.A. Morgan, S.M. Novak, S. Rusch-Gerdes, M. Acio, D.F. Dunbar, T.M. Holmes, C.H. Rexer, C. Savthyakumar and A.M. Vannier. 1999. Multicenter evaluation of the BACTEC MGIT 960 system for recovery of mycobacteria. J. Clin. Microbiol. 37: 748–752

Hawkins J.E., R.J. Wallace and B.A. Brown. 1991. Antibacterial drug susceptibility tests: mycobacteria. In: Balows A, Hausler WJ, Herrmann KL, Isenberg HD, Shadommy HJ, eds. Manual of clinical microbiology. 5th Edn. Washington DC, American Society for Microbiology, pp. 1138–1152

Heep M, B. Brandstatter, U. Rieger, N. Lehn, E. Richter, S. Rusch-Gerdes and S. Niemann. 2001. Frequency of rpoB mutations inside and outside the cluster I region in rifampin-resistant clinical Mycobacterium tuberculosis isolates. J Clin Microbiol, 39, 107-110.

Helb D., M. Jones, E. Story, C. Boehme, E. Wallace, K. Ho, J. Kop, M.R. Owens, R. Rodgers, P. Banada, H. Safi, R. Blakemore, N.T. Lan, E.C. Jones-López, M. Levi, M. Burday, I. Ayakaka, R.D. Mugerwa, B. McMillan, E. Winn-Deen, L. Christel, P. Dailey, M.D. Perkins, D.H. Persing and D Alland. 2010. Rapid detection of Mycobacterium tuberculosis and rifampin resistance by use of on-demand, near-patient technology. J Clin Microbiol. 48: 229-237.

Heym. B, B. Saint-Joanis, ST. Cole. 1999. The molecular basis of isoniazid resistance in *Mycobacterium tuberculosis*. Tuber. Lung Dis. 79: 267–271.

Hillemann D, S. Ruesch-Gerdes, C. Boehme and E. Richter. 2011. Rapid molecular detection of extrapulmonary tuberculosis by automated GeneXpert(R) MTB/RIF system. J Clin Microbiol. 49 : 1202-1205.

Hillemann, D., S. Rusch-Gerdes and E. Richter. 2007. Evaluation of the GenoType MTBDRplus assay for rifampin and isoniazid susceptibility testing of Mycobacterium tuberculosis strains and clinical specimens. J. Clin. Microbiol. 45:2635–2640

Johnson, R., E.M. Streicher, G.E. Louw, R.M. Warren, P.D. van Helden and T.C. Victor. 2006. Drug Resistance in *Mycobacterium tuberculosis* .Curr. Issues Mol. Biol. 8: 97–112.

Kalia A, N. Ahmad, A. Rattan. 1997. Diagnosis of multidrugresistant tuberculosis: comparaison of traditional, radiometric and molecular methods(abstract). In: Abstracts of the 20th International congress of chemotherapy; 29 Jun-3 Jul 1997; Sydney, Australia. Sydney: International Society of chemotherapy; p.211.

Kent P.A. and G.P. Kubica. 1985. Public Health Mycobacteriology. A guide for the Level III Laboratory. US Department of Healthand Human Services, Centers for Disease Control and Prevention, Atlanta

Kim B. J, S.Y. Kim, B.H. Park, M.A. Lyu, I.K. Park, G.H. Bai, S.J. Kim, C.Y. Cha and Y.H. Kook. 1997. Mutations in the rpoB gene of Mycobacterium tuberculosis that interfere with PCR-single-strand conformation polymorphism analysis for rifampin susceptibility testing. J Clin Microbiol. 35: 492-494.

Kim B.J., K.H. Lee, Y.J. Yun, E.M. Park, Y.G Park, G.H. Bai, C.Y. Cha and Y.H. Kook. 2004. Simultaneous identification of rifampin-resistant *Mycobacterium tuberculosis* and nontuberculous mycobacteria by polymerase chain reaction-single strand conformation polymorphism and sequence analysis of the RNA polymerase gene (rpoB). J. Microbiol. Methods. 58: 111–118.

Kourout M, I. Chaoui, R. Sabouni, O. Lahlou, M. El Mzibri, A.M. Jordaan, T.C. Victor, M. Akrim and R. El Aouad. 2009. Molecular characterisation of rifampicin-resistant Mycobacterium tuberculosis strains from Morocco. Int J Tuberc Lung Dis. 13: 1440-1442.

Kwoh D.Y., G.R. Davis, K.M. Whitefield, H.L. Chapelle, L.J. Di Michele and T.R. Gingeras. 1989. Transcription-based amplification system and detection of amplified human immunodeficiency virus type 1 with a bead-based sandwich hybridization format. Proc Natl Acad Sci U S A. 86: 1173-1177

Lee H, T.C. Victor, P.N. Suffys, U. singh, H.E. Bang, A.M. Jordaan, H.M. Gomes, V.N. Suresh, S.C. Kim, B.K. Khan, S.N. cho. 2003. Evaluation of polymerase Chain Reaction-Single Strand Conformation Polymorphism (PCR-SSCP) Analysis for the detection of the *rpoB* mutations associated with resistance to Rifampicin in *Mycobacterium tuberculosis*. World Journal of Nuclear Medicine. 2: 45-51

Lee H.Y, H.J. Myoung, H.E. Bang, G.H. Bai, S.J. Kim, J.D, Kimand S.N. Cho, S.N. 2002. Mutations in the embB locus among Korean clinical isolates of *Mycobacterium tuberculosis* resistant to ethambutol. Yonsei Med. J. 43: 59–64.

Lee, A.S., A.S. Teo, and S.Y. Wong. 2001. Novel mutations in ndh in isoniazid-resistant *Mycobacterium tuberculosis* isolates. Antimicrob. Agents Chemother. 45, 2157–2159.

Lee, A.S., I.H. Lim, L.L. Tang, L.L., A. Telenti, and S.Y. Wong. 1999. Contribution of kasA analysis to detection of isoniazid-resistant *Mycobacterium tuberculosis* in Singapore. Antimicrob.Agents Chemother. 43: 2087–2089.

Lienhardt C. and J.A. Ogden. 2004. Tuberculosis control in resource-poor countries: have we reached the limits of the universal paradigm? Trop. Med. Int. Health. 9: 833–841.

Ling D.I., A.A. Zwerling and M. Pai. 2008. GenoType MTBDR assays for the diagnosis of multidrug resistant tuberculosis: a meta-analysis. Eur Respir J. 32: 1165–1174.

Little M.C., J. Andrews, R. Moore, S. Bustos, L. Jones, C. Embres, G. Durmowicz, J. Harris, D. Berger, K. Yanson, C. Rostkowski, D. Yursis, J. Price, T. Fort, A. Walters, M. Collins, O. Llorin, J. Wood, F. Failing, C. O'Keefe, B. Scrivens, B. Pope, T. Hansen, K. Marino, K. Williams and M. Boenisch. 1999. Strand displacement amplification and homogeneous real-time detection incorporated in a second-generation DNA probe system, BDProbeTec ET. Biol. Chem. 45:777-784.

Mani, C., N. Selvakumar, S. Narayanan, and P.R. Narayanan. 2001. Mutations in the rpoB gene of multidrug-resistant Mycobacterium tuberculosis clinical isolates from India. J Clin Microbiol. 39: 2987-2990.

Marlowe EM, S.M. Novak Weekley, J. Cumpio, S.E. Sharp, M.A. Momeny, A. Babst, J.S. Carlson, M. Kawamura and M. Pandori. 2011. Evaluation of the Cepheid Xpert MTB/RIF assay for the Direct Detection of Mycobacterium tuberculosis Complex from Respiratory Specimens. J Clin Microbiol. 49: 1621-3

Martin A, N. Morcillo, D. Lemus, E. Montoro, M.A. Telles, N. Simboli, M. Pontino, T. Porras, C. León, M. Velasco, L. Chacon, L. Barrera, V. Ritacco, F. Portaels and J.C.

Palomino. 2005. Multicenter study of MTT and resazurin assays for testing susceptibility to first-line anti-tuberculosis drugs. Int J Tuberc Lung Dis. 9: 901–906.

Mazzarelli G., L. Rindi, P. Piccoli, C. Scarparo, C. Garzelli and E. Tortoli. 2003. Evaluation of the BDProbeTec ET System for Direct Detection of *Mycobacterium tuberculosis* in Pulmonary and Extrapulmonary Samples: a Multicenter Study. J. Clin Microbiol. 41: 1779–1782.

Mdluli K., R.A. Slayden, Y. Zhu, S. Ramaswamy, X. Pan, D. Mead, D.D. Crane, J.M. Musser and C.E. Barry, 1998. Inhibition of a *Mycobacterium tuberculosis* beta-ketoacyl ACP synthase by isoniazid. Science. 280: 1607–1610.

Meier A, P. Sander, K.J. Schaper, M. Scholz, and E.C. Bottger. 1996. Correlation of molecular resistance mechanisms and phenotypic resistance levels in streptomycin-resistant *Mycobacterium tuberculosis*. Antimicrob. Agents Chemother. 40, 2452–2454

Mello F.C., M.S. Arias, S. Rosales, A.G. Marsico, A. Pavón, C. Alvarado-Gálvez, C.L. Pessôa, M. Pérez, M.K. Andrade, A.L. Kritski, L.S. Fonseca, R.E. Chaisson, M.E. Kimerling and S.E. Dorman. 2007. Clinical evaluation of the microscopic observation drug susceptibility assay for detection of Mycobacterium tuberculosis resistance to isoniazid or rifampin. J Clin Microbiol. 45: 3387-3389.

Middlebrook. G. 1954. Isoniazid-resistance and catalase activity of tubercle bacilli. Am. Rev. Tuberc. 69: 471- 472.

Minion J., E. Leung, D. Menzies and M. Pai. 2010. Microscopic-observation drug susceptibility and thin layer agar assays for the detection of drug resistant tuberculosis: a systematic review and meta-analysis. Lancet Infect Dis. 10: 688-698

Moghazeh S. L, X. Pan, T. Arain, C.K. Stover, J.M. Musser and B.N. Kreiswirth. 1996. Comparative antimycobacterial activities of rifampin, rifapentine, and KRM-1648 against a collection of rifampin-resistant Mycobacterium tuberculosis isolates with known rpoB mutations. Antimicrob Agents Chemother. 40: 2655-2657.

Mokrousov I, NV Bhanu , PN Suffys , GV Kadival , SF Yap , SN Cho , AM Jordaan , O. Narvskaya , UB Singh , HM Gomes , H Lee , SP Kulkarni , KC Lim , BK Khan , D van Soolingen D, TC Victor , LM Schouls . 2004. Multicenter evaluation of reverse line blot assay for detection of drug resistance in Mycobacterium tuberculosis clinical isolates. J Microbiol Methods. 57: 323-335.

Montoro E, D. Lemus, M. Echemendia, A. Martin, F. Portaels, J.C. Palomino. 2005. Comparative evaluation of the nitrate reduction assay, the MTT test, and the resazurin microtitre assay for drug susceptibility testing of clinical isolates of ycobacterium tuberculosis. J Antimicrob Chemother. 55: 500–5.

Moore D.A., C.A. Evans, R.H. Gilman, L. Caviedes, J. Coronel, A. Vivar, E. Sanchez, Y. Piñedo, J.C. Saravia, C. Salazar, R. Oberhelman, M.G. Hollm-Delgado, D. LaChira, A.R. Escombe and J.S. Friedland. 2006. Microscopic-observation drug-susceptibility assay for the diagnosis of tuberculosis. N Engl J Med. 355: 1539-550.

Morcillo N, M. Zumarraga, A. Alito, A. Dolmann, L. Schouls, A. Cataldi, K. Kremer, D. van Soolingen. 2002. A low cost, home-made, reverse-line blot hybridisation assay for rapid detection of rifampicin resistance in Mycobacterium tuberculosis. Int. J. Tuberc. Lung Dis. 6: 959- 965.

Morlock G.P, B. Metchock, D. Sikes, J.T.Crawford and R.C. Cooksey, R.C. 2003. ethA, inhA, and katG loci of ethionamide-resistant clinical *Mycobacterium tuberculosis* isolates. Antimicrob. Agents Chemother. 47: 3799–3805.

Moure R, L. Munoz, M. Torres, M. Santin, R. Martin and F. Alcaide. 2010. Rapid Detection of Mycobacterium tuberculosis complex and Rifampin Resistance in Smear-negative Clinical Samples using an Integrated Real Time PCR Method. J Clin Microbiol. 49 : 1137 - 1139

Musser, J.M., V. Kapur, D.L. Williams, B.N. Kreiswirth, D. van Soolingen, and J.D. van Embden. 1996. Characterization of the catalase-peroxidase gene (katG) and inhA locus in isoniazid-resistant and - susceptible strains of *Mycobacterium tuberculosis* by automated DNA sequencing: restricted array of mutations associated with drug resistance. J. Infect. Dis. 173: 196–202.

Neville K, A. Bromberg, R. Bromberg, S. Bonk, B.A. Hanna and W.N. Rom. 1994. The third epidemic: multidrug-resistant tuberculosis. Chest. 105: 45–48

Othmani S.E., M. Zignol, N. Bencheikh, L. Laasri, N. Chaouki and J. Mahjour. 2006. Results of cohort analysis by category of tuberculosis retreatment cases in Morocco from 1996 to 2003. Int J Tuberc Lung Dis. 10: 1367-1372.

Ozkutuk, A., S. Kirdar, S. Ozden and N. Esen. 2006. Evaluation of Cobas Amplicor MTB test to detect Mycobacterium tuberculosis in pulmonary and extrapulmonary specimens. New Microbiol. 29: 269–273

Paramasivan CN, S. Sulochana, G. Kubendiran, P. Venkatesan and D.A. Mitchison. 2005. Bactericidal action of gatifloxacin, rifampin, and isoniazid on logarithmic- and stationary-phase cultures of Mycobacterium tuberculosis. Antimicrob Agents Chemother. 49: 627-631.

Piatek A.S., A. Telenti, M.R. Murray, H el Hajj, W.R. Jacobs, Jr., F.R. Kramer, and D. Alland. 2000. Genotypic analysis of *Mycobacterium tuberculosis* in two distinct populations using molecular beacons: implications for rapid susceptibility testing. Antimicrob. Agents Chemother. 44: 103–110.

Prammananan T., W. Cheunoy, D. Taechamahapun, J. Yorsangsukkamol, S. Phunpruch, P. Phdarat, M. Leechawengwong and A. Chaiprasert, 2008. Distribution of rpoB mutations among multidrug-resistant Mycobacterium tuberculosis (MDRTB) strains from Thailand and development of a rapid method for mutation detection. Clin Microbiol Infect. 14: 446-453.

Pretorius G.S., P.D. van Helden, F. Sirgel, K.D. Eisenach and T.C. Victor. 1995. Mutations in katG gene sequences in isoniazid-resistant clinical isolates of Mycobacterium tuberculosis are rare. Antimicrob Agents Chemother. 39: 2276-2281.

Rachow A., A. Zumla, N. Heinrich, G. Rojas-Ponce, B. Mtafya, K. Reither, E.N. Ntinginya, J. O'Grady, J. Huggett, K. Dheda, C. Boehme, M. Perkins, E. Saathoff and M. Hoelscher. 2011. Rapid and Accurate Detection of *Mycobacterium tuberculosis* in Sputum Samples by Cepheid Xpert MTB/RIF Assay—A Clinical Validation Study. PLoS One. 2011; 6: e20458

Ramaswamy S. and J.M. Musser, 1998. Molecular genetic basis of antimicrobial agent resistance in Mycobacterium tuberculosis: 1998 update. Tuber. Lung Dis. 79: 3-29.

Ramaswamy S.V., A.G. Amin, S. Göksel, C.E. Stager, S.J. Dou, H. El Sahly, S.L. Moghazeh, B.N. Kreiswirth and J.M. Musser. 2000. Molecular genetic analysis of nucleotide polymorphisms associated with ethambutol resistance in human isolates of Mycobacterium tuberculosis. Antimicrob Agents Chemother. 44: 326-336.

Rigouts, L., O. Nolasco, P. de Rijk, E. Nduwamahoro, A. Van Deun, A. Ramsay, J. Arevalo and F. Portaels. 2007. Newly developed primers for comprehensive amplification of the rpoB gene and detection of rifampin resistance in Mycobacterium tuberculosis. J Clin Microbiol. 45, 252-254.

Riska P.F, Jacobs W.R.Jr and D. Alland. 2000. Molecular determinants of drug resistance in tuberculosis. Int J Tuberc Lung Dis. 4: S4-10.

Roberts G.D., N.L. Goodman, L. Heifets, H.W. Larsh, T.H. Lindner, J.K. McClatchy, M.R. McGinnis, S.H. Siddiqi and P. Wright. 1983. Evaluation of the BACTEC radiometric method for recovery of mycobacteria and drug susceptibility testing of Mycobacterium tuberculosis from acid-fast smear-positive specimens. J Clin Microbiol 18: 689-396

Rossau R., H. Traore, H. De Beenhouwer, W. Mijs, G. Jannes, P. De Rijk and F. Portaels. 1997. Evaluation of the INNO-LiPA Rif. TB assay, a reverse hybridization assay for the simulta. neous detection of Mycobacterium tuberculosis complex an its resistance to rifampin. Antimicrob Agents Chemother. 41: 2093-2098.

Rozwarski, D.A., G.A. Grant, D.H. Barton, W.R. Jacobs, Jr., and J.C. Sacchettini. 1998. Modification of the NADH of the isoniazid target (InhA) from *Mycobacterium tuberculosis*. Science. 279: 98–102.

Ruffino-Netto A. 1970. Epidemiologia da Tuberculose - Estudode Alguns Aspectos Mensuráveis na Prova Tuberculínica,PhD Thesis, Faculdade de Medicina de Ribeirão Preto,Universidade de São Paulo, São Paulo, 55 pp.

Rusch-Gerdes S, C. Domehl, G. Nardi, M.R. Gismondo, H.M. Welscher and G.E. Pfyffer. 1999. Multicenter evaluation of the mycobacteria growth indicator tube for testing susceptibility of Mycobacterium tuberculosis to first-line drugs. J Clin Microbiol. 37: 45-48.

Sabouni, R., M. Kourout, I. Chaoui, A. Jordaan, M. Akrim, T.C. Victor, A. Filali Maltouf, M. El Mzibri, O. Lahlou and R. El Aouad. 2008. Molecular analysis of multidrug resistant Mycobacterium tuberculosis isolates from Morocco. Annals of Microbiology. 58: 749-754.

Scarparo C., P. Piccoli, A. Rigon, G. Ruggiero, M. Scagnelli and C. Piersimoni. 2000. Comparison of enhanced Mycobacterium tuberculosis amplified direct test with Cobas Amplicor Mycobacterium tuberculosis assay for direct detection of Mycobacterium tuberculosis complex in respiratory and extrapulmonary specimens. J Clin Microbiol. 38: 1559-1562.

Schilke K., K. Weyer, G. Bretzel, B. Amthor, J. Brandt, V. Sticht-Groh, P.B. Fourie, W.H. Haas. 1999. Universal pattern of RpoB gene mutations among multidrug-resistant isolates of Mycobacterium tuberculosis complex from Africa. Int J Tuberc Lung Dis. 3: 620-626.

Scorpio A. and Y. Zhang. 1996. Mutations in pncA, a gene encoding pyrazinamidase/nicotinamidase, cause resistance to the antituberculous drug pyrazinamide in tubercle bacillus. Nat. Med. 2: 662–667.

Scorpio A., P. Lindholm-Levy, L. Heifets, R. Gilman, S. Siddiqi, M. Cynamon and Y. Zhang. 1997. Characterization of pncA mutations in pyrazinamide resistant *Mycobacterium tuberculosis*. Antimicrob.Agents Chemother. 41: 540–543.

Sekiguchi J, Miyoshi-Akiyama, T, Augustynowicz-Kopec E., Zwolska Z, Kirikae F, Toyota E, Kobayashi I, Morita K, Kudo. K, Kato. S, Kuratsuji. T, Mori. T. and Kirikae. T. 2007. Detection of multidrug resistance in Mycobacterium tuberculosis. J Clin Microbiol. 45: 179-192.

Senna S.G., H.M. Gomes, M.O. Riberio, A.L. Kristki, M.L.R. Rossetti, P.N. Suffys. 2006. In house reverse line hybridization assay for rapide detection of susceptibility to rifampicin in isolates of Mycobacterium tuberculosis. Journal of Microbiological methods. 67: 385-389

Shamputa I.C., L. Rigouts and F. Portaels. 2004. Molecular genetic methods for diagnosis and antibiotic resistance detection of mycobacteria from clinical specimens. APMIS. 112: 728-752.

Sherman D.R., K. Mdluli, M.J. Hickey, T.M. Arain, S.L. Morris, C.E. Barry, III, and C.K. Stover, C.K. 1996. Compensatory ahpC gene expression in isoniazid resistant *Mycobacterium tuberculosis*. Science. 272: 1641–1643.

Slayden, R.A. and C.E. Barry, 2000. The genetics and biochemistry of isoniazid resistance in *Mycobacterium tuberculosis*. Microbes. Infect. 2: 659–669.

Smith M.B., J.S. Bergmann, M. Onoroto, G. Mathews and G.L. Woods. 1999. Evaluation of the enhanced amplified Mycobacterium tuberculosis direct test for direct detection of *Mycobacterium tuberculosis* complex in respiratory specimens. Arch Pathol Lab Med. 123: 1101-1103.

Soini H and J.M. Musser. 2001. Molecular Diagnosis of Mycobacteria. Clinical Chemistry. 47: 809-814.

Somoskovi A, L.M. and M. Salfinger. 2001. The molecular basis of resistance to isoniazid, rifampin, and pyrazinamide in Mycobacterium tuberculosis. Respir Res. 2: 164-168.

Spargo C.A., P.D. Haaland, S.R. Jurgensen, D.D. Shank and G.T. Walker. 1993. Chemiluminescent detection of strand displacement amplified DNA from species comprising the Mycobacterium tuberculosis complex. Mol Cell Probes. 7: 395-404.

Sreevatsan S., X. Pan, Y. Zhang, B.N. Kreiswirth and J.M Musser. 1997a. Mutations associated with pyrazinamide resistance in pncA of *Mycobacterium tuberculosis* complex organisms. Antimicrob. Agents Chemother. 41: 636–640.

Sreevatsan S., K.E. Stockbauer, X. Pan, B.N. Kreiswirth, S.L. Moghazeh, W.R. Jr.Jacobs, A. Telenti and J.M. Musser. 1997b. Ethambutol resistance in *Mycobacterium tuberculosis*: critical role of embB mutations. Antimicrob. Agents Chemother. 41: 1677- 1681.

Sreevatsan S., X. Pan, K.E. Stockbauer, N.D.Connell, B.N. Kreiswirth, T.S. Whittam and J.M. Musser. 1997c. Restricted structural gene polymorphism in the *Mycobacterium tuberculosis* complex indicates evolutionarily recent global dissemination. Proc. Natl. Acad. Sci. USA. 94: 9869–9874.

Srisuwanvilai L.O., P. Monkongdee, L.J. Podewils, K. Ngamlert, V. Pobkeeree, P. Puripokai, P. Kanjanamongkolsiri, W. Subhachaturas, P. Akarasewi, C.D. Wells, J.W. Tappero and J.K. Varma. 2008. Performance of the BACTEC MGIT 960 compared with solid media for detection of Mycobacterium in Bangkok, Thailand. Diagn Microbiol Infect Dis. 61: 402-427

Stauffer F., R. Mutschlechner, P. Hasenberger, S. Stadlbauer and H. Schinko. 1995. Detection of *Mycobacterium tuberculosis* complex in clinical specimens by a commercial polymerase chain reaction kit. Eur J Clin Microbiol Infect Dis. 14: 1046-1051

Sterling T.R., H.P. Lehmann and T.R. Frieden. 2003. Impact of DOTS compared with DOTS-plus on multidrug resistant tuberculosis and tuberculosis deaths: decision analysis. Br. Med. J. 326: 574-579.

Takayama K. and J.O. Kilburn. 1989. Inhibition of synthesis of arabinogalactan by ethambutol in Mycobacterium smegmatis. Antimicrob. Agents Chemother. 33: 1493–1499.

Takiff H.E, L. Salazar, C. Guerrero, W. Philipp, W.M. Huang, B. Kreiswirth, S.T. Cole, W.R.Jr. Jacobs and A. Telenti. 1994. Cloning and nucleotide sequence of *Mycobacterium tuberculosis* gyrA and gyrB genes and detection of quinolone resistance mutations. Antimicrob. Agents Chemother. 38: 773–780.

Taniguchi H, H. Aramaki, Y. Nikaido, Y. Mizuguchi, M. Nakamura, T. Koga and S. Yoshida. 1996. Rifampicin resistance and mutation of the rpoB gene in Mycobacterium tuberculosis. FEMS Microbiol Lett. 144: 103-108.

Telenti A, W.J. Philipp, S. Sreevatsan, C. Bernasconi, K.E. Stockbauer, B. Wieles, J.M. Musser, and W.R., Jr Jacobs. 1997. The emb operon, a gene cluster of *Mycobacterium tuberculosis* involved in resistance to ethambutol. Nat. Med. 3: 567–570.

Telenti, A.,P. Imboden, F. Marchesi, D. Lowrie, S. Cole, M.J. Colston, L. Matter, K. Schopfer and T Bodmer. 1993. Detection of rifampicin-resistance mutations in *Mycobacterium tuberculosis*. Lancet. 341: 647–650.

Tevere V.J., P.L. Hewitt, A. Dare, P. Hocknell, A. Keen, J.P. Spadoro and K. Young. 1996. Detection of *Mycobacterium tuberculosis* by PCR amplification with pan-*Mycobacterium* primers and hybridization to an *M. tuberculosis*-specific probe. J Clin Microbiol. 34: 918-923.

Vaccarezza R.F. 1965. Robert Koch - La Etiologia de la Tuberculosis y Otros Trabajos, Eudeba, Buenos Aires, p. 109- 124.

van Rie A., R. Warren, L. Mshanga, A.M. Jordaan, G.D. van der Spuy, M. Richardson, J. Simpson, R.P. Gie, D.A. Enarson, N. Beyers, P.D. van Helden, and T.C. Victor. 2001. Analysis for a limited number of gene codons can predict drug resistance of Mycobacterium tuberculosis in a high-incidence community. J. Clin. Microbiol. 39: 636- 641.

Vannelli T.A, A.Dykman and P.R. Ortiz de Montellano. 2002. The antituberculosis drug ethionamide is activated by a flavoprotein monooxygenase. J. Biol. Chem. 277: 12824–12829.

Victor T.C, A. van Rie, A.M. Jordaan, M. Richardson, G.D. Der Spuy, N. Beyers, P.D. van Helden, and R. Warren. 2001. Sequence polymorphism in the *rrs* gene of

Mycobacterium tuberculosis is deeply rooted within an evolutionary clade and is not associated with streptomycin resistance. J. Clin. Microbiol. 39: 4184- 4186.

Victor T.C, A.M. Jordaan, A Van Rie G.D. Van der Spuy, M. Richardson, P.D. van Helden, R. Warren. 1999. Detection of mutations in drug resistance genes of Mycobacterium tuberculosis by a dot-blot hybridization strategy. Tubercli and Lung disease. 79: 343-348.

Victor T.C, P.D. van Helden P.D and R. Warren. 2002. Prediction of drug resistance in *M. tuberculosis*: molecular mechanisms, tools, and applications. IUBMB. Life. 53: 231–237.

Walley J. 1997. DOTS for TB: it's not easy. Afr. Health *20*, 21–22.

WHO. 2001. World Health Organization. Guidelines for drug susceptibility testing for second-line anti-tuberculosis drugs for DOTS-plus. 2001.

WHO. 2003. World Health Organization. WHO report 2003: Global Tuberculosis Control.

WHO. 2008. World Health Organization: Anti-tuberculosis resistance in the world: WHO/ IUATLD global project on anti-tuberculosis drug surveillance 2002-2007, Report number 4.

WHO. 2008. World Health Organization. Moving research findings into new WHO policies. Geneva: World Health Organization.

WHO. 2009. World Health Organization. The WHO Global Laboratory Initiative.

WHO. 2010. World Health Organisation. Multidrug and extensively drug-resistant TB (M/XDR-TB). Global report on surveillance and response,

Wilson. M.L. 2011. Recent Advances in the Laboratory Detection of Mycobacterium tuberculosis Complex and Drug Resistance, Clinical Infectious Diseases. 52 :1350–1355

Xu C, B.N. Kreiswirth, S. Sreevatsan, J.M. Musser, and K. Drlica. 1996. Fluoroquinolone resistance associated with specific gyrase mutations in clinical isolates of multidrug-resistant *Mycobacterium tuberculosis*. J. Infect. Dis. 174: 1127–1130.

Yang B., H. Koga, H. Ohno, K. Ogawa, M. Fukuda, Y. Hirakata, S. Maesaki, K. Tomono, T. Tashiro and S. Kohno. 1998. Relationship between antimycobacterial activities of rifampicin, rifabutin and KRM-1648 and rpoB mutations of Mycobacterium tuberculosis. J. Antimicrob Chemother. 42: 621-628.

Yuen L.K., D. Leslie and P.J. Coloe. 1999. Bacteriological and molecular analysis of rifampin resistant Mycobacterium tuberculosis strains isolated in Australia. J Clin Microbiol. 37: 3844-3850.

Zakham F., H. Bazoui, M. Akrim, S. Lamrabet, O. Lahlou, M. El Mzibri, A Benjouad, R. El Aouad and M.M. Ennaji. 2011. evaluation of conventional polymerase chain reaction for the diagnosis of *mycobacterium tuberculosis* in the clinical specimens from Morocco. Journal of Infection in Developing Countries.

Zhang Y and D. Mitchison. 2003. The curious characteristics of pyrazinamide: a review. Int. J. Tuberc. Lung Dis. 7: 6–21.

Zhang Y. and W.W. Yew. 2009. Mechanisms of drug resistance in Mycobacterium tuberculosis. Int J Tuberc Lung Dis. 13: 1320-1330.

Zhang Y., C. V., and Jacobs W.R.Jr. 2005. Mechanisms of Drug Resistance in Mycobaterium tuberculosis. In Tuberculosis and the Tubercle Bacillus, Vol. Chapter 8 (Ed, al., S. T. C. e.) ASM Press, Washington, D.C., pp. 115-140.

Zhang, Y., Garbe, T., and Young, D. 1993. Transformation with katG restores isoniazid-sensitivity in *Mycobacterium tuberculosis* isolates resistant to a range of drug concentrations. Mol. Microbiol. 8: 521–524.

Zhang. Y., B. Heym, B. Allen, D. Young and S. Cole. 1992. The catalase-peroxidase gene and isoniazid resistance of *Mycobacterium tuberculosis*. Nature 358: 591–593.

Zimhony O, C. Vilcheze, and W.R.,Jr Jacobs. 2004. Characterization of Mycobacterium smegmatis expressing the *Mycobacterium tuberculosis* fatty acid synthase I (fas1) gene. J. Bacteriol. 186: 4051–4055.

24

Pattern of Circulating *Mycobacterium tuberculosis* Strains in Sri Lanka

Dhammika Magana-Arachchi
Institute of Fundamental Studies
Sri Lanka

1. Introduction

Historically tuberculosis (TB) has been and today it remains the leading cause of mortality in adults due to an infectious agent, and with the increasing prevalence of TB's resistance to the drugs of choice the problem posed by TB to public health should not be underestimated. The strain classification or sub typing is important epidemiologically for recognizing outbreaks of infection, detecting the cross transmission of nosocomial pathogens, determining the source of infection, recognizing the particularly virulent strains of organisms and in monitoring vaccination programs (Olive and Bean, 1999). Sub typing has been accomplished by a number of different approaches, and if the method to be successful it has to satisfy several criteria. Mainly all the organisms within a species must be type able by the method used and secondly, it must have high differentiation power and the methodologies should be reproducible (Olive and Bean, 1999).

Molecular epidemiology makes use of the genetic diversity within strains of infectious organisms to track the transmission of these organisms in human populations and to evaluate the host and parasite - specific risk factors for disease spread. In the past, efforts to type strains of *M. tuberculosis* in human hosts were hampered by the lack of a strain specific immune response and by an apparent lack of genetic polymorphism in the organism. However advances in the field of TB research paved the way in developing molecular techniques which allowed the identification and tracking of individual strains of *M. tuberculosis*.

1.1 Molecular epidemiology of tuberculosis

1.1.1 Organization and sequence of genome

It is thought that the progenitor of the *M. tuberculosis* complex comprising *M. tuberculosis, M. bovis, M. bovis BCG, M .microti* and *M. africanum* arose from a soil bacterium and that the human bacillus may have been derived from the bovine form following the domestication of cattle. The complex lacks inter strain genetic diversity, and nucleotide changes are very rare. The $H_{37}Rv$ strain of *M. tuberculosis* was isolated in 1905, and since then it has found extensive, world - wide application in biomedical research. It has retained full virulence in animal models of tuberculosis and also susceptible to drugs and amenable to genetic manipulation (Cole et al., 1998). The genome comprises 4,411,529 base pairs (bp) with a G + C content of 65.6%, which is relatively constant throughout the genome and the genome is rich in repetitive DNA, and several regions show higher than average G + C content which corresponds to sequences belonging to a large gene family that includes the polymorphic G + C rich sequences (PGRSs) (Cole et al., 1998).

1.1.2 Insertion sequences and prophages

The genome of $H_{37}Rv$ contains 16 copies of the insertion sequence IS*6110*, and 6 copies of the insertion element IS*1081* (Philipp et al., 1996). Cole et al in 1998 found another 32 different insertion sequences, and of the 13E12 family of repetitive sequences which exhibit some of the characteristics of mobile genetic elements. Most of the insertion sequences belong to the IS*3* and IS*256* families but six of them form a new group (Cole et al., 1998). Most of the insertion sequences in *M. tuberculosis* $H_{37}Rv$ are inserted in intergenic or non-coding regions (close to tRNA genes), with clustering suggesting the existence of insertion hot-spots that prevent genes from being inactivated (Cole et al., 1998). The chromosomal distribution of the insertion sequences is informative and shows selection against insertions in the quadrant encompassing *oriC* and an overrepresentation in the direct repeat region that contains the prototype IS*6110* (Cole et al., 1998). According to Cole et al, two prophages, phiRv1 and phiRv2 (both - 10 kb in length) have been detected in the $H_{37}Rv$ genome sequence and only IS*1532* exhibited significant variability indicating that most of the prophages and insertion sequences are currently stable (Cole et al., 1998).

1.1.3 Insertion sequence IS*6110*

Insertion sequence IS*6110* is a 1361 base pair long sequence that was detected exclusively in members of the TB complex and differences of only a few nucleotides have been detected between the sequenced copies. The sequence is flanked by two 28 base pair repeats and has two open reading frames (ORF) that show homology with genes coding for putative transposases of other elements of the IS3 family, which are typical features of mobile elements (Suffys et al., 1997). Though the transposition of IS*6110* has not been experimentally demonstrated in *M. tuberculosis*, mobility of IS*986* has been observed. The number of copies of IS*6110* present in the genome is species and strain specific (Suffys et al., 1997) and most strains of *M. tuberculosis* carry between 8 to 15 copies in different positions of the genome. Several single copy strains of *M. tuberculosis* had been reported, while other studies found some *M. tuberculosis* isolates, which were devoid of the IS*6110* sequence.

1.2 Genotyping methods

Mycobacterial strain typing by means of molecular methods has become an important instrument for tuberculosis surveillance, control and prevention (van Soolingen, 1998).

1.2.1 Restriction Fragment Length Polymorphism (RFLP)

Among DNA fingerprinting methods which restriction fragment length polymorphism (RFLP) typing is the most common method used has permitted novel investigations of the epidemiology and pathogenesis of tuberculosis. The use of IS*6110*, an insertion sequence which is present in *Mycobacterium tuberculosis*, is generally considered to be the gold standard for tuberculosis molecular epidemiology studies (van Embden et al., 1993), but other molecular typing techniques could be used as adjuncts in selected circumstances

(Cohn and O'Brien, 1998). Das et al., 1995 studied the utility of a standardized IS*6110* / *Pvu* II, RFLP typing method for distinguishing between isolates of *M. tuberculosis*, and assess the potential for distinguishing between relapse versus re infection rates. They concluded that despite the high frequency of single and zero band isolates in the population, the discriminatory power of RFLP typing with IS*6110* is sufficiently high to be useful for clinical and epidemiological studies (Das et al., 1995). Sahadevan et al., 1995 observed that *M. tuberculosis* isolates obtained from patients' sputa on diagnosis and during follow-up after short-course chemotherapy in Madras, had either no copy or only a single copy of IS*6110*. This posed a limitation for DNA fingerprinting with an IS*6110*-based probe to determine the frequency of exogenous re infection versus that of endogenous reactivation. They overcame this limitation by using an alternate probe, the direct-repeat element. Comparison of pre- and post treatment isolates by direct-repeat restriction fragment length polymorphism analysis indicated a high degree of endogenous reactivation among patients who had relapses after the successful completion of chemotherapy (Sahadevan et al., 1995). van Duin et al., investigated an episode of laboratory cross contamination using IS*6110* RFLP typing and it proved to be a useful tool to trace the source of contamination (van Duin et al., 1998).

1.2.2 Spoligotyping

Spoligotyping is a technique based on the polymorphism of the direct repeat (DR) locus present in *M. tuberculosis* DNA. The DR sequences are composed of multiple 36bp copies, interspersed by short non repetitive sequences (Kmerbeek et al., 1997). However, the spacer sequences between any two specific direct repeats are conserved among strains (Kmerbeek et al., 1997). The presence or absence of each non repetitive sequence creates a pattern for each strain when analyzed by spoligotyping. A database of spoligotypes of *M. tuberculosis* has been created (Sola et al., 2001) containing the global distribution and phylogenetic analysis of worldwide spoligotypes and this database is useful for comparing the patterns found in different regions of the world, enabling a better understanding of the dynamics of disease distribution. Simultaneous use of RFLP and spoligotyping methods increases understanding the epidemiological factors that facilitates the spread of tuberculosis inside a country. Studies have revealed that both transmission and reactivation are contributing to the spread of tuberculosis in the world. Another study result highlighted the importance of molecular epidemiology studies of tuberculosis in insufficiently studied regions with a high TB burden, in order to uncover the true extent of genetic diversity of the pathogen.

1.2.3 MIRU

Another genotyping technique which becoming popular is mycobacterial interspersed repeat units (MIRU). MIRU genotyping categorizes the number and size of the repeats in each of 12 independent MIRUs, with the use of a polymerase-chain-reaction (PCR) assay, followed by gel electrophoresis to categorize the number and size of repeats in 12 independent loci, each of which has a unique repeated sequence (Supply et al., 2001). The discriminatory power of MIRU genotyping is almost as great as that of IS*6110*-based genotyping (Supply et al., 2001). Unlike IS*6110*-based genotyping, MIRU analysis can be automated and can thus be used to evaluate large numbers of strains, yielding intrinsically digital results that can be easily catalogued on a computer data base (Supply et al., 2001). A Web site has been set up so that a worldwide data base of MIRU patterns can be created

(Supply et al., 2001). MIRU genotyping is technically simpler than IS*6110*-based genotyping and can be applied directly to *M. tuberculosis* cultures without DNA purification (Barnes and Cave, 2003).

Sri Lanka is an island in the Indian Ocean, located in Southern Asia, southeast of India, in a strategic location near major Indian Ocean sea lanes. Although India accounts for nearly one-third of the global TB burden, with a population of 19 million Sri Lanka is among the low TB prevalence countries in the region. Only a few studies have been performed in Sri Lanka applying modern molecular DNA fingerprint techniques that are able to directly trace routes of TB transmission e.g., to analyze the epidemiology of resistant *M. tuberculosis* strains in Sri Lanka.

Therefore, this chapter focus on Molecular Epidemiology of Tuberculosis including the two studies conducted in Sri Lanka on *M. tuberculosis* isolates with IS*6110* RFLP assays and spoligotyping.

2. Genotyping by RFLP & spoligotyping

2.1 Study population

One hundred and seventy sputum smear positive TB patients admitted for re-treatment to Chest Hospital, Welisara, Sri Lanka were enrolled for the first study. There were 24 patients among the chest clinic attendees having a history of imprisonment before being diagnosed as having TB (ex-prisoners). The study population consisted of 131 culture positive re treatment TB patients. Remaining patients were excluded, as their cultures were negative. The second study consisted of 121 mycobacterial isolates collected from first visit patients attending the Central Chest Clinic, Kandy, Sri Lanka who were positive for acid fast bacilli on direct examination of sputum by Ziehl- Neelsen stain and/or culture and/or had radiological findings suggestive of TB.

2.1.1 Specimen processing, culture and isolation of genomic DNA from mycobacteria

Sputum samples were decontaminated using the standard Sodium hydroxide - sodium citrate - N acetyl - L - cysteine method and were inoculated on Lowenstein-Jenson (LJ) medium and Middle brook 7H-10 agar medium to isolate the *M. tuberculosis* strains. The strains of *M. tuberculosis* obtained from these media were used for antibiotic sensitivity testing and RFLP analysis. Isolation of Genomic DNA was performed using standard protocols.

2.1.2 Antibiotic sensitivity testing

In the first study 12 drugs were tested and the criterion for resistance was based on the 1% survival level of the organism in comparison with a control medium without the drug. Resistance was defined as survival of the tubercle bacilli at the following drug concentrations (μg/ml); isoniazid (H), 0.2; rifampin (R), 1.0; streptomycin (S), 2.0; ethambutol (E), 5.0; pyrazinamide (Z), 25.0; *p*-amino salicylic acid (PASER), 2.0; ethionamide (Et), 5.0; cycloserine (Cs), 30.0; kanamycin (Km), 5.0; viomycin (Vm), 5.0; ciprofloxacin (Cx), 2.0 and rifabutin (Rb), 2.0 (Magana Arachchi et al., 2010). For the second study isoniazid and rifampin were tested.

2.2 IS*6110* – RFLP and spoligotyping

In the first study RFLP analysis of the 131 isolates by Southern blotting and DNA hybridization with IS*6110* was performed according to the standard fingerprinting method (van Embden et al., 1993). In the second study DNA fingerprinting using IS*6110* as a probe was performed for 120 *M. tuberculosis* strains according to standardized protocol of van Embden et al., 1993. The software GeneDirectory from SYNGENE was used to compare RFLP hybridization patterns, using the Dice Coefficient of similarity and the UPGMA algorithm, with a 1% band position tolerance. A total of 110 *M. tuberculosis* isolates were subjected to standard spoligotyping and the spoligo patterns were analyzed using MS Excel data sheets and grouped together for any similarity. The data was further analyzed by comparing with the SPOTCLUST data base

2.2.1 IS*6110* – RFLP

2.2.1.1 Digestion of chromosomal DNA for RFLP

Genomic DNA (5 µg) per each sample / isolate (obtained from above procedure) was digested with restriction enzyme *Pvu* II in a final volume of 25 µl as recommended by the manufacturer (Pharmacia Biotech).

2.2.1.2 Separation of DNA fragments by electrophoresis

The *Pvu* II digested chromosomal DNA from samples was size fractionated on 1% agarose gels. Along with the samples a DNA marker (λ cleaved *Hind* III/PhiX 174-*Hae* III) and DNA from the reference *M. tuberculosis* strain cleaved with *Pvu* II was included.

2.2.1.3 Southern blotting

Gel was soaked in HCl (0.25 M) for 20 minutes, followed by several volumes of gel soak I solution (1.5 M NaCl, 0.5 M NaOH) for 30 minutes and next in several volumes of gel soak II solution (1 M Tris HCl, pH 8.0, 1.5 M NaCl) for 1 hr at room temperature with constant shaking. The gel was then Southern blotted onto nylon filters.

2.2.1.4 Preparation of DNA probe by PCR

The IS*6110* - specific DNA probe of 245 bp was amplified by PCR using the oligonucleotide primers INS-1 (5'-CGTGAGGGCATCGAGGTGGC-3') and INS- 2 (5'-GCGTAGGCGTCGGT GAC AAA-3') corresponding to bp 631 to 650 and 856 to 875 which are based on the positions of the IS*6110* sequence, respectively.

2.2.1.5 Preparation of the labelled probe for RFLP

The probe was labelled by using a direct nucleic acid labelling and detection kit (ECL, Amersham, RPN 3001) according to the manufacturer's instructions. DNA to be labelled was diluted to a concentration of 10 ng/µl using water. DNA was denatured by heating for 5 min in a boiling water bath. The DNA sample was immediately cooled on ice for 5 min and centrifuged (2 sec, 12000 g). An equivalent volume of DNA labelling reagent was added to the cooled DNA and mixed thoroughly. An equivalent volume of glutaraldehyde was added to the solution, and spun briefly in a micro centrifuge. Next the DNA was incubated for 10 min at 37 ^{0}C. The labelled DNA probe was stored in 50% (v/v) glycerol at -20 ^{0}C until used.

2.2.1.6 Hybridization and detection

The nylon filter was pre hybridized with hybridization buffer (0.125 ml/cm^2) in a sealed plastic bag for 1 hour at 42 ^{0}C. Labelled probe was mixed with the hybridization buffer, and was added to the solution containing the filter. The nylon filter was hybridized overnight at 42 ^{0}C with shaking. Next the hybridized filter was removed from the plastic bag and placed in a clean plastic box and the filter was washed twice (2x10 min) with the pre warmed (55 ^{0}C) primary wash buffer at 55 ^{0}C. Then the filter was placed in a clean plastic box and washed twice with the secondary wash buffer for 5 min at room temperature on a shaking platform.

Next the filters were treated with detection reagents as per manufacturers instructions in a dark room and then exposed to Kodak XAR-5 film for overnight at room temperature. The nylon filters were stored under moist conditions at 4 ^{0}C for further use.

2.2.2 Spoligotyping

Spoligotyping was carried out as previously described by Kmerbeek et al., 1997.

2.2.2.1 Preparation of the membrane containing the spacer-oligonucleotides

Standard spacer oligonucleotides (n=43) were diluted to the optimized concentrations in 150 µl 500 mM $NaHCO_3$, pH 8.4. Next Biodyne C membrane was activated by 10 min incubation in 10 ml freshly prepared 16% (w/v) 1-ethyl -3-(3-dimethyl aminopropyl) carbodiimide (EDAC) in demineralized water, in a rolling bottle at room temperature. Membrane was rinsed with water for 2 min, placed on the mini blotter, and filled the slots with diluted oligonucleotides. Next membrane was incubated for 1 min at room temperature and then oligonucleotide solutions were removed by aspiration. Next blot was incubated in 100 mM NaOH for 10 min in a sealed bag to in activate the membrane. Membrane was washed in 250 ml 2x SSPE/ 0.1%SDS for 5 min at 60 ^{0}C and then in 100 ml 20 mM EDTA, pH 8.0 for 15 min at room temperature. Membrane was stored at 4 ^{0}C until used.

2.2.2.2 PCR for DR

PCR was performed with primers Dra (5′-GGTTTTGGGTCTGACGAC-3′) (biotinylated 3′end) and Drb (5′-CCGAGAGGGGACGGAAAC-3′). The PCR reaction contained 10 ng of DNA, 1U of *Taq* DNA polymerase, 20 pmol of each primer and 200 µm dNTPs. The cycling parameters were 3 min at 96 ^{0}C, followed by 1 min at 96 ^{0}C, 1 min at 55 ^{0}C and 30 sec at 72 ^{0}C for 30 cycles.

2.2.2.3 Hybridization with PCR product and detection

Membrane was washed in 250 ml 2x SSPE/ 0.1% SDS for 5 min at 60 ^{0}C and was placed in the mini blotter in a way that the slots were perpendicular to the line pattern of the applied oligonucleotides. 20 µl of the PCR product was added into 150 µl 2x SSPE/0.1% SDS and the diluted product was denatured by heating for 10 min at 100 ^{0}C and was immediately cooled on ice. Next residual fluid was removed from the slots and the slots were filled with diluted PCR product and incubated for 1hr at 60 ^{0}C. Next samples were removed and the membrane was washed twice in 250 ml 2x SSPE/ 0.5% SDS for 10 min at 60 ^{0}C. Membrane was placed in a sealed bag and allowed it cool to prevent inactivation of the peroxidase. Membrane was incubated in 1:4000 diluted streptavidin-peroxidase conjugate: (2.5 µl streptavidin-peroxidase conjugate in 10 ml of 2x SSPE/ 0.5% SDS for 45-60 min in a sealed bag). Next membrane was washed twice in 250 ml 2x SSPE/ 0.5% SDS for 10 min at 42 ^{0}C. Then membrane was rinsed twice in 250 ml 2x SSPE for 5 min at room temperature. For chemiluminescence detection of hybridizing DNA the membrane was incubated for 1 min in 20 ml ECL detection liquid. Membrane was covered with a Saran-wrap and was exposed to an X-ray film overnight at room temperature. Finally, the X-ray film was developed using Kodak developer (1 min) and fixer (3 min).

3. Transmission of tuberculosis

3.1 Pattern of TB transmission in first study

In the first study the persistence of *M. tuberculosis* strains in a population was examined. To estimate the degree of transmission of TB within the general population (Colombo district) and among the prison population, analysis of the RFLP data were carried out in three ways: (I) determination of the degree of clustering of matching DNA types as a measure of transmission within the general population (ii) determination of the clustering and matching DNA types among the prisoners and (iii) degree of clustering and matching types among the prisoners , ex-prisoners and the patients from the general population.

The study showed that the majority of circulating *M. tuberculosis* strains in Sri Lanka belongs to a limited number of families, but the degree of IS*6110* DNA polymorphism among strains was high. Dendogram analysis showed 41 distinct IS*6110* banding patterns (Magana Arachchi et al., 2000). A close relationship between prison isolates and those from the general population was observed in this study (Magana Arachchi et al., 2000). Of the 20 strains isolated from prisoners, none of the strains displayed identical fingerprints (Magana Arachchi et al., 2000). In bacterial isolates of prisoners and ex-prisoners from the general population, there were two strains, which had identical banding patterns, while there were clear similarities between several isolates (Magana Arachchi et al., 2000). Comparative analysis of the study populations, observed five pairs showing identical banding patterns. One pair had a strain from prisoner and the other ex prisoner while another pair had identical banding patterns between an ex-prisoner and a patient from general population (Magana Arachchi et al., 2000). This indicates the spread of TB between prisoners and general population. Analysis of the data showed that ex-prisoners contributed to a substantial population of TB patients in the general population (Magana Arachchi, 2001). Therefore persons entering prison, carry the risk of being exposed to TB and when they leave could potentially carry the TB bacillus (Magana Arachchi, 2001). Reactivation of the latent disease among some will result in many new cases for many years to come. Compounding the tragedy is the fact that the prison is a perfect environment to produce drug resistant strains (MDR TB). Most prisoners in Sri Lanka do not receive follow up medical treatment, as they are lost for further follow up after discharge from prison. Inconsistent drug supplies can lead to strains of TB that are resistant to drugs. Thus inmates when released to their home communities pose a risk to public health as well as to themselves. Therefore continuity of medical care after release should take place in such instances.

Previous studies showed that *M. tuberculosis* strains carrying one or few IS*6110* copies are often difficult to differentiate by IS*6110* standard RFLP analysis because of a site specific preference for insertion of the IS element. Therefore to further differentiate the strains other genetic markers such as polymorphic rich GC repetitive sequence (PGRS) and direct repeats (DR) have been used (van Soolingen et al., 1998). In the first study for DNA fingerprinting restriction enzyme *Pvu* II was used to cleave the chromosomal DNA of the mycobacterial strains (Magana Arachchi, 2001). The enzyme cleaves the 1.35 – kb IS*6110* element at a single site. In the first study the 541 bp DNA probe used for the hybridization corresponds to a piece of the IS*6110* element and the *Pvu* II site is located within that region. By using this DNA probe all of the possible IS*6110* containing restriction fragments were visualised (Magana Arachchi, 2001) and when analysing the fingerprints 2 bands were considered as a single copy. Therefore *M. tuberculosis* strains carrying one or few IS*6110* copies could be differentiated by the DNA probe used (Magana Arachchi, 2001). There were 6 strains among the prisoners who had a single copy of the IS*6110* and among the general population there were 13 strains which had a single IS copy (Magana Arachchi et al., 2010). In this study 68% of the isolates had less than five copies which were similar to that of other countries in the Asian region, such as India, Malaysia, Oman and Hong Kong (Magana Arachchi et al., 2010). According to previous studies, the strains from countries with a high prevalence of TB exhibited less DNA polymorphism than do strains in countries with a low prevalence of infection (van Soolingen et al., 1998). However strains analysed in study I showed an extensive polymorphism in the banding patterns even though the numbers of copies were less.

Number of IS*6110* copies	Number of strains among prisoners, n= 20 (%)	Number of strains among ex-prisoners, n=24 (%)	Number of strains among general population, n=106 (%)
1	6 (30)	6 (25)	13 (10.32)
2	4 (20)	5 (20.83)	11 (8.73)
3	2 (10)	5 (20.83)	24 (19.05)
4	4 (20)	2 (8.33)	22 (17.46)
5	3 (15)	4 (16.67)	20 (15.87)
6	1 (5)	2 (8.33)	10 (7.94)
7	0 (0)	0 (0)	06 (4.76)

Table 1. Comparison of the IS element copies (IS*6110*) found among the different categories from Study I

3.1.1 Pattern of TB transmission in second study

The data included in this section are based on a study conducted over a period of 2 years in which total 121 *M. tuberculosis* isolates were analyzed from the first visit (n=178) and recurrent patients (n=12) who attended the Central Chest Clinic, Kandy, for pulmonary treatment. Two of the isolates from the first visit patients in this study (who were treated as having tuberculosis in the Central Chest Clinic, Kandy) were identified as mycobacteria other than tuberculosis (MOTT) biochemically. This finding is comparable to a previous study in which mycobacterial isolates obtained from patients throughout Sri Lanka where MOTT accounted for 3.27% of the total isolates. The isolate from the recurrent tuberculosis patient was found to be a MOTT strain with rifampin resistance, which explained the reason for the treatment failure in that patient (Magana Arachchi, et al unpublished data). In RFLP analysis all three strains did not produce any banding pattern with IS*6110* confirming their species variation.

3.1.1.1 RFLP analysis

The epidemiological analysis of TB using IS*6110* is based on the observation that the polymorphism of IS*6110* RFLP patterns among unrelated clinical isolates is high, where as epidemiologically related *M. tuberculosis* strains show identical or similar (one band variation) finger prints (Barnes and Cave, 2003). In this study RFLP analysis was successfully carried out to differentiate *Mycobacterium tuberculosis* complex from mycobacteria other than tuberculosis in 100 of 122 isolates from the first visit patients. A high degree of DNA polymorphism in both banding patterns and number of copies of IS*6110* among strains were observed. None of the isolates had an identical banding pattern except for the three strains with a single copy of IS*6110*. The number of IS*6110* DNA containing *Pvu* II fragments in strains varied between 1 and 17 indicating that these strains contain 1 to 17 copies of the IS*6110* element (Magana Arachchi et al., 2011). Table 2 summarizes the number of IS copies found in the strains that were investigated among the study group. Strains containing a single copy of IS*6110* were predominant among the study population (12) and except for three strains, the location of the bands in fingerprints were different and therefore the location of IS*6110* elements in the chromosomal DNA. Therefore *M. tuberculosis* strains carrying one or few IS*6110* copies were differentiated without difficulty (Magana Arachchi et al., 2011). In this study 52% of the isolates had five or less

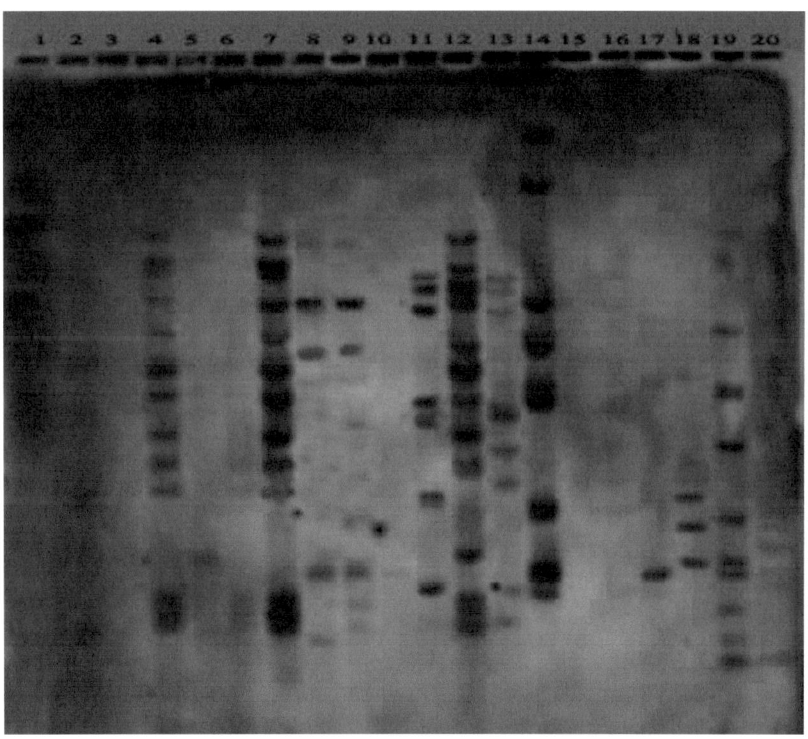

Fig. 1. IS*6110* DNA finger prints of *M. tuberculosis* isolates from study population of Kandy

Number of IS*6110* copies	Number of strains	% of strains
0	15[a]+2[b]+10[c] = 27	27
1	12	12
2	3	3
3	3	3
4	5	5
5	4	4
6	9	9
7	3	3
8	4	4
9	6	6
10	6	6
11	8	8
12	2	2
13	1	1
14	3	3
15	1	1
16	2	2
17	1	1

[a] = MTC / MTb *Mycobacterium tuberculosis,* [b] = MOTT confirmed, [c] = to be identified

Table 2. IS element copies observed in *M. tuberculosis* isolates from Kandy

than five copies and pattern is similar to the previous study in which 68% was recorded from recurrent TB patients (Magana Arachchi et al., 2011).

The fingerprints of the 73 strains were subjected to similarity analysis by using the software programme GeneDirectory from SYNGENE. This study showed that the majority of circulating *M. tuberculosis* strains in Kandy belongs to a single family, but the degree of IS*6110* DNA polymorphism among strains was high. In total 71 distinct IS*6110* patterns were found with strains clustering into one main family (63) and 10 distinct strains. Within the main family three isolates were grouped into one cluster, with closely related isolates while rests of the bacterial strains (60) were grouped into one. Sub clustering pattern of the main family was interesting with total 57 bacterial strains clustering into 3 main groups with 19, 27 and 11 strains respectively (Magana Arachchi et al., 2011). Interpretation of the clustering of the isolates in the family is complex and the explanation for the high degree of polymorphism in DNA fingerprints can be due to the different origins. Without performing DNA sequencing analysis definite conclusions cannot be made whether the isolates underwent any genetic changes within a given time (Magana Arachchi et al., 2011).

3.1.1.2 Spoligotyping

In this study, the used the algorithm SPOTCLUST incorporates biological information on spoligotype evolution, without attempting to derive the full phylogeny of *M. tuberculosis* complex. A total of 110 *M. tuberculosis* isolates were analyzed by spoligotyping. When spoligo patterns were compared from SPOTCLUST which was based on the SpolDB3 model, 24 distinct families were identified including the nine major spoligotyping-based families;

Mycobacterium africanum, M. bovis, East African-Indian (EAI) Beijing, Haarlem, Latin American and Mediterranean (LAM), Central and Middle Eastern Asian (CAS), a European family X, and a default family T (Table 3). The most predominant group among the isolates of *M. tuberculosis* corresponded to Family33. In this family, only spacers 33-34 are absent and recently described clade MANU of Indian origin belongs to the same family (Magana Arachchi et al., 2011). When compared to the single publication of spoligotyping patterns from Sri Lanka similarity was observed in only five clades namely Beijing, T1, EAI5, T2 and T3 (Magana Arachchi et al., 2011). According to the analysis, bacterial strains were distributed among all three principal genetic groups PGG1, PGG2 and PGG3. Segregation of *M. tuberculosis* into 'ancestral' versus 'modern' lineages based on PGG indicates that isolates from Kandy have originated from both lineages. In the spoligotyping patterns high strain diversity was observed and except for two strains 000000000003771 (ST1) and 000000000000031(ST 585) the tested strains were not defined in the latest spoligotype data bases SpolDB4/SITVIT (Magana Arachchi et al., 2011). The cluster analysis on spoligotyping are being carried out and after completing it in due course identifying the risk factors associated with TB transmission as well as the evolution of *M. tuberculosis* in Sri Lanka could be achieved.

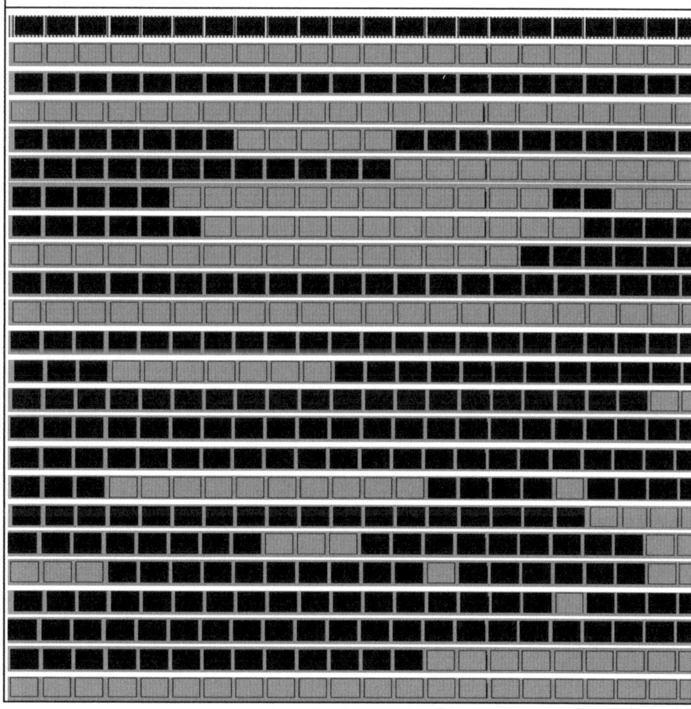

Spacer 1 5 10 15 20 25 30 35 40 43	Family	T
	Family 33	45
	Family36	13
	*M.tuberculosis*EAI1	07
	M. tuberculosis Beijing	07
	M. africanum	05
	Family 35	05
	*M. tuberculosis*LAM7	05
	M. tuberculosis T3	03
	M. bovis - BCG	02
	M. tuberculosis T1	02
	M. microti	02
	M. tuberculosis T2	02
	M. tuberculosis CAS	01
	M. tuberculosis LAM8	01
	M. tuberculosis Haarlem3	01
	M. tuberculosis Haarlem1	01
	M. tuberculosis X3	01
	M. tuberculosis H37Rv	01
	M. tuberculosis LAM 3	01
	M. tuberculosis LAM 1	01
	M. tuberculosis X2	01
	M. tuberculosis EAI-5	01
	M. tuberculosis T4	01
	M. tuberculosis Haarlem2	01

Table 3. Spoligotyping - based families that observed in *M. tuberculosis* isolates in patients with tuberculosis in Kandy by SPOTCLUST (n=110)

3.2 Evaluation of drug susceptibility

It has also been noted that the DNA polymorphism could be made use of to identify transmission rates of drug resistance and drug sensitive strains. RFLP typing can be carried out on primary isolates to determine drug resistance. By comparison of these isolates with the existing RFLP patterns of the drug resistance isolates the time taken for determining drug resistance may be much shorter compared to the conventional antibiotic sensitivity testing which takes more than four weeks. Genotyping also permits the evaluation of isolates with different patterns of drug susceptibility. Such an evaluation may helpful in cases in which the original organism developed resistance during or after antituberculosis therapy, the patient was reinfected with a different *M. tuberculosis* strain or cross contamination is suspected (Barnes and Cave, 2003). According to literature higher number of susceptible *M. tuberculosis* strains tends to be in clusters, where as only 22% of the isoniazid (INH) mono resistant strains were found to be clustered. But some studies did not find differences in clustering between susceptible and streptomycin mono-resistant strains (Soolingen et al., 1993). In the first study no difference in clustering was observed among the drug resistance and susceptible isolates, while analysis is being performed for the second study. Most studies have shown that acquisition of drug resistance of *M. tuberculosis in vivo* did not result in any observable IS mediated genetic rearrangements. But in contrast to the findings of others the relative, instability of IS*6110* was found in one of two MDR out break strains, and also four of the nine tested IS*6110* RFLP patterns showed a minor and different alteration. According to them the transposition rate may be strongly related to the *M. tuberculosis* genotype represented. In study I there were 2 pairs of isolates, which had identical banding patterns. However the pattern of drug resistance in the two strains was different and these isolates were collected from patients coming from different districts but from same Western province. Although they come to the same hospital for treatment, the strains were unlikely to be epidemiologically related. The findings of other research showed that non-random association of IS*6110* with *M .tuberculosis* could result in false positive clustering in unselected collections of isolates.

3.3 IS*6110* as a diagnostic tool

Among the strains tested in the first study there were two strains (one strain from general population and the other from DNA amplification studies) that lacked the IS*6110* element. In the second study among the strains tested there were 25 strains that lacked the IS*6110* element. Among these, 15 strains were confirmed as *M. tuberculosis* while three were identified as MOTT with DNA sequencing and biochemical analysis. This has implications for diagnosis of infection when IS*6110* is used as the sequence for DNA amplification.

3.4 Insights into transmission of TB

Clustered cases of TB are defined as those in which have identical or closely related genotypes with recent transmission while isolates with distinct genotypes generally represent a reactivation or infection acquired in the distant past (Barnes and Cave, 2003). However there are limitations to this concept (Barnes and Cave, 2003). Both studies showed that the majority of circulating *M. tuberculosis* strains in Sri Lanka belongs to a limited number of families, but the degree of IS*6110* DNA polymorphism among strains was high. Interpretation of the clustering of the isolates in the family is complex and the explanation for the high degree of polymorphism in DNA fingerprints can be due to the different origins. Molecular epidemiologic studies have shown that the dynamics of the transmission of TB vary greatly geographically (Barnes and Cave, 2003). Findings of the two studies indicate the differences observed in two provinces in both banding patterns and number of copies of IS*6110* among strains with Colombo district having 0-7 IS copies while Kandy having 0-17 copies of IS*6110* (Tables 1 and 2).

4. Future use of genotyping

Although the number of copies of IS*6110* can range from 0-25, population based molecular epidemiological studies report that most strains contain 8-18 copies a number sufficient to discrimination between the majority of strains (Burgos and Pym, 2002) and the findings of the two studies clearly emphasize the value of RFLP and spoligotyping in molecular epidemiology. However both studies included only culture-positive patients to enhance the possibility of typing actively transmitting strains. Although the exclusion of culture-negative cases could potentially have introduced a bias in the strain composition, due to study constraints RFLP and spoligotyping were not performed on all patients. Additionally by performing both RFLP and spoligotyping on culture positives high strain diversity was observed with a large number of small clusters, as well as a significant proportion of strains hitherto unreported in the global databases. But performing spoligotyping alone has advantageous over IS*6110* RFLP typing. As the technique needs only small amounts of DNA the test can be performed on clinical samples directly or on strains of *M. tuberculosis* shortly after their inoculation into liquid cultures (Kmerbeek et al., 1997). Presently the gold standard for molecular epidemiological studies on tuberculosis is changing towards MIRU-VNTR typing because this technique generates easily analyzed numerical results and it is less labour intensive and has a discriminative power comparable to that of IS*6110*-based RFLP (Barnes and Cave, 2003).

Genotyping has been used to study the transmission dynamics of TB in both developed and developing countries. However, only the developed nations are using it to guide tuberculosis control efforts (Barnes and Cave, 2003). This is the first study in Sri Lanka in which both the RFLP pattern of *M. tuberculosis* strains and the spoligotyping in a population has been examined. In this study the feasibility of establishing molecular typing methods in a developing country like Sri Lanka has been demonstrated specially in spoligotyping without using any commercial kits.

5. Conclusions

Typing of *Mycobacterium tuberculosis* isolates is of great potential value for basic and epidemiological studies on tuberculosis. Results obtained from restriction fragment length polymorphism typing and spoligotyping show that the majority of circulating *Mycobacterium tuberculosis* strains in Sri Lanka belong to a limited number of families, but the degree of IS*6110* DNA polymorphism among strains were high. By using the genetic marker of IS*6110* it was possible to differentiate most of the *M. tuberculosis* isolates. The preliminary inferences from these studies plead for a more extensive analysis of the data, to study the variability of *M. tuberculosis* strains and their transmission dynamics. The goal of molecular epidemiology is to quantify the extent of ongoing transmission of infectious agents and to identify host and strain specific risk factors for disease spread. Molecular methods in epidemiology require the development of both appropriate epidemiologic study design and analytical tools to yield meaningful assessments of disease transmission. Therefore the interpretation of molecular epidemiological studies should largely depend on the study question, the geographical area under study and the typing methods used to prevent the sampling bias in the molecular epidemiology of TB.

6. Acknowledgement

The research works on TB were supported by three grants RG/95/BT/08 NARESA, RG/2006/HS/07 NSF and 07-47 of NRC Sri Lanka. I am expressing my sincere gratitude to Professor Jennifer Perera and Dr. N.V. Chandrasekharan for their valuable guidance and Dr. D. Medagedara and Professor V. Thevanesam for their support in tuberculosis research and to Ms. R. P. Wanigatunge and Ms. S. Maheswaran for technical support in preparation of manuscript.

7. References

Burgos, M.V., & Pym, A.S. (2002). Molecular epidemiology of tuberculosis. *Eur Respir J*, 20, Suppl. 36, pp. 54-65, ISSN 0904-1850.

Barnes, P.F., & Cave, D.M. (2003). Molecular epidemiology of tuberculosis. *N Engl J Med*, 349, pp. 1149-1156.

Cole, S.T., Brosch, R., Parkhill, J., Garnier, T., Churcher, C., Harris, D., Gordon, S.V., Eiglmeier, K., Gas, S., Barry III, C.E., Tekaia, F., Badcock, K., Basham, D., Brown, D., Chillingworth, T., Connor, R., Davies, R., Devlin, K., Feltwell, T., Gentles, S., Hamlin, N., Holroyd, S., Hornsby, T., Jagels, K., Krogh, A., McLean, J., Moule, S., Murphy, L., Oliver, K., Osborne, J., Quail, M.A., Rajandream, M.-A., Rogers, J., Rutter, S., Seeger, K., Skelton, J., Squares, R., Squares, S., Sulston, J.E., Taylor, K., Whitehead, S., & Barrell, B.G. (1998). Deciphering the biology of *Mycobacterium tuberculosis* from the complete genome sequence. *Nature*, 393, pp. 537-544.

Cohn, D.L., & O'Brien, R.J. (1998). The use of restriction fragment length polymorphism (RFLP) analysis for epidemiological studies of tuberculosis in developing countries. *Int J Tuberc Lung Dis*, 2, 1, pp. 16-26.

Das, S., Paramasivan, C.N., Lowrie, D.B., Prabhakar, R., & Narayanan, P.R. (1995). IS*6110* restriction fragment length polymorphism typing of clinical isolates of *Mycobacterium tuberculosis* from patients with pulmonary tuberculosis in Madras, South India. *Tubercle and Lung Disease*, 76, 6, pp. 550-554.

Kamerbeek, J., Schouls, L., Kolk, A., Van Agterveld, M., Van Soolingen, D., Kuijper, S., Bunschoten, A., Molhuizen, H., Shaw, R., Goyal, M., & Van Embden, J. (1997). Simultaneous detection and strain differentiation of *M. tuberculosis* for diagnosis and epidemiology. *Journal of Clinical Microbiology*, 35, 4, pp. 907-914.

Magana Arachchi, D.N., Perera. J., Gamage, S., & Chandrasekharan, N.V. (2000). DNA fingerprinting of *M. tuberculosis* using restriction fragment length polymorphism (RFLP) with special reference to the prison population. *Proceedings of the Sri Lanka*

Association for the Advancement of Science, 56th Annual Session, 1391-023X, Colombo, Sri Lanka, 27th November- 1st December, p. 34.

Magana Arachchi, D.N. (2001). PCR based detection techniques and DNA fingerprinting by restriction fragment analysis of *Mycobacterium tuberculosis*. University of Colombo, PhD Thesis.

Magana Arachchi, D.N., Perera, A.J., Senaratne, V., & Chandrasekaran, N.V. (2010). Pattern of drug resistance and RFLP analysis on *Mycobacterium tuberculosis* strains isolated from recurrent tuberculosis patients. *Southeast Asian Journal of Tropical Medicine and Public Health*, 41, 3, pp. 583-589.

Magana Arachchi, D.N., Medagedara, D., & Thevanesam, V. (2011). Molecular characterization of *Mycobacterium tuberculosis* isolates from Kandy, Sri Lanka. *Asian Pacific Journal of Tropical Diseases*, 1, pp. 181-186, (In press).

Olive, D.M., & Bean, P. (1999). Principles and applications of methods for DNA based typing of microbial organisms. *Journal of Clinical Microbiology*, 37, 6, pp. 1661-1669.

Philipp, W.J., Poulet, S., Eiglmeier, K., Pascopellat, L., Balasubramaniant, V., Heym, B., Bergh, S., Bloomt, B.R., Jacobs, W.R., Jr., & Cole, S.T. (1996). An integrated map of the genome of the tubercle bacillus, *Mycobacterium tuberculosis* H37Rv and comparison with *Mycobacterium leprae. Proc Natl Acad Sci, USA*, 93, pp. 3132-3137.

Sahadevan, R., Narayanan, S., Paramasivan, C.N., Prabhakar, R., & Narayanan, P.R. (1995). Restriction fragment length polymorphism typing of clinical isolates of *Mycobacterium tuberculosis* from patients with pulmonary tuberculosis in Madras, India, by use of direct-repeat probe. *Journal of Clinical Microbiology*, 33, 11, pp. 3037-3039.

Sola, C., Filliol, I., Gutierrez, M.C., Mokrousov, I., Vincent, V., & Rastogi, N. (2001). Spoligotype database of *Mycobacterium tuberculosis*: biogeographic distribution of shared types and epidemiologic and phylogenetic perspectives. *Emerg Infect Dis*, 7, 3, pp. 390-396.

Suffys, P.N., de Araujo, M.E.I., & Degrave, W.M. (1997). The changing face of the epidemiology of tuberculosis due to molecular strain typing- A review. Memorias Do Instituto Oswaldo Cruz, Rio de Janeiro, 92, 3, pp. 297-316.

Supply, P., Lesjean, S., Savine, E., Kremer, K., van Soolingen, D., & Locht, C. (2001). Automated high-throughput genotyping for study of global epidemiology of *Mycobacterium tuberculosis* based on mycobacterial interspersed repetitive units. *Journal of Clinical Microbiology*, 39, 10, pp. 3563-3571.

van Duin, J.M., Pijnenburg, J.E., van Rijswoud, C.M., de Haas, P.E., Hendriks, W.D., & van Soolingen, D. (1998). Investigation of cross contamination in a *Mycobacterium tuberculosis* laboratory using *IS6110* DNA fingerprinting. *International Journal of Tuberculosis and Lung Disease*, 2, 5, pp. 425-429.

van Embden, J.D.A.,Cave, M.D., Crawford, J.T., Dale, J.W., Eisenach, K.D., Gicquel, B., Hermans, P., Martin, C., Mcadam, R., Shinnick, T.M., & Small, P.M. (1993). Strain identification of *Mycobacterium tuberculosis* by DNA fingerprinting:

Recommendation for a standardized methodology. *J Clin Microbiol*, 31, 2, pp. 406-409.

van Soolingen, D. (1998). Utility of molecular epidemiology of tuberculosis. *Eur Respir J*, 11, 795-797.

25

Health Interventions to Improve the Medication Efficacy in Tuberculosis Treatment

Jean Leandro dos Santos, Chung Man Chin, Ednir de Oliveira Vizioli, Fernando Rogério Pavan and Luiz Antonio Dutra
Universidade Estadual Paulista "Júlio de Mesquita Filho"
Faculdade de Ciências Farmacêuticas – UNESP Araraquara
Brazil

1. Introduction

Tuberculosis (TB) is an infectious disease caused by Mycobacterium tuberculosis. According to the World Health Organization (WHO), there are an estimated of 8.8 million new cases annually -including 200.000 HIV-infected individuals- and 1.6 million deaths (WHO, 2008). Despite some reports demonstrates reduction of new cases, it is extensive in literature data showing the problem of drug-resistance and the consequence of this one to the effective treatment (FAUCI, 2008). The drug resistance can be caused by several factors such as: 1) antibiotic selective pressure characterized by inadequate selection or dosage; 2) immune status of the individuals; 3) No compliance by patients; 4) natural selection or any pre-existing resistances in the infecting clone, among others (Figure 1).

Nowadays, HIV co-morbidity treatment is a challenge. It has been reported that HIV is a potent risk factor to TB disease development. Some studies showed that HIV/TB co-infection increase 100 times the risk to develop TB disease when compared to people infected only with TB (HAVLIR & BARNES, 1999; PITCHENIK et al., 1988). In addition, the probability to develop drug resistance is higher in patients under HIV infection treatment due mainly drug related problems (Frieden et al. 1993; Gordin et al., 1996).

One of the first randomized studies about antitubercular drug was performed with streptomycin. This drug reduces 50% the mortality of infected patients after 6 months of treatment. However, it was observed high rate of resistance in cases of monotherapy. The combination of drugs reduces the resistance to TB drugs, therefore the current treatment of tuberculosis involves multidrug therapy (Herzog, 1998).

WHO recommends the use of rifampicin (or rifabutin), isoniazid, pyrazinamide and ethambutol by two months followed by rifampicin and isoniazid for four months. The first phase of the treatment aims eliminates the bacilli in mutiplicate and semi dormant stage. The second stage called the maintenance phase aims eliminate dormant bacilli reducing the number of failures and relapses (Bisaglia, 2003). The scheme of treatment is prolonged (6 months) contributing to no-therapy compliance by some patients.

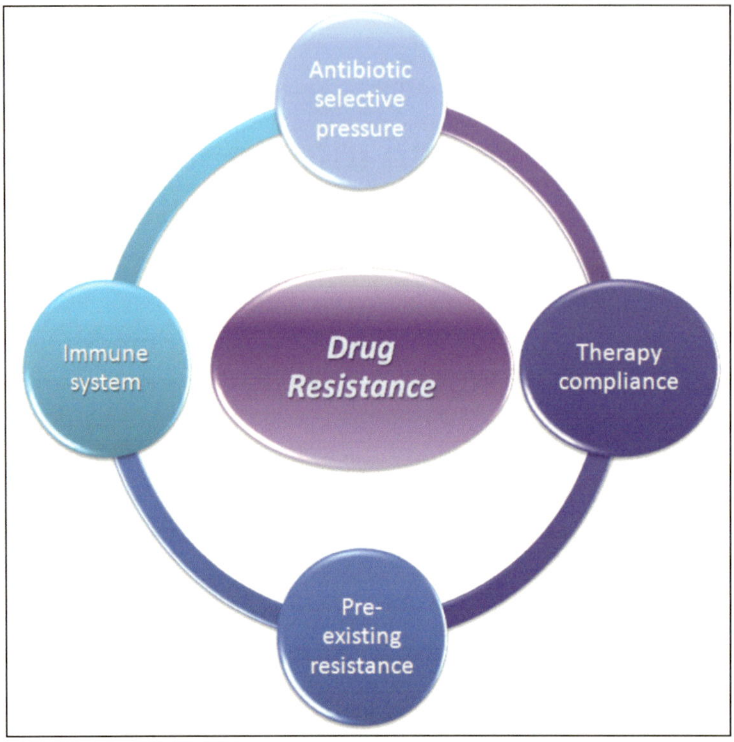

Fig. 1. Some causes of TB drug resistance.

The lack of therapy adherence is a serious problem to eliminate TB mainly in developing countries. Several aspects are related to this problem such as: adverse effects of TB drugs, long-term therapy, damage to certain organs (i.e. liver), lack of available drugs and co-morbidities.

Another important aspect to be considered in tuberculosis treatment is the unavailability of new drugs. The last discovery drug to TB was rifampicin in the 60's. Despite TB drug development efforts have emerged in the last years few advances were reached. Currently, there are some drugs, obtained by molecular modification, being evaluated in clinical trials. An ideal drug against TB must possess some characteristics that include: broad spectrum of action with possibility to be use in resistant strains; adequate pharmacokinetic profile increasing the concentration in some tissues target and reduce drug-drug interaction; adequate and shorten treatment duration reducing pill burden in order to reduce numbers of pills taken increasing the patients compliance (Koul et al, 2011).

The combination of all these factors discussed above makes difficult TB treatment. Not only strategies to discovery new drugs, but rational approach to improve the use of old drugs are essential to improve the efficacy of the treatment. This chapter aiming discusses some factors to improve medication efficacy in tuberculosis treatment. Some aspects of TB such as disease development, resistance and treatment will be discussed. Furthermore therapeutical aspects such as drug-drug interaction, patient compliance and some health interventions will be present.

TB Treatment

According to WHO new patients is recommended the treatment to receive a daily intensive phase of the two months of the isoniazid (H), rifampicin (R), pyrazinamid (P) and ethambutol (E); followed by 4 months for the maintenance phase of the H and R [2HRZE/4HR] (WHO, 2009). This treatment is highly efficient for the drug-susceptible TB patients, but, the questions is what about the latent and MDR (multi-drug resistant) or XDR (extremely drug-resistant) TB treatment?

Latent tuberculosis is individuals infected with M. tuberculosis but has no active disease. Although this state not is completely clear, there are two main hypothesis to explain this condition: 1) M. tuberculosis persists in a lazy state within granulomatous lesions, but periodically recrudesces; 2) the bacterium persisting in a dormant state resides within alveolar epithelial cells in the lung apices and adipocytes (Ma et al., 2010). Epidemiologically latent infection is responsible to contaminated 1/3 of the world population, and there is no specific treatment for it (Koul et al., 2011). However H has been used as preventive therapy (IPT) has long been known to markedly reduce the risk of reactivation of latent M. tuberculosis infection, but this affirmation not is completely proved and clear (Golub et al., 2008).

MDR-TB occurs when the TB mycobacteria are resistant to at least H, R and XDR-TB occur when the mycobacteria has the same resistant characteristic than MDR-TB plus resistant to any fluoroquinolone, and at least one of three injectable second-line drugs (capreomycin, kanamycin, and amikacin). The resistant bacteria are selected due to mainly to failure of the treatment. Failures attributed mainly to the desistance of treatment by the patient. To understand how the bacteria become resistant is not completely understood, but various biochemical pathways to escape the lethal action of drugs can be assigned: (i) decreased intracellular accumulation of the antibiotic by an alteration of outer membrane permeability, diminished transport across the inner membrane, (ii) alteration of the target by mutation or enzymatic modification; (iii) enzymatic detoxification of the drug; and (iv) bypass of the drug target. The coexistence of several of these mechanisms in the same host can lead to MDR and XDR-TB. (Piddock et al., 2006; De Rossi et al., 2006). Another important question that needs to be highlighted is the association of these biochemical resistant pathways with the efflux pump system. Efflux is a ubiquitous mechanism responsible for intrinsic and acquired drug resistance in prokaryotic and eukaryotic cells. M. tuberculosis presents one of the largest numbers of putative drug efflux pumps compared with its genome size. Antimicrobial resistance in an efflux mutant is due to one of two mechanisms: (i) expression of the efflux pump protein is increased or (ii) the protein contains an amino acid substitution(s) that makes the protein more efficient at export (Piddock, 2006).

MDR treatment, anti-TB drugs are grouped according to efficacy, experience of use and drug class. There are five groups and only the group 1 can receive the first line drugs, all others groups will receive the second-line drugs namely: kanamycin (Km), amikacin (Am), capreomycin (Cm), streptomycin (S), Levofloxacin (Lfx), Moxifloxacin (Mfx), Ofloxacin (Ofx), para-aminosalicylic acid (PAS), cycloserine (Cs), terizidone (Trd), ethionamide (Eto), protionamide (Pto), clofazimine (Cfz), linezolid (Lzd), amoxicillin/clavulanate (Amx/Clv), thioacetazone (Thz), imipenem/cilastatin (Ipm/Cln), clarithromycin (Clr) (WHO, 2009).

2. TB therapy problems

TB treatment presents several challenges to be overcome. The treatment abandonment is one of them which contribute to development of resistance by mycobacterium to available drugs. The abandonment or lack of adherence occurs when the patient does not attend to receive medication for a month or more (Pablós-Méndez et al., 1997). Several factors contribute to this situation such as socio-economic factors, adverse effects of drugs, co-morbidities, environmental factors (familiar, social behavior). In developing countries the access to adequate health system is one of the most problems to TB therapy. It is very common situation that the population has not medical service neither education level to comprehend the therapy. There is a relation between poverty and predisposition to disease difficult the TB control. Malnutrition, increased expensive to take medicines and stigmatization are some intrinsic factors related to the inadequate control of TB in poor countries (Cegielski & McMurray, 2004; Atre et al., 2009; Dhingra et al., 2010; WHO, 2005; Hargreaves et al., 2011). Educational levels and employment are conditions related to abandonment of therapy. It has been reported that a worker, provider of family without adequate financial support present high abandonment rate (64%). An interesting relation is also observed when someone analyses the educational level of the patients. Those which possess higher education (university) demonstrate high level of adherence despite those with low educational level. Low level of knowledge is directed relate to inadequate treatment (Grace & Chenhall, 2006). The Table 1 shows the main reasons related to treatment abandonment.

The adverse effect of antitubercular drugs is one the main causes of therapy abandonment. Some adverse effects of antitubercular drugs are described above:

Socio-economic	Worker, a provider of family, lack of financial sources for feeding and locomotion: 64% abandonment. Unemployed: 36% abandonment (finantial problems and low self steem) Education: illiteracy (20% abandonment), less than 8 years of study (72 % abandonment), between 8 and 12 years of study (8% abandonment) and more than 13 years (0% abandonment).
Therapeutical	Adverse effects relate to antitubercular drugs: nausea, vomiting, hyperthermia and edema. Denial and oblivion. Regimens: - 2 months: R/I/P + 4 months R/I = 88% abandonment; - 6 months: S/P/E/Et = 8% abandonment; - 6 months S/I/Et = 4% abandonment. R – rifampicin; I – isoniazid; P- pyrazinamide; S- streptomycin; E – ethambutol; Et – ethionamide.

Disease related problems	Non-acceptance of diagnosis, riot with the illness. No knowledge of the existence of extra-pulmonary forms. No symptoms after initial treatment interpreted by patients as a cure (Uplekar et al 2001).
Health related problems	Fractures, improvement of symptoms, mental Illness; Hepatitis (do not show tolerance to treatment); *Patients with co-morbidity* Diabetes / TB = TB infections have more severe, with treatment failure rate of 8.5 x higher, which generates most abandoned, because this patient needs a longer treatment (Gupta et al, 2011). HIV / TB: The patient focuses on the treatment of HIV, at least tolerate the associated treatment. It is discouraged when after diagnosis of HIV, or vice versa (53% abandonment).
Familiar	Death and other diseases in the family, motivation, recommendation to stop (by others); Living away from family; Overpopulation in a single family home (sleeping more than two in same bed); Absence of familiar support.
Social behavior and sex	An anthropological phenomenon is observed with male younger, unmarried and/or separated which seek to preserve their particular way of life believing that they are not susceptible to TB disease. This group has not a tendency to modify some habits to contribute for the TB treatment during the 6 months of treatment (Gonçalves et al., 1999).
Risk groups	A community in contact with contagious TB or focus intra-household is recommended prophylaxis with isoniazid, however, is not accepted by individuals. Typically, these individuals end up contaminating and seek treatment lately; Alcoholic: 24% abandonment; Smokers: 40% (Mendes & Fensterseifer, 2004) 48.8% (Christmas 1997) abandoned; Drinker and smoker: 86.6% abandonment (Lima et al., 2001); Drug addict: 12% abandonment;
Others	Patient does not trust in the treatment, doctors or the health system itself. Wait for the health service; Distance from health service; System health bureaucracy.

Table 1. Main reasons related to treatment abandonment.

- Isoniazid: Peripheral neuritis (prevent with the use of pyridoxine); may occur again, optic neuritis, ataxia, mental disturbances and incoordination. Hypersensitivity to isoniazid can cause fever, various skin rashes, hepatitis and skin rashes, hematologic reactions may occur (agranulocytosis, eosinophilia, thrombocytopenia, anemia); neuritis and optic atrophy. Twitches, dizziness, ataxia, paresthesias, numbness, toxic encephalopathy are other manifestations of neurotoxicity of isoniazid. It may also appear several mental abnormalities. May precipitate seizures in patients with previous history of seizures.
- Rifampicin: Facial flushing, generalized itching and skin rash, purpura, epistaxis, menorrhagia, gingival bleeding and hemolytic anemia. Pseudogripal syndrome with fever, malaise, headache, chills and myalgia, which may progress to interstitial nephritis, acute tubular necrosis, thrombocytopenia and shock. In the digestive tract: Malaise, loss of appetite, nausea, vomiting, jaundice, liver failure and diarrhea.
- Pirazinamide: Liver damage with elevation of plasmatic AST and ALT is the main adverse effect. Furthermore it is observed arthralgia, anorexia, nausea and vomiting, dysuria, malaise and fever.
- Ethambutol: The observed adverse reactions include itching, joint pain, gastrointestinal disorders, abdominal pain, malaise, headache, dizziness, mental confusion, disorientation and possible hallucinations, acute gout or hyperuricemia. Although rare the peripheral neuritis and retrobulbar optic neuritis (blurred vision, eye pain, red-gray images, decreased vision) are reported. The retrobulbar optic neuritis is dose-dependent, occurring more frequently with daily doses of 25 mg / kg and after two months of therapy, in many cases is reversible after several weeks or several months.

In general, the adverse effects related to first line antitubercular drugs include skin rash, itch, nausea and vomiting, thrombocytopenia, symptoms influenza-símile, arthralgias and neuropsychiatric manifestations (Yee et al., 2003; Fekih et al., 2011; Fountain et al., 2005).

It has been reported that the rate of adverse effects during the treatment could reach 30% of the patients or 7,3 per 100 patients/month. Therapy with four drugs increase the incidence to 23,3 events by 100-patients/month. In addition, the adverse effects are used to appear during the first 100 days of treatment and the most common effects observed were hepatitis (28%), gastrointestinal disorders (19%), skin rash (15%), weakness or tiredness (7%) and joint pain (6%) (Yee et al., 2003).

The hepatotoxicity is a deleterious adverse effect responsible to determine changes in therapy. TB first line drugs such as rifampicin, rifabutin, isoniazid and pyrazinamide can cause hepatotoxicity, alone isoniazid is responsible to 20% of reported cases. The combination of drugs increases the probability to develop hepatotoxicity. Risk factors such as HIV co-infection, hepatitis B and/or C, alcohol abuse or the use of some medicines (i.e. anticonvulsant) should be taken in consideration due the due to the increased likelihood of causing liver toxicity.

In situation which patients present previous diagnosis of advance liver disease, when the doctor wants to keep only one hepatotoxic drug, rifampicin is usually selected. However, other agents should be added the therapy such as fluorquinolone, cycloserine and aminoglycoside. The treatment time of these schemes can vary from 12-18 months (American Thoracic Society, 2003).

It is important to note that the assessment of adverse effects should be performed throughout therapy, and compared with pre-treatment parameters. The patient should be prepared to identify adverse effects related to the use of anti-TB drugs.

Environment factors are determinants for TB treatment. The family has a crucial role to the treatment. The knowledge of the disease by all familiar members is an important factor to control TB. After the first phase of the treatment, when some symptoms decrease, is common identify problems with adherence by patients. So, educational interventions by health professionals are important to improve the TB treatment management. Some studies demonstrated that previous cases in the family increase the knowledge and the adherence by patients (Costa et al., 2011). However, some factors such live away from family, absence of familiar support and overpopulation in a single family home (with more than two people sleeping in the same bed) is a risk factor to abandon TB treatment.

Gender is another factor relate to TB. Worldwide, more men than women are diagnosed with TB. This higher TB notification in men is relate to epidemiological differences such as risk of exposure, infection and progression to disease. However, it has been reported that women have higher case of fatalities in the early reproductive ages and higher rates of progression from infection to disease (Holmes et al., 1998).

The association of TB with co-morbidities is a complicated factors related to increase of adverse effects and high rate of abandonment treatment by patients. It has been reported that treatment fail is increased 8.5 times in diabetic patients with TB, general relate to abandonment. In diabetic group infection with TB seems to be more severe that in people no-diabetic (Gupta et al., 2011).

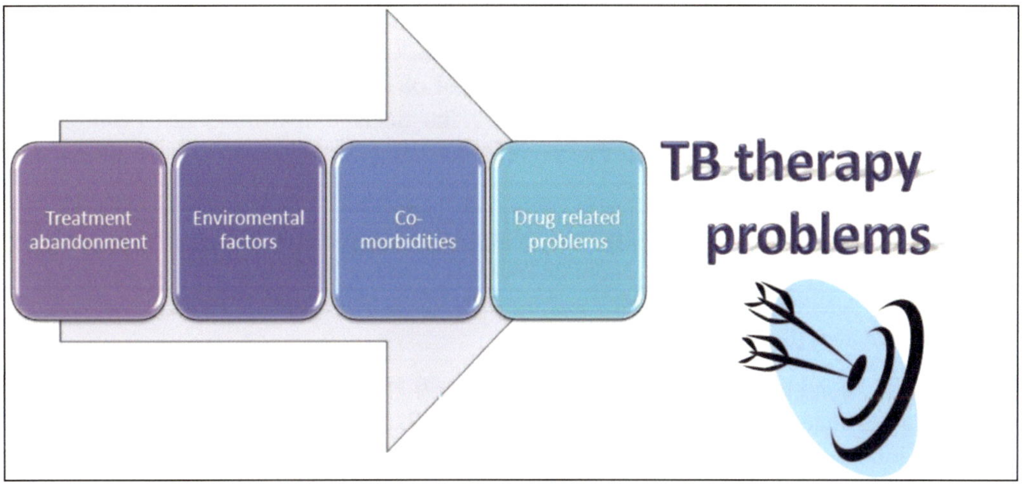

Fig. 2. Some TB therapy problems.

The abandonment of HIV co-infection patients could reach 53% (Table 1). The recommended TB treatment of HIV-negative people is the same of HIV-positive people but sometimes the therapy is extended to 9 months or more in patients with extra-pulmonar TB. However, some management of the therapy is complicated due to paradoxical reaction, drug interactions and the difficulty to ingest a large number of tablets (Yew, 2002). The paradoxical reactions, is an exacerbation of TB symptoms, due to due to immune recovery, called immune reconstitution syndrome. Although the mechanism is not totally clear it is presumed to represent an interaction between the host responses and effects produced by mycobacterial products leading to inflammatory lesions (Orlovic & Smego, 2001). Some symptoms include restart or worsening of fever, lymphadenopathy, dyspnea, worsening of brain injury (Navas et al., 2002).

3. Anti-TB drug interactions

Concurrent treatment of TB and HIV is associated with a higher risk of adverse reactions compared to treatment of either infection alone. The first-line anti-TB drugs isoniazid, rifampin, and pyrazinamide may each cause hepatotoxicity, which may be compounded by concomitant use of protease inhibitors (PI) and nonnucleoside reverse transcriptase inhibitors (NRTI). Pharmacokinetic interactions between HIV and TB regimens can have a significant impact on the therapeutic efficacy of each regimen.

Rifamycin antibiotics, the main drug in TB therapy induce the synthesis of drug metabolizing enzymes (cytochrome P450 emzyme system, particulary the CYP 3A4, CYP 2C8/9 isoenzymes and to a lesser extent CYP2C19 and CYPD6 isozymes; the rifamycins vary in their potential as CYP450 inducers. Potency of induction: Rifampin > rifapentine > rifabutin. Rifampin also upregulates the synthesis of cytosolic drug-metabolizing enzymes, including glucuronosyl transferase, an enzyme involved in the metabolism of zidovudine and raltegravir. Potent induction of the cytochrome p450 system by rifampin can lead to subtherapeutic levels of the protease inhibitors accompanied by virological failure

Antiretroviral treatment (ART) improves survival in co-infected TB patients and vice-versa, however, these concomitant drug therapy in the early stage can increase risk of paradoxal TB- immune reconstitution inflammatory syndrome, risk of overlapping drug toxicities with possibility in drug treatment interruption, high pill burden that can impact in adherence and increased potential drug-drug interactions. The delayed treatment can promote the advancing immunosuppression and the development of others opportunist conditions that may increase mortality.

The estimated cumulative probability to develop an adverse event was significantly higher in HIV/TB co-infected in Ruanda patients: 20.9% within the first month of antituberculous treatment (vs. 3.0% in HIV-uninfected) and up to 29.9% at two months of treatment (vs. 6.9% in HIV-uninfected) (Gordin et al., 1996)

Rifamycin is related to interact with four classes of anti-HIV drugs (protease inhibitors, non-nucleoside reverse-transcriptase inhibitors [NNRTI], CCR5-receptor antagonistis and integrase inhibitors. Zidovudine, the nucleoside analogues and enfuvirtide do not have significant interactions with rifamycins.

The initial ATR regimens in areas with high rates of TB use efavirenz (in combination with nucleoside analogues), because of its potency and durability on randomized clinical trials.

The co-adminstration rifampin decrease plasma concentration of efavirenz but not in a significant way. Some expertise suggested an increase of efavirenz to 800 mg in TB/HIV concomitant treatment to patients weighing more than 60 kg (WHO guidelines). However, Cohen and Meinttjes (2010), do not recommend these proceedings based on the fact that the CYP 450 2B6 516 G>T polymorphism, which impairs the function of the primary pathway of efavirenz metabolism (2B6) is present in African populations. So, the consequence of even

		Cmax	AUC	Cmin	
nevirapine + **RIFAMPIN**	Decrease plasma Concentration Caution: Sub-therapeutic dosage found	↓50%	↓58%	↓68%	The standard dose of neveriapine should be used among patients taking rifampin (200 mg daily for 2 weeks, followed by 200 mg twice daily *Increasing nevirapine dose by 50% to 300 mg twice/daily would achieve therapeutic concentration but safety has not been adequately explored as a routine clinical practice and my result in hypersensivity reactions.
nevirapine + **RIFABUTIN**	Not significant changes in plasma concentration				300 mg rifabutin daily or thrice weekly **no changes recommended**
Efavirenz + **RIFAMPIN**	not significant decrease plasma concentration	↓24%	↓25%	↓22%	Rifampin 600 mg once/day 200 mg efanvirenz twice/day No changes recommended
	Increase clinical toxicity : anxiety, depression, hepatitis (mainly in African descendent) * efavirenz has been associated with hepatotoxicity during postmarketing use. **-co-administration of drugs with caution**: drugs that induces liver damages such as acetaminophen, kava-kava, statins, metformin				(600 mg once daily) in combination with an anti-TB regimen containing rifampin (480 to 720 mg/day based on body weight) for 7 days

Efavirenz + RIFABUTIN	↓rifabutin plasma concentration		↓ 38%		**Recommendation:** ↑ to 450-600 mg of rifabutin (daily or intermittent)
Delavirdine + RIFAMPIN	Strongly ↓ delavirdine plasma concentration **NOT RECOMMEND CONCOMITANT USE**	↓90%,	↓97%	↓100%	rifampin (600 mg once daily for 15 days) ↓ plasma concentration of delavirdine (400 mg 3x/ day for 30 days)
Delavirdine + RIFABUTIN	Strongly ↓ delavirdine plasma concentration and ↑rifabutin concentration by 100% (AUC) **NOT RECOMMEND CONCOMITANT USE**	↓72%	↓82%	↓94%	300 mg once daily for 15 days
Etravirine + **RIFAMPIN**	Strongly ↓ etravirine plasma concentration **NOT RECOMMEND CONCOMITANT USE**				Predicted (etravirine is a substrate of CYP450 2C19, 2C9, and 3A4).
	The risk of peripheral neuropathy may be increased during concurrent use of two or more agents that are associated with this adverse effect. In some cases, the neuropathy may progress or become irreversible despite discontinuation of the medications				**+ ETHABUTOL + ISONIAZIDE (same effect can be observed when use ethambutol + isoniazide only)**

Etravirine + **RIFAMPIN**	**+ food**		↓50%		Food increase bioavailabitily of etravirine (unknown mechanism, but ranging from 345 kilocalories containing 17 grams fat to 1160 kilocalories containing 70 grams fat did not impact on etravirine bioavailability
Etravirine + **RIFABUTIN**	Decrease etravirine Cmin			↓ 45%	No clinical experience. (300 mg rifabutin daily or 3 x weekly) **No changes recommended**
Atazanavir * + **RIFAMPIN**	Strongly ↓ atazanavir plasma concentration **NOT RECOMMEND CONCOMITANT USE**		↓95%		* with etravirine may ↓ atazanavir, with or without low-dose ritonavir as a pharmacokinetic booster. The mechanism is etravirine induction of CYP450 3A4, the isoenzyme responsible for the metabolic clearance of atazanavir and other protease inhibitors
Atazanavir + RIFABUTIN	Increase rifabutin plasma concentration		↑250%		Recommendation: ↓ribatutin dose to 150 mg/ day or 3 x week
	+ food **Recommendation:** To ensure maximal oral absorption of atazanavir, it should be administered with or immediately after a meal	↑57%	↑70%		administration with a light meal ↑increased AUC of a single 400 mg dose of atazanavir relative to the fasting state.
Fos-amprenavir + **RIFAMPIN**	Strongly decrease fosamprenavir plasma concentration – NOT RECOMMEND CONCOMITANT USE		↓75-95%		the mechanism is rifampin induction of CYP450 3A4, the isoenzyme responsible for the metabolic clearance of PIs.

Fos-amprenavir + RIFABUTIN	Increase significantly rifabutin plasma and 25-) desacetylrifabutin in 7.39 fold(Cmax) 13.35 fold (AUC) 32.9 fold (Cmin) **Use with caution**	↑119%	↑193%	↑271%	The mechanism is amprenavir inhibition of CYP450 3A4, the isoenzyme responsible for the metabolic clearance of rifabutin and 25-O-desacetylrifabutin **Recommendation:** ↓ribatutin dose to 150 mg/day or 3 x week
saquinavir /indinavir or nelfinavir + RIFAMPIN	Strongly decrease of protease inhibitors (PIs) plasma concentration **NOT RECOMMEND CONCOMITANT USE**		↓75% to 95%		The mechanism is rifampin induction of CYP450 3A4, the isoenzyme responsible for the metabolic clearance of PIs.
Indinavir + RIFABUTIN	↑ RIFABUTIN concentration and ↓ indinavir by 34%		↑170%		**Recommendation:** ↓ribatutin dose to 150 mg/day or 3 x week
nelfinavir + RIFABUTIN	↑ RIFABUTIN concentration		↑207%		Not significant change in nelfinavir concentration. **Recommendation:** ↓ribatutin dose to 150 mg/day or 3 x week.
Ritonavir + RIFAMPIN	**Use with caution**		↓35%		no change in rifampin concentration (600 mg/day) rifampin will decrease the level or effect of ritonavir by P-glycoprotein (MDR1) efflux transporter **Recommedantion:** Monitor for antiretroviral activity of ritonavir
Ritonavir + saquinavir + RIFAMPIN	Hepatotoxicity. Transaminase elevations up to or even exceeding 20 times the upper limit of normal.(38 %) **Use with caution**				Drug-induced hepatitis with marked ↑ transaminase has been observed in healthy volunteers receiving rifampin 600 mg once daily with ritonavir 100 mg and saquinavir 1000 mg twice daily (i.e., ritonavir-boosted saquinavir). The mechanism has not been described.

Ritonavir + lopinavir + rifampin	Hepatotoxicity. **Use with caution**				Lopinavir / ritonavir– 2 tablets (200 mg of lopinavir with 50 mg of ritonavir) + 300 mg of ritonavir twice-daily + 600 mg rifampin/day Have favorable pharmacokinetic and clinical data among young children
Ritonavir + lopinavir + rifampin	Rifampin decrease plasma concentration of lopinavir **Use with caution:**				Increase the dose of lopinavir / ritonavir to 4 tablets (200 mg of lopinavir with 50 mg of ritonavir) twice-daily. This combination resulted in hepatitis in all adult healthy volunteers in an initial study.
Ritonavir + lopinavir Rifabutin	↑ RIFABUTIN and 25-o-desacetil rifabutin (47,5 fold) concentration		303%		**Recommendation**: ↓ribatutin dose to 150 mg/day or 3 x week
atazanavir/ tipranavir or darunavir + ritonavir + rifampin	Rifampin strongly decrease of protease inhibitors (PIs) plasma concentration – **NOT RECOMMEND CONCOMITANT USE**				The mechanism is rifampin induction of CYP450 3A4, the isoenzyme responsible for the metabolic clearance of PIs.
Ritonavir + saquinavir/indinavir/amprenavir/fos - amprenavir/ atazanavir/tipranavir or darunavir + RIFABUTIN	↑ RIFABUTIN and 25-o-desacetil rifabutin concentration (varyng degreee)				**Recommendation:** ↓ribatutin dose to 150 mg/day or 3 x week

Maraviroc + rifampin	↓ maraviroc plasma concentration	↓66%	↓63%	↓ 78%	No clinical experience with increased dose of maraviroc + rifampin Recommendation: no changes in rifampin dose (600 mg/day)
Maraviroc + rifampin	Patients with severe renal impairment or end-stage renal disease (CrCl <30 mL/min) given maraviroc may have an increased risk of postural hypotension due to increased maraviroc exposure. Moreover, these patients often have cardiovascular comorbidities that could predispose them to adverse cardiovascular events triggered by postural hypotension.				No studies have been performed in subjects with severe renal impairment or ESRD co-treated with maraviroc and potent CYP450 3A4 inducers. Hence, no dosage recommendation for maraviroc is available for these patients.
Maraviroc + rifabutin	Not studied				
Raltegravir + rifampin	↓ **Raltegravir** plasma concentration		↓ 40-61%		No clinical experience with increased dose of raltegravir + rifampin Recommendation: no changes in rifampin dose (600 mg/day)
Raltegravir + rifabutin	No studied				
Isoniazid + indinavir	↑		↑13%		The mechanism probably is competitive inhibition of isoniazid metabolism **Recommendation:** monitor isoniazide-related toxicity

Isoniazid + lopinavir	The magnitude and clinical significance of this interaction are unknown				Coadministration with inhibitors of CYP450 3A4 may increase the plasma concentrations of lopinavir, which is metabolized by the isoenzyme
Streptomycin + tenofovir	Coadministration of tenofovir with other nephrotoxic agents may increase the risk and severity of renal impairment due to additive effects on the kidney. Additionally, renal impairment secondary to the use of these agents may reduce the clearance of tenofovir, which is primarily eliminated by renal excretion.				the risk is low in patients with adequate renal function receiving the normally recommended dosage but may increase in patients with underlying renal impairment
Zidovudine + rifampin	↓ zidovudine plasma concentration not significantly rifabutin also reportedly decreased zidovudine AUC by 32% and increased its clearance by 43%				rifampin (600 mg orally once a day for 14 days) recomemmendation Monitor for antiretroviral activity of zidovudine

Table 2. Antitubercular Drug Interactions.

No changes were observed when use nevirapine and rifabutin. Others some important considerations area presented below:

TB/HIV treatment need to avoid co-administration: with potent inducers of CYP450 isoenzymes such as carbamazepine, phenobarbital, phenytoin, rifampin and rifapentine due the risk of reduced viral susceptibility and resistance development associated with sub-therapeutic antiretroviral drug levels.

The use of tenofovir in HIV/TB need avoid the co-administration: with other potentially nephrotoxic agents (e.g., aminoglycosides; polypeptide, glycopeptide, and polymyxin antibiotics; amphotericin B; adefovir; cidofovir; foscarnet; cisplatin; deferasirox; gallium nitrate; lithium; mesalazine; certain immunosuppressants; intravenous bisphosphonates; intravenous pentamidine; high intravenous dosages of methotrexate; high dosages and/or chronic use of nonsteroidal anti-inflammatory agents. Renal function should be evaluated prior to and during therapy with tenofovir. Patients with renal insufficiency at baseline or during treatment may require dosage adjustment in accordance with the manufacturer's product labeling.

The use of efavirenz in HIV/TB need avoid the co-administration: with potentially hepatotoxicity agents: pyrazinamide, isoniazid, acetaminophen; alcohol; androgens and anabolic steroids; azole antifungal agents; ACE inhibitors; endothelin receptor antagonists; interferons; other nucleoside reverse transcriptase inhibitors; retinoids; thiazolidinediones; anticonvulsants such as carbamazepine, hydantoins, felbamate, and valproic acid; lipid-lowering medications such as fenofibrate, HMG-CoA reductase inhibitors, and niacin; herbals and nutritional supplements such as chaparral, comfrey, DHEA, kava, pennyroyal oil, and red yeast rice. Patients should be advised to seek medical attention if they experience potential signs and symptoms of hepatotoxicity such as fever, rash, itching, anorexia, nausea, vomiting, fatigue, right upper quadrant pain, dark urine, light-colored stools, and jaundice. Monitoring of liver function should occur before and during treatment, especially in patients with other hepatic disease (including hepatitis B or C co-infection) or marked transaminase elevations. The benefit of continued therapy with efavirenz should be considered against the unknown risks of significant liver toxicity in patients who develop persistent elevations of serum transaminases greater than five times the upper limit of normal.

The use of tenofovir in HIV/TB treatment with streptomycin: Caution for renal function impairment due to additive effects on the kidney. The deleterious effect on the kindney can occur with concomitant use of others nephrotoxic drugs such as aminoglycosides; polypeptide, glycopeptide, and polymyxin antibiotics; amphotericin B; adefovir; cidofovir; foscarnet; cisplatin; deferasirox; gallium nitrate; lithium; mesalamine; certain immunosuppressants; intravenous bisphosphonates; intravenous pentamidine; high intravenous dosages of methotrexate; high dosages and/or chronic use of nonsteroidal anti-inflammatory agents. Renal function should be evaluated prior to and during therapy. Patients with renal insufficiency at baseline or during treatment may require dosage adjustment in accordance with the manufacturer's product labeling.

The use of maraviroc in HIV/TB treatment with rifampin and others CYP 450 3A4 inhibitors: maraviroc should be administered at a dosage of 600 mg twice daily during coadministration with potent CYP450 3A4 inducers such as efavirenz, rifampin, carbamazepine, phenobarbital, and phenytoin. However, if a potent CYP450 3A4 inhibitor such as itraconazole, ketoconazole, delavirdine, clarithromycin, telithromycin, nefazodone, or any protease inhibitor (except tipranavir + ritonavir) is also used in combination with the inducer, then maraviroc dosage should be reduced to 150 mg twice daily. Maraviroc is contraindicated for use in combination with potent CYP450 3A4 inducers in patients with severe renal impairment or end-stage renal disease (CrCl <30 mL/min).

The use of Isoniazid in HIV/TB treatment with ritonavir/lopinavir and others PIs: The isoniazid will increase the level or effect of PIs by affecting hepatic/intestinal enzyme CYP3A4 metabolism. Avoid co-administration with others inhibitors of the hepatic/intestinal enzyme CYP3A4 metabolism such as macrolide antibiotics, itraconazole, ketoconazole, nefazodone, fluconazole, verapamil, diltiazen, grapefruit juice.

Isoniazid + ethambutol: increase the risk of peripheral neuropathy: burning, tingling, pain, or numbness in the hands and feet

Isoniazid + rifampin/rifabutin: The risk of hepatotoxicity is greater when rifampin and isoniazid are given concomitantly than when either drug is given alone. Rifampin alters the metabolism of isoniazid and increase the amount of toxic metabolites. Similar reaction may occur with rifabutin and isoniazid. Patients who are elderly, have hepatic impairment, are slow acetylators of isoniazid, drink alcohol daily, are female, or are taking other CYP450-inducing agents may be at greater risk of hepatotoxicity. Recommend the monitoring for clinical or laboratory evidence of hepatic function during the treatment. Discontinuation of either or both drugs may be necessary when simptoms of hepatite such as fatigue, weakness, malaise, anorexia, nausea, or vomiting appears.

Isoniazid + food: Food significantly reduces isoniazid absorption, increasing the risk of therapeutic failure or resistance. The mechanism is unknown. In addition, the ingestion of certain histamine-rich fish (e.g., tuna) and cheeses during isoniazid therapy may cause a flushing reaction in some patients. The proposed mechanism is inhibition of monoamine oxidase and histaminase by isoniazid, resulting in histamine intoxication. The associated symptoms is: flushing, tachycardia, chills, headache, nausea, vomiting, diarrhea, burning sensation, sweating, or shortness of breath after eating certain foods. Isoniazid cause depletion of B6 vitamin during the treatment. Since HIV-infected persons are at increased risk for isoniazid-induced peripheral neuropathy, these patients should take vitamin B6 and avoid antiretroviral drugs with potential peripheral neurotoxicity (e.g., stavudine and didanosine).

4. Adherence to therapy – Process to improve medication efficacy

It has been reported that treatment abandonment rate reaches until 25% of all patients during the treatment (Veronesi & Focaccia, 1996). In developing countries such as Brazil, this rates decreased in the last years to 4,5%, but it is possible to find out in some regions values until 20,3% (Costa, Gonçalves & Menezes, 1998; Lima et al., 2001). The WHO's recommendation is that abandonment rates must be until 5%, however, it is possible to find in some countries such as Colombia abandonment rates of 65,6% (Mateus-Solarte & Carvajal-Barona, 2008).

In order to reduce the abandonment of therapy and ensure the correct treatment of patients some strategies have been adopted to improve adherence to therapy. According to WHO "Adherence corresponds to the behavior of one person - in terms of taking a drug, a diet or executing lifestyle changes - that is in accordance with recommendations arising from health professionals" (WHO, 2003).

Adherence to therapy is a serious problem responsible for the evolution of diseases and complications, loss of quality of life and even death. In the United States it is estimated that the cost of low compliance reach over $ 147 billion (Council on Patient Information and Education, 2007). WHO estimate that rate of adherence of patients which treat chronic diseases is only 50% (WHO, 2003). These same values were found in a study with TB patients (Cuneo, 1989).

Literature reports show that interventions to promote adherence are effective in short treatments, but these same interventions are less effective in prolonged treatments. In the latter situation it requires a combination of strategies, becoming more complex the interventions performed by health professionals (Haynes et al., 2009).

Several methods are available in the literature to assess adherence to treatment. These methods can be divided into direct and indirect. In direct methods is possible to quantify the drug in the body. These methods are expensive, invasive and not available for all drugs, however are suitable methods to say whether or not adherence to therapy allowing include adjust the dose. The indirect methods allow assessing the use of medicines by health professionals. These methods are usually overestimated and with low sensitivity. Among the indirect methods can include: patient's self-report; prescriber's report; pill count; measurement of prescription replacement (allowing indirect evaluation of non-compliance by the lack of access to medication). Strategies using devices of separation and counting of medicines may be useful for patients who do not understand the regimen. These devices can be purchased at pharmacies and separate properly in accordance with the therapy the patient by the pharmacist.

However, in the therapy of tuberculosis, one of the strategies most used and recommended by the World Health Organization (WHO) treatment involves supervised therapy (DOTS - Directly Observed Therapy). DOTS strategy includes the delivery of a short course of standard drugs, lasting 6 months for new Patients (and 8 months for retreatment Patients). The delivery includes the direct observation of therapy (DOT), either by a health worker or by caregiver (WHO, 2002).

During the promotion of strategies to increase adherence is important to consider some factors related to therapy adherence that may be related to: patient, health professional, the disease condition, treatment and health care system (and the policies government).

With regard to the patient an important strategy to be adopted is empowerment. This strategy is an educational intervention that aims to transfer responsibilities to patients which is tone of the most important person responsible to conduct the therapy, based in the principle that the decision to follow or not the treatment is only taken by the patient. The patient must know about the disease and treatment to participate in the process of using the medicine. Factors such as social stigma are common in patients with tuberculosis, however, this factor must be worked in the intervention. Economic factors and access to health services are factors that also interfere with the patient's decision to adhere to therapy or not.

With regard to health professionals, active participation is required in treating patients, because is often the situation that them cannot understand the proper way to use the anti-tubercular drugs. The treatment cannot be seen as the sole responsibility of the patient. Health professionals have a large portion of the contribution of adherence to treatment. With regard to health status, disease severity and the observation of improvement with the medicines use is important for maintenance adherence. In situations where the goal of therapy is not immediately improve the main symptoms, should be established an accord with the patients which should be aware of the goals of therapy. Treatment should be simplified to suit the patient's situation. Complex dosing regimens tend have higher dropout rates. The health system has an important role in the adherence. Access to professional and medicines is a determining factor for treatment. There is no possibility to discuss adherence even if the patients do not have access to health care. In this case, it is essential to adopt policies to control diseases such as tuberculosis ensuring access to the entire population.

Several strategies have been described in the literature to promote adherence to therapy. Educational interventions may involve pedagogical strategies (oral or written) aiming increase the knowledge. This strategy can be used individually or collectively. The uses of written or audiovisual materials help the patient to understand the strategy.

Behavioral interventions aimed changing certain habits. They are guided by theories about behavior change. In these strategies the role of health professionals is essential in promoting adherence. This one can work with combinations of rewards and communication strategies, such as reminders to join the proposed therapy. Praise for the efforts is the reward commonly used. The possibility of monitoring the condition at home is also very useful and enables patient involvement in the action plan proposed.

Interventions with affective character take into account social relationships and may be done with the patient or the family. Family visits provide a good opportunity for this type of intervention. The professional can intervene, in educational way, with all the family doing them to understand the situation and help the patient. In TB intervention the combination of strategies seems to be more appropriate to increase therapy adherence.

5. Pharmacotherapeutic monitoring

Some care should be taken into account in monitoring patients for tuberculosis to detect adverse effects or ineffective therapy since the beginning of treatment. After 3 months of treatment, most patients (90-95%) will have negative smears (American Thoracic Society, 2003). Thus, situations of therapeutical inefficacy will be characterized with smear-positive after this period. Among factors responsible for ineffective treatment can be mentioned: bacterial resistance, poor absorption of drugs, inadequate adherence to treatment and drug interactions (Figure 3).

Some adverse effects such as peripheral neuritis induced by isoniazid can be prevented by supplementation with vitamin B6 (pyridoxine). This approach should be considered in special situations such as malnutrition, pregnancy, HIV co-infection and alcohol abuse.

Monitoring liver function is especially important for patients with any risk factor. About 20% of patients will have elevated levels of liver transaminases without symptoms. In such cases, after treatment the enzymes return to levels considered normal. Hepatitis should be suspected only when the elevation of transaminases is three to five times higher than considered normal associated with symptoms such as nausea, vomiting and abdominal pain. Some risk factors for hepatotoxicity are: chronic liver disease or hepatitis, alcohol abuse, use of isoniazid, female, HIV infection, low body mass index and age over 60 years

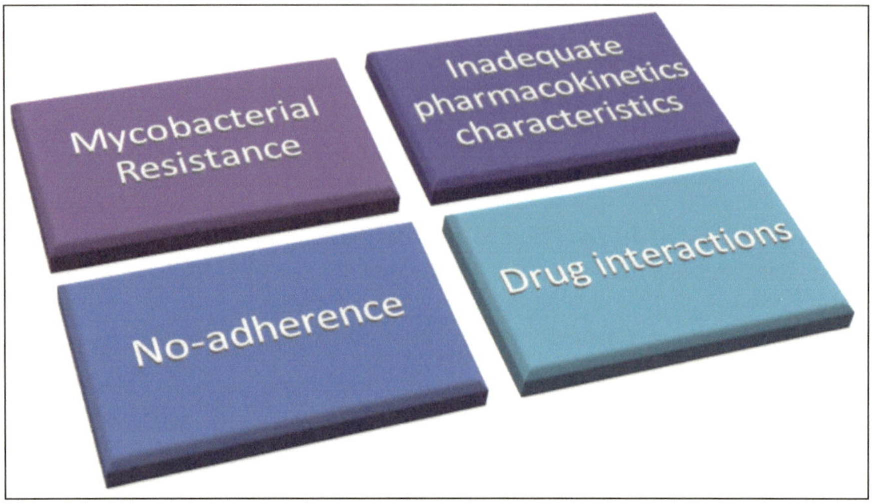

Fig. 3. Some factors responsible to inefficacy.

The action plan for monitoring patients with hepatotoxicity during the treatment includes withdrawal of all medicines. After the reduction of transaminases levels, reintroduction of individual drug must be re-thinking. It is recommended to start treatment with rifampicin (less hepatotoxic), and between 3-7 days to introduce a new drug. Treatment regimens without isoniazid are possible. In this last case, one possibility is treating the patient with rifampicin, ethambutol and pyrazinamide for six months.

Drug interactions should be identified and prevented. Beyond the hepatotoxic effect already discussed, some antituberculosis drugs like rifampicin are metabolic enzymatic inducers and may interfere with the metabolism of many drugs. One example is the oral contraceptive whose effectiveness can be compromised with concomitant use of rifampicin. In these situations alternative reproductive control methods should be used. Isoniazid may increase serum levels of drugs of narrow therapeutic index such as theophylline used by asthma patients.

Regimen that includes rifabutin is generally preferred, as rifabutin appears to be as effective as rifampin but is a much less potent inducer of CYP450 3A4. Non rifamycin-containing regimens is related to higher rates of treatment relapse and failure; longer treatment duration with increased adverse effects and higher mortality rates. This regimen is only recommended to patients who are intolerant of rifamycins or are infected with rifamycin-resistant strains.

Usual dosages of rifampin may be used in patients receiving ritonavir 600 mg twice/day or ritonavir 400 mg twice/day in combination with another PI at reduced dosage (e.g., saquinavir 400 mg twice/ day). If the patients have not begun antiretroviral therapy at the time TB treatment is initiated, clinicians may also consider using rifampin and postponing ATR therapy, because in the early HIV stage of the disease, there is low risk of HIV disease progression or death. During this period the physician may monitor CD4 cell count and postpone antiretroviral therapy until TB treatment is complete. However, the optimal time for starting ATR therapy should be individualized based on initial response to TB treatment and occurrence of adverse effects such as IRIS.

A patient who cannot take efavirenz, and when rifabutin is not available, the alternative is nevirapine - with rifampin. The pharmacokinetic effect of the rifamycin is moderate in this regimen. When used with isoniazid, rifampin, and pyrazinamide, there is some concern about hepatotoxicity. However, given the risk of reduced viral susceptibility and resistance development associated with subtherapeutic antiretroviral drug levels of nevirapine, some experts recommend that alternative antimycobacterial agents be considered in patients already receiving effective nevirapine-containing antiretroviral therapy.

Other alternatives for patients who cannot take efavirenz, and when rifabutin is not available, are as follows: rifampin with a) zidovudine/lamivudine/abacavir/tenofovir treatment; b) zidovudine/lamivudine/tenofovir or c) zidovudine/lamivudine/abacavir. The toxicity of these alternative regimens is primarily anemia. Pharmacokinetic concerns are a 50% decrease in zidovudine and the effect on abacavir is not yet evaluated. For the treatment of latent TB infection, a nine-month regimen of isoniazid may be considered.

In general, treatment of TB /HIV in the context of ATR therapy is complex and requires an individualized approach. Experts in the treatment of HIV-related tuberculosis should be consulted, and TB and HIV care providers should work in close coordination throughout the best treatment considering patient quality of life.

Additional care should be conducted with patients who have resistant infection. To decrease the resistance some principles should be adopted: a) the scheme more effective should be adopted, b) the therapeutic regimen should include at least three antimycobacterial drugs, c) the treatment should be daily and preferably monitorate by health professional and d) medicines should not be left for possible "future use".

In situations of resistance to isoniazid, one possibility is the use of rifampicin, pyrazinamide, ethambutol (and some fluoroquinolone) for a period of 6 months. For resistance to rifampicin and isoniazid regimen can be use fluoroquinolone, pyrazinamide and ethambutol associated with some other drug for a period of 18-24 months. In situations of resistance to rifampin, isoniazid, pyrazinamide (or ethambutol) the scheme would be to use a fluoquinolone (ethambutol or pyrazinamide depending on the susceptibility) and two alternative agents for a period of 24 months.

In cases of latent infection, correctly detected, should be assessed the risk and benefit of treatment. People living with HIV, immunocompromised, malnourished, drug users and from endemic regions with positive test to TB are considered at risk of developing tuberculosis. A study by Wilkinson and colleagues (1998) demonstrated that treatment for latent infection in HIV people decreased by 43% the risk of developing tuberculosis (Wilkinson et al., 1998). Among the schemes that have been proposed that it should be noted: a) isoniazid for 6-9 months in the absence of active infection b) rifampicin and isoniazid for 3 months and others (Balcells et al. 2006; Ena et al., 2005).

All these factors must be taken into account during the pharmacotherapeutic monitoring of tuberculosis patients to adequate the therapy and improve quality of life of patients with tuberculosis.

6. Conclusion

The current TB treatment presents several challenges. The absence of development new drugs is the cruelest face of this disease. This fact associated with inadequate treatment and TB-drug resistance contributes to survival of the disease today. Anti-TB therapy has several problems relate to noncompliance, lack of adherence to therapy, patients with co-morbidity, socio-economic factors, environmental factors and problems related to drugs such as adverse effects and drug interactions. Health interventions can improve the medication efficacy, reduce the resistance and improve patients quality of life. Pharmacotherapeutic follow-up and adequate strategies to increase therapy adherence are important factors to be monitored during TB therapy. It is important to keep in mind that interventions that guarantee the adequate use of the medication are the first step to improve TB treatment.

7. References

American Thoracic Society, CDC, Infections Disease Society of America. Treatment of tuberculosis. MMWR Recomm Rep 2003; 52:1-77.

Atre, S.; Kudale, A.; Morankar, S.; Gosoniu, D.; Weiss, M. G. Gender and community views of stigma and tuberculosis in rural Maharashtra, India. Global Public Health. (2009). Vol. 13, pp. 1-16.

Balcells, M. E.; Thomas, S. L.; Godfrey-Fausset, P.; Grant, A. D. Isoniazid preventive therapy and risk for resistance tuberculosis. Emerging Infectious Disease, (2006). Vol. 12, pp. 744-751.

Bisaglia, J. B. Atualização terapêutica em tuberculose: principais efeitos adversos dos fármacos. Boletim de Pneumologia Sanitária, (2003). Vol. 11, pp. 53-59.

Brasil, Ministerio da Saúde/ FNS/ CNPS. Plano nacional de controle da tuberculose: manual de normas. 5° ed. Brasília, 2000.

Cegielski, J. P.; McMurray, D. N. The relationship between malnutrition and tuberculosis: evidence from studies in humans and experimental animals. International Journal of Tuberculosis Lung Disease. (2004). Vol 8, pp. 286–298.

Center of Disease Control and Prevention. (2011). http://www.cdc.gov/tb/TB_HIV_Drugs/default.htm. Cited 01 Sept. 2011.

Costa, J. S. D.; Gonçalves, H.; Menezes, A. M. B. et al. Controle epidemiológico da tuberculose na cidade de Pelotas, Rio Grande do Sul, Brasil: Adesão ao tratamento. Caderno de Saúde Pública, (1998). Vol. 14, pp. 409-415.

Costa, S. M.; Mendoza-Sassi, R. A.; Teixeira, T. P.; Leivas, V. A.; Cézar-Vaz, M. R. Conhecimento dos clientes com tuberculose pulmonar e seus familiares sobre adesão ao tratamento e fatores associados, no município do Rio Grande (RS). Ciência & Saúde Coletiva, (2011). Vol.16, pp. 1427-1435.

Council on Patient Information and Education (NCPIE) Enhancing prescription medicine adherence: a national action plan. Bethesha : NCPIE; 2007. Avaiable in: www.talkaboutrx.org/documents/enhancing_prescription_medicine_adherence.pdf [accessed in 01/09/2011].

Cuneo WD, Snider DE (1989) Enhancing patient compliance with tuberculosis therapy. Clinics In Chest Medicine, (1989). Vol. 10, pp. 375–380.

De Rossi, E.; Aínsa, J.A.; Riccardi, G. Role of mycobacterial efflux transporters in drug resistance: an unresolved question. FEMS Microbiology Reviews, (2006). Vol. 30, pp. 36-52.

Dhingra, V. K.; Khan, S. A sociological study on stigma among TB patients in Delhi. Indian Journal of Tuberculosis. (2010). Vol. 57, pp. 12–18.

Drug. Com (2011). http://www.drugs.com/drug_interactions.php. Cited 01 Sept. 2011.

Ena, J.; Valls, V. Short-course therapy with rifampicin plus isoniazid, compared with standard therapy with isoniazid, for latent tuberculosis infection: a meta-analysis. Clinical Infectious Diseases, (2005). Vol. 40, pp. 670-676.

Fauci, A. S. The NIAID Tuberculosis Working Group, Multidrug-resistant and extensively drug-resistant tuberculosis: the National Institute of Allergy and Infectious Diseases Research agenda and recommendations for priority research. Journal Infectious Diseases (2008). Vol. 197, pp. 1493–1498.

Fekih, L.; Boussoffara, L.; Fenniche, S.; Abdelghaffar, H.; Megdiche, M. L. Neuropsychiatric side effects of antituberculosis agents. Revue Medicale Liege. (2011). Vol. 66, pp. 82-85.

Fiuza de Melo, F. A. & Afiune, J. B. Quimitorepia da tuberculose: bases, condutas e procedimentos. Jornal Brasileiro Pneumologia, (1993). Vol. 19, pp. 42-49.

Fountain, F. F.; Tolley, E.; Chrisman, C. R.; Self, T. H. Isoniazid hepatotoxicity associated with treatment of latente tuberculosis infection: a 7-year evaluation from a public health tuberculosis clinic. Chest, (2005). Vol. 128, pp. 116-123.

Frieden, T. R.; Sterling, T. Pablos-Mendez, A.; Kilburn, J. O.; Cauthen, G. M.; Dooley, S. W. The emergence of drug-resistant tuberculosis in New York City. New England Journal of Medicine, (1993). Vol. 328, pp. 521–526.

Golub, J.E.; Astemborski, J.; Ahmed, M.; Cronin, W.; Mehta, S.H.; Kirk, G.D.; Vlahov, D.; Chaisson, R.E. Long-term effectiveness of diagnosing and treating latent tuberculosis infection in a cohort of HIV-infected and at-risk injection drug users. Journal Acquired Immune Deficiency Syndrome, (2008). Vol. 49, pp. 532-537.

Gonçalves, H.; Costa, J. S. D.; Menezes, A. M. B.; Knauth, D.; Leal, O. F. Adesão à Terapêutica da Tuberculose em Pelotas, Rio Grande do Sul: na Perspectiva do Paciente. Caderno de Saúde Pública, (1999). Vol. 15, pp. 777-87.

Gordin, F. M.; Nelson, E. T.; Matts, J. P. The impact of human immunodeficiency virus infection on drug-resistant tuberculosis. American Journal of Respiratory and Critical Care Medicine, (1996). Vol. 154, pp. 1478–1483.

Grace, J.; Chenhall, R. A. Rapid Anthropological Assessment of Tuberculosis in a Remote Aboriginal Community in Northern Australia. Human Organization. (2006). Vol. 65, pp.387-399.

Gupta, S.; Shenoy, V. P.; Bairy, I.; Srinivasa, H.; Mukhopadhyay, C. Diabetes mellitus and HIV as co-morbidities in tuberculosis patients of rural south India. J Journal of Infection and Public Health, (2011). Vol. 4, pp. 140-144.

Hargreaves, J. R.; Boccia, D.; Evans, C. A.; Adato, M.; Petticrew, M.; Porter, J. D. The social determinants of tuberculosis: from evidence to action. American Journal of Public Health. (2011). Vol. 101, pp. 654-662.

Havlir, D. V and Barnes, P. F. Tuberculosis in patients with human immunodeficiency virus infection. New England Journal of Medicine, (1999). Vol. 340, pp. 367-373.

Haynes, R.B.; Ackloo, E.; Sahota, N.; McDonald, H.P.; Yao, X. Interventions for enhancing medication adherence. Cochrane Database of Systematic Reviews. In: The Cochrane Library, issue 3, 2009. Art. No. CD000011.

Herzog, H. History of tuberculosis. Respiration, (1998). Vol. 65, pp5-15.

Holmes, C. B.; Hausler, H.; Nunn, P. A. Review of sex differences in the epidemiology of tuberculosis. Internation Journal of Tuberculosis Lung Disease. (1998). Vol. 2, pp. 96–104.

Koul, A.; Arnoult, E.; Lounis, N.; Guillemont, J.; Andries, K. The challenge of new drug discovery for tuberculosis. Nature, (2011). Vol. 469, pp. 483-490.

Koul, A.; Arnoult, E.; Lounis, N.; Guillemont, J.; Andries, K. The challenge of new drug discovery for tuberculosis. Nature, (2011). Vol. 469, pp. 483-490.

Lima, M. B.; Mello, D. A.; Morais, A. P. P.; Silva, W. C. Estudo de casos sobre abandono do tratamento da tuberculose: Avaliação do atendimento, percepção e conhecimentos sobre a doença na perspectiva dos clientes (Fortaleza, Ceará, Brasil). Caderno de Saúde Pública, (2001). Vol. 17, pp. 877-885.

Lorent, N.; Sebatunzi, O.; Mukeshimana, G.; Van den Ende, J.; Clerinx, J. Incidence and risk factors of serious adverse events during antituberculous treatment in Rwanda: a prospective cohort study. PLoS One, (2011) Vol. 6, 1956–1966.

Ma, Z.; Lienhardt, C.; McIlleron, H.; Nunn, A.J.; Wang X. Global tuberculosis drug development pipeline: the need and the reality. Lancet, (2010). Vol 375, pp. 2100-2109.

Mateus-Solarte, J. C.; Carvajal-Barona, R. Factors predictive of adherence to tuberculosis treatment, Valle Del Cauca, Colombia. International Journal of Tuberculosis Lung Disesase, (2008). Vol. 12, pp. 520-526.

Medscape (2011). Drug, Disease & Procedures. http://reference.medscape.com/drug-interactionchecker. Cited 01 Sept. 2011.

Mendes, A. M.; Fensterseifer, L. M. Tuberculose: porque os pacientes abandonam o tratamento? Boletim de Pneumologia Sanitária, (2004). Vol.12, pp. 25-36.

Natal, S. Tratamento da Tuberculose: Causas da Não-Aderência. Boletim de Pneumologia Sanitária, (1997). Vol. 5, pp. 51-68.

Navas, E.; Martín-Dávila, P.; Moreno, L.; Pintado, V.; Casado, J. L.; Fortún, J.; Pérez-Elías, M. J.; Gomez-Mampaso, E.; and Moreno, S. Paradoxical Reactions of Tuberculosis in Patients With the Acquired Immunodeficiency Syndrome Who Are Treated With

Highly Active Antiretroviral Therapy. Archives of Internal Medicine, (2002). Vol. 162, pp. 97-99.

Orlovic, D.; Smego Jr, R. A. Paradoxical tuberculous reactions in HIV-infected patients. International Journal of Tuberculosis Lung Disease, (2001). Vol. 5, 370-375.

Pablos-Méndez, A.; Cnirsch, C. A.; Barr, R. G.; Lerner, B. H.; Frieden, T. R. Nonadherence in tuberculosis treatment: Predictors and consequences in New York City. American Journal of Medicine, (1997). Vol. 102, pp. 164-170.

Piddock, L.J. Clinically relevant chromosomally encoded multidrug resistance efflux pumps in bacteria. Clinical Microbiology Reviews, (2006). Vol.19, pp.382-402.

Piggott, D. A.; Karakousis, P. C. Timing of antiretroviral therapy for HIV in the setting of TB treatment. Clinical and Developmental Immunology, (2011). Vol. 2011, pp. 1039-1047.

Pitchenik, A. E.; Fertel, D. and Bloch, A. B. Mycobacterial disease: epidemiology, diagnosis, treatment, and prevention. Clincs In Chest Medicine, (1988). Vol. 9, pp. 425-441.

Sabaté, E. Adherence to long-term therapies: evidence for action. Geneva (Switzerland): WHO, 2003, ISBN 92 4 154599 2. Available in: http://www.who.int/chp/knowledge/publications/adherence_full_report.pdf [accessed in 01 september, 2011].

Uplekar, M. W.; Rangan, S.; Weiss, M.; G.; Ogden, J.; Borgdorff, M. W.; Hudelson, P. Attention to gender issues in tuberculosis control. International Journal of Tuberculosis Lung Disease, (2001). Vol. 5, pp. 220-224.

Venkatesh, K. K.; Swaminathan, S.; Andrews, J. R.; Mayer, K. H. Tuberculosis and HIV co-infection: screening and treatment strategies. Drugs, (2011). Vol. 71, pp. 1133-1152.

Veronesi, R. & Focaccia, R. Tuberculose in: Veronesi: tratado de infectologia, ed Atheneu São Paulo, 1996.

WHO (2002). An expanded DOTS framework for effective tuberculosis control. WHO/CDS/TB/2002.297. Geneva: World Health Organization. 23 p.

WHO (2005) Addressing poverty in TB control: options for national TB control programmes. WHO/HTM/TB/2005.352.Geneva, Switzerland, 80p.

WHO (2008). Global Tuberculosis Control—Surveillance, Planning, Financing: WHO Report 2008. Geneva, Switzerland. WHO/HTM/TB/2008.393.

WHO (2009) Treatment of tuberculosis: guidelines. 4 ed. WHO/HTM/TB/2009.420. Geneva, Switzerland. 160 p.

Wilkinson, D.; Squire, S. B.; Garner, P. Effect of preventive treatment for tuberculosis in adults infected with HIV: systematic review of randomized placebo controlled trials. BMJ, (1998). Vol. 317, pp. 625-629.

Yee, D.; Valiquette, C.; Pelletier, M.; Parisien, I.; Rocher, I.; Menzies, D. Incidence of serious side effects from first-line antituberculosis drugs among patients treated for active tuberculosis. American Journal of Respiratory and Critical Care Medicine, (2003). Vol. 167, pp. 1472-1477.

Yew, W. W. Clinically significant interactions with drugs used in the treatment of tuberculosis. Drug Safety, (2002). Vol. 25, pp. 111-133.

Zhang, J.; Zhu, L.; Stonier, M.; Coumbis, J.; Xu, X.; Wu, Y.; Arikan, D.; Farajallah, A.; Bertz, R. Determination of rifabutin dosing regimen when administered in combination with ritonavir-boosted atazanavir. Journal of Antimicrobial Chemotherapy, (2011). Vol. 66, pp. 2075–2082.